Evidence-based
Physical
Diagnosis

Evidence-based
Physical
Diagnosis

Steven McGee, M.D.
Professor of Medicine
University of Washington School of Medicine

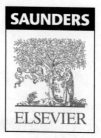

SAUNDERS

ELSEVIER

SAUNDERS
ELSEVIER

11830 Westline Industrial Drive
St. Louis, Missouri 63146

EVIDENCE-BASED PHYSICAL DIAGNOSIS
Copyright © 2007 by Saunders, an imprint of Elsevier Inc.

Notice

Neither the Publisher nor the Author assume any responsibility for any loss or injury and/or damage to persons or property arising out of or related to any use of the material contained in this book. It is the responsibility of the treating practitioner, relying on independent expertise and knowledge of the patient, to determine the best treatment and method of application for the patient.

The Publisher

Library of Congress Cataloging-in-Publication Data

McGee, Steven R.
    Evidence-based physical diagnosis / Steven McGee. – 2nd ed.
      p. cm.
    Includes bibliographical references.
    ISBN-13: 978-1-4160-2898-7   ISBN-10: 1-4160-2898-6
      1. Physical diagnosis. 2. Evidence-based medicine. I. Title.
RC76.M347 2007
616.07'54–dc22
                                            2006050471

ISBN-13: 978-1-4160-2898-7
ISBN-10: 1-4160-2898-6

Printed in the United States of America.

Last digit is the print number: 9 8 7 6 5 4 3 2

DEDICATION

To Rosalie, Connor, and Matt

PREFACE TO THE SECOND EDITION

The purpose of the second edition of *Evidence-based Physical Diagnosis* is to enrich our understanding of physical diagnosis by further exploring its origins, pathogenesis, and diagnostic accuracy. Special effort has been made to compare classic physical signs to modern technologic standards, thereby identifying those signs that remain accurate and valuable to us today. In addition to updating each chapter and "Diagnostic Accuracy" table from the first edition, this edition includes new material addressing the value of physical signs in patients with shock; coma; lymphadenopathy; coronary artery disease and myocardial infarction; cirrhosis; bacteremia and fever; aortic dissection; tremor and Parkinson's disease; and shoulder, knee, and ankle pain. Also, this edition includes many new illustrations that depict important aspects of examination technique or explain pathogenesis of difficult-to-understand findings, such as the Trendelenburg gait, Pemberton's sign, or pivot shift sign. Finally, this edition includes new "Evidence based Medicine rules," figures that convey at a glance the meaning of likelihood ratios and quickly identify those physical findings that are most accurate.

I am indebted to several investigators who provided me with information unavailable in their published work: Drs. George Murrell and Judie Walton (rotator cuff tears), Masayuki Ikeda (vital signs and coma), Sharon Strauss (forced expiratory time), and Eduardo Garcia-Pachon (Hoover's sign). I am also grateful to Dr. Guy de Bruyn, who brought to my attention several studies on the diagnosis of cirrhosis, and to Drs. Howard Chansky, Ali Samii, James Orcutt, Greg Gardner, Greg Nakamoto, and Brad Anawalt, who reviewed portions of the book and provided important comment. Also, I want to thank my editor, Rolla Couchman, who provided unflagging support and assistance throughout the preparation of this edition.

My hope is that this book will help all clinicians adopt an evidence-based approach to physical diagnosis, an approach that emphasizes signs with proven accuracy and reliability and that gives clinicians a level of diagnostic confidence that otherwise accrues only after decades of clinical experience. Physical examination remains a fundamental diagnostic tool, and my hope is that this book will help to preserve its value in the care of patients.

Steven McGee, M.D.
February 2007

INTRODUCTION TO
THE FIRST EDITION

The purpose of this book is to explore the origins, pathophysiology, and diagnostic accuracy of many of the physical signs used today in adult patients. We have a wonderfully rich tradition of physical diagnosis, and my hope is that this book will help to square this tradition, now almost two centuries old, with the realities of modern diagnosis, which often rely more on technologic tests such as clinical imaging and laboratory testing. The tension between physical diagnosis and technologic tests has never been greater. Having taught physical diagnosis for 20 years, I frequently observe medical students purchasing textbooks of physical diagnosis during their preclinical years to study and master traditional physical signs, but then neglecting or even discarding this knowledge during their clinical years, after observing that modern diagnosis often takes place at a distance from the bedside. One can hardly fault a student who, caring for a patient with pneumonia, does not talk seriously about crackles and diminished breath sounds when all of his teachers are focused on the subtleties of the patient's chest radiograph. Disregard for physical diagnosis also pervades our residency programs, most of which have formal x-ray rounds, pathology rounds, microbiology rounds, and clinical conferences addressing the nuances of laboratory tests. Very few have formal physical diagnosis rounds.

Reconciling traditional physical diagnosis with contemporary diagnostic standards has been a continuous process throughout the history of physical diagnosis. In the 1830s, the inventor of topographic percussion, Professor Pierre Adolphe Piorry, taught that there were nine distinct percussion sounds which he used to outline the patient's liver, heart, lungs, stomach, and even individual heart chambers or lung cavities. Piorry's methods flourished for more than a century and once filled 200-page manuals,[1] although today, thanks to the introduction of clinical imaging in the early 1900s, the only vestige of his methods is percussion of the liver span. In his 1819 *A Treatise on Diseases of the Chest*,[2] Laennec wrote that lung auscultation could detect "every possible case" of pneumonia. It was a matter of only 20 years before other careful physical diagnosticians tempered Laennec's enthusiasm and pointed out that the stethoscope had diagnostic limitations.[3] And, for most of the twentieth century expert clinicians believed that all late systolic murmurs were benign, until Barlow in 1963 showed that they often represented mitral regurgitation, sometimes of significant severity.[4]

There are two contemporary polar opinions of physical diagnosis. Holding the less common position are clinicians who believe that all traditional physical signs remain accurate today, and these clinicians continue to quiz students about Krönig's isthmus and splenic percussion signs. A more common position is that physical diagnosis has little to offer the modern clinician and that traditional signs, though interesting, cannot compete with the accuracy of our more technologic diagnostic tools. Neither position, of course, is completely correct. I hope that this book, by examining the best evidence comparing physical signs to current diagnostic standards, will bring clinicians to a more appropriate middle-ground: that physical diagnosis is a reliable diagnostic tool that can still help clinicians with many, but not all, clinical problems.

Although some regard evidence-based medicine as "cookbook medicine," this is incorrect, because there are immeasurable subtleties in our interaction with patients that clinical studies cannot address (at least, not as yet) and because the diagnostic power of any physical sign (or any test, for that matter) depends in part on our ideas about disease prevalence, which in turn depend on our own personal interviewing skills and clinical experience.[a] Instead, evidence-based physical diagnosis simply summarizes the best evidence available whether a physical sign is accurate or not. The clinician who understands this evidence can then approach his own patients with the confidence and wisdom that would have developed had he personally examined and learned from the thousands of patients reviewed in the studies of this book.

Sometimes, comparing physical signs with modern diagnostic standards reveals that the physical sign is outdated and perhaps best discarded (e.g., capillary refill time, topographic percussion of diaphragm excursion). Other times the comparison reveals that physical signs are extremely accurate and probably underused (e.g., early diastolic murmur at the left lower sternal area for aortic regurgitation, conjunctival rim pallor for anemia, or a palpable gallbladder for extrahepatic obstruction of the biliary ducts). And still other times, the comparison reveals that the physical sign *is* the diagnostic standard, just as most of physical examination was a century ago (e.g., systolic murmur and click of mitral valve prolapse, hemiparesis for stroke, neovascularization for proliferative diabetic retinopathy). For some diagnoses, a tension remains between physical signs and technologic tests, making it still unclear which should be the diagnostic standard (e.g., the diagnoses of cardiac tamponade or carpal tunnel syndrome). And for still other others, the comparison is impossible because clinical studies comparing physical signs to traditional diagnostic standards do not exist.

My hope is that the material in this book will allow clinicians of all levels—students, house officers, and seasoned clinicians alike—to examine patients more confidently and accurately, thus restoring physical diagnosis to its appro-

---

[a]These subjects are discussed fully in Chapters 1 and 3.

priate, and often pivotal, diagnostic role. Once well-versed in evidence-based physical diagnosis, clinicians can then settle most important clinical questions at the time and place they should be first addressed—the patient's bedside.

Steven McGee, M.D.
July 1, 2000

REFERENCES

1. Weil A. Handbuch und Atlas der topographischen Perkussion. Leipzig: F. C. W. Vogel, 1880.
2. Laennec RTH. A treatise on the diseases of the chest (facsimile edition by Classics of Medicine library). London: T. and G. Underwood, 1821.
3. Addison T. The difficulties and fallacies attending physical diagnosis of the chest. In: Wilks, Daldy (eds): A collection of the published writings of the late Thomas Addison (facsimile edition by Classics of Medicine library). London: The New Sydenham Society, 1846, p 242.
4. Barlow JB, Pocock WA, Marchand P, Denny M. The significance of late systolic murmurs. *Am Heart J.* 1963;66:443-452.

TABLE OF CONTENTS

UNDERSTANDING THE EVIDENCE

Diagnostic Accuracy of Physical Findings

I. INTRODUCTION

If a physical sign characteristic of a suspected diagnosis is present (i.e., **positive** finding), that diagnosis becomes more likely; if the characteristic finding is absent (i.e., **negative** finding), the suspected diagnosis becomes less likely. How much these positive and negative results modify probability, however, is distinct for each physical sign. Some findings, when positive, shift probability upward greatly, but they change it little when negative. Other signs are more useful if they are absent, because the negative finding practically excludes disease, although the positive one changes probability very little.

Much of this book consists of tables that specifically describe how positive or negative findings change the probability of disease, a property called "diagnostic accuracy." Understanding these tables first requires review of four concepts: pretest probability, sensitivity, specificity, and likelihood ratios (LRs).

II. PRETEST PROBABILITY

Pretest probability is the probability of disease (i.e., prevalence) before application of the results of a physical finding. Pretest probability is the starting point for all clinical decisions. For example, the clinician may know that a certain physical finding shifts the probability of disease upward 40%, but this information alone is unhelpful unless the clinician also knows the starting point: If the pretest probability for the particular diagnosis was 50%, the finding is diagnostic (i.e., post-test probability 50% + 40% = 90%); if the pretest probability was only 10%, the finding is less helpful, because the probability of disease is still the flip of a coin (i.e., post-test probability 10% + 40% = 50%).

Published estimates of disease prevalence, given a particular clinical setting, are available for most clinical problems (Table 1-1), although the clinician must adjust these estimates with information from his or her own practice. For example, large studies based in emergency departments show that 12% to 30% of patients presenting with cough and fever have pneumonia (see Table 1-1). The probability of pneumonia, however, is certainly lower in patients presenting with cough and fever to an office-based practice in the community, and it may be higher if cough and fever develop in patients with cancer or human immunodeficiency virus (HIV) infection. In fact, because the best estimate of pretest probability incorporates information from the clinician's own practice—how specific underlying diseases, risks, and exposures make disease more or less likely—the practice of evidence-based medicine is never "cookbook"

Table 1-1	Pretest Probability	
Setting (Ref)	**Diagnosis**	**Probability (%)**
Acute abdominal pain[1-3]	Small bowel obstruction	4
Aortic flow murmur[4]	Severe aortic stenosis	5
Cough and fever[5]	Pneumonia	12–30
Acute calf pain or swelling[6-14]	Proximal deep vein thrombosis	13–43
Pleuritic chest pain, dyspnea, or hemoptysis[15-18]	Pulmonary embolism	9–43
Murmur of mitral regurgitation, referred for echocardiography[19]	Moderate-to-severe mitral regurgitation	33
Murmur of aortic regurgitation, referred for echocardiography or angiography[19-21]	Moderate-to-severe aortic regurgitation	49

medicine but instead consists of decisions based on the unique characteristics of the patients the clinician sees.

III. SENSITIVITY AND SPECIFICITY

A. DEFINITIONS

Sensitivity and specificity describe the discriminatory power of physical signs. **Sensitivity** is the proportion of patients *with* the diagnosis who *have* the physical sign (i.e., have the *positive* result). **Specificity** is the proportion of patients *without* the diagnosis who *lack* the physical sign (i.e., have the *negative* result).

Calculation of sensitivity and specificity requires construction of a 2 × 2 table (Fig. 1-1) that has two columns (one for "diagnosis present" and another for "diagnosis absent") and two rows (one for "physical sign present" and another for "physical sign absent"). These rows and columns create four boxes: one for the "true positives" (cell a, sign and diagnosis present), one for "false positives" (cell b, sign present but disease absent), one for the "false negatives" (cell c, sign absent but disease present), and one for the "true negatives" (cell d, sign and disease absent).

Figure 1-1 presents data from a hypothetical study of 100 patients presenting with pulmonary hypertension. The clinician knows that tricuspid regurgitation is a complication of pulmonary hypertension and wonders how accurately a single physical sign—the presence of a holosystolic murmur at the left lower sternal border—detects this complication.* In this study, 42 patients have significant tricuspid regurgitation (the sum of column 1) and 58 patients do not (the sum of column 2). The **sensitivity** of the holosystolic murmur is the proportion of patients with disease (i.e., tricuspid regurgitation, 42 patients) who have the characteristic murmur (i.e., the *positive* result, 22 patients), which is 22/42 = 0.52 or 52%. The **specificity** of the holosystolic murmur is the proportion of patients *without* disease (i.e., no tricuspid regurgitation, 58 patients) who *lack* the murmur (i.e., the *negative* result, 55 patients), which is 55/58 = 0.95 or 95%.

To recall how to calculate sensitivity and specificity, Sackett and others have suggested helpful mnemonics: sensitivity is "pelvic inflammatory disease" (or "PID," meaning "positivity in disease") and specificity is "National Institutes of Health" (or "NIH," meaning "negativity in health").[23,24]

B. USING SENSITIVITY AND SPECIFICITY TO DETERMINE PROBABILITY OF DISEASE

The completed 2 × 2 table can be used to determine the accuracy of the holosystolic murmur, which is how well its presence or absence discriminates between

---

*The numbers used in this example are very close to those in reference 22. See also Chapter 42.

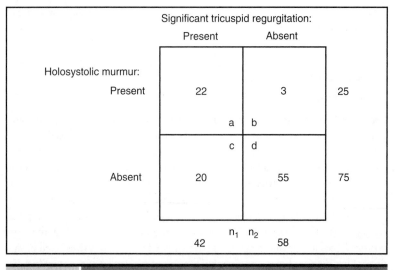

| FIGURE 1-1 | 2 × 2 TABLE. |

The total number of patients with disease (tricuspid regurgitation in this example) is the sum of the first column, or $n_1 = a + c$. The total number of patients without disease is the sum of the second column, or $n_2 = b + d$. The *sensitivity* of a physical finding (holosystolic murmur at the left lower sternal edge, in this example) is the proportion of patients with disease who have the finding (i.e., $a/(a + c)$ or a/n_1). The *specificity* of a physical finding is the proportion of patients without disease who lack the finding (i.e., $d/(b + d)$ or d/n_1). The *positive likelihood ratio (LR)* is proportion of patients with disease who have a positive finding (a/n_1) divided by the proportion of patients without disease who have a positive finding (b/n_2), or sensitivity/(1 – specificity). The *negative LR* is the proportion of patients with disease who lack the finding (c/n_1) divided by the proportion of patients without disease who lack the finding (d/n_1), or (1 – sensitivity)/specificity. In this example, the sensitivity is 0.52 (22/42), the specificity is 0.95 (55/58), the positive LR is 10.1 ((22/42)/(3/58)), and the negative LR is 0.5 ((20/42)/(55/58)).

those with tricuspid regurgitation and those without it. In Fig. 1-1, the first row includes all 25 patients with the murmur (i.e., the positive results). Of these 25 patients, 22 have tricuspid regurgitation; therefore the probability of tricuspid regurgitation, if the murmur is present (*positive* finding), is 22/25 or 88% (i.e., the "post-test probability" if the murmur is present). The second row includes all 75 patients without the murmur. Of these 75 patients, 20 have tricuspid regurgitation; therefore, the post-test probability of tricuspid regurgitation, if the murmur is absent (i.e., *negative* finding) is 20/75 or 27%.

In this example, the pretest probability of tricuspid regurgitation is 42%. The presence of the murmur (positive result) shifts the probability of disease upward considerably more (i.e., 46%, from 42% to 88%) than the absence of the murmur (negative result) shifts it downward (i.e., 15%, from 42% to 27%). This illustrates an important property of physical signs with a high specificity: When present, physical signs with *high specificity* greatly *increase* the probability of disease. A corollary to this applies to findings with high sensitivity: When *absent*, physical signs with a high *sensitivity* greatly *decrease* the probability of disease. The holosystolic murmur has a high specificity (95%) but only a meager sensitivity (52%), meaning that, at the bedside, a positive result (the presence of a murmur) has greater diagnostic importance than the negative result (the absence of the murmur). The presence of the characteristic murmur argues compellingly for tricuspid regurgitation, but its absence is less helpful simply because many patients with significant regurgitation lack the characteristic murmur.

Sackett and others have suggested mnemonics for these characteristics as well: "SpPin" (i.e., a *Sp*ecific test, when *P*ositive, rules *in* disease) and "SnNout" (i.e., a *S*e*n*sitive test, when *N*egative, rules *out* disease).[24]

IV.   LIKELIHOOD RATIOS

LRs, like sensitivity and specificity, describe the discriminatory power of physical signs. Although they have many advantages, the most important is how simply and quickly they can be used to estimate post-test probability.

A.   DEFINITION

The LR of a physical sign is the proportion of patients *with* disease who have a particular finding divided by the proportion of patients *without* disease who also have the same finding.

$$LR = \frac{\text{Probability of finding in patients } \textit{with} \text{ disease}}{\text{Probability of same finding in patients } \textit{without} \text{ disease}}$$

The adjectives "positive" or "negative" indicate whether that LR refers to the presence of the physical sign (i.e. "positive" result) or to the absence of the physical sign (i.e., the "negative" result).

A **positive LR**, therefore, is the proportion of patients *with* disease who *have* a physical sign divided by the proportion of patients *without* disease who also *have* the same sign. The numerator of this equation—proportion of patients with disease who have the physical sign—is the sign's sensitivity. The denominator—proportion of patients without disease who have the sign—is the complement of specificity, or (1 − specificity). Therefore,

$$\text{Positive LR} = \frac{(\text{sens})}{(1 - \text{spec})}$$

In our hypothetical study (see Fig. 1-1), the proportion of patients with tricuspid regurgitation who have the murmur is 22/42 or 52.4% (i.e., the finding's sensitivity) and the proportion of patients without tricuspid regurgitation who also have the murmur is 3/58 or 5.2% (i.e., 1 − specificity). The ratio of these proportions [i.e., (sensitivity)/(1 − specificity)] is 10.1, which is the positive LR for a holosystolic murmur at the lower sternal border. This number means that patients *with* tricuspid regurgitation are 10.1 times more likely to have the holosystolic murmur than those *without* tricuspid regurgitation.

Similarly, the **negative LR** is the proportion of patients *with* disease *lacking* a physical sign divided by the proportion of patients *without* disease also *lacking* the sign. The numerator of this equation—proportion of patients with disease *lacking* the finding—is the complement of sensitivity, or (1 − sensitivity). The denominator of the equation—proportion of patients without disease *lacking* the finding—is the specificity. Therefore,

$$\text{Negative LR} = \frac{(1 - \text{sens})}{(\text{spec})}$$

In our hypothetical study, the proportion of patients with tricuspid regurgitation lacking the murmur is 20/42 or 47.6% (i.e., 1 − sensitivity) and the proportion of patients without tricuspid regurgitation lacking the murmur is 55/58 or 94.8% (i.e., the specificity). The ratio of these proportions [i.e. (1 − sensitivity)/ (specificity)] is 0.5, which is the negative LR for the holosystolic murmur. This number means that patients *with* tricuspid regurgitation are 0.5 times less likely to lack the murmur than those *without* tricuspid regurgitation (the inverse statement is less confusing: patients *without* tricuspid regurgitation are 2 times more likely to lack a murmur than those *with* tricuspid regurgitation).

Although these formulae are difficult to recall, the interpretation of LRs is straightforward. Findings with LRs greater than 1 increase the probability of disease; the greater the LR, the more compelling the argument *for* disease. Findings whose LRs lie between 0 and 1 decrease the probability of disease; the closer the LR is to zero, the more convincing the finding argues *against* disease. Findings whose LRs equal 1 lack diagnostic value because they do not change probability at all. "Positive LR" describes how probability changes when the finding is *present*. "Negative LR" describes how probability changes when the finding is *absent*.

LRs, therefore, are nothing more than diagnostic weights, whose possible values range from 0 (i.e., excluding disease) to infinity (i.e., pathognomic for disease, see Fig, 1-2).

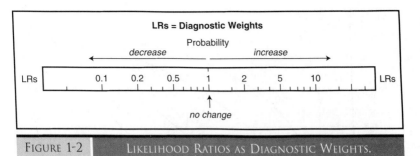

FIGURE 1-2   LIKELIHOOD RATIOS AS DIAGNOSTIC WEIGHTS.

The relationship between a specific physical sign and a specific disease is described by a unique number—its likelihood ratio (LR)—which is nothing more than a diagnostic weight describing how much that sign argues for or against that specific disease. The possible values of LRs range from zero to infinity (∞). Findings with LRs greater than 1 argue *for* the specific disease (the greater the value of the LR, the more the probability of disease increases). Findings with LRs less than 1 argue *against* the disease (the closer the number is to zero, the more the probability of disease decreases). LRs that equal 1 do not change probability of disease at all.

B.   USING LRS TO DETERMINE PROBABILITY

The clinician can use the LR of a physical finding to estimate probability of disease in three ways: (1) using graphs or other easy-to-use nomograms[25, 26]; (2) using bedside approximations; or (3) using formulae.

1.   Using Graphs
a.   Parts of the Graph

Fig. 1-3 is an easy-to-use graph that illustrates the relationship between pretest probability (x-axis) and post-test probability (on the y-axis), given the finding's LR. The straight line bisecting the graph into an upper left half and lower right half describes the LR of 1, which has no discriminatory value because, for findings with this LR, post-test probability always equals pretest probability. Physical findings that argue *for* disease (i.e., LRs > 1) appear in the upper left half of the graph; the larger the LR the more the curve approaches the upper left corner. Physical findings that argue *against* disease (i.e., LRs < 1) appear in the lower right half of the graph; the closer the LR is to zero the more the curve approaches the lower right corner.

In Fig. 1-3, the three depicted curves with LRs greater than 1 (i.e., LR = 2, 5, and 10) are mirror images of the three curves with LRs less than 1 (i.e., LR = 0.5, 0.2, and 0.1) (This assumes the "mirror" is the line LR = 1.) This symmetry

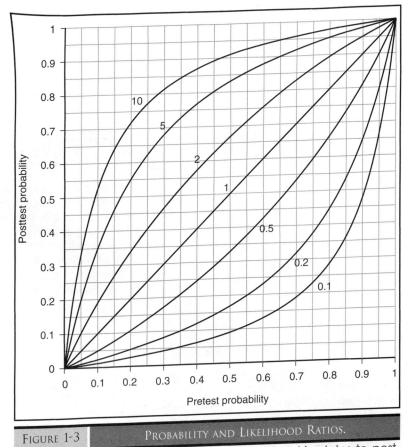

| FIGURE 1-3 | PROBABILITY AND LIKELIHOOD RATIOS. |

The curves describe how pretest probability (x-axis) relates to post-test probability (y-axis), given the likelihood ratio (LR) for the physical finding. Only the curves for seven likelihood ratios are depicted (from LR = 0.1 to LR = 10). See text.

indicates that findings with an LR of 10 argue as much *for* disease as those with an LR = 0.1 argue *against* disease (although this is true only for the intermediate pretest probabilities). Similarly, LR = 5 argues as much for disease as LR = 0.2 argues against it, and LR = 2 mirrors LR = 0.5. Keeping these companions curves in mind will help the clinician interpret the LRs throughout this book.*

---

*These companion pairs are easy to recall because they are the inverse of each other: The inverse of 10 is 1/10 = 0.1; the inverse of 5 is 1/5 = 0.2; the inverse of 2 is 1/2 = 0.5.

If a finding has an LR other than one of these depicted seven curves, its position can be estimated with little loss in accuracy. For example, the curve for LR = 4 lies between LR = 5 and LR = 2, although closer to LR= 5 than to LR = 2.

b.   Using the Graph to Determine Probability

To use this graph, the clinician identifies on the x-axis the patient's pretest probability, derived from published estimates and clinical experience, and extends a line upward from that point to meet the LR curve for the physical finding. The clinician then extends a horizontal line from this point to the y-axis to identify post-test probability.

Figure 1-4 depicts this process for the lower sternal holosystolic murmur and tricuspid regurgitation. The pretest probability of tricuspid regurgitation is 42%. If the characteristic murmur is present (positive LR = 10), a line is drawn upward from 0.42 on the x-axis to the LR = 10 curve; from this point, a horizontal line is drawn to the y-axis to find the post-test probability (88%). If the murmur is absent (negative LR = 0.5), the post-test probability is the y-value where the vertical line intersects the LR = 0.5 curve (i.e., post-test probability of 27%).

These curves illustrate an additional important point: Physical signs are diagnostically most useful when they are applied to patients who have pretest probabilities in the intermediate range (i.e., 20% to 80%), because in this range the different LR curves diverge the most from the LR = 1 curve (thus, shifting probability up or down a large amount). If instead the pretest probability is already very low or very high, all the LR curves cluster close to the line LR = 1 curve in either the bottom left or upper right corners, thus changing probability relatively little.

2.   Approximating Probability

The clinician can avoid using graphs and instead approximate post-test probability by remembering the following two points: (1) the companion LR curves in Fig. 1-3 are LR = 2 and LR = 0.5, LR = 5 and LR = 0.2, and LR = 10 and LR = 0.1; and (2) the first three multiples of 15 are 15, 30, and 45. Using this rule, the LRs of 2, 5, and 10 increase probability about 15%, 30%, and 45%, respectively (Fig. 1-5), the LRs of 0.5, 0.2, and 0.1 decrease probability about 15%, 30%, and 45%, respectively.[27] These estimates are accurate to within 5% to 10% of the actual value, as long the clinician rounds estimates greater than 100 to an even 100% and estimates below zero to an even 0%.

Therefore, in our hypothetical patient with pulmonary hypertension, the finding of a holosystolic murmur (LR = 10) increases the probability of tricuspid regurgitation from 42% to 87% (i.e., 42% + 45% = 87%, which is only 1% lower than the actual value). The absence of the murmur (LR = 0.5) decreases the probability of tricuspid regurgitation from 42% to 27% (i.e., 42% − 15% = 27%, which is identical to actual value).

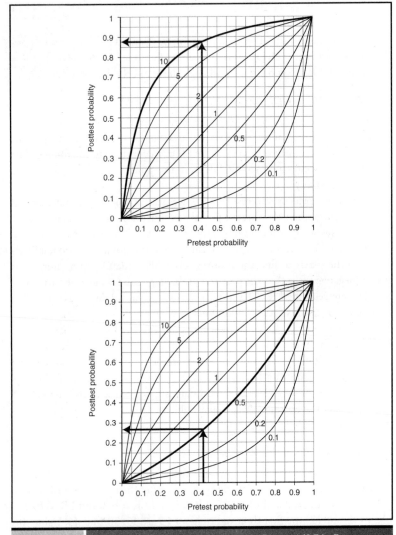

FIGURE 1-4

PROBABILITY AND LIKELIHOOD RATIOS (LR): PATIENTS WITH PULMONARY HYPERTENSION.

In our hypothetical clinician's practice, 42% of patients with pulmonary hypertension have the complication of tricuspid regurgitation (i.e., pretest probability is 42%). To use the curves, the clinician finds 0.42 on the x-axis and extends a line upward. The post-test probability of tricuspid regurgitation is read off the y-axis where the vertical line intersects the curve of the appropriate LR. The probability of tricuspid regurgitation if a holosystolic murmur is present at the left lower sternal edge is 88%; the probability if the finding is absent is 27%.

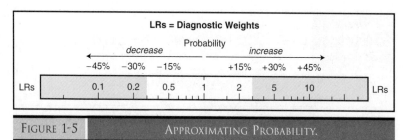

LRs = Diagnostic Weights

FIGURE 1-5   APPROXIMATING PROBABILITY.

Clinicians can estimate changes in probability by recalling the likelihood ratios (LRs) 2, 5, and 10 and the first three multiples of 15 (i.e., 15, 30, 45). A finding whose LR is 2 increases probability about 15%, one of 5 increases it 30%, and one of 10 increases it 45% (these changes are *absolute* increases in probability). LRs whose values are 0.5, 0.2, and 0.1 (i.e., the reciprocals of 2, 5, and 10) decrease probability 15%, 30%, and 45%, respectively. Throughout this book, LRs with values ≥3 or ≤0.3 (represented by the shaded part of the diagnostic weight "ruler") are presented in boldface type to indicate those physical findings that change probability sufficiently to be clinically meaningful (i.e., they increase or decrease probability at least 20% to 25%).

Table 1-2 summarizes similar bedside estimates for all LRs between 0.1 and 10.0.

3. Calculating Probability

The post-test probability also can be calculated by first converting pretest probability (P_{pre}) into pretest odds (O_{pre}):

$$O_{pre} = \frac{P_{pre}}{(1 - P_{pre})}$$

The pretest odds (O_{pre}) is multiplied times the LR of the physical sign to determine the post-test odds (O_{post}):

$$O_{post} = O_{pre} \times LR$$

The post-test odds (O_{post}) converts back to post-test probability (P_{post}), using:

$$P_{post} = \frac{O_{post}}{(1 + O_{post})}$$

Table 1-2 — Likelihood Ratios and Bedside Estimates

Likelihood Ratio	Approximate Change in Probability*
0.1	−45%
0.2	−30%
0.3	−25%
0.4	−20%
0.5	−15%
1	No change
2	+15%
3	+20%
4	+25%
5	+30%
6	+35%
7	
8	+40%
9	
10	+45%

*These changes describe absolute increases or decreases in probability. For example, a patient with pretest probability of 20% and physical finding whose likelihood ratio is 5 would have a post-test probability of 20% + 30% = 50%. The text describes how to easily recall these estimates.
From McGee S. Simplifying likelihood ratios. J Gen Intern Med. 2002;17:646-649.

Therefore, in our hypothetical example of the patients with pulmonary hypertension, the pretest odds for tricuspid regurgitation is $[(0.42)/(1 − 0.42)]$ or 0.72. If the murmur is present (LR = 10), the post-test odds is (0.72×10) or 7.2, which translates to a post-test probability of $[(7.2)/(1 + 7.2)]$ or 0.88 (i.e., 88%). If the murmur wave is absent (LR = 0.5), the post-test odds is (0.72×0.5) or 0.36, which translates to a post-test probability of $[(0.36)/(1 + 0.36)]$ or 0.27 (i.e., 27%).

Clinical medicine, however, is rarely as precise as these calculations suggest, and for most decisions at the bedside, the approximations described in "Approximating test Probability" are more than adequate.

C. ADVANTAGES OF LIKELIHOOD RATIOS

1. Simplicity

In a single number, the LR conveys to clinicians how convincingly a physical sign argues for or against disease. If the LR of a finding is large, disease is likely, and if the LR of a finding is close to zero, disease is doubtful. This advantage allows clinicians to quickly compare different diagnostic strategies and thus refine clinical judgment.[27]

2. Accuracy

Using LRs to describe diagnostic accuracy is superior to sensitivity and specificity, because the earlier described mnemonics, SpPin and SnNout, are sometimes misleading. For example, according to the mnemonic SpPin, a finding with a specificity of 95% should argue conclusively for disease, but it does so only if the positive LR for the finding is a high number. If the finding's sensitivity is 60%, the positive LR is 12.0 and the finding does argue convincingly for disease (i.e., consistent with the SpPin mnemonic); if the finding's sensitivity is only 10%, however, the positive LR is 2.0 and post-test probability changes only slightly (i.e., inconsistent with SpPin mnemonic). Similarly, a highly sensitive finding argues convincingly against disease (i.e., SnNout) only when its calculated negative LR is a number close to zero.

3. Levels of Findings

Another advantage of LRs is that a physical sign measured on an ordinal scale (e.g., 0, 1+, 2+, 3+) or continuous scale (e.g., blood pressure) can be categorized into different levels to determine the LR for each level, thereby increasing the accuracy of the finding. Other examples include continuous findings such as heart rate, respiratory rate, temperature, and percussed span of the liver and ordinal findings such as intensity of murmurs and degree of edema.

For example, in patients with chronic obstructive lung disease (i.e., emphysema, chronic bronchitis), breath sounds are typically faint. If the clinician grades the intensity of breath sounds on a scale from 0 (absent) to 24 (very loud), based on the methods discussed in Chapter 27, he or she can classify the patient's breath sounds into one of four groups: scores of 9 or less (very faint), 10 to 12, 13 to 15, or greater than 15 (loud). Each category then has its own LR (Table 1-3): Scores of 9 or less argue strongly for obstructive disease (LR = 10.2), whereas scores greater than 15 argue convincingly against it (LR = 0.1). Scores from 10 to 12 argue somewhat for disease (LR = 3.6), and scores from 13 to 15 provide no diagnostic information (LR not significantly different from 1.0). If the clinician had instead identified breath sounds as simply "faint" or "normal/increased" (i.e. the traditional positive or negative finding), the finding may still discriminate between patients with and without obstructive disease, but it misses the point that the discriminatory power of the sign resides mostly with scores less than 10 and greater than 15.

When findings are categorized into levels, the term specificity becomes meaningless. For example, the specificity of a breath sound score of 13 to 15 is 80%, which means that 80% of patients without chronic airflow limitation have values other than 13 to 15, although the 80% does not convey whether most of

Table 1-3	Breath Sound Intensity and Chronic Airflow Limitation	
Breath Sound Score		Likelihood Ratio
9 or less		10.2
10–12		3.6
13–15		NS
>15		0.1

NS, *not significant.*
From References 28 and 29.

these other values are greater than 15 or less than 13. Similarly, when findings are put in more than two categories, the LR descriptor negative is no longer necessary, because all LRs are positive ones for their respective category.

4. Combining Findings

A final advantage of LRs is that clinicians can use them to combine findings, which is particularly important for those physical signs with positive LRs around 2.0 or negative LRs around 0.5, signs that by themselves change probability little but when combined change probability a greater amount. Individual LRs can be combined, however, only if the findings are "independent."

a. Independence of Findings

"Independence" means that the LR for second finding does not change once the clinician determines whether the first finding is present or absent. For a few diagnostic problems, investigators have identified which findings are independent of each other. These findings appear as components of "diagnostic scoring schemes" in the tables throughout this book. For most physical findings, however, very little information is available about independence, and the clinician must judge whether combining findings is appropriate.

One important clue is that most independent findings have unique pathophysiology. For example, when considering pneumonia in patients with cough and fever, the clinician could combine the findings of abnormal mental status and diminished breath sounds, using the individual LRs of each finding because abnormal mental status and diminished breath sounds probably have separate pathophysiology. Similarly, when considering heart failure in patients with dyspnea, the clinician could combine the findings of elevated neck veins and third heart sound because these findings also have different pathophysiology.

Examples of findings whose individual LRs should *not* be combined (because the findings share the same pathophysiology) are flank dullness and shifting dullness in the diagnosis of ascites (both depend on intra-abdominal contents dampening the vibrations of the abdominal wall during percussion), neck stiffness and Kernig's sign in the diagnosis of meningitis (both are caused by meningeal irritation), and edema and elevated neck veins in the diagnosis of heart failure (both depend on elevated right atrial pressure).

Until more information is available, the safest policy for the clinician to follow, when combining LRs of individual findings, is to combine no more than three findings, all of which have distinct pathophysiology.

b. How to Combine Findings

The clinician can use any of the methods previously described to combine findings, simply by making the post-test probability from the first finding the pretest probability for the second finding. For example, a hypothetical patient with acute fever and cough has two positive findings that we believe have separate pathophysiology and therefore are independent: abnormal mental status (LR = 1.9 for pneumonia) and diminished breath sounds (LR = 2.3 for pneumonia). The pretest probability of pneumonia, derived from published estimates and clinical experience, is estimated to be 20%. Using the graph, the finding of abnormal mental status increases the probability form 20% to 32%; this post-test probability then becomes the pretest probability for the second finding, diminished breath sounds, which increases probability from 32% to 52%—the overall probability after application of the two findings. Using the approximating rules, both findings (LRs ≈ 2.0) increase the probability about 15%; the post-test probability is thus 20% + 15% + 15% = 50% (an error of only 2%). Using formulas to calculate probability, the LRs of the separate findings are multiplied together and the product is used to convert pretest into post-test odds. The product of the two LRs is 4.4 (1.9×2.3); the pretest odds is 0.2/0.8 = 0.25; the post-test odds is $0.25 \times 4.4 = 1.1$, which equals a probability of 1.1/2.1 = 52%.

REFERENCES

1. Eskelinen M, Ikonen J, Lipponen P. Contributions of history-taking, physical examination, and computer assistance to diagnosis of acute small-bowel obstruction: A prospective study of 1333 patients with acute abdominal pain. *Scand J Gastroenterol.* 1994;29:715-721.
2. Brewer RJ, Golden GT, Hitch DC, et al. Abdominal pain: An analysis of 1000 consecutive cases in a university hospital emergency room. *Am J Surg.* 1976;131:219-223.

3. Böhner H, Yang Z, Franke C, et al. Simple data from history and physical examination help to exclude bowel obstruction and to avoid radiographic studies in patients with acute abdominal pain. *Eur J Surg.* 1998;164:777-784.

4. Aronow WS, Kronzon I. Correlation of prevalence and severity of valvular aortic stenosis determined by continuous-wave Doppler echocardiography with physical signs of aortic stenosis in patients aged 62 to 100 years with aortic systolic ejection murmurs. *Am J Cardiol.* 1987;60:399-401.

5. Heckerling PS, Tape TG, Wigton RS, et al. Clinical prediction rule for pulmonary infiltrates. *Ann Intern Med.* 1990;113:664-670.

6. Wells PS, Anderson DR, Bormanis J, et al. Value of assessment of pretest probability of deep-vein thrombosis in clinical management. *Lancet.* 1997;350:1795-1798.

7. Miron MJ, Perrier A, Bounameaux H. Clinical assessment of suspected deep vein thrombosis: Comparison between a score and empirical assessment. *J Intern Med.* 2000;247:249-254.

8. Anderson DR, Wells PS, MacLeod B, et al. Thrombosis in the emergency department. *Arch Intern Med.* 1999;159:477-482.

9. Aschwanden M, Labs KH, Jeanneret C, et al. The value of rapid D-dimer testing combined with structured clinical evaluation for the diagnosis of deep vein thrombosis. *J Vasc Surg.* 1999;30:929-935.

10. Funfsinn N, Caliezi C, Baiasiutti FD, et al. Rapid D-dimer testing and pre-test clinical probability in the exclusion of deep venous thrombosis in symptomatic outpatients. Blood Coagul Fibrinolysis. 2001;12(3):165-170.

11. Kearon C, Ginsberg JS, Douketis J, et al. Management of suspected deep venous thrombosis in outpatients by using clinical assessment and D-dimer testing. *Ann Intern Med.* 2001;135:108-111.

12. Oudega R, Hoes AW, Moons KGM. The Wells rule does not adequately rule out deep venous thrombosis in primary care patients. *Ann Intern Med.* 2005;143:100-107.

13. Schutgens REG, Ackermark P, Haas FJLM, et al. Combination of a normal D-dimer concentration and a non-high pretest clinical probability score is a safe strategy to exclude deep venous thrombosis. *Circulation.* 2003;107:593-597.

14. Tick LW, Ton E, van Voorthuizen T, et al. Practical diagnostic management of patients with clinically suspected deep vein thrombosis by clinical probability test, compression ultrasonography, and D-dimer test. *Am J Med.* 2002;113:630-635.

15. Chagnon I, Bounameaux H, Aujesky D, et al. Comparison of two clinical prediction rules and implicit assessment among patients with suspected pulmonary embolism. *Am J Med.* 2002;113:269-275.

16. Miniati M, Bottai M, Monti S. Comparison of 3 clinical models for predicting the probability of pulmonary embolism. *Medicine.* 2005;84:107-114.

17. Wells PS, Anderson DR, Rodger M, et al. Excluding pulmonary embolism at the bedside without diagnostic imaging: Management of patients with suspected pulmonary embolism presenting to the emergency department by using a simple clinical model and D-dimer. *Ann Intern Med.* 2001;135:98-107.

18. Wolf SJ, McCubbin TR, Feldhaus KM, et al. Prospective validation of Wells criteria in the evaluation of patients with suspected pulmonary embolism. *Ann Emerg Med.* 2004;44:503-510.

19. Desjardins VA, Enriquez-Sarano M, Tajik J, et al. Intensity of murmurs correlates with severity of valvular regurgitation. *Am J Med.* 1996;100:149-156.

20. Frank MJ, Casanegra P, Migliori AJ, Levinson GE. The clinical evaluation of aortic regurgitation. *Arch Intern Med.* 1965;116:357-365.

21. Linhart JW. Aortic regurgitation: Clinical, hemodynamic, surgical, and angiographic correlations. *Ann Thorac Surg.* 1971;11:27-37.

22. Rahko PS. Prevalence of regurgitant murmurs in patients with valvular regurgitation detected by Doppler echocardiography. *Ann Intern Med.* 1989;111:466-472.

23. Sackett DL, Richardson WS, Rosenberg W, Haynes RB. *Evidence-based medicine: How to practice and teach EBM.* New York: Churchill Livingstone; 1997.

24. Sackett DL, Haynes RB, Tugwell P. *Clinical epidemiology: A basic science for clinical medicine,* 1st ed. Boston: Little, Brown and Co.; 1985.

25. Fagan TJ. Nomogram for Bayes' theorem. *N Engl J Med.* 1975;293:257.

26. Grimes DA, Schulz KF. Refining clinical diagnosis with likelihood ratios. *Lancet.* 2005;365:1500-1505.

27. McGee S. Simplifying likelihood ratios. *J Gen Intern Med.* 2002;17:646-649.

28. Bohadana AB, Peslin R, Uffholtz H. Breath sounds in the clinical assessment of airflow obstruction. *Thorax.* 1978;33:345-351.

29. Pardee NE, Martin CJ, Morgan EH. A test of the practical value of estimating breath sound intensity: Breath sounds related to measured ventilatory function. *Chest.* 1976;70:341-344.

2

Using the Tables in This Book

I. INTRODUCTION

Information about the diagnostic accuracy of physical findings is presented in two types of tables in this book: (1) "Frequency of Findings" tables, which display only the sensitivity of physical signs, and (2) "Diagnostic Accuracy" tables, which present the sensitivity, specificity, and likelihood ratios (LRs) of various physical signs.

II. FREQUENCY OF FINDINGS TABLES

A. DEFINITION

Frequency of findings tables summarize multiple studies of patients with a specific diagnosis and present the sensitivity of physical signs found in that disorder. These tables provide no information about a sign's specificity. An example is Table 2-1, listing the frequency of findings in constrictive pericarditis, a disorder in which a diseased and unyielding pericardium interferes with diastolic filling of the heart.

| Table 2-1 | Constrictive Pericarditis* |

Physical Finding	Frequency (%)†
Neck Veins	
Elevated neck veins	98
Prominent Y descent (Friedrich's sign)	57–94
Kussmaul's sign	50
Arterial Pulse	
Irregularly irregular (atrial fibrillation)	36–70
Blood Pressure	
Pulsus paradoxus > 10 mm Hg	17–43
Auscultation of Heart	
Pericardial knock	28–94
Pericardial rub	4
Other	
Hepatomegaly	87–100
Edema	63
Ascites	53–89

*Data from 181 patients from References 1–8
Diagnostic standard: For constrictive pericarditis, surgical and postmortem findings,[1,2,5,6] sometimes in combination with hemodynamic findings.[3,4,7,8]
†Results are overall mean frequency or, if statistically heterogenous, the range of values.

B. PARTS OF THE TABLE

1. Finding

The first column lists the various physical signs, organized by organ system, with the findings of each organ system listed from most to least frequent.

2. Frequency

The second column lists the sensitivity (or frequency) of the physical signs. If the sensitivity from every study is statistically similar, the overall mean frequency is presented (e.g., in Table 2-1, 98% of patients with constrictive pericarditis have elevated neck veins). If the sensitivities from the different studies are statistically diverse ($P < .05$ by the Chi-squared test), the range of values instead is presented (e.g., in Table 2-1, 28% to 94% have a pericardial knock— a loud heart sound heard near the apex during early diastole).

3. Footnotes

The footnotes to these tables present the source of the information and the diagnostic standards used. For example, the information in Table 2-1 is based on 181 patients from eight different studies, which based the diagnosis of constrictive pericarditis on surgical, postmortem, or hemodynamic findings.

C. INTERPRETATION

Because the frequency of findings tables provide just information about a sign's sensitivity, they can only be used to support a statement that a physical sign, when *absent*, argues *against* disease. The absence of any finding whose sensitivity (or frequency) is greater than 95% is a compelling argument against that diagnosis (i.e., the negative LR is 0.1 or less, even if the specificity of the finding, which is unknown, is as low as 50%). In Table 2-1, elevated venous pressure is such a finding (sensitivity 98%): If the clinician is considering the diagnosis of constrictive pericarditis, but the patient's bedside estimate of venous pressure is normal, the diagnosis becomes very unlikely.

Similarly, the absence of two or three independent findings having sensitivities greater than 80% is also a compelling argument against disease* (Chapter 1 defines independent findings).

III. DIAGNOSTIC ACCURACY TABLES

A. DEFINITION

Diagnostic accuracy tables summarize information from large numbers of patients who present with similar symptoms but different diagnoses. The tables present the physical sign's sensitivity, specificity, and positive and negative LRs, which then indicate how well that physical sign discriminates between patients with a particular diagnosis of interest and those without it. The criteria for selecting these studies appear in "Criteria for Selecting Studies Used in Diagnostic Accuracy Tables" (see Section IV, p. 25).

EBM Box 2-1 presents an example that summarizes the diagnostic accuracy of physical signs for pneumonia, as applied to a large number of patients with cough and fever (see Chapter 29 for complete table). In these studies, only about 20% of patients had pneumonia; the remainder had other causes of cough and fever such as sinusitis, bronchitis, or rhinitis.

B. PARTS OF THE TABLE

1. Finding

The first column presents the physical signs, organized by organ system, and the source of the information. Validated scoring schemes that combine findings appear in the bottom rows of these tables.

---

*This statement assumes that the product of the LRs being combined is less than 0.1. Therefore, $LR^n = \left[\dfrac{(1 - sens)}{(spec)} \right]^n \leq 0.1$, where n = number of findings being combined. If the specificity of the findings is as low as 50%, each of two findings being combined must have a sensitivity greater than 84%, and each of three findings being combined must have a sensitivity greater than 77%.

Box 2-1   Pneumonia*

Finding (Ref)[†]	Sensitivity (%)	Specificity (%)	Likelihood Ratio if Finding	
			Present	Absent
General Appearance				
Cachexia [9]	10	97	**4.0**	NS
Abnormal mental status[10-12]	12–14	92–95	1.9	NS
Lung Findings				
Percussion dullness[9-11,13,14]	4–26	82–99	**3.0**	NS
Diminished breath sounds[10,11,13,14]	15–49	73–95	2.3	0.8
Bronchial breath sounds[10]	14	96	**3.3**	NS
Egophony[9-11]	4–16	96–99	**4.1**	NS
Crackles[9-15]	19–67	36–94	1.8	0.8
Wheezing[10-15]	15–36	50–85	0.8	NS
Diagnostic Score (Heckerling et al.)[10,16]				
0 or 1 findings	7–29	33–65	**0.3**	...
2 or 3 findings	48–55	...	NS	...
4 or 5 findings	38–41	92–97	**8.2**	...

NS, not significant.
Likelihood ratio (LR) if finding present = positive LR; LR if finding absent = negative LR
*Diagnostic standard: For pneumonia, infiltrate on chest radiograph.
†Definition of findings: For Heckerling's diagnostic score, the clinician scores 1 point for each of the following five findings that are present: temperature > 37.8°C, heart rate > 100/min, crackles, diminished breath sounds, and absence of asthma.

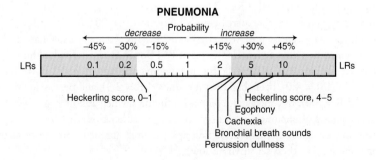

PNEUMONIA

2. Sensitivity and Specificity

The second and third columns present the range of a physical sign's sensitivity and specificity observed in these studies.

3. Likelihood Ratios

The third and fourth columns present the physical sign's positive and negative LR (for clarity, "likelihood ratio if finding *present*" refers to the positive LR, and "likelihood ratio if finding *absent*" refers to the negative LR). In contrast to sensitivity and specificity, which are presented as a range of values, LRs are described by a single number, derived by using a statistical technique called the random effects model (see "Summarizing Likelihood Ratios" later).[17] Only statistically significant LRs are presented in these tables. If the 95% confidence intervals (CIs) for an LR, positive or negative, include the value of 1.0, that result of the physical finding does not statistically discriminate between patients with disease and those without it, and the notation NS for "not significant" is recorded in the table.

4. Footnote

The footnotes to these tables describe the diagnostic standards used in the studies and, if necessary, definitions of findings that appear in the table. The footnote for EBM Box 2-1, for example, indicates that the diagnostic standard for pneumonia was the chest radiograph; it also describes the components of Heckerling's diagnostic scoring scheme presented in the bottom rows of the table.

5. Rules

Evidence-based medicine rules appear with each table, visually displaying those findings that are the most compelling arguments *for* disease and those that are the most compelling arguments *against* disease.

C. INTERPRETATION OF TABLE AND RULES

To use these tables and rules, the clinician must only glance at the LR columns to appreciate the discriminatory power of different findings. LRs with the highest value argue the most *for* disease; LRs with the value closest to zero argue the most *against* disease. The boldface type in the table and the gray shading on the rules highlight all findings with LRs ≥ 3.0 or ≤ 0.3, thus allowing quick identification of those physical signs that increase probability more that 20% to 25% (LR ≥ 3.0) and those that decrease it more that 20% to 25% (LR ≤ 0.3; see also Chapter 1).

In patients with cough and fever (see EBM Box 2-1), the individual findings arguing the most convincingly for pneumonia are egophony (LR = 4.1), cachexia (LR = 4.0), bronchial breath sounds (LR = 3.3), and percussion dullness (LR = 3.0). In contrast, no *individual* findings, when absent, argue *against* the diagnosis of pneumonia (all negative LRs are either close to 1.0 or not significant), primarily because these findings are often absent in proven cases of pneumonia (i.e., their sensitivity is low).

EBM Box 2-1 also shows that 4 or more points using Heckerling's diagnostic scheme argues strongly *for* pneumonia (LR = 8.2), whereas the presence of 0 or 1 point argues *against* the diagnosis (LR = 0.3).

IV. CRITERIA FOR SELECTING STUDIES USED IN DIAGNOSTIC ACCURACY TABLES

All studies of adult patients that met the following four criteria were included in the tables of this book.

A. PATIENTS WERE SYMPTOMATIC

The study had to enroll patients presenting to clinicians with symptoms or other problems. Therefore, studies using asymptomatic controls, which tend to inflate the specificity of physical signs, were excluded. Clinicians do not need a physical sign to help them distinguish patients with pneumonia from healthy persons (who would not be consulting the doctor); instead, they are interested in those physical signs distinguishing pneumonia from other causes of cough and fever.

B. DEFINITION OF PHYSICAL SIGN

The physical sign in the study had to be clearly defined.

C. INDEPENDENT COMPARISON TO A DIAGNOSTIC STANDARD

There had to be an independent comparison to an acceptable diagnostic standard. "Independent comparison" means that the physical sign was not used to select patients for testing with the diagnostic standard. Acceptable diagnostic standards include laboratory testing, clinical imaging, surgical findings, or postmortem analysis.

D. 2 × 2 TABLE COULD BE CONSTRUCTED

The studies had to provide figures or tables from which numbers could be extracted to construct 2 × 2 tables and calculate sensitivity, specificity, and LRs. If any cell of the 2 × 2 table contained the value of zero, 0.5 was added to all cells, to avoid creating the unlikely LRs of 0 or infinity.

V. SUMMARIZING LIKELIHOOD RATIOS

The random effects model by Dersimonian and Laird,[17] which considers both within study and between study variance to calculate a pooled LR, was used to summarize the LRs from the various studies. Table 2-2 illustrates how this model works. In the top rows of this table are the individual data from all studies of egophony that appeared in EBM Box 2-1, including the finding's sensitivity, specificity, positive and negative LRs, and LRs 95% CIs. The bottom row of Table 2-2 shows how all of this information is summarized throughout the book.

In each of the studies, egophony was very specific (96% to 99%) but insensitive (4% to 16%), and the positive LRs were all greater than 1, indicating that the finding of egophony argues for pneumonia. For one of the three studies (i.e., Gennis, Gallagher, Falvo, et al.[11]), the positive LR was not significant because the 95% CI includes the value of 1 (i.e., the LR value of 1 has no discriminatory value). For the other two studies, the 95% CI of the positive LR excluded the value of 1, thus making them statistically significant. The summary measure for the positive LR (fourth row of this table) is both clinically significant (4.08, a large positive number) and statistically significant (its 95% CI excludes 1.0). All of this information is summarized, in the notation used in this book (last row), by simply presenting the pooled LR of 4.1 (Interested readers may consult the Appendix for the 95% CIs of all LRs in this book.)

In contrast, the negative LRs from each study have both meager clinical significance (i.e. 0.87 to 0.96, values close to 1) and, for two of the three studies, no statistical significance (i.e., the 95% CI includes 1). The pooled negative LR also lacks clinical and statistical significance. Because statistically it is no different from 1.0 (i.e., the 95% CI of the pooled value, 0.88 to 1.01, includes 1), it is summarized using the notation NS.

Presenting the single pooled result for statistically significant LRs and NS for the statistically insignificant ones simplifies the table and makes it much simpler to grasp the point that the finding of egophony in patients with cough

Table 2-2	Egophony and Pneumonia— Individual Studies			
Reference	Sensitivity (%)	Specificity (%)	Positive LR (95% CI)	Negative LR (95% CI)
Heckerling et al.[10]	16	97	4.91 (2.88, 8.37)	0.87 (0.81, 0.94)
Gennis et al.[11]	8	96	2.07 (0.79, 5.41)	0.96 (0.90, 1.02)
Diehr et al.[9]	4	99	7.97 (1.77, 35.91)	0.96 (0.91, 1.02)
Pooled result			4.08 (2.14, 7.79)	0.93 (0.88, 1.01)
Notation used in book	4–16	96–99	4.1	NS

CI, confidence interval; LR, likelihood ratio; NS, not significant.

and fever argues for pneumonia (LR = 4.1), but the absence of egophony changes probability very little or not at all.

REFERENCES

1. Paul O, Castleman B, White PD. Chronic constrictive pericarditis: A study of 53 cases. *Am J Med Sci.* 1948;216:361-377.
2. Mounsey P. The early diastolic sound of constrictive pericarditis. *Br Heart J.* 1955; 17:143-152.
3. Tyberg TI, Goodyer AVN, Langou RA. Genesis of pericardial knock in constrictive pericarditis. *Am J Cardiol.* 1980;46:570-575.
4. Schiavone WA. The changing etiology of constrictive pericarditis in a large referral center. *Am J Cardiol.* 1986;58:373-375.
5. Lange RL, Botticelli JT, Tsagaris TJ, et al. Diagnostic signs in compressive cardiac disorders: Constrictive pericarditis, pericardial effusion, and tamponade. *Circulation* 1966;33:763-777.
6. Evans W, Jackson F. Constrictive pericarditis. *Br Heart J.* 1952;14:53-69.
7. Wood P. Chronic constrictive pericarditis. *Am J Cardiol.* 1961;7:48-61.
8. El-Sherif A, El-Said G. Jugular, hepatic, and praecordial pulsations in constrictive pericarditis. *Br Heart J.* 1971;33:305-312.
9. Diehr P, Wood RW, Bushyhead J, et al. Prediction of pneumonia in outpatients with acute cough: a statistical approach. *J Chron Dis.* 1984;37(3):215-225.
10. Heckerling PS, Tape TG, Wigton RS, et al. Clinical prediction rule for pulmonary infiltrates. *Ann Intern Med.* 1990;113:664-670.
11. Gennis P, Gallagher J, Falvo C, et al. Clinical criteria for the detection of pneumonia in adults: Guidelines for ordering chest roentgenograms in the emergency department. *J Emerg Med.* 1989;7:263-268.
12. Mehr DR, Binder EF, Kruse RL, et al. Clinical findings associated with radiographic pneumonia in nursing home residents. *J Fam Pract.* 2001;50:931-937.
13. Melbye H, Straume B, Aasebo U, Dale K. Diagnosis of pneumonia in adults in general practice. *Scand J Prim Health Care.* 1992;10:226-233.
14. Melbye H, Straume B, Aasebo U, Brox J. The diagnosis of adult pneumonia in general practice. *Scand J Prim Health Care.* 1988;6:111-117.
15. Singal BM, Hedges JR, Radack KL. Decision rules and clinical prediction of pneumonia: Evaluation of low-yield criteria. *Ann Emerg Med.* 1989;18:13-20.
16. Emerman CL, Dawson N, Speroff T, et al. Comparison of physician judgment and decision aids for ordering chest radiographs for pneumonia in outpatients. *Ann Emerg Med.* 1991;20:1215-1219.
17. DerSimonian R, Laird N. Meta analysis in clinical trials. *Control Clin Trials.* 1986;7:177-188.

Reliability of Physical Findings

"Reliability" refers to how often multiple clinicians, examining the same patients, agree that a particular physical sign is present or absent. As characteristics of a physical sign, reliability and accuracy are distinct qualities, although significant interobserver disagreement tends to undermine the finding's accuracy and prevents clinicians from applying it confidently to their own practice. Disagreement about physical signs also contributes to the growing sense among clinicians, not necessarily justified, that physical examination is less scientific than more technologic tests, such as clinical imaging and laboratory testing, and that physical examination lacks their diagnostic authority.

The most straightforward way to express reliability, or interobserver agreement, is "simple agreement," which is the proportion of total observations in which clinicians agree about the finding. For example, if two clinicians examining 100 patients with dyspnea agree that a third heart sound is present in 5 patients and is absent in 75 patients, simple agreement would be 80% (i.e., (5 + 75)/100 = 0.80; in the remaining 20 patients, only one of the two clinicians heard a third heart sound). Simple agreement has advantages, including being easy to calculate and understand, but a significant disadvantage is that agreement may be quite high by chance alone. For example, if one of the clinicians in our hypothetical study heard a third heart sound in 10 of the 100 dyspneic patients and the other heard it in 20 of the patients (even though they agreed about the presence of the heart sound in only 5 patients), simple agreement *by chance alone* would be 74%.* With chance agreement this high, the observed 80% agreement no longer seems so impressive.

To address this problem, most clinical studies now express interobserver agreement using the kappa (κ)-statistic, which usually has values between 0 and 1 (The appendix at the end of this chapter shows how to calculate the κ-statistic). A κ-value of 0 indicates that observed agreement is the same as that expected by chance, and a κ-value of 1 indicates perfect agreement. According to convention, a κ-value 0 to 0.2 indicates *slight* agreement, 0.2 to 0.4 *fair* agreement, 0.4 to 0.6 *moderate* agreement, 0.6 to 0.8 *substantial* agreement, and 0.8 to 1.0 almost *perfect* agreement.† Rarely, physical signs have κ-values less than 0 (theoretically as low as −1), indicating the observed agreement was worse than chance agreement.

Table 3-1 presents the κ-statistic for most of the physical signs discussed in this book, demonstrating that, with rare exceptions, observed agreement is better than chance agreement (i.e., κ-statistic exceeds 0). About 60% of findings have a κ-statistic of 0.4 or more, indicating that observed agreement is moderate or better.

Clinical disagreement occurs for many reasons—some causes clinicians can control, but others are inextricably linked to the very nature of clinical medicine and human observation in general. The most prominent reasons include the following: (1) The physical sign's definition is vague or ambiguous. For example, experts recommend about a dozen different ways to perform auscultatory percussion of the liver, thus making the sign so nebulous that significant interobserver disagreement is guaranteed. Ambiguity also results if signs are defined with terms that are not easily measurable. For example, clinicians assessing whether a peripheral pulse is present or absent demonstrate moderate-to-almost perfect agreement (κ = 0.52 to 0.92, see Table 3-1), but when the same clinicians are asked to record whether the palpable pulse is normal or diminished, they have great difficulty agreeing about the sign (κ = 0.01 to 0.15)

---

*Agreement by chance approaches 100% as the percentage of positive observations for both clinicians approaches 0% or 100% (i.e., both clinicians agree that a finding is very uncommon or very common) Appendix 1 shows how to calculate chance agreement.
†No measure of reliability is perfect, especially for findings whose prevalence clinicians agree approaches 0% or 100%. For these findings, simple agreement tends to overestimate reliability, and the κ-statistic tends to underestimate the reliability.

Table 3-1	Interobserver Agreement and Physical Signs	
Finding (Ref)	**κ-Statistic***	

Finding (Ref)	κ-Statistic*
GENERAL APPEARANCE	
Mental status examination	
Mini-Mental Status Examination[1]	0.28–0.80
Clock-drawing test (Wolf-Klein method)[2]	0.73
Confusion Assessment Method for delirium[3,4]	0.81
Altered mental status[5]	0.71
Stance and gait	
Abnormal gait[6,7]	0.11–0.71
Skin	
Patient appears anemic[8,9]	0.23–0.48
Nailbed pallor[10]	0.19–0.34
Conjunctival pallor (rim method)[11]	0.54–0.75
Ashen or pale skin[5]	0.34
Cyanosis[8,12]	0.36–0.70
Jaundice[13]	0.65
Vascular spiders[13,14]	0.64–0.73
Palmar erythema[13,14]	0.37–0.49
Hydration status	
Patient appears dehydrated[8]	0.44–0.53
Axillary dryness[15]	0.50
Increased moisture on skin[8]	0.31–0.53
Capillary refill > 3 seconds[5]	0.29
Nutritional assessment	
Abnormal nutritional state[8]	0.27–0.36
Other	
Consciousness impaired[8]	0.65–0.88
Patient appears older than age[8]	0.38–0.42
Patient appears in pain[8]	0.43–0.75
Generally unwell in appearance[8]	0.52–0.64
VITAL SIGNS	
Tachycardia (heart rate > 100/min)[16]	0.85
Bradycardia (heart rate < 60/min)[16]	0.87
Systolic hypertension (SBP > 160 mm Hg)[16]	0.75
Hypotension (SBP < 90 mm Hg)[16,17]	0.27–0.90
Osler's sign[18–20]	0.26–0.72
Elevated body temperature, palpating the skin[8]	0.09–0.23
Tachypnea[5,12,16]	0.25–0.60
HEAD AND NECK	
Diabetic retinopathy	
Microaneurysms[21,22]	0.58–0.66

Table 3-1 Interobserver Agreement and Physical Signs—Cont'd

Finding (Ref)	κ-Statistic*
Intraretinal hemorrhages[21,22]	0.89
Hard exudates[21,22]	0.66–0.74
Cotton wool spots[21,22]	0.56–0.67
Intraretinal microvascular abnormalities (IRMA)[21,22]	0.46
Neovascularization near disc[21,22]	0.21–0.48
Macular edema[21,22]	0.21–0.67
Overall grade[21,22]	0.65
Hearing	
Whispered voice test[23]	0.16–1.0
Thyroid	
Thyroid gland diffuse, multinodular or solitary nodule[24]	0.25–0.70
Goiter[25]	0.38–0.77
Meninges	
Nuchal rigidity, present or absent[26]	0.76
LUNGS	
Inspection	
Clubbing[12,27]	0.33–0.45
Breathing difficulties[8]	0.54–0.69
Gasping respirations[5]	0.63
Reduced chest movement[12,28]	0.14–0.38
Scalene or sternocleidomastoid muscle contraction[5,29]	0.52–0.53
Kyphosis[27]	0.37
Displaced trachea[12]	0.01
Palpation	
Tracheal descent during inspiration[29]	0.62
Impalpable apex beat[12,27]	0.33–0.44
Decreased tactile fremitus[12]	0.24
Increased tactile fremitus[12]	0.01
Subxiphoid point of maximal cardiac impulse[30]	0.30
Paradoxical costal margin movement[29]	0.56
Percussion	
Hyper-resonant percussion note[12,28,30]	0.26–0.50
Dull percussion note[12,28,31]	0.16–0.52
Diaphragm excursion more or less than 2 cm, by percussion[30]	−0.04
Diminished cardiac dullness[30]	0.49
Auscultatory percussion abnormal[32]	0.18–0.39

Continued

Table 3-1	Interobserver Agreement and Physical Signs—Cont'd	

Finding (Ref)	κ-Statistic*
Auscultation	
Reduced breath sound intensity[12,28,30,31,33,34]	0.16–0.51
Bronchial breathing[12,28]	0.19–0.32
Whispering pectoriloquy[12]	0.11
Crackles[12,31,33,35]	0.21–0.63
Wheezes[12,30,31,33,34]	0.43–0.93
Rhonchi[28,34]	0.38–0.55
Pleural rub[12]	0.51
Special tests	
Snider test < 10 cm[30]	0.39
Forced expiratory time[30,36,37]	0.27–0.70
Hoover sign[34]	0.74
Wells simplified rule for pulmonary embolism[38]	0.54–0.62
HEART	
Neck veins	
Neck veins, elevated or normal[35,39]	0.38–0.69
Abdominojugular test[39]	0.92
Palpation	
Palpable apical impulse present[40–42]	0.68–0.82
Palpable apical impulse measureable[43]	0.56
Palpable apical impulse displaced lateral to midclavicular line[35,40,41]	0.43–0.64
Percussion	
Cardiac dullness > 10.5 cm from midsternal line[44,45]	0.57
Auscultation	
S2 diminished or absent, vs. normal[46]	0.54
S_3 sound[35,39,47–49]	−0.17–0.75
S_4 sound[48]	0.15–0.52
Systolic murmur, present or absent[46]	0.19
Systolic murmur radiates to right carotid[46]	0.33
Systolic murmur, long systolic or early systolic[50]	0.78
Murmur intensity (Levine grade)[51]	0.43–0.60
Systolic murmur grade > 2/6[52]	0.59
Carotid pulsation	
Delayed carotid upstroke[46]	0.26
Reduced carotid volume[46]	0.24
ABDOMEN	
Inspection	
Abdominal distension[53,54]	0.35–0.42
Abdominal wall collateral veins, present vs. absent[13]	0.47

| Table 3-1 | Interobserver Agreement and Physical Signs—Cont'd |

Finding (Ref)	κ-Statistic*
Palpation and percussion	
Ascites[13,14]	0.63–0.75
Abdominal tenderness[53–55]	0.31–0.68
Surgical abdomen[54]	0.27
Abdominal wall tenderness test[56]	0.52
Rebound tenderness[53]	0.25
Guarding[53,54]	0.36–0.49
Rigidity[53]	0.14
Abdominal mass palpated[54]	0.82
Palpable spleen[13,14]	0.33–0.75
Palpable liver edge[57]	0.44–0.53
Liver consistency, normal or abnormal[13]	0.40
Liver firm to palpation[58]	0.72
Liver, nodular or not[13]	0.29
Liver, tender or not[14]	0.49
Liver, span > 9 cm by percussion[35]	0.11
Spleen palpable or not[59]	0.56–0.70
Spleen percussion sign (Traube's), positive or not[60]	0.19–0.41
Abdominal aortic aneurysm, present vs. absent[61]	0.53
Auscultation	
Normal bowel sounds[54]	0.36
EXTREMITIES	
Peripheral vascular disease	
Peripheral pulse, present vs. absent[62,63]	0.52–0.92
Peripheral pulse, normal or diminished[62]	0.01–0.15
Diabetic foot	
Monofilament sensation, normal or abnormal[64–66]	0.48–0.83
Edema and deep venous thrombosis	
Dependent edema[35]	0.39
Well's pretest probability for DVT[67]	0.75
Musculoskeletal system-shoulder	
Shoulder tenderness[68]	0.32
Painful arc[68]	0.64
External rotation of shoulder < 45 degrees[68]	0.68
Supraspinatus test (empty can)[68]	0.49
Infraspinatus test (resisted external rotation)[68]	0.49
Impingement sign (Hawkins-Kennedy)[68]	0.29
Drop arm test[68]	0.28

Continued

Table 3-1	Interobserver Agreement and Physical Signs—Cont'd

Finding (Ref)	κ-Statistic*
Musculoskeletal system-knee	
Ottawa knee rules[69]	0.77
Knee effusion visible[69–71]	0.28–0.59
Knee flexion < 90 degrees[69]	0.74
Patellar tenderness[69,70]	0.69–0.76
Head of fibula tenderness[69]	0.64
Inability to bear weight immediately and emergency room after knee injury[69,70]	0.75–0.81
Bony swelling of knee[72]	0.55
Medial joint line tenderness of knee[71,72]	0.21–0.40
Lateral joint line tenderness of knee[71,72]	0.25–0.43
Patellofemoral crepitus[72]	0.24
Mediolateral instability of knee[72]	0.23
McMurray sign[71,73]	0.16–0.35
Musculoskeletal system-ankle	
Inability to walk 4 steps immediately and in emergency room after ankle injury[74,75]	0.71–0.97
Medial malleolar tenderness[75]	0.82
Lateral malleolar tenderness[75]	0.80
Navicular tenderness[75]	0.91
Base of fifth metatarsal tenderness[75]	0.94
Ottawa ankle/midfoot rule[76]	0.61
NEUROLOGIC EXAMINATION	
Cranial nerves	
Pharyngeal sensation, present or absent[77]	1.0
Facial palsy, present or absent[78,79]	0.57
Dysarthria, present or absent[80]	0.61–0.77
Water swallow test (50 mL)[81]	0.60
Oxygen desaturation test (for aspiration risk)[81]	0.60
Abnormal tongue strength[80]	0.55–0.63
Motor examination	
Muscle strength, MRC scale[82–84]	0.69–0.93
Muscle atrophy[85]	0.32–0.81
Spasticity, 6-point scale[86]	0.21–0.61
Rigidity, 4-point scale[87]	0.64
Asterixis[13]	0.42
Sensory examination	
Light touch sensation, normal, diminished, or increased[85]	0.63
Pain sensation, normal, diminished, or increased[83,85]	0.41–0.57
Vibratory sensation, normal or diminished[85]	0.45–0.54

Table 3-1	Interobserver Agreement and Physical Signs—Cont'd

Finding (Ref)	κ-Statistic*
Reflex examination	
Reflex amplitude, NINDS scale[88]	0.51–0.61
Ankle jerk, present or absent[83,89,90]	0.34–0.94
Asymmetric knee jerk[83]	0.42
Primitive reflexes, amplitude and persistence[91]	0.46–1.0
Babinski response[78,79,92]	0.17–0.54
Coordination	
Finger-nose test[78,79]	0.55
Dysmetria, finger-to-nose test, rated 0 to 3[93]	0.36–0.40
Peripheral nerve	
Spurling's test[94]	0.60
Flick sign[95]	0.90
Hypalgesia index finger[95]	0.50
Tinel's sign[95]	0.47
Phalen's sign[95]	0.79
Straight-leg raising test[83,96–98]	0.21–0.68
Crossed-leg raising test[83]	0.49

DVT, deep vein thrombosis; MRC, Medical Research Council; NINDS, National Institute of Neurological Disorders; SBP, systolic blood pressure.
*Interpretation of the κ-statistic: 0–0.2 slight agreement, 0.2–0.4 fair agreement, 0.4–0.6 moderate agreement, 0.6–0.8 substantial agreement, and 0.8–1.0 almost perfect agreement.

simply because they have no idea what the next clinician means by "diminished." (2) The clinician's technique is flawed. For example, common mistakes are using the diaphragm instead of the bell of the stethoscope to detect the third heart sound, or stating a muscle stretch reflex is absent without first trying to elicit it using a reinforcing maneuver (e.g., Jendrassik maneuver). (3) Biologic variation of the physical sign. The pericardial friction rub, pulsus alternans, cannon A waves, Cheyne-Stokes respirations, and many other signs are notoriously evanescent, tending to come and go over time. (4) The clinician is careless or inattentive. The bustle of an active practice may lead clinicians to listen to the lungs while conducting the patient interview or to search for a subtle murmur in a noisy emergency room. Reliable observations require undistracted attention and an alert mind. (5) The clinician's biases influence the observation. When findings are equivocal, expectations influence perceptions. For example, in a patient who just started blood pressure medications, borderline hypertension may become normal blood pressure; in a patient with increasing bilateral edema, borderline distended neck veins may become clearly elevated venous pressure, or, in a patient with new weakness, the equivocal Babinski sign may become clearly positive. Sometimes, biases actually create the finding: if the clinician holds a flashlight too long over an eye with suspected optic nerve disease, he or she may temporarily bleach the retina of that eye and produce the Marcus Gunn pupil, thus confirming the original suspicion.

The lack of perfect reliability with physical diagnosis is sometimes regarded as a significant weakness, a reason that physical diagnosis is less reliable and scientific than clinical imaging and laboratory testing. Nonetheless, Table 3-2 shows that, for most of our *diagnostic standards*— chest radiography, computed tomography, screening mammography, angiography, magnetic resonance imaging, ultrasonography, endoscopy, and pathology—interobserver agreement is also less than perfect, with κ-statistics similar to those observed with physical signs. Even with laboratory tests, which present the clinician with a single, indisputable number, interobserver disagreement is still possible and even common, simply because the clinician has to interpret the laboratory test's *significance*. For example, in one study of three endocrinologists reviewing the same thyroid function tests and other clinical data of 55 consecutive outpatients with suspected thyroid disease, the endocrinologists disagreed about the final diagnosis 40% of the time.[24] Computerized interpretation of test results performs no better: In a study of pairs of electrocardiograms taken only 1 minute apart from 92 patients, the computer interpretation was significantly different 40% of the time, even though the tracings showed no change.[114]

By defining abnormal findings precisely, by studying and mastering examination technique, and by observing every detail at the bedside attentively and without bias or distraction, we can minimize interobserver disagreement and make physical diagnosis more precise. However, it is simply impossible to abstract every detail of our observations of patients into exact physical signs, and in this way physical diagnosis is no different from any of the other tools we use to categorize disease. So long as both the material and the observers of clinical medicine are human beings, a certain amount of subjectivity always will be with us.

APPENDIX: CALCULATION OF THE κ-STATISTIC

The observations of two observers who are examining the same N patients independently are customarily displayed in a 2×2 table, similar to that in Fig. 3-1. Observer A finds the sign to be present in w_1 patients and absent in w_2 patients; observer B finds the sign to be present in y_1 patients and absent in y_2

Table 3-2 Interobserver Agreement—Diagnostic Standards

Finding (Ref)	κ-Statistic*
Chest radiography	
Cardiomegaly[39]	0.48
Interstitial edema[39]	0.83
Pulmonary vascular redistribution[39]	0.50
Grading pulmonary fibrosis, 4-point scale[99]	0.45
Contrast venography	
Deep vein thrombosis in leg[100]	0.53
Screening mammography	
Suspicious lesion, present vs. absent[101]	0.47
Digital subtraction angiography	
Renal artery stenosis[102]	0.65
Coronary arteriography	
Classification of coronary artery lesions[103]	0.33
Computed tomography of head	
Normal or abnormal, patient with stroke[104]	0.60
Lesion on right or left side, patient with stroke[104]	0.65
Mass effect, present or absent[104]	0.52
Computed tomography of the chest	
Lung cancer staging[105]	0.40–0.60
Magnetic resonance imaging of head	
Compatible with multiple sclerosis[106]	0.57–0.87
Magnetic resonance imaging of lumbar spine	
Intervertebral disc extrusion, protrusion, bulge, or normal[107]	0.59
Lumbar nerve root compression[108]	0.83
Ultrasonography	
Calf deep vein thrombosis, present or absent[109]	0.69
Thyroid nodule, present or absent[110,111]	0.57–0.66
Endoscopy	
Grade of reflux esophagitis[112]	0.55
Pathologic examination of liver biopsy	
Cholestasis[113]	0.40
Alcoholic liver disease[113]	0.49
Cirrhosis[113]	0.59

*Interpretation of the κ-statistic: 0–0.2 slight agreement, 0.2–0.4 fair agreement, 0.4–0.6 moderate agreement, 0.6–0.8 substantial agreement, and 0.8–1.0 almost perfect agreement.

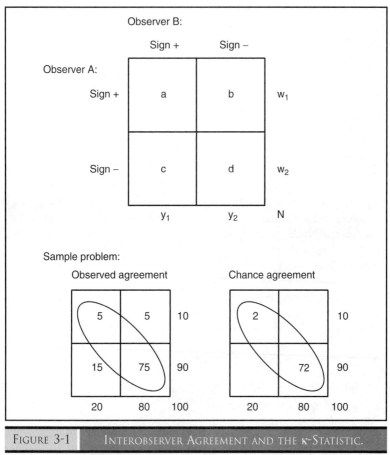

FIGURE 3-1   INTEROBSERVER AGREEMENT AND THE κ-STATISTIC.

Top half, Conventional 2 × 2 table displaying data for calculation of κ-statistic. *Bottom half,* A sample case, in which observed agreement is 80%, chance agreement is 74%, and the κ-statistic is 0.23 (see Appendix for discussion).

patients. The two observers agree the sign is present in *a* patients and absent in *d* patients. Therefore, the observed agreement (P_O) is:

$$P_O = (a + d)/N$$

Calculation of the κ-statistic first requires calculation of the agreement that would have occurred by chance alone. Among all the patients, observer A found the fraction w_1/N to have the sign; therefore, by chance alone, among the y_1 patients with the sign according to observer B, observer A would find the sign in (w_1/N) times y_1 or (w_1y_1/N) patients (i.e., this is the *number* of patients in which both observers agree the sign is present, by chance alone). Similarly, both observers would agree the sign is absent by chance alone in (w_2y_2/N) patients. Therefore, the expected chance agreement (P_E) is their sum, divided by N:

$$P_E = (w_1y_1 + w_2y_2)/N^2$$

This equation shows that agreement by chance alone (P_E) approaches 100% as both w_1 and y_1 approach 0 or N (i.e., both clinicians agree that a finding is rare or that it is very common).

The κ-statistic is the increment in observed agreement beyond that expected by chance $(P_O - P_E)$, divided by the maximal increment that could have been observed had the observed agreement been perfect $(1 - P_E)$:

$$\kappa = \frac{(P_O - P_E)}{(1 - P_E)}$$

For example, Fig. 3-1 depicts the observations of two observers in a study of 100 patients with dyspnea. Both agree the third heart sound is present in 5 patients and absent in 75 patients; therefore simple agreement is $(5 + 75)/100$ or 0.80. By chance alone, they would have agreed about the sound being present in $(10 \times 20)/100$ patients (i.e., 2 patients) and absent in $(90 \times 80)/100$ patients (i.e., 72 patients); therefore, chance agreement is $(2 + 72)/100$ patients or 0.74. The κ-statistic for this finding becomes $(0.80 - 0.74)/(1 - 0.74) = (0.06)/(0.26) = 0.23$.

REFERENCES

1. O'Connor DW, Pollitt PA, Hyde JB, et al. The reliability and validity of the mini-mental state in a British community survey. *J Psychiatr Res.* 1989;23(1):87-96.
2. Ainslie NK, Murden RA. Effect of education on the clock-drawing dementia screen in non-demented elderly persons. *J Am Geriatr Soc.* 1993;41:249-252.
3. Inouye SK, Van Dyck CH, Alessi CA, et al. Clarifying confusion: The confusion assessment method. A new method for detection of delirium. *Ann Intern Med.* 1990;113:941-948.
4. Gonzalez M, de Pablo J, Fuente E, et al. Instrument for detection of delirium in general hospitals: Adaptation of the confusion assessment method. *Psychosomatics.* 2004;45:426-431.
5. Jones AE, Aborn LS, Kline JA. Severity of emergency department hypotension predicts adverse hospital outcome. *Shock.* 2004;22:410-414.

6. Eastlack ME, Arvidson J, Snyder-Mackler L, et al. Interrater reliability of video-taped observational gait-analysis assessments. *Phys Ther.* 1991;71:465-472.

7. Verghese J, Lipton RB, Hall CB, et al. Abnormality of gait as a predictor of non-Alzheimer's dementia. *N Engl J Med.* 2002;347:1761-1768.

8. Gjorup T, Hendriksen C, Bugge PM, Jensen AM. Global assessment of patients: a bedside study. II. Interobserver variation and frequency of clinical findings. *J Intern Med.* 1990;228:147-150.

9. Gjorup T, Bugge PM, Hendriksen C, Jensen AM. A critical evaluation of the clinical diagnosis of anemia. *Am J Epidemiol.* 1986;124:657-665.

10. Nardone DA, Roth KM, Mazur DJ, McAfee JH. Usefulness of physical examination in detecting the presence or absence of anemia. *Arch Intern Med.* 1990;150:201-204.

11. Sheth TN, Choudhry NK, Bowes M, Detsky AS. The relation of conjunctival pallor to the presence of anemia. *J Gen Intern Med.* 1997;12:102-106.

12. Spiteri MA, Cook DG, Clarke SW. Reliability of eliciting physical signs in examination of the chest. *Lancet.* 1988;2:873-875.

13. Espinoza P, Ducot B, Pelletier G, et al. Interobserver agreement in the physical diagnosis of alcoholic liver disease. *Dig Dis Sci.* 1987;32:244-247.

14. Theodossi A, Knill-Jones RP, Skene A, et al. Inter-observer variation of symptoms and signs in jaundice. *Liver.* 1981;1:21-32.

15. Eaton D, Bannister P, Mulley GP, Connolly MJ. Axillary sweating in clinical assessment of dehydration in ill elderly patients. *Br Med J.* 1994;308:1271.

16. Edmonds ZV, Mower WR, Lovato LM, Lomeli R. The reliability of vital sign measurements. *Ann Emerg Med.* 2002;39:233-237.

17. Lemeshow S, Teres D, Klar J, et al. Mortality probability models (MPM II) based on an international cohort of intensive care unit patients. *JAMA.* 1993;270: 2478-2486.

18. Hla KM, Samsa GP, Stoneking HT, Feussner JR. Observer variability of Osler's maneuver in detection of pseudohypertension. *J Clin Epidemiol.* 1991;44:513-518.

19. Belmin J, Visintin JM, Salvatore R, et al. Osler's maneuver: Absence of usefulness for the detection of pseudohypertension in an elderly population. *Am J Med.* 1995; 98:42-49.

20. Tsapatasaris NP, Napolitana BT, Rothchild J. Osler's maneuver in an outpatient clinic setting. *Arch Intern Med.* 1991;151:2209-2211.

21. Milton RC, Ganley JP, Lynk RH. Variability in grading diabetic retinopathy from stereo fundus photographs: comparison of physician and lay readers. *Br J Ophthalmol.* 1977;61:192-201.

22. Early Treatment Diabetic Retinopathy Study Research Group. Grading diabetic retinopathy from stereoscopic color fundus photographs: An extension of the modified Airlie House Classification. ETDRS report number 10. *Ophthalmology.* 1991;98:786-806.

23. Eekhof JAH, de Bock GH, de Laat JAPM, et al. The whispered voice: The best test for screening for hearing impairment in general practice? *Br J Gen Pract.* 1996;46:473-474.

24. Jarlov AE, Nygaard B, Hegedus L, et al. Observer variation in the clinical and laboratory evaluation of patients with thyroid dysfunction and goiter. *Thyroid.* 1998;8:393-398.

25. Siminoski K. The rational clinical examination: Does this patient have a goiter? *JAMA.* 1995;273:813-817.

26. Lindsay KW, Teasdale GM, Knill-Jones RP. Observer variability in assessing the clinical features of subarachnoid hemorrhage. *J Neurosurg.* 1983;58:57-62.

27. Schilling RSF, Hughes JPW, Dingwall-Fordyce I. Disagreement between observers in an epidemiological study of respiratory disease. *Br Med J.* 1955;1:65-68.

28. Gjorup T, Bugge PM, Jensen AM. Interobserver variation in assessment of respiratory signs: Physicians' guesses as to interobserver variation. *Acta Med Scand.* 1984;216:61-66.

29. Stubbing DG, Mathur PN, Roberts RS, Campbell EJM. Some physical signs in patients with chronic airflow obstruction. *Am Rev Respir Dis.* 1982;125:549-552.

30. Badgett RG, Tanaka DJ, Hunt DK, et al. Can moderate chronic obstructive pulmonary disease be diagnosed by historical and physical findings alone? *Am J Med.* 1993;94:188-196.

31. Mulrow CD, Dolmatch BL, Delong ER, et al. Observer variation in the pulmonary examination. *J Gen Intern Med.* 1986;1:364-367.

32. Nelson RS, Rickman LS, Mathews WC, et al. Rapid clinical diagnosis of pulmonary abnormalities in HIV-seropositive patients by auscultatory percussion. *Chest.* 1994;105:402-407.

33. Holleman DR, Simel DL, Goldberg JS. Diagnosis of obstructive airways disease from the clinical examination. *J Gen Intern Med.* 1993;8:63-68.

34. Garcia-Pachon E. Paradoxical movement of the lateral rib margin (Hoover sign) for detecting obstructive airway disease. *Chest.* 2002;122:651-655.

35. Gadsboll N, Hoilund-Carlsen PF, Nielsen GG, et al. Symptoms and signs of heart failure in patients with myocardial infarction: Reproducibility and relationship to chest X-ray, radionuclide ventriculography and right heart catheterization. *Eur Heart J.* 1989;10:1017-1028.

36. Schapira RM, Schapira MM, Funahashi A, et al. The value of the forced expiratory time in the physical diagnosis of obstructive airways disease. *JAMA.* 1993;270: 731-736.

37. Badgett R, Tanaka D. The diagnostic value of the forced expiratory time. *JAMA.* 1994;271:25.

38. Wolf SJ, McCubbin TR, Feldhaus KM, et al. Prospective validation of Wells criteria in the evaluation of patients with suspected pulmonary embolism. *Ann Emerg Med.* 2004;44:503-510.

39. Butman SM, Ewy GA, Standen JR, et al. Bedside cardiovascular examination in patients with severe chronic heart failure: Importance of rest or inducible jugular venous distension. *J Am Coll Cardiol.* 1993;22:968-974.

40. O'Neill TW, Smith M, Barry M, Graham IM. Diagnostic value of the apex beat. *Lancet.* 1989;1:410-411.

41. O'Neill TW, Barry MA, Smith M, Graham IM. Diagnostic value of the apex beat. *Lancet*. 1989;2(8661):499.

42. Mulkerrin E, Saran R, Dewar R, et al. The apex cardiac beat: Not a reliable clinical sign in elderly patients. *Age Ageing*. 1991;20:304-306.

43. Dans AL, Bossone EF, Guyatt GH, Fallen EL. Evaluation of the reproducibility and accuracy of apex beat measurement in the detection of echocardiographic left ventricular dilation. *Can J Cardiol*. 1995;11:493-497.

44. Heckerling PS, Wiener SL, Moses VK, et al. Accuracy of precordial percussion in detecting cardiomegaly. *Am J Med*. 1991;91:328-334.

45. Heckerling PS, Wiener SL, Wolfkiel CJ, et al. Accuracy and reproducibility of precordial percussion and palpation for detecting increased left ventricular end-diastolic volume and mass: A comparison of physical findings and ultrafast computed tomography of the heart. *JAMA*. 1993;270:1943-1948.

46. Etchells E, Glenns V, Shadowitz S, et al. A bedside clinical prediction rule for detecting moderate or severe aortic stenosis. *J Gen Intern Med*. 1998;13:699-704.

47. Ishmail AA, Wing S, Ferguson J, et al. Interobserver agreement by auscultation in the presence of a third heart sound in patients with congestive heart failure. *Chest*. 1987;91:870-873.

48. Lok CE, Morgan CD, Ranganathan N. The accuracy and interobserver agreement in detecting the "gallop sounds" by cardiac auscultation. *Chest*. 1998;114:1283-1288.

49. Tribouilloy CM, Enriquez-Sarano M, Mohty D, et al. Pathophysiologic determinants of third heart sounds: A prospective clinical and Doppler echocardiographic study. *Am J Med*. 2001;111:96-102.

50. Forssell G, Jonasson R, Orinius E. Identifying severe aortic valvular stenosis by bedside examination. *Acta Med Scand*. 1985;218:397-400.

51. Keren R, Tereschuk M, Luan X. Evaluation of a novel method for grading heart murmur intensity. *Arch Pediatr Adolesc Med*. 2005;159:329-334.

52. Reichlin S, Dieterle T, Camli C, et al. Initial clinical evaluation of cardiac systolic murmurs in the ED by noncardiologists. *Am J Emerg Med*. 2004;22:71-75.

53. Bjerregaard B, Brynitz S, Holst-Christensen J, et al. The reliability of medical history and physical examination in patients with acute abdominal pain. *Meth Inform Med*. 1983;22:15-18.

54. Pines J, Pines LU, Hall A, et al. The interrater variation of ED abdominal examination findings in patients with acute abdominal pain. *Am J Emerg Med*. 2005;23:483-487.

55. Priebe WM, DaCosta LR, Beck IT. Is epigastric tenderness a sign of peptic ulcer disease? *Gastroenterol*. 1982;82:16-19.

56. Srinivasan R, Greenbaum DS. Chronic abdominal wall pain: A frequently overlooked problem. Practical approach to diagnosis and management. *Am J Gastroenterol*. 2002;97:824-830.

57. Rajnish J, Amandeep S, Namita J, et al. Accuracy and reliability of palpation and percussion for detecting hepatomegaly: A rural hospital-based study. *Indian J Gastroenterol.* 2004;23:171-174.

58. Tine F, Caltagirone M, Camma C, et al. Clinical indicants of compensated cirrhosis: a prospective study. In: Dianzani MU, Gentilini P, eds. *Chronic liver damage: Proceedings of the Annual Meeting of the Italian national programme on liver cirrhosis, San Miniato, Italy 11-13 January 1990.* Amsterdam: Excerpta Medica; 1990:187-198.

59. Barkun AN, Camus M, Green L, et al. The bedside assessment of splenic enlargement. *Am J Med.* 1991;91:512-518.

60. Barkun AN, Camus M, Meagher T, et al. Splenic enlargement and Traube's space: How useful is percussion? *Am J Med.* 1989;87:562-566.

61. Fink HA, Lederle FA, Roth CS, et al. The accuracy of physical examination to detect abdominal aortic aneurysm. *Arch Intern Med.* 2000;160:833-836.

62. Myers KA, Scott DF, Devine TJ, et al. Palpation of the femoral and popliteal pulses: A study of the accuracy as assessed by agreement between multiple observers. *Eur J Vasc Surg.* 1987;1:245-249.

63. Brearley S, Shearman CP, Simms MH. Peripheral pulse palpation: An unreliable physical sign. *Ann Roy Coll Surg Eng.* 1992;74:169-171.

64. Diamond JE, Mueller MJ, Delitto A, Sinacore DR. Reliability of diabetic foot evaluation. *Physical Ther.* 1989;69:797-802.

65. Smieja M, Hunt DL, Edelman D, et al. Clinical examination for the detection of protective sensation in the feet of diabetic patients. *J Gen Intern Med.* 1999;14:418-424.

66. Edelman D, Sanders LJ, Pogach L. Reproducibility and accuracy among primary care providers of a screening examination for foot ulcer risk among diabetic patients. *Prevent Med.* 1998;27:274-278.

67. Wells PS, Anderson DR, Bormanis J, et al. Value of assessment of pretest probability of deep-vein thrombosis in clinical management. *Lancet.* 1997;350:1795-1798.

68. Ostor AJK, Richards CA, Prevost AT, et al. Interrater reproducibility of clinical tests for rotator cuff lesions. *Ann Rheum Dis.* 2004;63:1288-1292.

69. Stiell IG, Greenberg GH, Wells GA, et al. Prospective validation of a decision rule for the use of radiography in acute knee injuries. *JAMA.* 1996;275:611-615.

70. Stiell IG, Greenberg GH, Wells GA, et al. Derivation of a decision rule for the use of radiography in acute knee injuries. *Ann Emerg Med.* 1995;26:405-413.

71. Dervin GF, Stiell IG, A WG, Grabowski J. Physicians' accuracy and interrator reliability for the diagnosis of unstable meniscal tears in patients having osteoarthritis of the knee. *Can J Surg.* 2001;44:267-274.

72. Cushnagham J, Cooper C, Dieppe P, et al. Clinical assessment of osteoarthritis of the knee. *Ann Rheum Dis.* 1990;49:768-770.

73. Evans PJ, Bell GD, Frank C. Prospective evaluation of the McMurray test. *Am J Sports Med.* 1993;21:604-608.

74. Stiell IG, Greenberg GH, McKnight RD, et al. Decision rules for the use of radiography in acute ankle injuries: Refinement and prospective validation. *JAMA.* 1993;269:1127-1132.

75. Springer BA, Arciero RA, Tenuta JJ, Taylor DC. A prospective study of modified Ottawa ankle rules in a military population: Interobserver agreement between physical therapists and orthopaedic surgeons. *Am J Sports Med.* 2000;28: 864-868.

76. Pigman EC, Klug RK, Sanford S, Jolly BT. Evaluation of the Ottawa clinical decision rules for the use of radiography in acute ankle and midfoot injuries in the emergency department: An independent site assessment. *Ann Emerg Med.* 194;24:41-45.

77. Davies AE, Kidd K, Stone SP, MacMahon J. Pharyngeal sensation and gag reflex in healthy subjects. *Lancet.* 1995;345:487-488.

78. Hansen M, Christensen PB, H. SS, et al. Inter-observer variation in the evaluation of neurological signs: Patient-related factors. *J Neurol.* 1994;241:492-496.

79. Hansen M, Sindrup SH, Christensen PB, et al. Interobserver variation in the evaluation of neurologic signs: Observer dependent factors. *Acta Neurol Scand.* 1994;90:145-149.

80. McCullough GH, Wertz RT, Resenbek JC, et al. Inter- and intrajudge reliability of a clinical examination of swallowing in adults. *Dysphagia.* 2000;15:58-67.

81. Lim SHB, Lieu PK, Phua SY, et al. Accuracy of bedside clinical methods compared with fiberoptic endoscopic examination of swallowing (FEES) in determining the risk of aspiration in acute stroke patients. *Dysphagia.* 2001;16:1-6.

82. Segatore M. Determining the interrater reliability of motor power assessments using a spinal cord testing record. *J Neurosci Nurs.* 1991;23:220-223.

83. Vroomen PCAJ, De Krom MCTFM, Knottnerus JA. Consistency of history taking and physical examination in patients with suspected lumbar nerve root involvement. *Spine.* 2000;25:91-97.

84. Brandsma JW, Schreuders TAR, Birke JA, et al. Manual muscle strength testing: Intraobserver and interobserver reliabilities for the intrinsic muscles of the hand. *J Hand Ther.* 1995;8:185-190.

85. Viikari-Juntura E. Interexaminer reliability of observations in physical examinations of the neck. *Phys Ther.* 1987;67:1526-1532.

86. Haas BM, Bergstrom E, Jamous A, Bennie A. The inter rater reliability of the original and of the modified Ashworth scale for the assessment of spasticity in patients with spinal cord injury. *Spin Cord.* 1996;34:560-564.

87. van Dillen L, Roach KE. Interrater reliability of a clinical scale of rigidity. *Phys Ther.* 1988;68:1679-1681.

88. Litvan I, Mangone CA, Werden W, et al. Reliability of the NINDS myotatic reflex scale. *Neurology* 1996;47:969-972.

89. O'Keeffe STO, Smith T, Valacio R, et al. A comparison of two techniques for ankle jerk assessment in elderly subjects. *Lancet.* 1994;344:1619-1620.

90. Clarke CE, Davies P, Wilson T, Nutbeam T. Comparison of the tendon and plantar strike methods of eliciting the ankle reflex. *J Neurol Neurosurg Psychiatry.* 2005;74:1351-1352.

91. Vreeling FW, Jolles J, Verhey FRJ, Houx PJ. Primitive reflexes in healthy, adult volunteers and neurological patients: Methodological issues. *J Neurol.* 1993;240:495-504.

92. Maher J, Reilly M, Daly L, Hutchinson M. Plantar power: Reproducibility of the plantar response. *Br Med J.* 1992;304:482.

93. Swaine BR, Sullivan SJ. Reliability of the scores for the finger-to-nose test in adults with traumatic brain injury. *Phys Ther.* 1993;73:71-78.

94. Wainner RS, Fritz JM, Irrgang JJ, et al. Reliability and diagnostic accuracy of the clinical examination and patient self-report measures for cervical radiculopathy. *Spine.* 2003;28:52-63.

95. Wainner RS, Fritz JM, Irrgang JJ, et al. Development of a clinical prediction rule for the diagnosis of carpal tunnel syndrome. *Arch Phys Med Rehabil.* 2005;86:609-618.

96. McCombe PF, Fairbank JCT, Cockersole BC, Pynsent PB. Reproducibility of physical signs in low-back pain. *Spine.* 1989;14:909-918.

97. Van den Hoogen HJM, Koes BW, Deville W, et al. The inter-observer reproducibility of Lasegue's sign in patients with low back pain in general practice. *Br J Gen Pract.* 1996;46:727-730.

98. Poiraudeau S, Foltz V, Drape JL, et al. Value of the bell test and the hyperextension test for diagnosis in sciatica associated with disc herniation: Comparison with Lasegue's sign and the crossed Lasegue's sign. *Rheumatology.* 2001;40:460-466.

99. Baughman RP, Shipley RT, Loudon RG, Lower EE. Crackles in interstitial lung disease: Comparison of sarcoidosis and fibrosing alveolitis. *Chest.* 1991;100:96-101.

100. Illescas FF, Lerclerc J, Resenthall L, et al. Interobserver variability in the interpretation of contrast venography, technetium-99m red blood cell venography and impedance plethysmography for deep vein thrombosis. *J Can Assoc Radiol.* 1990;41:264-269.

101. Elmore JG, Wells CK, Lee CH, et al. Variability in radiologists' interpretations of mammograms. *N Engl J Med.* 1994;331:1493-1499.

102. DeVries AR, Engels PHC, Overtoom TT, et al. Interobserver variability in assessing renal artery stenosis by digital subtraction angiography. *Diagn Imag Clin Med.* 1984;53:277-281.

103. Herrman JPR, Azar A, Umans VAWM, et al. Inter- and intra-observer variability in the qualitative categorization of coronary angiograms. *Int J Card Imag.* 1996;12:21-30.

104. Shinar D, Gross CR, Hier DB, et al. Interobserver reliability in the interpretation of computed tomographic scans of stroke patients. *Arch Neurol.* 1987;44:149-155.

105. Webb WR, Sarin M, Zerhouni EA, et al. Interobserver variability in CT and MR staging of lung cancer. *J Comput Assist Tomogr.* 1993;17:841-846.

106. Barkhof F, Filippi M, van Waesberghe JHTM, et al. Interobserver agreement for diagnostic MRI criteria in suspected multiple sclerosis. *Neuroradiology.* 1999;41:347-350.

107. Jensen MC, Brant-Zawadzki MN, Obuchowski N, et al. Magnetic resonance imaging of the lumbar spine in people without back pain. *N Engl J Med.* 1994;331:69-73.

108. Vroomen PCAJ, de Krom MCTFM, Wilmink JT, et al. Diagnostic value of history and physical examination in patients suspected of lumbosacral nerve root compression. *J Neurol Neurosurg Psychiatry.* 2000;72:630-634.

109. Atri M, Herba MJ, Reinhold C, et al. Accuracy of sonography in the evaluation of calf deep vein thrombosis in both postoperative surveillance and symptomatic patients. *AJR.* 1996;166:1361-1367.

110. Jarlov AE, Nygard B, Hegedus L, et al. Observer variation in ultrasound assessment of the thyroid gland. *Br J Radiol.* 1993;66:625-627.

111. Schneider AB, Bekerman C, Leland J, et al. Thyroid nodules in the follow-up of irradiated individuals: Comparison of thyroid ultrasound with scanning and palpation. *J Clin Endocrinol Metab.* 1997;82:4020-4027.

112. Bytzer P, Havelund T, Moeller Hansen J. Interobserver variation in the endoscopic diagnosis of reflux esophagitis. *Scand J Gastroenterol.* 1993;28:119-125.

113. Theodossi A, Skene AM, Portmann B, et al. Observer variation in assessment of liver biopsies including analysis by kappa statistics. *Gastroenterology.* 1980;79: 232-241.

114. Spodick DH, Bishop RL. Computer treason: Intraobserver variability of an electrocardiographic computer system. *Am J Cardiol.* 1997;80:102-103.

2

GENERAL APPEARANCE OF THE PATIENT

Mental Status Examination

I. INTRODUCTION

Dementia is a clinical syndrome characterized by deteriorating cognition, behavior, and autonomy that affects 3% to 11% of adults older than 65 years living in the community.[1] Before making the diagnosis of dementia, the clinician must exclude delirium (i.e., acute confusion; see "Diagnosis of Delirium" later).

Of the many simple and rapid bedside tests developed to diagnose dementia, the most extensively investigated ones are the clock-drawing test and Mini-Mental Status Examination (MMSE).

II. CLOCK-DRAWING TEST

The clock-drawing test was originally developed in the early 1900s to evaluate soldiers who had suffered head wounds to the occipital or parietal lobes, which often caused subsequent difficulty composing images correctly with the appropriate number of parts of the correct size and orientation (i.e., constructional apraxia).[2] To correctly depict a clock, patients must be able to follow directions, comprehend language, visualize the proper orientation of an object, and execute normal movements, all tasks that may be disturbed in dementia.[3]

A.   TECHNIQUE AND SCORING

There are at least a dozen different methods for performing and scoring the clock-drawing test,[2,4,5] some of which have intricate grading systems that defeat the test's simplicity.[3,6-8] A simple and well-investigated method is that by Wolf-Klein.[9] In this method, the clinician gives the patient a piece of paper with a preprinted circle four inches in diameter and asks the patient to "draw a clock." If the patient has any questions, the clinician only repeats the same instructions and gives no other guidance. The patient may take as long as he wants to complete the task.

Figure 4-1 describes how to score the patient's drawing.

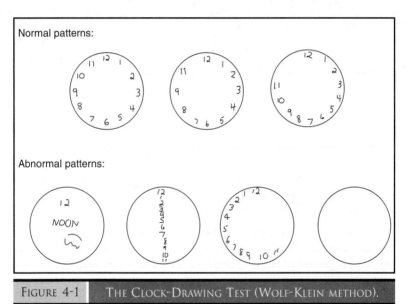

| FIGURE 4-1 | THE CLOCK-DRAWING TEST (WOLF-KLEIN METHOD). |

The clock-drawing is normal if the patient has included most of the 12 numbers in the correct clockwise orientation. The patient does not need to draw the hands of the clock, and abnormal spacing of the numbers, however inappropriate, is still regarded normal as long as the numbers are in correct order and near the rim. Normal clock-drawing patterns, from left to right, are "normal," "missing one number," and "inappropriate spacing." Abnormal clock-drawing patterns, from left to right, are "irrelevant figures," "unusual arrangement" (i.e., vertical orientation of numbers), "counterclockwise rotation," and "absence of numbers." (Adapted from Wolf-Klein GP, Silverstone FA, Levy AP, et al. Screening for Alzheimer's disease by clock drawing. *J Am Geriatr Soc.* 1989;37:730-734.)

B. CLINICAL SIGNIFICANCE

In patients without other known causes of constructional apraxia (e.g., parietal lobe lesion), a positive clock-drawing test argues for the diagnosis of dementia [likelihood ratio (LR) = 5.3, EBM Box 4-1]. A normal clock-drawing test is not as useful, being elicited from up to half of patients having dementia as defined by other measures. The clock-drawing test differs from the MMSE in that the clock-drawing test is not affected by the patient's level of education.[10] Also, the clock-drawing test accurately predicts decline of the patient's MMSE score, as measured 4 years later, independent of the patient's age and the baseline MMSE score.[31]

Box 4-1 Dementia and Delirium*

Finding (Ref)	Sensitivity (%)	Specificity (%)	Likelihood Ratio if Finding	
			Present	Absent
DEMENTIA[†]				
Abnormal clock drawing test[9–13]	36–75	72–98	**5.3**	0.5
Mini-Mental Status Examination: Traditional Threshold				
23 or less[14–22]	69–100	78–99	**8.1**	**0.2**
Mini-Mental Status Examination: 3 Levels				
20 or less[16,18–20]	39–69	93–99	**14.5**	...
21 to 25[18–20]	26–51	...	2.2	...
26 or more[18–20]	4–10	14–27	**0.1**	...
DELIRIUM				
Positive test using "Confusion Assessment Method"[†23–28]	46–94	83–98	**10.3**	**0.2**

Likelihood ratio (LR) if finding present = positive LR; LR if finding absent = negative LR
*Diagnostic standards: for dementia, dementia by the NINCDS-ADRDA criteria,[9,10,29,30] the DMS criteria,[12–15,17,18,20,22] the CAMDEX instrument,[16] AGECAT,[21] or a neurologist's opinion[19]; for delirium, the DMS criteria.[21,23–28]
†Definition of findings: for abnormal clock drawing test, see Fig. 4-1; for Confusion Assessment Method, see text.

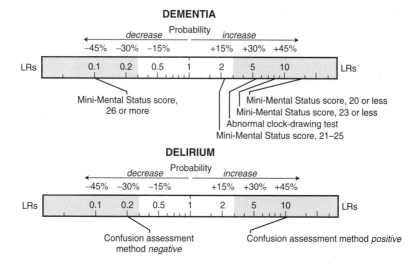

III. THE MINI-MENTAL STATUS EXAMINATION

A. INTRODUCTION

The MMSE (Table 4-1) was introduced in 1975 by Folstein and others, as an 11-part bedside test requiring only 5 to 10 minutes to administer, compared with the 1 to 2 hours of time demanded by more formal tests for dementia.[32] The MMSE combines questions that are highly specific but not sensitive (i.e., questions about orientation) with questions that are highly sensitive but not specific (i.e., poor recall or inability to perform serial 7s).[33]

B. CLINICAL SIGNIFICANCE

EBM Box 4-1 illustrates that the traditional threshold for the MMSE (abnormal being scores of 23 or lower) performs very well: assuming there is no evidence of delirium (see "Diagnosis of Delirium" later), scores from 0 to 23 argue strongly for the diagnosis of dementia (LR = 8.1), and scores from 24 to 30 argue against it (LR = 0.2). Nonetheless, because false-positive results become a concern when such a threshold is applied to large populations with a low incidence of dementia, such as persons living independently in the community, some experts prefer interpreting the MMSE score in three ranges (see EBM Box 4-1): A score of 20 or less rules-in dementia (LR = 14.5), one of 26 or more rules-out dementia (LR = 0.1), and scores between 21 to 25 are regarded as less conclusive (LR = 2.2), indicating further investigation of the patient is necessary.

Table 4-1	The Mini-Mental Status Examination	
	Test	Maximum Score
Orientation		
	1. What is the year? Season? Date? Day? Month?*	5
	2. Where are we? State? County? City? Hospital? Floor?*	5
Registration		
	3. Name 3 objects. Ask patient to name the items* Repeat the answers until the patient learns all three	3
Attention and Calculation		
	4. Serial 7s (ask the patient to begin with 100 and count backward by 7s, stopping after 5 substractions: 93, 86, 79, 72, 65)* or Spell "world" backward*	5
Recall		
	5. Ask the patient to name the three objects learned under "registration" above*	3
Language		
	6. Point to a pencil and watch, asking the patient to name them*	2
	7. Have the patient repeat "no ifs, ands, or buts"	1
	8. Have the patient follow a three-stage command (e.g., Take a paper in your right hand. Fold the paper in half. Put the paper on the floor")*	3
	9. Have the patient read and obey the following sentence, written in large letters: "Close your eyes"	1
	10. Have the patient write a sentence†	1
	11. Have the patient copy a picture of two intersecting pentagons	1
	Total	30

Adapted from references 20 and 32.
*Give 1 point for each correct answer.
†The sentence should make sense and contain a subject and object to earn the 1 point; spelling errors are ignored.

The MMSE score may be used to follow patients over time, but only changes of 4 points or more indicate a significant change of cognition (this is based on the standard deviation of results in stable patients).[15,34] The level of the patient's education also affects the MMSE score, whether or not dementia is present,[15,17,30,35,36] and some have suggested adjusting the threshold for a positive test downward slightly in more poorly educated persons.[15,30]

IV. DIAGNOSIS OF DELIRIUM ("CONFUSION ASSESSMENT METHOD")

Delirium is an acute and reversible confusional state, which affects up to 20% of elderly patients hospitalized with acute medical illnesses.[24,37] Of the several screening tools available to diagnose delirium,[24] one simple and well-investigated one is the Confusion Assessment Method.[23]

A. SCORING

The clinician looks for the following four clinical features: (1) change in mental status (compared with the patient's baseline) that is *acute* and *fluctuating*, (2) difficulty focusing attention or trouble keeping track of what is being said, (3) disorganized thinking (e.g., rambling or irrelevant conversation, unpredictable switching between subjects, illogical flow of ideas), and (4) altered level of consciousness (e.g., lethargic, stuporous, or hyperalert).

A positive test requires both features (1) and (2) *and* either (3) or (4).

B. CLINICAL SIGNIFICANCE

As illustrated in EBM Box 4-1, a positive test argues strongly *for* delirium (LR = 10.3) and a negative test argues *against* delirium (LR = 0.2). Another version of this test, adapted for use in mechanically ventilated patients who cannot talk, has similar accuracy.[38,39] In any patient with delirium, positive bedside tests for *dementia* are meaningless because of the high false-positive rate.

REFERENCES

1. Knopman DS. The initial recognition and diagnosis of dementia. *Am J Med.* 1998;104(4A):2S-12S.
2. Watson YI, Arfken CL, Birge SJ. Clock completion: An objective screening test for dementia. *J Am Geriatr Soc.* 1993;41:1235-1240.
3. Mendez MF, Ala T, Underwood KL. Development of scoring criteria for the clock drawing task in Alzheimer's disease. *J Am Geriatr Soc.* 1992;40:1095-1099.
4. Sunderland T, Hill JL, Mellow AM, et al. Clock drawing in Alzheimer's disease: A novel measure of dementia severity. *J Am Geriatr Soc.* 1989;37:725-729.
5. Agrell A, Dehlin O. The clock-drawing test. *Age Ageing.* 1998;27:399-403.
6. Tuokko H, Hadjistavropoulos T, Miller JA, Beattie BL. The clock test: A sensitive measure to differentiate normal elderly from those with Alzheimer disease. *J Am Geriatr Soc.* 1992;40:579-584.
7. Esteban-Santillan C, Praditsuwan R, Ueda H, Geldmacher DS. Clock drawing test in very mild Alzheimer's disease. *J Am Geriatr Soc.* 1998;46:1266-1269.

8. Lin KN, Wang PN, Chen C, et al. The three-item clock-drawing test: a simplified screening test for Alzheimer's disease. *Eur Neurol.* 2003;49:53-58.

9. Wolf-Klein GP, Silverstone FA, Levy AP, et al. Screening for Alzheimer's disease by clock drawing. *J Am Geriatr Soc.* 1989;37:730-734.

10. Ainslie NK, Murden RA. Effect of education on the clock-drawing dementia screen in non-demented elderly persons. *J Am Geriatr Soc.* 1993;41:249-252.

11. Brodaty H, Moore CM. The Clock Drawing Test for dementia of the Alzheimer's type: A comparison of three scoring methods in a memory disorders clinic. *Int J Geriatr Psychiatry.* 1997;12:619-627.

12. Storey JE, Rowland JTJ, Basic D, Conforti DA. A comparison of five clock scoring methods using ROC (receiver operating characteristic) curve analysis. *Int J Geriatr Psychiatry.* 2001;16:394-399.

13. Tuokko H, Hadjistavropoulos T, Rae S, O'Rourke N. A comparison of alternative approaches to the scoring of clock drawing. *Arch Clin Neuropsychol.* 2000;15:137-148.

14. Grut M, Fratiglioni L, Viitanen M, Winblad B. Accuracy of the mini-mental status examination as a screening test for dementia in a Swedish elderly population. *Acta Neurol Scand.* 1993;87:312-317.

15. Tangalos EG, Smith GE, Ivnik RJ, et al. The mini-mental state examination in general medical practice: clinical utility and acceptance. *Mayo Clin Proc.* 1996;71:829-837.

16. O'Connor DW, Pollitt PA, Hyde JB, et al. The reliability and validity of the mini-mental state in a British community survey. *J Psychiatr Res.* 1989;23:87-96.

17. Gagnon M, Letenneur L, Dartigues JF, et al. Validity of the mini-mental state examination as a screening instrument for cognitive impairment and dementia in French elderly community residents. *Neuroepidemiology.* 1990;9:143-150.

18. Kay DWK, Henderson AS, Scott R, et al. Dementia and depression among the elderly living in the Hobart community: The effect of the diagnostic criteria on the prevalence rates. *Psychol Med.* 1985;15:771-788.

19. Dick JPR, Guiloff RJ, Stewart A, et al. Mini-mental state examination in neurological patients. *J Neurol Neurosurg Psychiatry.* 1984;47:496-499.

20. Anthony JC, LeResche L, Niaz U, et al. Limits of the 'Mini-Mental State' as a screening test for dementia and delirium among hospital patients. *Psychol Med.* 1982;12:397-408.

21. Cullen B, Fahy S, Cunningham CJ, et al. Screening for dementia in an Irish community sample using MMSE: A comparison of norm-adjusted versus fixed cut-points. *Int J Geriatr Psychiatry.* 2005;20:371-376.

22. Heinik J, Solomesh I, Lin R, et al. Clock Drawing Test-Modified and Integrated Approach (CDT-MIA): description and preliminary examination of its validity and reliability in dementia patients referred to a specialized psychogeriatric setting. *J Geriatr Psychiatry Neurol.* 2003;17:73-80.

23. Inouye SK, Van Dyck CH, Alessi CA, et al. Clarifying confusion: The confusion assessment method. A new method for detection of delirium. *Ann Intern Med.* 1990;113:941-948.

24. Pompei P, Foreman M, Cassel CK, et al. Detecting delirium among hospitalized older patients. *Arch Intern Med.* 1995;155:301-307.

25. Zou Y, Cole MG, Primeau FJ, et al. Detection and diagnosis of delirium in the elderly: Psychiatrist diagnosis, confusion assessment method, or consensus diagnosis? *Int Psychoger.* 1998;10:303-308.

26. Gonzalez M, de Pablo J, Fuente E, et al. Instrument for detection of delirium in general hospitals: Adaptation of the confusion assessment method. *Psychosomatics.* 2004;45:426-431.

27. Laurila JV, Pitkala KH, Standberg TE, Tilvis RS. Confusion assessment method in the diagnostics of delirium among aged hospital patients: Would it serve better in screening than as a diagnostic instrument? *Int J Geriatr Psychiatry.* 2002;17:1112-1119.

28. Rolfson DB, McElhaney JE, Jhangri GS, Rockwood K. Validity of the confusion assessment method in detecting postoperative delirium in the elderly. *Int Psychogeriatr.* 1999;11:431-438.

29. McKhann G, Drachman D, Folstein M, et al. Clinical diagnosis of Alzheimer's disease: Report of the NINCDS-ADRDA Work Group under the auspices of Department of Health and Human Services Task Force on Alzheimer's Disease. *Neurology.* 1984;34:939-944.

30. Uhlmann RF, Larson EB. Effect of education on the mini-mental state examination as a screening test for dementia. *J Am Geriatr Assoc.* 1991;39:876-880.

31. Ferrucci L, Cecchi F, Guralnik JM, et al. Does the clock drawing test predict cognitive decline in older persons independent of the mini-mental state examination? *J Am Geriatr Soc.* 1996;44:1326-1331.

32. Folstein MF, Folstein SE, McHugh PR. "Mini-mental state": A practical method for grading the cognitive state of patients for the clinician. *J Psychiatr Res.* 1975;12:189-198.

33. Klein LE, Roca RP, McArthur J, et al. Diagnosing dementia: Univariate and multivariate analyses of the mental status examination. *J Am Geriatr Soc.* 1985;33:483-488.

34. Bowie P, Branton T, Holmes J. Should the mini mental state examination be used to monitor dementia treatments? *Lancet.* 1999;354:1527-1528.

35. O'Connor DW, Pollitt PA, Treasure FP, et al. The influence of education, social class and sex on Mini-Mental State scores. *Psychol Med.* 1989;19:771-776.

36. Brayne C, Calloway P. The association of education and socioeconomic status with the Mini Mental State examination and the clinical diagnosis of dementia in elderly people. *Age Ageing.* 1990;19:91-96.

37. Lewis LM, Miller DK, Morley JE, et al. Unrecognized delirium in ED geriatric patients. *Am J Emerg Med.* 1995;13:142-145.

38. Ely EW, Inouye SK, Bernard GR, et al. Delirium in mechanically ventilated patients: Validity and reliability of the confusion assessment method for the intensive care unit (CAM-ICU). *JAMA.* 2001;286:2703-2710.

39. Ely EW, Margolin R, Francis J, et al. Evaluation of delirium in critically ill patients: Validation of the confusion assessment method for the intensive care unit (CAM-ICU). *Crit Care Med.* 2001;29:1370-1379.

Stance and Gait

I. INTRODUCTION

Observation of the patient's gait not only uncovers important neurologic problems (e.g. Parkinson's disease, hemiparesis) and musculoskeletal problems (e.g., spinal stenosis, hip disease) but also provides information otherwise unavailable from the conventional examination, such as clues to the patient's emotions, overall function, and even prognosis. For example, the slowness of an elderly person's gait accurately predicts falls, future disability, and risk of institutionalization.[1-7] In patients with congestive heart failure, the gait's speed and stride predict cardiac index, future hospitalization, and mortality as well as the ejection fraction and better than performance on a treadmill.[8-10] Even depressed patients have a characteristic gait, marked by a shorter stride and weaker push-off with the heel, when compared with non-depressed persons.[11]

This chapter reviews both the musculoskeletal and neurologic causes of the abnormal gait. The phases of the normal gait are depicted in Fig. 5-1.

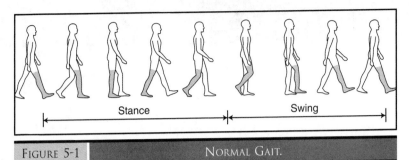

Stance	Swing

FIGURE 5-1	NORMAL GAIT.

This figure illustrates the phases of normal gait, focusing on the right leg (colored gray). Normal gait consists of the "stance phase" (the period during which the leg bears weight) and "swing phase" (the period during which the leg advances and does not bear weight). The stance and swing make up the "stride," which is the interval from the time one heel strikes the ground to when it again strikes the ground. During the normal stance phase, it is the *extensor* muscles that contract—the gluteus maximus in early stance, the quadriceps in midstance, and the plantar flexors (soleus and gastrocnemius) in terminal stance pushing off the heel. The healthy swing, in contrast, requires contraction of the *flexor* muscles, all of which are activated early in the swing phase—hip flexors (iliopsoas), knee flexors (hamstrings), and ankle flexors (tibialis anterior and toe extensors).[12,13] (Figure adapted from The Pathokinesiology Service and the Physical Therapy Department of Ranchos Los Amigos Medical Center. *Observational gait analysis.* Downey, CA: Los Amigos Research and Education Institute, Inc; 1993.)

II. ETIOLOGY OF GAIT DISORDERS

Which gait abnormalities a clinician is likely to see depends on the nature of his or her practice. Among patients presenting to neurologists, the most common causes of gait disorder are stroke and Parkinson's disease, followed by frontal gait disorder, myelopathy (e.g., cervical spondylosis, B_{12} deficiency), peripheral neuropathy, and cerebellar disease.[14,15] Among patients presenting to general clinicians, most gait abnormalities are caused by arthritis, followed by orthostatic hypotension, stroke, Parkinson's disease, and intermittent claudication.[16]

III. TYPES OF GAIT DISORDERS AND THEIR SIGNIFICANCE

Disorders of gait may occur because of any of four fundamental problems: pain, immobile joints, muscle weakness, or abnormal limb control. Abnormal limb control, in turn, may result from spasticity, rigidity, problems with proprioception, cerebellar diseases, or problems with cerebral control.

When analyzing disturbances of gait, the most important initial question is to ask whether the gait is symmetric or asymmetric. Pain, immobile joints, and muscle weakness are usually unilateral and therefore cause *asymmetric* abnormalities of the gait. Rigidity, proprioceptive and cerebellar diseases, and problems with central control all cause *symmetric* abnormalities of the gait. Spasticity may cause *asymmetric* abnormalities (i.e., hemiplegia) or *symmetric* abnormalities (i.e., paraplegia) of the gait.

A. PAINFUL GAIT ("ANTALGIC GAIT")

If putting weight on one limb causes pain, patients adopt unusual gaits to minimize this pain (the word antalgic derives from the Greek *an* and *algesis*, meaning "against pain"). All antalgic gaits have one characteristic feature: the short contralateral step.

1. The Short Contralateral Step

After bearing weight on the affected leg, patients with pain quickly step onto the sound leg. The short contralateral step produces an uneven cadence, which is identical to the gait persons adopt when there is a rock in one shoe.

2. Other Characteristic Features

Other features of the antalgic gait depend on whether the pain is located in the foot, knee, or hip. Each of these gaits has distinctive features, which allow diagnosis from a distance, although it is sometimes more efficient to simply ask the patient which joint is painful.

a. Foot Pain

In patients with foot pain, the foot contacts the ground abnormally. For example, patients may bear weight during stance on their heel only, forefoot only, or along the lateral edge of the foot.

b. Knee Pain

Patients with knee pain display a stiff knee that does not extend or flex fully during stride.[17,18]

c. Hip Pain ("Coxalgic Gait")

Patients with hip pain limit the amount of hip extension toward the end of stance (normally, the hip extends 20 degrees). The most characteristic feature of the coxalgic gait, however, is an asymmetric and excessive lateral shift of the patient's upper body toward the weight-bearing side when standing on the painful limb (i.e., the trunk leans and ipsilateral arm abducts, Fig. 5-2).[19,20] This unusual movement is called "lateral lurch."

Lateral lurch reduces the pain of patients with hip disease, because it minimizes the need to activate the ipsilateral hip abductor muscles. These muscles

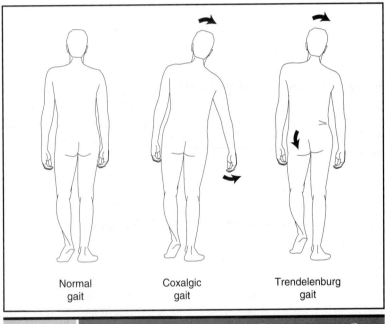

| Normal gait | Coxalgic gait | Trendelenburg gait |

FIGURE 5-2   COMPARISON OF COXALGIC AND TRENDELENBURG GAIT.

In both abnormal gaits (middle and right figures), the trunk may lean over the abnormal leg during stance *(arrow)*, but in patients with hip pain (coxalgic gait, middle figure), the trunk lean and accompanying ipsilateral arm movement *(arrow)* is more dramatic ("lateral lurch") and the opposite pelvis does not fall excessively. In the Trendelenburg gait (from ineffective or weak hip abductors, right figure), the opposite pelvis falls excessively *(arrow)*, and the conspicuous but opposing swings of the upper body and pelvis create the impression of a hinge between the sacral and lumbar spine. In these figures, the patient is bearing weight on the affected side, that is, *right* hip pain (coxalgic gait) and ineffective *right* hip abductors (Trendelenburg gait).

normally support the upper body during swing of the other leg, but when activated can easily put 400 pounds of pressure on the femoral head, a force that patients with hip disease cannot tolerate. By leaning over the painful limb during stance, patients effectively balance their center of gravity over the painful limb and thus avoid activation of the hip abductors.

B. IMMOBILE JOINTS

Most clinicians do not consider immobile joints as a cause of abnormal gait, but the condition is well known to physiatrists. A common example is plantar flexion contracture, which may occur after prolonged periods of plaster immobilization or confinement to a chair or bed. Patients with a plantar flexion contracture may place their weight abnormally on the forefoot during initial stance, or, during midstance, lift their heel too early or lean their trunk forward. During swing phase, the abnormally flexed foot has difficulty clearing the floor, and the patient may drag the foot or develop an unusual movement to clear it, such as contralateral trunk lean or contralateral vaulting.[12,13]

The clinician can easily identify immobile joints as the cause of abnormal gait by testing the range of motion of hips, knees, and ankles of both legs.

C. WEAKNESS OF SPECIFIC MUSCLES

Weakness of the hip extensor and abductor muscles (i.e., gluteus maximus and medius/minimus), knee extensors (quadriceps), and foot and toe dorsiflexors (tibialis anterior and toe extensors) all cause specific abnormalities of gait. The gluteus maximus and quadriceps gait are much less prevalent today than they were in the days of poliomyelitis and diphtheria.

1. Trendelenburg Gait and Sign (Abnormal Gluteus Medius and Minimus)

a. Definition of Trendelenburg Gait (or Trendelenburg's Symptom; Friedrich Trendelenburg 1844-1924)

The Trendelenburg gait occurs when the gluteus medius and minimus do not function properly. These two muscles abduct the hip, an action that supports the opposite pelvis and prevents it from dropping excessive amounts during the normal single-limb stance.[21] During walking, a slight dip of the opposite pelvis is normal during stance phase on one limb. The finding of *excessive drop* of the opposite pelvis, however, is the abnormal Trendelenburg gait. When the abnormality is bilateral, the pelvis waddles like that of a duck.

Like patients with the coxalgic gait (see previous "Hip Pain ['Coxalgic Gait']"), patients with Trendelenburg gait may lean their trunk over the abnormal leg during stance, but the lean lacks the dramatic lurch seen in coxalgic gait, and the opposing sways of the ipsilateral shoulder and opposite pelvis make it appear as if patients with the Trendelenburg gait have a hinge between their sacral and lumbar spine (see Fig. 5-2).[19,22]

b. Etiology of Trendelenburg Gait

Causes include the following: (**1**) **neuromuscular weakness of the hip abductors.** Although poliomyelitis and progressive muscular atrophy were important causes historically, this gait now occurs as a complication of hip arthroplasty using a lateral approach, which risks damage to the superior gluteal nerve or gluteus medius muscle[23–25] and (**2**) **hip disease,** especially congenital dislocation of the hip and coxa vara (i.e., "bent hip," a deformity in which the angle between femoral neck and body is significantly decreased). In both of these disorders, the abnormal upward displacement of the greater trochanter shortens the fibers of the gluteus medius and makes them more horizontal instead of vertical, thus abolishing their role as abductors.

c. Trendelenburg Sign

In 1895, before use of roentgenography, Friedrich Trendelenburg was the first to show that the waddling gait of patients with congenital dislocation of the hip was due to weak abductor function not the upward movement of the femur during stance (which was what his contemporaries believed). He successfully argued this by inventing a simple test, now known as Trendelenburg's sign. In this test, the patient is asked to stand on one leg with the other hip flexed to 90 degrees (the clinician may help the patient balance by supporting the ipsilateral arm to align the ipsilateral shoulder over the hip being tested).[26] In patients with normal abductor strength, the contralateral buttock rises, but if the abductor muscles are weak, the contralateral buttock falls (the buttock falls until the ipsilateral femur and pelvis come into contact).

It is important to remember that the side being tested is the one bearing the weight. Some deformities of the leg, such as severe genu varum, may cause a false-positive result.[27]

2. Gluteus Maximus Gait

When the hip extensors are weak, the patient develops a characteristic abnormal backward trunk lean during early stance, which places the patient's center of gravity behind the hip joint line and removes the need for the gluteus maximus to contract (Fig. 5-3).

3. Weak Quadriceps Gait

When the knee extensors are weak, two different abnormalities of gait may appear. Some patients develop a characteristic hyperextension of the knee during stance (see Fig. 5-3). This at first seems paradoxical because the normal action of the quadriceps is knee extension, which should therefore be weak in these patients.

However, the main role of the quadriceps during gait is to support the flexed knee during stance, and patients with weak quadriceps avoid bearing weight on a flexed knee by hyperextending the joint (i.e., "genu recurvatum"). They can fully extend the knee because their hip flexes strongly during swing and then decelerates abruptly, which whips the tibia forward.[13] Alternatively, other patients with a weak quadriceps may place their hand just above the knee to support the weak leg and prevent the knee from buckling during stance (see Fig. 5-3).

Most patients with weak quadriceps muscles have great difficulty walking on uneven ground.

4.   Foot Drop (Weak Tibialis Anterior and Toe Extensors)

The characteristic features in these patients are: (1) "foot slap," which is the uncontrolled slap of the forefoot immediately after the heel makes contact; this causes two sounds instead of one when the abnormal foot contacts the ground, producing a the characteristic cadence (in a patient with *unilateral* foot drop) of "dada . . . da. . . . dada. . . . da," and (2) "steppage gait," in which the patient excessively flexes the hip and knee of the abnormal side during the swing phase to clear the foot from the ground (see Fig. 5-3).[12]

D.   SPASTICITY

Spasticity is a feature of weakness of the upper motor neuron type (see Chapter 57). Characteristic gaits are the hemiplegic gait and diplegic (paraplegic) gait.

1.   Hemiplegic Gait[28-30]

The characteristic gait occurs because of poor control of the flexor muscles during swing phase and spasticity of the extensor muscles acting to lengthen the affected leg (compared with the healthy side). The ankle is abnormally flexed downward and inward (equinovarus deformity), and initial contact during stance is abnormal, along the lateral edge of the foot or forefoot. The knee is stiff, hyperextends during stance, and does not flex normally during swing. The contralateral step often advances just to meet the position of the paralyzed limb, instead of advancing normally beyond it.

Because the paralyzed leg is hyperextended, and therefore longer than the sound leg, the patient may drag the toe of the affected leg during swing or adopt abnormal movements to clear that limb during the swing phase. These movements include contralateral trunk lean, which raises the ipsilateral pelvis to clear the paralyzed leg, and circumduction, which describes the toe tracing a semicircle on the floor, first moving outward and then inward as it advances, instead of the normal straight forward movement (Fig. 5-4).

According to classic teachings, the clinician may sometimes suspect mild hemiplegia because of asymmetric swinging of the arms, although one study has shown that asymmetric arm swinging occurs in 70% of normal persons.[31]

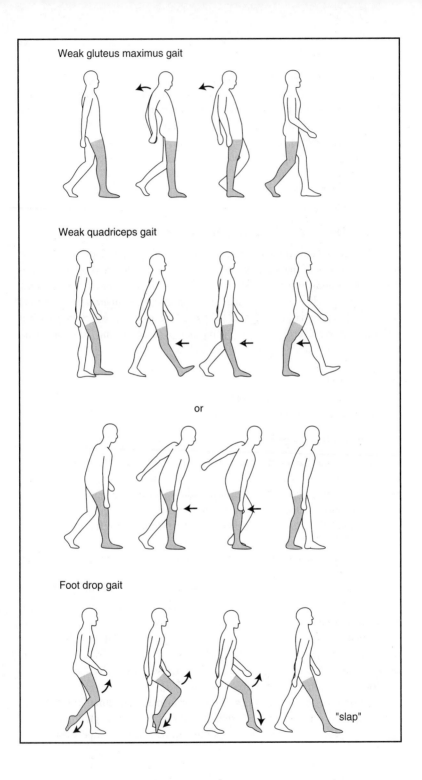

Weak gluteus maximus gait

Weak quadriceps gait

or

Foot drop gait

"slap"

2. Diplegic Gait

Diplegic gait affects patients with spinal cord disease (e.g., spinal cord trauma, cervical spondylosis, B_{12} deficiency), in whom both spasticity and abnormal proprioception cause a characteristic slow, laborious, and stiff-legged gait. In some spastic diplegias of childhood, adductor spasm causes the feet to cross in front of each other, a finding sometimes called "scissors gait."

E. RIGIDITY

Chapter 57 describes the characteristic features of rigidity and how it differs from spasticity. The most common gait abnormality resulting from rigidity is the Parkinsonian gait.

1. The Parkinsonian Gait (Fig. 5-5)[32,33]

The characteristic features are (1) flexed posture of the arms, hips, trunk, and neck; (2) rigidity of movement (en bloc turning, difficulty initiating gait); (3) steps that are flat-footed, small, and shuffling and have a narrow base; (4) diminished arm swing (the normal excursion, measured at the wrist, averages 16 inches; the average value for patients with Parkinson's disease is 5 inches); (5) involuntary hastening of gait (festination); and (6) poor postural control (retropulsion).

2. Differential Diagnosis

Patients with spinal stenosis superficially resemble those with Parkinson's disease in that they have a flexed stance ("simian stance"), which reduces the

FIGURE 5-3	CHARACTERISTIC GAITS OF WEAK MUSCLES.

In each figure, the shading indicates the limb with the weak muscle and the black arrows indicate the diagnostic movements. Because both the gluteus maximus and quadriceps muscles are *extensor* muscles, abnormalities of these muscles produce characteristic findings during the *stance* phase. Because the foot dorsiflexors (i.e., the weak muscles causing foot drop) are *flexor* muscles, abnormalities produce characteristic findings during the *swing* phase. In the weak gluteus maximus gait *(top row)*, there is an abnormal backward lean during stance. In the weak quadriceps gait *(middle rows)*, patients may hyperextend their knee during stance (i.e., genu recurvatum, *second row*) or place their ipsilateral arm on the leg to prevent the knee from buckling *(third row)*. In the foot drop gait *(bottom row)*, the actual foot weakness is conspicuous *(bottom arrows)*, and there is excessive flexion of the hip and knee during the swing phase *(upper arrow)* and a slapping sound of the foot when it strikes the ground. See text.

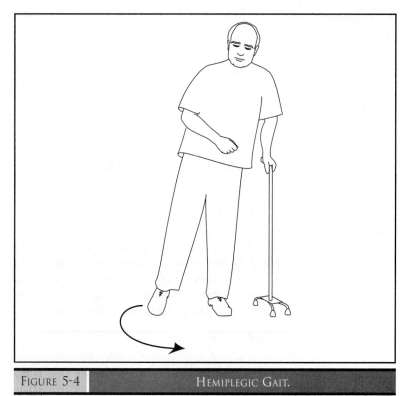

FIGURE 5-4	HEMIPLEGIC GAIT.

In a patient with right hemiparesis, the paretic arm is flexed and paretic leg is hyperextended. To clear the extended right leg from the floor, the patient leans over the healthy left leg and slowly advances the stiffened, paralyzed right leg with a circumducting movement *(arrow)*.

tension on the lumbosacral nerves.[34] Patients with spinal stenosis, however, complain of pain and otherwise have a normal gait.

The distinguishing features of the frontal gait disorder, which also may superficially resemble the Parkinsonian gait, is discussed in the "Definition" section of "Frontal Gait Disorder."

F. ATAXIA

The characteristic features of the ataxic gait are a wide-based gait with irregular, uneven, and sometimes staggering steps (the normal base, measured when one limb swings past the other at midstance, is 2 to 4 inches). There are two types of ataxia, sensory ataxia and cerebellar ataxia.

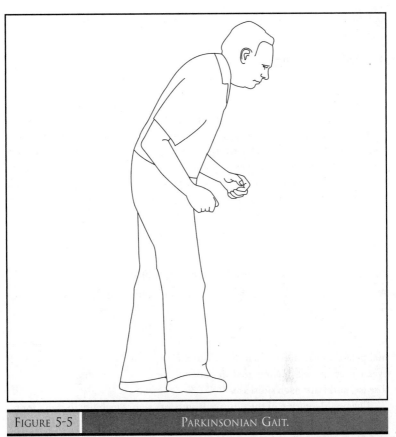

| FIGURE 5-5 | PARKINSONIAN GAIT. |

The characteristic features are flexed posture (trunk, neck, and arms), diminished arm swing, narrow-based gait, and shuffling steps.

1. Sensory Ataxia

Sensory ataxia affect patients with significant proprioceptive loss (see Chapter 58). Characteristically, the patient looks down and walks as if throwing his or her feet, which tend to slap on the ground. Smooth, familiar routes cause less trouble than uneven, rough ones.

2. Cerebellar Ataxia

Patients place their feet too far apart or too close together irregularly and sway, stagger, and reel in all directions as if intoxicated by alcohol.[35,36] In contrast to sensory ataxia, patients with cerebellar ataxia have other cerebellar signs, including dysmetria, hypotonia, intention tremor, dysarthria, and nystagmus (see Chapter 61).

3.   Romberg's Sign
a.   Introduction

In his famous textbook, written between 1840 and 1846, Moritz Romberg described the sign now bearing his name, as a finding in patients with tabes dorsalis who have severe sensory ataxia from syphilitic damage to the dorsal columns of the spinal cord. Romberg wrote that, when a patient with tabes dorsalis stands and closes his eyes, "he immediately begins to move from side to side, and the oscillations soon attain such a pitch that unless supported, he falls to the ground."[37] Most authors claim that Romberg's sign is negative in patients with cerebellar ataxia, although it is important to know that Romberg did not make this claim, cerebellar disease having not yet been defined during his time (Duchenne and Babinski later added this diagnostic point).[38]

b.   Definition of a Positive Romberg's Sign

A problem with Romberg's sign is that various authors differ on what constitutes a positive test: Some state it is the increased swaying that occurs when the eyes close, whereas others require the patient to be on the verge of falling down.[37] Increased swaying alone seems to be a poor choice, because most normal persons sway more when they close their eyes, and increased swaying with eyes closed is well documented in patients with vestibular disease, cerebellar disease, and Parkinson's disease.[39-42]

The best definition of the positive Romberg's sign is inability to stand for 60 seconds with feet together and eyes closed. In one study, every healthy person and more than half of the patients with cerebellar ataxia could maintain this position for 60 seconds, whereas half of the patients with sensory ataxia lasted only 10 seconds before beginning to topple over.[43]

A related sign, the sharpened Romberg's sign,[44] in which patients must stand with one foot in front of the other with eyes closed, has little proven diagnostic value. Many normal persons, especially elderly ones, are unable to stand like this for very long.[43,45]

G.   FRONTAL GAIT DISORDER
1.   Definition

"Frontal gait disorder" is an imprecise term describing a combination of findings seen in patients with cerebral tumors, subdural hematomas, dementing illness, normal pressure hydrocephalus, and multiple lacunar infarcts.[46-48] The characteristic findings are (1) slow, shuffling, wide-based gait ("marche a petit pas"); (2) hesitation in starting to walk ("ignition failure"); (3) difficulty picking feet off the floor ("magnetic foot" response); and (4) poor postural control. Motor function of the legs is sometimes much better when these patients are seated or lying, suggesting an element of gait apraxia.

Some of these findings resemble parkinsonism, but the distinguishing features of the frontal gait disorder are its wide base, normal arm swing, lack of other features of parkinsonism, more upright posture, and higher incidence of dementia and urinary incontinence.

2. Clinical Significance

In studies of elderly patients undergoing computed tomography of the head because of neurologic problems, the finding of a frontal gait disorder* correlates strongly with the computed tomography finding of ventricular enlargement.[15,49,50] Only a minority of these patients, however, met the criteria for normal pressure hydrocephalus, suggesting that the findings of ventricular enlargement and gait disturbance are general ones occurring in many different forebrain disorders.[15,49]

IV. EVALUATION OF GAIT DISORDERS

The methods of evaluating gait range from very simple tests that require minutes to complete, which are most appropriate when screening elderly patients for their risk of falls, to the much more comprehensive observational gait analysis, which physiatrists use to break down complicated gait abnormalities into smaller components to direct treatment.[13] Most clinicians adopt an intermediate approach and ask the patient first to walk back and forth several strides at a time, and then again on the toes, heels, and using tandem steps, all maneuvers that may bring out weak muscles or difficulties with balance.

Testing gait is essential, whatever the method, because it is common to find patients who have normal findings during conventional tests of motor, sensory, musculoskeletal, and visual function, yet who, when asked to stand and walk, demonstrate an abnormal gait.[51]

A. OBSERVATIONAL GAIT ANALYSIS[12,13]

Using this method, the clinician watches the patient walk and focuses on one limb at a time, first observing the ankle, then the knee, hip, pelvis, and trunk. At each joint, the clinician considers each of the possible causes that contribute to abnormal gait: pain, immobile joints, muscle weakness, and abnormal limb control.

---

*The specific definition of abnormal gait in these studies was a gait disturbance not attributable to muscle weakness, Parkinson's disease, or musculoskeletal problems.

Each abnormal movement has a differential diagnosis. For "abnormal ipsilateral trunk lean during stance," possible causes include ipsilateral hip pain, ipsilateral short limb (more than 1½ inches shorter), or intentional attempts to clear the contralateral limb during swing (e.g., foot drop or extended limb). For "dragging of the foot or toe during swing," causes are weak ipsilateral ankle dorsiflexor muscles, ipsilateral plantar flexion contractures, inadequate ipsilateral hip or knee flexion, or impaired proprioception.

An excellent manual of observational gait analysis has been published.[12]

B. SIMPLE TESTS OF GAIT

These tests are especially useful in elderly patients to evaluate the risk of falls and to determine functional independence. Validated tests include the "timed 8-foot walk" test, the "timed up and go" test, and the "stops talking when walking" test.

1. Timed 8-Foot Walk Test[1]

The clinician measures the time it takes the patient to walk 8 feet using his or her normal pace. The measured time predicts future disability, as determined 4 years later.

2. Timed "Up and Go" Test[3]

The clinician measures the time it takes the patient to rise from a standard chair, walk to a line on the floor 3 m away, turn, return, and sit down again. The measured time correlates with other accurate but more complex measures of functional independence.

3. Stops Talking When Walking

In one study of elderly nursing home residents, the finding that the patient stopped walking when initiating conversation predicted subsequent falls during 6-month follow-up with a sensitivity of 48%, specificity of 95%, positive likelihood ratio of 8.8, and negative likelihood ratio of 0.6.[2] In this study, all falls were observed and recorded by nursing home staff. Other studies have failed to duplicate these results,[52,53] but these studies enrolled patients living in the community and measured only those falls recalled by the patient. Whether these differences are important is unknown.

V. CANES

Physical examination of gait is not complete without considering the length of the patient's cane and which arm the patient uses to hold the cane.

A. LENGTH OF CANE

Twenty-three percent to 42% of the time, the cane is too long or too short by 5 cm or more.[54,55] An appropriately fitted cane should extend the distance from the distal wrist crease to the ground, when the patient is wearing everyday shoes and placing his or her arms at the sides.[56]

B. CONTRALATERAL VERSUS IPSILATERAL USE OF CANE

In patients with hip and knee arthritis, the conventional teaching is for the patient to hold the cane in the contralateral hand, although compelling evidence for contralateral cane use exists only for patients with hip arthritis.[57–59] By placing just 20, 33, or 38 pounds of pressure on a cane contralateral to a diseased hip when standing on that hip, the patient can *reduce* the pressure on the diseased femoral head by 165, 272, or 319 pounds, respectively.[57]

REFERENCES

1. Guralnik JM, Ferrucci L, Simonsick EM, et al. Lower-extremity function in persons over the age of 70 years as a predictor of subsequent disability. *N Engl J Med.* 1995;332:556-561.
2. Lundin-Olsson L, Nyberg L, Gustafson Y. "Stops walking when talking" as a predictor of falls in elderly people. *Lancet.* 1997;349:617.
3. Podsiadlo D, Richardson S. The timed "up and go": A test of basic functional mobility for frail elderly persons. *J Am Geriatr Soc.* 1991;39:142-148.
4. Tinetti ME, Speechley M, Ginter SF. Risk factors for falls among elderly persons living in the community. *N Engl J Med.* 1988;319:1701-1707.
5. Friedman PJ, Richmond DE, Baskett JJ. A prospective trial of serial gait speed as a measure of rehabilitation in the elderly. *Age Ageing.* 1988;17:227-235.
6. Bootsma-van der Wiel A, Gussekloo J, De Craen AJM, et al. Walking and talking as predictors of falls in the general population: The Leiden 85-plus study. *J Am Geriatr Soc.* 2003;51:1466-1471.
7. Verghese J, Lipton RB, Hall CB, et al. Abnormality of gait as a predictor of non-Alzheimer's dementia. *N Engl J Med.* 2002;347:1761-1768.
8. Bittner V, Weiner DH, Yusuf S, et al. Prediction of mortality and morbidity with a 6-minute walk test in patients with left ventricular dysfunction. *JAMA.* 1993;270:1702-1707.
9. Cowley AJ, Fullwood LJ, Muller AF, et al. Exercise capability in heart failure: Is cardiac output important after all. *Lancet.* 1991;337:771-773.
10. Davies SW, Greig CA, Jordan SL, et al. Short-stepping gait in severe heart failure. *Br Heart J.* 1992;55:469-472.
11. Sloman L, Berridge M, Homatidis S, et al. Gait patterns of depressed patients and normal subjects. *Am J Psychiatry.* 1982;139:94-97.

12. The Pathokinesiology Service and the Physical Therapy Department of Ranchos Los Amigos Medical Center. *Observational gait analysis*. Downey, CA: Los Amigos Research and Education Institute, Inc.; 1993.

13. Perry J. *Gait analysis: Normal and pathological function*. Thorofare, NJ: SLACK, Inc; 1992.

14. Fuh JL, Lin KN, Wang SJ, et al. Neurologic diseases presenting with gait impairment in the elderly. *J Geriatr Psych Neurol*. 1994;7:89-92.

15. Sudarsky L, Ronthal M. Gait disorders among elderly patients. *Arch Neurol*. 1983;40:740-743.

16. Hough JC, McHenry MP, Kammer LM. Gait disorders in the elderly. *Am Fam Phys*. 1987;35:191-196.

17. Murray MP, Gore DR, Sepic SB, Mollinger LA. Antalgic maneuvers during walking in men with unilateral knee disability. *Clin Ortho Rel Res*. 1985;199:192-200.

18. Messier SP, Loeser RF, Hoover JL, et al. Osteoarthritis of the knee: Effects on gait, strength, and flexibility. *Arch Phys Med Rehabil*. 1992;73:29-36.

19. Calve J, Galland M, de Cagny R. Pathogenesis of the limp due to coxalgia: The antalgic gait. *J Bone Joint Surg*. 1939;21:12-25.

20. Murray MP, Gore DR, Clarkson BH. Walking patterns of patients with unilateral hip pain due to osteoarthritis and avascular necrosis. *J Bone Joint Surg Am*. 1971;53:259-274.

21. Gottschalk F, Kourosh S, Leveau B. The functional anatomy of tensor fasciae latae and gluteus medius and minimus. *J Anat*. 1989;166:179-189.

22. Peltier LF. Trendelenburg's test: 1895. *Clin Ortho Rel Res*. 1998;355:3-7.

23. Pai VS. Significance of the Trendelenburg test in total hip arthroplasty. *J Arthroplasty*. 1996;11:174-179.

24. Ramesh M, O'Byrne JM, McCarthy N, et al. Damage to the superior gluteal nerve after the Hardinge approach to the hip. *J Bone Joint Surg Br*. 1996;78:903-906.

25. Baker AS, Bitounis VC. Abductor function after total hip replacement. *J Bone Joint Surg Br*. 1989;71:47-50.

26. Hardcastle P, Nade S. The significance of the Trendelenburg test. *J Bone Joint Surg Br*. 1985;67:741-746.

27. Vasudevan PN, Vaidyalingam KV, Nair PB. Can Trendelenburg's sign be positive if the hip is normal? *J Bone Joint Surg Br*. 1997;79:462-466.

28. Brandstater ME, De Bruin H, Gowland C, Clark BM. Hemiplegic gait: Analysis of temporal variables. *Arch Phys Med Rehabil*. 1983;64:583-587.

29. Knutsson E, Richards C. Different types of disturbed motor control in gait of hemiparetic patients. *Brain*. 1979;102:405-430.

30. Perry J. The mechanics of walking in hemiplegia. *Clin Orthop*. 1969;63:23-31.

31. Riley TL, Ray WF, Massey EW. Gait mechanisms: Asymmetry of arm motion in normal subjects. *Military Med*. 1977;142:467-468.

32. Knutsson E. An analysis of parkinsonian gait. *Brain*. 1972;95:475-486.

33. Rogers MW. Disorders of posture, balance, and gait in Parkinson's disease. *Clin Geriatr Med.* 1996;12:825-845.
34. Simpkin PA. Simian stance: A sign of spinal stenosis. *Lancet.* 1982;2:652-653.
35. Gilman S, Bloedel JR, Lechtenberg R. *Disorders of the cerebellum.* Philadelphia: F. A. Davis, Co.; 1981.
36. Holmes G. Clinical symptoms of cerebellar disease and their interpretation. Lecture 3. *Lancet.* 1922;2:59-65.
37. Rogers JH. Romberg and his test. *J Laryngol Otol.* 1980;94:1401-1404.
38. Schiller F. Staggering gait in medical history. *Neurology.* 1995;37:127-135.
39. Ojala M, Matikainen E, Juntunen J. Posturography and the dizzy patient: A neurological study of 133 patients. *Acta Neurol Scand.* 1989;80:118-122.
40. Baloh RW, Jacobson KM, Beykirch K, Honrubia V. Static and dynamic posturography in patients with vestibular and cerebellar lesions. *Arch Neurol.* 1998;55:649-654.
41. Bronstein AM, Hood JD, Gresty MA, Panagi C. Visual control of balance in cerebellar and Parkinsonian syndromes. *Brain.* 1990;113:767-779.
42. Lanska DJ, Goetz CG. Romberg's sign: Development, adoption, and adaptation in the 19th century. *Neurology.* 2000;55:1201-1206.
43. Notermans NC, van Dijk GW, van der Graaff Y, et al. Measuring ataxia: quantification based on the standard neurological examination. *J Neurol Neurosurg Psychiatry.* 1994;57:22-26.
44. Graybiel A, Fregly AR. A new quantitative ataxia test battery. *Acta Otolaryngol (Stockh).* 1966;61:292-312.
45. Heitmann DK, Gossman MR, Shaddeau SA, Jackson JR. Balance performance and step width in noninstitutionalized, elderly, female fallers and nonfallers. *Phys Ther.* 1989;69:923-931.
46. Nutt JG, Marsden CD, Thompson PD. Human walking and higher-level gait disorders, particularly in the elderly. *Neurology.* 1993;43:268-279.
47. Alexander NB. Gait disorders in older adults. *J Am Geriatr Soc.* 1996;44:434-451.
48. Thompson PD. Gait disorders accompanying diseases of the frontal lobes. *Adv Neurol.* 2001;87:235-241.
49. Koller WC, Wilson RS, Glatt SL, et al. Senile gait: Correlation with computed tomographic scans. *Ann Neurol.* 1983;13:343-344.
50. Fisher CM. Hydrocephalus as a cause of disturbances of gait in the elderly. *Neurology.* 1982;32:1358-1363.
51. Tinetti ME, Ginter SF. Identifying mobility dysfunctions in elderly patients: Standard neuromuscular examination or direct assessment? *JAMA.* 1988;259:1190-1193.
52. Bloem BR, Cramer M, Valkenburg VV. "Stops walking when talking" does not predict falls in Parkinson's disease. *Ann Neurol.* 2000;48:268-269.
53. Hyndman D, Ashburn A. "Stops walking when talking" as a predictor of falls in people with stroke living in the community. *J Neurol Neurosurg Psychiatry.* 2004;75:994-997.

54. George J, Binns VE, Clayden AD, Mulley GP. Aids and adaptations for the elderly at home: Underprovided, underused, and undermaintained. *Br Med J.* 1988;296:1365-1366.

55. Sainsbury R, Mulley GP. Walking sticks used by the elderly. *Br Med J.* 1982;284:1751.

56. Mulley GP. Walking sticks. *Br Med J.* 1988;296:475-476.

57. Blount WP. Don't throw away the cane. *J Bone Joint Surg Am.* 1956;38A:695-708.

58. Edwards BG. Contralateral and ipsilateral cane usage by patients with total knee or hip replacement. *Arch Phys Med Rehabil.* 1986;67:734-740.

59. Vargo MM, Robinson LR, Nicholas JJ. Contralateral vs. ipsilateral cane use: Effects on muscles crossing the knee joint. *Am J Phys Med Rehabil.* 1992;71(3):170-176.

Jaundice

I. INTRODUCTION

Jaundice is an abnormal yellowish discoloration of the skin and mucous membranes caused by accumulation of bile pigment. There are three forms of jaundice: (1) hemolytic (resulting from increased bilirubin production from excessive breakdown of red cells), (2) hepatocellular (resulting from disease of the liver parenchyma, sometimes referred to as "nonobstructive jaundice" or "medical jaundice"), and (3) obstructive (resulting from mechanical obstruction of the biliary ducts outside the liver, sometimes referred to as "surgical jaundice"). The most common causes of hepatocellular jaundice are viral hepatitis and alcoholic cirrhosis; the most common causes of obstructive jaundice are gallstone disease (i.e., choledocholithiasis) and pancreatic carcinoma.[1,2]

Because hemolytic disorders cause less than 2% of all jaundice[1,3] and because hemolysis usually causes obvious hematologic abnormalities and no other signs of liver disease, the clinician's usual task at the bedside of a jaundiced patient is to differentiate nonobstructive hepatocellular jaundice from obstructive jaundice.

II. THE FINDINGS

A. JAUNDICE

Jaundice is usually first noted in the conjunctiva of the eyes. Although the traditional term for this is "scleral icterus," this is a misnomer because pathologic studies reveal most of the pigment to be deposited in the conjunctiva, not the avascular sclera.[4] As jaundice progresses and the serum bilirubin increases, the face, mucous membranes, and eventually the entire skin acquires a yellow or orange hue.

Prominent yellowish subconjunctival fat may be mistaken for conjunctival jaundice, but fat usually is limited to the conjunctival folds and, unlike jaundice, spares the area near the cornea. Patients with carotenemia (from excess carrot or multivitamin ingestion) also develop a yellowish discoloration of the skin, especially the palms, soles, and nasolabial fold; however, in contrast to jaundice, the conjunctiva are spared.[5]

B. ASSOCIATED FINDINGS

Several findings traditionally distinguish hepatocellular from obstructive disease.

1. Hepatocellular Jaundice

Findings characteristic of hepatocellular jaundice are spider telangiectasia, palmar erythema, dilated abdominal wall veins, splenomegaly, asterixis, and fetor hepaticus.

a. Spider Telangiectasia ("Spider Angiomata")

Spider telangiectasia are dilated cutaneous blood vessels that have three components: (1) a central arteriole (the "body" of the spider), which, when compressed slightly with a glass slide, can be seen to pulsate; (2) multiple radiating "legs"; and (3) surrounding erythema, which may encompass the entire lesion or only its central portion.[6] After blanching, the returning blood fills the central arteriole first before traveling to the peripheral tips of each leg. Spiders are most numerous on the face and neck, followed by the shoulders, thorax, arms, and hands. They are rare on the palms, scalp, and below the umbilicus.[6] This peculiar distribution may reflect the neurohormonal properties of the microcirculation, because this distribution is also where blushing is most intense.[6]

Acquired vascular spiders are associated with three clinical conditions: liver disease, pregnancy, and malnutrition.[7] In patients with liver disease, the spiders advance and regress with disease severity, and their appearance correlates somewhat with an abnormally increased ratio of serum estradiol to testosterone levels.[8] In pregnant women, vascular spiders typically appear between the second and fifth months and usually disappear within days after delivery.[7] Vascular spiders also have been described in normal persons, but these lesions, in contrast to those of liver disease, are always small in number (average three) and size.[6]

Vascular spiders were first described by the English physician Erasmus Wilson in 1867.[6]

b. Palmar Erythema

Palmar erythema is a symmetric reddening of the surfaces of the palms, most pronounced over the hypothenar and thenar eminences.[7] Palmar erythema occurs in the same clinical conditions as vascular spiders, and the two lesions tend to come and go together.[7,9]

c. Dilated Abdominal Veins

In some patients with cirrhosis, high portal vein pressures lead to the development of collateral vessels connecting the portal venous and systemic venous systems. One group of collateral vessels develops around the umbilicus, connecting the left portal vein via paraumbilical vessels to abdominal wall veins.[10] These abdominal wall veins may become so prominent and numerous that they resemble a cluster of serpents, thus earning the name "caput medusae."[11] Dilated abdominal veins of portal hypertension may generate a continuous humming murmur heard during auscultation between the xiphoid and umbilicus.[12]

Dilated abdominal veins also occur in the superior vena cava syndrome (if the obstruction also involves the azygous system)[13] and inferior vena cava syndrome.[14] In these disorders, however, the collateral veins tend to appear on the lateral aspects of the abdominal wall. A traditional test to distinguish vena caval obstruction from portal hypertension is to strip abdominal wall veins below the umbilicus and see which way blood is flowing (in portal-systemic collateral veins, flow should hypothetically flow away from the umbilicus, whereas in collateral veins from inferior vena cava obstruction, flow is reversed and toward the head).[15] This test is unreliable, however, because most dilated abdominal vessels lack competent valves and the clinician can "demonstrate" blood to flow in both directions in patients with both disorders.

d. Palpable Spleen

Because a principal cause of splenomegaly is portal hypertension from severe hepatocellular disease,[16,17] a traditional teaching is that the finding of splenomegaly in a jaundiced patient argues for hepatocellular disease.

e. Asterixis

Asterixis, originally described by Adams and Foley in 1949[18,19] is one of the earliest findings of hepatic encephalopathy and is thus typical of hepatocellular jaundice. To elicit the sign, the patient holds his or her arms outstretched with fingers spread apart. After a short latent period, both fingers and hands commence to "flap" with abrupt movements occurring at irregular intervals of a fraction of a second to seconds (thus earning the name "liver flap"). The fundamental problem in asterixis is the inability to maintain a fixed posture ("asterixis" comes from the Greek *sterigma* meaning "to support"), and consequently, asterixis also can be demonstrated at other sites by having the patient elevate the leg and dorsiflex the foot, close the eyelids forcibly, or protrude the tongue.[18,20] Because some voluntary contraction of the muscles is necessary to elicit asterixis, the sign disappears once coma ensues (although in some comatose patients the finding appears during the grasp reflex; see Chapter 59).[18]

Electromyograms reveal that the actual flap of asterixis is caused by an abrupt disappearance of electrical activity in the muscle.[20] Asterixis is therefore a form of negative myoclonus.

Asterixis is not a specific sign of liver disease and also appears in encephalopathy from hypercapnia, uremia, and other disorders.[21,22] Unilateral asterixis indicates structural disease in the contralateral brain.[23,24]

f. Fetor Hepaticus

Fetor hepaticus is the characteristic breath of patients with severe parenchymal disease, which has been likened to "a mixture of rotten eggs and garlic."[25,26] Gas chromatography reveals that the compound causing the odor is dimethylsulfide. Fetor hepaticus is a sign of severe portal-systemic shunting, not encephalopathy per se, because levels of dimethylsulfide correlate best with the degree of portal-systemic shunting[27] and because alert patients with severe portal-systemic shunting also have the characteristic breath.[27]

2. Obstructive Jaundice: Palpable Gallbladder (Courvoisier's Sign)

The presence of a smooth, nontender, distended gallbladder in a patient with jaundice is a traditional sign of obstructive jaundice. Courvoisier's sign refers to the association of the palpable gallbladder and extrahepatic obstruction, a sign whose accuracy is discussed fully in Chapter 47.

III. CLINICAL SIGNIFICANCE

A. DETECTION OF JAUNDICE

Although the traditional teaching is that jaundice becomes evident once the serum bilirubin exceeds 2.5 to 3 mg/dL, clinical studies reveal that only 70% to 80% of observers detect jaundice at this threshold.[28,29] The sensitivity of examination increases to 83% if the serum bilirubin exceeds 10 mg/dL and 96% if the bilirubin exceeds 15 mg/dL.

B. HEPATOCELLULAR VERSUS OBSTRUCTIVE JAUNDICE

Several studies have shown that, just using the bedside and basic laboratory findings (i.e., before clinical imaging), clinicians accurately distinguish hepatocellular from obstructive jaundice more than 80% of the time.[30-32] Easy-to-use and accurate scoring charts that combine symptoms, signs, and laboratory values have been developed.[1]

EBM Box 6-1 presents how well physical signs distinguish hepatocellular from obstructive jaundice. Because "disease" in this table was defined as hepa-

Box 6-1 Findings Predicting Hepatocellular Jaundice in Patients with Jaundice*

Finding (Ref)†	Sensitivity (%)	Specificity (%)	Likelihood Ratio if Finding	
			Present	Absent
General appearance				
Weight loss[31,33]	10–49	21–97	NS	NS
Skin				
Spider angiomata[31,33]	35–47	88–97	**4.7**	0.6
Palmar erythema[31]	49	95	**9.8**	0.5
Dilated abdominal veins[31]	42	98	**17.5**	0.6
Abdomen				
Ascites[31]	44	90	**4.4**	0.6
Palpable spleen[31,33]	29–47	83–90	2.9	0.7
Palpable gallbladder[31]	0†	69	**0.04**	1.4
Palpable liver[31,33]	71–83	15–17	NS	NS
Liver tenderness[31,33]	37–38	70–78	NS	NS

NS, not significant; likelihood ratio (LR) if finding present = positive LR; LR if finding absent = negative LR.

*Diagnostic standard: For nonobstructive (vs. obstructive) jaundice, needle biopsy of liver, surgical exploration, or autopsy.

†None of the 41 patients with medical jaundice in this study had a palpable gallbladder; for calculation of the LRs, 0.5 was added to all cells of the 2 × 2 table.

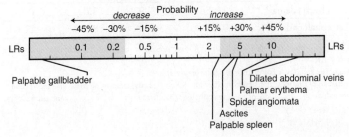

tocellular jaundice, likelihood ratios (LRs) with a large positive number argue for hepatocellular jaundice and those with an LR close to zero argue against hepatocellular jaundice and thus for obstructive jaundice.

These studies show that, in patients presenting with jaundice, the physical signs of portal hypertension (dilated abdominal veins, LR = 17.5; ascites, LR = 4.4;

Box 6-2 Findings Predicting Cirrhosis in Patients with Chronic Liver Disease*

Finding (Ref)[†]	Sensitivity (%)	Specificity (%)	Likelihood Ratio if Finding	
			Present	Absent
Skin				
Spider angiomata[34–41]	33–66	48–98	**3.7**	0.6
Palmar erythema[35,37,38,40]	12–63	49–98	2.6	0.7
Jaundice[35,39,41,42]	21–44	83–93	2.6	0.8
Dilated abdominal wall veins[35,40]	24–51	80–98	**5.4**	0.7
Abdomen				
Hepatomegaly[35,38–41,43]	31–96	20–96	2.0	0.6
Palpable liver in epigastrium[41]	86	68	2.6	**0.2**
Liver edge firm to palpation[38,43]	71–78	71–74	2.7	0.4
Splenomegaly[34,36–43]	5–85	35–98	2.3	0.8
Ascites[34,35,37,39–42]	14–52	82–99	**6.6**	0.8
Other				
Peripheral edema[35,39,40]	24–56	87–92	**3.0**	0.7
Encephalopathy[34,35,37]	9–29	98–99	**8.8**	NS

NS, not significant; likelihood ratio (LR) if finding present = positive LR; LR if finding absent = negative LR.

*Diagnostic standard: For cirrhosis, needle biopsy of liver.

[†]Definition of findings: For hepatomegaly and splenomegaly, examining clinician's impression using palpation, percussion, or both; encephalopathy, disordered consciousness, and asterixis[18]

CIRRHOSIS

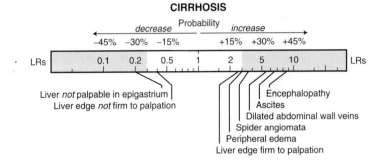

and palpable spleen, LR = 2.9), palmar erythema (LR = 9.8), and spider angiomata (LR = 4.7) all argue *for* hepatocellular jaundice. The only finding arguing strongly *against* hepatocellular jaundice is the palpable gallbladder (LR = 0.04; in other words, the finding of a palpable gallbladder argues *for* obstructed bile ducts with an LR of 26.0, the inverse of 0.04).

In these studies, weight loss occurred in all etiologies and did not discriminate well between hepatocellular and obstructive etiologies. Also unhelpful were the findings of liver tenderness and a palpable liver. The palpable liver remains unhelpful even when it is defined as a liver edge extending more than 4 to 5 fingerbreaths below the right costal margin.[31]

C. DIAGNOSIS OF CIRRHOSIS

The diagnosis of cirrhosis in patients with liver disease has important prognostic and therapeutic implications. EBM Box 6-2 displays the diagnostic accuracy of physical examination for cirrhosis, determined from study of hundreds of patients presenting with chronic liver disorders of widely varying etiologies. According to this table, the findings that increase the probability of cirrhosis the most are encephalopathy (irrational behavior, disordered consciousness and asterixis; LR = 8.8, see EBM Box 6-2), ascites (LR = 6.6), dilated abdominal veins (LR = 5.4), spider angiomata (LR = 3.7), and peripheral edema (LR = 3.0). Other findings also argue for cirrhosis, but to a lesser degree: jaundice (LR = 2.6), palmar erythema (LR = 2.6), a liver edge that is firm to palpation (LR = 2.7) or found in the epigastrium (LR = 2.6), and splenomegaly (LR = 2.3). The only findings arguing against cirrhosis are the *absence* of a palpable liver in the epigastrium (LR = 0.2) and the *absence* of a firm liver edge (LR = 0.4).

In one study of patients with chronic liver disease and known esophageal varices, the number and size of spider angiomata correlated with the patient's risk of subsequent variceal bleeding.[44]

REFERENCES

1. Lindberg G, Thomsen C, Malchow-Moller A, et al. Differential diagnosis of jaundice: Applicability of the Copenhagen Pocket Chart proved in Stockholm patients. *Liver.* 1987;7:43-49.

2. Theodossi A, Spiegelhalter D, Portmann B, et al. The value of clinical, biochemical, ultrasound and liver biopsy data in assessing patients with liver disease. *Liver.* 1983;3:315-326.

3. Matzen P. Diagnosis in jaundice: A contemporary approach. *Dig Dis.* 1986;4:220-230.

4. Tripathi RC, Sidrys LA. 'Conjunctival icterus,' not 'scleral icterus'. *JAMA.* 1979; 242:2558.

5. Monk B. Carotenemia. *Int J Dermatol.* 1983;22:376-377.

6. Bean WB. *Vascular spiders and related lesions of the skin.* Springfield, IL: Charles C. Thomas; 1958.

7. Bean WB. Acquired palmar erythema and cutaneous vascular "spiders". *Am Heart J.* 1943;25:463-477.

8. Pirovino M, Linder R, Boss C, et al. Cutaneous spider nevi in liver cirrhosis: Capillary microscopical and hormonal investigations. *Klin Wochenschr.* 1988;66: 298-302.

9. Morrison GR. Causative factors in palmar erythema. *Geriatrics.* 1975;30:59-61.

10. Lafortune M, Constantin A, Breton G, et al. The recanalized umbilical vein in portal hypertension: A myth. *AJR.* 1985;114:549-553.

11. Cohen SM. Caput medusae. *N Engl J Med.* 1999;341:419.

12. Armstrong EL, Adams WL, Tragerman LJ, Townsend EW. The Cruveilhier-Baumgarten syndrome: Review of the literature and report of two additional cases. *Ann Intern Med.* 1942;16:113-151.

13. Nieto AF, Doty DB. Superior vena cava obstruction: Clinical syndrome, etiology, and treatment. *Curr Prob Canc.* 1986;10:442-484.

14. Missal ME, Robinson JA, Tatum RW. Inferior vena cava obstruction: Clinical manifestations, diagnostic methods, and related problems. *Ann Intern Med.* 1965;62:133-161.

15. Coetzee T. Clinical anatomy of the umbilicus. *S Afr Med J.* 1980;57:463-466.

16. Lipp WF, Eckstein EH, Aaron AH. The clinical significance of the palpable spleen. *Gastroenterology.* 1944;3:287-291.

17. O'Reilly RA. Splenomegaly at a United States county hospital: Diagnostic evaluation of 170 patients. *Am J Med Sci.* 1996;312:160-165.

18. Adams RD, Foley JM. The neurological disorder associated with liver disease. *Res Pub Assoc Nerv Ment Dis.* 1953;32:198-237.

19. Adams RD, Foley JM. The neurological changes in the more common types of severe liver disease. *Trans Am Neurol Assoc.* 1949;74:217-219.

20. Leavitt S, Tyler HR. Studies in asterixis. *Arch Neurol.* 1964;10:360-368.

21. Conn HO. Asterixis in non-hepatic disorders. *Am J Med.* 1960;29:647-661.

22. Conn HO. Asterixis: Its occurrence in chronic obstructive pulmonary disease, with a commentary on its general mechanism. *N Engl J Med.* 1958;259:564-569.

23. Reinfeld H, Louis S. Unilateral asterixis: Clinical significance of the sign. *N Y State J Med*. 1983;83:206-208.

24. Kim JS. Asterixis after unilateral stroke: Lesion location of 30 patients. *Neurology*. 2001;56:533-536.

25. Davidson LSP. Mercaptan in the breath of patients with severe liver disease. *Lancet*. 1949;2:197-198.

26. Challenger F, Walshe JM. Foetor hepaticus. *Lancet*. 1955;1:1239-1241.

27. Tangerman A, Meuwese-Arends MT, Jansen JBM. Cause and composition of foetor hepaticus. *Lancet*. 1994;343:483.

28. Hung OL, Kwon NS, Cole AE, et al. Evaluation of the physician's ability to recognize the presence or absence of anemia, fever, and jaundice. *Acad Emerg Med*. 2000; 7:146-156.

29. Ruiz MA, Saab S, Rickman LS. The clinical detection of scleral icterus: Observations of multiple examiners. *Mil Med*. 1997;162:560-563.

30. Martin WB, Apostolakos PC, Roazen H. Clinical versus actuarial prediction in the differential diagnosis of jaundice. *Am J Med Sci*. 1960;240:571-578.

31. Schenker S, Balint J, Schiff L. Differential diagnosis of jaundice: Report of a prospective study of 61 proved cases. *Am J Dig Dis*. 1962;7:449-463.

32. O'Connor KW, Snodgrass PJ, Swonder JE, et al. A blinded prospective study comparing four current noninvasive approaches in the differential diagnosis of medical versus surgical jaundice. *Gastroenterology*. 1983;84:1498-1504.

33. Burbank F. A computer diagnostic system for the diagnosis of prolonged undifferentiating liver disease. *Am J Med*. 1969;46:401-415.

34. Czaja AJ, Wolf AM, Baggenstoss AH. Clinical assessment of cirrhosis in severe chronic active liver disease: Specificity and sensitivity of physical and laboratory findings. *Mayo Clin Proc*. 1980;55:360-364.

35. Hamberg KJ, Carstenesen B, Sorensen TIA, Eghoje K. Accuracy of clinical diagnosis of cirrhosis among alcohol-abusing men. *J Clin Epidemiol*. 1996;49:1295-1301.

36. Hay CRM, Preston FE, Triger DR, et al. Predictive markers of chronic liver disease in hemophilia. *Blood*. 1987;69:1595-1599.

37. Lashner BA, Jonas RB, Tang HS, et al. Chronic hepatitis: Disease factors at diagnosis predictive of mortality. *Am J Med*. 1988;85:609-614.

38. Marmo R, Romano M, Peduto A, et al. Decision-making model for a non-invasive diagnosis of compensated liver cirrhosis. *Ital J Gastroenterol*. 1993;25:1-8.

39. Nakamura T, Nakamura S, Aikawa T, et al. Clinical studies of alcoholic hepatic diseases. *Tohoku J Exp Med*. 1967;93:179-189.

40. Rankin JGD, Orrego-Matte H, Deschenes J, et al. Alcoholic liver disease: The problem of diagnosis. *Alcohol Clin Exp Res*. 1978;2:327-338.

41. McCormick PA, Nolan N. Palpable epigastric liver as a physical sign of cirrhosis: A prospective study. *Eur J Gastroenterol Hepatol*. 2004;16:1331-1334.

42. Cozzolino G, Lonardo A, Francica G, et al. Differential diagnosis between hepatic cirrhosis and chronic active hepatitis: Specificity and sensitivity of physical and

laboratory findings in a series from the Mediterranean area. *Am J Gastroenterol.* 1983;78:442-445.

43. Tine F, Caltagirone M, Camma C, et al. Clinical indicants of compensated cirrhosis: A prospective study. In: Dianzani MU, Gentilini P, eds. *Chronic liver damage: Proceedings of the Annual Meeting of the Italian national programme on liver cirrhosis, San Miniato, Italy 11-13 January 1990.* Amsterdam: *Excerpta Medica;* 1990:187-198.

44. Foutch PG, Sullivan JA, Gaines JA, Sanowski RA. Cutaneous vascular spiders in cirrhotic patients: Correlation with hemorrhage from esophageal varices. *Am J Gastroenterol.* 1988;83:723-726.

Cyanosis

I. DEFINITIONS

Cyanosis is an abnormal bluish discoloration of the skin and mucous membranes, caused by blue-colored blood circulating in the superficial capillaries and venules. The blue color usually represents excessive amounts of deoxygenated hemoglobin, although in some patients it results from increased amounts of methemoglobin or sulfhemoglobin. Cyanosis may be "central" or "peripheral." In **central cyanosis** the blood leaving the heart is colored blue; in **peripheral cyanosis,** the blood leaving the heart is red, although it becomes blue by the time it reaches the fingers and toes. **Pseudocyanosis,** in contrast, refers to a permanent bluish discoloration caused by deposition of blue pigments in the skin.

Cyanosis was first described in 1761 by Morgagni, who attributed it to pulmonic stenosis.[1] In 1869, Claude Bernard described the qualitative difference in blood gases between blue venous blood and red arterial blood. The first person to quantify how much deoxygenated hemoglobin was necessary to produce the blue color was Lundsgaard in 1919.[1]

II. PATHOGENESIS

A. THE BLUE COLOR

Blood becomes blue when an absolute amount of blue pigment (usually deoxy-hemoglobin) accumulates, probably because only then is the blue color deep enough to be seen through the opaque epidermis.[1-4] Once this minimal amount of deoxyhemoglobin accumulates and cyanosis appears, the amount of additional red blood (or oxyhemoglobin) matters little to the overall skin color.

The color of the skin depends on the color of blood flowing through the dermal capillaries and subpapillary venous plexus, not the arteries and veins, which lie too deep to contribute to skin color.[1,5] There has been much confusion over the absolute concentration of deoxyhemoglobin required for cyanosis, primarily because some investigators have mistakenly equated arterial levels of deoxyhemoglobin, which are easy to measure, with capillary levels, which impart the blue color but must be higher than the measured arterial levels. In patients with central cyanosis, the *average* amount of *arterial* deoxyhemoglobin is 3.48 ± 0.55 g/dL (or 5.3 g/dL in the capillaries and small venules). The *minimal* amount of *arterial* deoxyhemoglobin causing cyanosis is 2.38 g/dL (or 4.24 g/dL in the capillaries and small venules).[*, 4]

Because cyanosis depends on the absolute quantity of deoxyhemoglobin, not the relative amount, the level of oxygen saturation at which the finding appears depends on the patient's total hemoglobin concentration (i.e., 5 g/dL of deoxyhemoglobin in the capillaries represents a higher percent of oxygen desaturation for an anemic patient, who has less total hemoglobin, than it does for a polycythemic patient). This relationship is displayed in Table 7-1, showing that polycythemic patients may become cyanotic with only mild hypoxemia (i.e., oxygen saturation of 88% if the total hemoglobin is 20 g/dL, which is an oxygen tension of 56 mm Hg), yet anemic patients do not develop the finding until hypoxemia is severe (i.e., oxygen saturation of 70% if the total hemoglobin is 8 g/dL, which is an oxygen tension of 36 mm Hg).[†]

B. PERIPHERAL CYANOSIS

In peripheral cyanosis, blood leaving the heart is red, but because of increased extraction of oxygen by peripheral tissues, enough deoxyhemoglobin accumulates to turn it blue in the subepidermal blood vessels of the feet and hands. The

---

*Levels of capillary deoxyhemoglobin were calculated assuming that the difference in oxygen content between the arteries and veins is 5 mL of oxygen/dL of blood and that the amount of deoxyhemoglobin in the capillaries is midway between that of the arteries and veins.

†These figures are calculated as follows: for the polycythemic patient (total hemoglobin of 20 g/dL), 2.38 g/dL of arterial deoxyhemoglobin indicates that there is 20 – 2.38 or 17.62 g/dL of oxyhemoglobin. Oxygen saturation, therefore, is (17.62)/(20) = 0.88, or 88%. For the anemic patient, the calculation is (8–2.38)/8 = 0.7, or 70% saturation.

Table 7-1	Cyanosis and Hemoglobin Concentration	

	Cyanosis Appears at*	
Hemoglobin Concentration (g/dL)	Oxygen Saturation (%) Less Than	Arterial pO_2 (mm Hg) Less Than
6	60	31
8	70	36
10	76	40
12	80	45
14	83	47
16	85	50
18	87	54
20	88	56

*These figures assume that central cyanosis begins to appear when 2.38 g/dL of deoxygenated hemoglobin accumulates in arterial blood (see text for calculations). The corresponding pO_2 was obtained from standard hemoglobin dissociation curves for oxygen.

clinician can easily demonstrate the phenomenon of peripheral cyanosis by wrapping a rubber band around a finger: Oxygen continues to be extracted from the stagnant blood, and within a minute or two, the distal digit turns blue.

III. THE FINDING

Cyanosis is best appreciated in areas of the body where the overlying epidermis is thin and subepidermal vessels are abundant, such as the lips, nose, cheeks, ears, hands, feet, and the mucous membranes of the oral cavity.[1,6] Cyanosis is more easily appreciated with fluorescent lighting than with incandescent lighting or daylight.[4]

A. CENTRAL CYANOSIS

Patients with central cyanosis have blue discoloration of the lips, tongue, and sublingual tissues in addition to the hands and feet. In patients with central cyanosis, the correlation between different levels of oxygen desaturation and severity of cyanosis is best when the color is determined from examination of the lips and buccal mucosa.[7,8] Some patients with longstanding central cyanosis also have clubbing of the digits.

When central cyanosis is suspected, yet administration of oxygen fails to diminish the blue color, the clinician should consider methemoglobinemia or sulfhemoglobinemia. Many patients with methemoglobinemia are described as having a characteristic brownish or "chocolate" hue ("chocolate cyanosis").[9]

Because cyanosis depends on blue blood being present in the underlying blood vessels, maneuvers that express blood out of the vessels, such as pressure on the skin, make the blue color temporarily disappear.

B. PERIPHERAL CYANOSIS

Peripheral cyanosis causes blue hands and feet, although the mucous membranes of the mouth are pink. Warming the patient's limb skin often lessens the blue color of peripheral cyanosis because it improves flow of blood to that area, whereas in central cyanosis, warming of the skin causes either no change or makes the blue color deeper.

C. PSEUDOCYANOSIS

In patients with pseudocyanosis, the mucous membranes of the mouth are pink, and blanching of the skin by pressure does not make the color disappear.[6]

D. CYANOSIS AND OXIMETRY

Cyanosis affects co-oximetry (i.e., blood gas analysis in the laboratory) differently than it affects pulse oximetry (i.e., equipment used at the bedside; see Chapter 18). Co-oximetry is able to distinguish deoxyhemoglobin from other abnormal hemoglobins and therefore indicates hypoxemia only in patients with central cyanosis (i.e., because it samples *arterial* blood, oxygen levels are normal in peripheral cyanosis). Pulse oximetry, in contrast, detects the *color* of the pulsatile waveform in the digit. Although it also indicates hypoxemia in patients with central cyanosis and high deoxyhemoglobin levels, pulse oximetry sometimes falsely indicates arterial hypoxemia in patients with peripheral cyanosis or with abnormal hemoglobins (see Chapter 18). Both co-oximetry and pulse oximetry indicate normal oxygen levels in pseudocyanosis.

IV. CLINICAL SIGNIFICANCE

A. CENTRAL CYANOSIS

Any disorder causing hypoxemia may cause enough deoxyhemoglobin to accumulate in the blood leaving the heart, thus producing central cyanosis. Typical etiologies are pulmonary edema, pneumonia, and intracardiac right-to-left shunts.

The finding of central cyanosis detects an arterial deoxyhemoglobin level of 2.38 g/dL or more with a sensitivity of 79% to 95%, specificity of 72% to 95%, positive likelihood ratio (LR) of 7.4, and negative LR of 0.2.[2,4] With knowledge of the patient's hemoglobin concentration, therefore, the clinician can be reasonably confident that the finding of central cyanosis indicates an arterial oxygen level below that indicated in Table 7-1.

B. PERIPHERAL CYANOSIS

In clinical practice, common causes of peripheral cyanosis are low cardiac output, arterial disease or obstruction (e.g., Raynaud's disease), and venous disease.

C. PSEUDOCYANOSIS

Pseudocyanosis may occur after exposure to metals ("chrysiasis" of gold therapy; "argyria" from topical silver compounds) or drugs (amiodarone, minocycline, chloroquine, or phenothiazines).[6,10,11]

REFERENCES

1. Lundsgaard C, Van Slyke DD. Cyanosis. *Medicine.* 1923;2:1-76.
2. Goss GA, Hayes JA, Burdon JGW. Deoxyhaemoglobin concentrations in the detection of central cyanosis. *Thorax.* 1988;43:212-213.
3. Martin L, Khalil H. How much reduced hemoglobin in necessary to generate central cyanosis? *Chest.* 1990;97:182-185.
4. Barnett HB, Holland JG, Josenhans WT. When does central cyanosis become detectable? *Clin Invest Med.* 1982;5:39-43.
5. Lewis T. *The blood vessels of the human skin and their responses.* London: Shaw and Sons; 1927.
6. Carpenter KD. A comprehensive review of cyanosis. *Crit Care Nurs.* 1993;13:66-72.
7. Kelman GR, Nunn JF. Clinical recognition of hypoxaemia under fluorescent lamps. *Lancet.* 1966;1:1400-1403.
8. Medd WE, French EB, Wyllie VM. Cyanosis as a guide to arterial oxygen desaturation. *Thorax.* 1959;14:247-250.
9. Whelan JF. Methemoglobin as a cause of cyanosis. *Can Med Assoc J.* 1984;130:1260.
10. Familton MJG, Armstrong RF. Pseudo-cyanosis: Time to reclassify cyanosis? *Anaesthesia* 1989;44:257.
11. Timmins AC, Morgan GAR. Argyria or cyanosis. *Anaesthesia* 1988;43:755-756.

Anemia

I. INTRODUCTION

Anemia refers to an abnormally low number of circulating red cells, caused by blood loss, hemolysis, or underproduction of cells by the bone marrow. In patients with acute blood loss, physical signs reflect the changing vital signs of hypovolemia (see Chapter 15). In chronic anemia, the subject of this chapter, physical examination focuses instead on the color of skin and conjunctiva. Chronic anemia is a feature of almost all chronic diseases.

II. THE FINDINGS

In chronic anemia, the skin and conjunctiva may appear abnormally pale because the amount of red-colored oxyhemoglobin circulating in the dermal and subconjunctival capillaries and venules is reduced.[1] This finding, however, is not always reliable, because the color of the skin also depends on the diameter of these minute vessels, the amount of circulating deoxyhemoglobin, and the patient's natural skin pigments.[1] Vasoconstriction from cold exposure or sympathetic stimulation also may cause pallor, and the pallor of anemia may be obscured by other colors, such as the red color of vasodilation (inflammatory response or permanent vascular injury from ischemia, cold, or radiation), the blue color of cyanosis (see Chapter 7), or the brown color of natural pigments of dark-skinned persons. Theoretically, examination of the conjunctiva, nailbeds, and palms minimizes the effects of the patient's natural skin pigments.

Most clinicians assess for pallor subjectively, by comparing the patient's skin color with their own color or with some recollection of normal skin color. One definition of pallor, however, is more objective: **conjunctival rim pallor** is present if examination of the inferior conjunctiva reveals the color of the anterior rim to be the same pale fleshy color of the deeper posterior aspect of the palpebral conjunctiva.[2] Normally, in persons without anemia, the anterior rim has a bright red color that contrasts with the fleshy color of the posterior portion.

III. CLINICAL SIGNIFICANCE

EBM Box 8-1 presents the diagnostic accuracy of physical signs for chronic anemia as applied to hundreds of patients. These studies all excluded patients

 Box 8-1   Anemia*

Finding (Ref)[†]	Sensitivity (%)	Specificity (%)	Likelihood Ratio if Finding	
			Present	Absent
Pallor at any site[3-5]	38–77	66–92	**4.1**	0.4
Facial pallor[4]	46	88	**3.8**	0.6
Nail bed pallor[4,5]	59–60	66–93	NS	0.5
Palmar pallor[4,5]	58–64	74–96	**5.6**	0.4
Palmar crease pallor[4]	8	99	**7.9**	NS
Conjunctival pallor[4-7]	31–62	82–97	**4.7**	0.6
Conjunctival rim pallor[2]				
Pallor present	10	99	**16.7**	...
Pallor borderline	36	...	2.3	...
Pallor absent	53	16	0.6	...

NS, not significant; likelihood ratio (LR) if finding present = positive LR; LR if finding absent = negative LR.
*Diagnostic standard: For anemia, hematocrit <35%,[4] hemoglobin <11 g/dL,[2, 5-7] or hemoglobin <11 g/dL in women and <13 g/dL in men.[3]
[†]Definition of findings: For pallor at any site, examination of skin, nailbeds, and conjunctiva[3-5]; for facial pallor, the study excluded black patients; for palmar crease pallor, examination after gentle extension of the patient's fingers; for conjunctival rim pallor, see text.

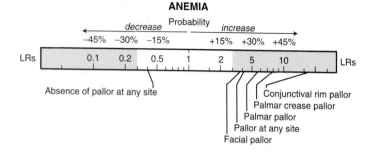

ANEMIA

with acute bleeding and those who had received recent transfusions. As much as possible, the color of skin and conjunctiva was determined under natural lighting.

According to these studies, the most compelling findings arguing *for* anemia are conjunctival rim pallor [likelihood ratio (LR) = 16.7], palmar crease pallor (LR = 7.9), palmar pallor (LR = 5.6), conjunctival pallor (i.e., not specifically of the conjunctival rim, LR = 4.7), pallor at any site (LR = 4.1), and facial pallor (light-skinned persons only, LR = 3.8).* Nailbed pallor has no diagnostic value (LR not significant), and another study† showed that nail bed pallor as determined by simple inspection and by "absence of nail bed blanching" were equivalent.[8] Importantly, no physical sign convincingly argues *against* the diagnosis of anemia (i.e., no LR < 0.4).

REFERENCES

1. Lewis T. *The blood vessels of the human skin and their responses.* London: Shaw and Sons; 1927.
2. Sheth TN, Choudhry NK, Bowes M, Detsky AS. The relation of conjunctival pallor to the presence of anemia. *J Gen Intern Med.* 1997;12:102-106.
3. Gjorup T, Bugge PM, Hendriksen C, Jensen AM. A critical evaluation of the clinical diagnosis of anemia. *Am J Epidemiol.* 1986;124:657-665.
4. Nardone DA, Roth KM, Mazur DJ, McAfee JH. Usefulness of physical examination in detecting the presence or absence of anemia. *Arch Intern Med.* 1990;150:201-204.
5. Stoltzfus RJ, Edward-Raj A, Dreyfuss ML, et al. Clinical pallor is useful to detect severe anemia in populations where anemia is prevalent and severe. *J Nutr.* 1999;129: 1675-1681.

---

*In these studies, the definition of "conjunctival pallor" (overall assessment of conjunctival color) is distinct from "conjunctival rim pallor" (see Section II).
†This study was excluded from the table because the clinicians were aware of the patient's red cell count.

6. Kent AR, Elsing SH, Hebert RL. Conjunctival vasculature in the assessment of anemia. *Ophthalmology*. 2000;107:274-277.

7. van den Broek NR, Ntonya C, Mhango E, White SA. Diagnosing anaemia in pregnancy in rural clinics: Assessing the potential of the haemoglobin colour scale. *Bull World Health Org*. 1999;77:15-21.

8. Strobach RS, Anderson SK, Doll DC, Ringenberg QS. The value of the physical examination in the diagnosis of anemia: Correlation of the physical findings and the hemoglobin concentration. *Arch Intern Med*. 1988;148:831-832.

9

Hypovolemia

I. INTRODUCTION

The term "hypovolemia" refers collectively to two distinct disorders: (1) "volume depletion," which is the loss of sodium from the extracellular space (intravascular and interstitial fluid) that occurs after gastrointestinal hemorrhage, vomiting, diarrhea, and diuresis and (2) "dehydration," which refers to losses of intracellular water that ultimately cause cellular desiccation and elevate the plasma sodium concentration and osmolality.[1] Chapter 15 discusses the accuracy of abnormal vital signs in patients with volume depletion; this chapter discusses assorted additional findings.

II. THE FINDINGS AND THEIR PATHOGENESIS

Many of the traditional signs of hypovolemia—dry mucous membranes, sunken eyes, shriveled skin and tongue, confusion—originate in classic descriptions of cholera as findings of patients near vascular collapse.[2] Presumably, cellular dehydration, interstitial space dehydration, and poor perfusion contribute to these signs; however, studies of their pathogenesis are unavailable.

Poor skin turgor refers to the slow return of skin to its normal position after being pinched between the examiner's thumb and forefinger.[3,4] The protein elastin is responsible for the recoil of skin, and *in vitro* experiments show that its recoil time increases 40-fold after loss of as little as 3.4% of its wet weight.[3] Elastin also deteriorates with age, however, suggesting that poor skin turgor may be a less specific finding of hypovolemia in elderly patients.

III.   CLINICAL SIGNIFICANCE

EBM Box 9-1 presents clinical studies comparing traditional signs to laboratory tests of hypovolemia (i.e., serum urea-to-creatinine level, osmolarity, or sodium level). These studies enrolled elderly patients presenting to emergency departments with vomiting, decreased oral intake, or diarrhea. Few if any were as desperately hypovolemic as patients with classic cholera.

Box 9-1   Hypovolemia*

Finding (Ref)	Sensitivity (%)	Specificity (%)	Likelihood Ratio if Finding	
			Present	Absent
Skin, eyes, and mucous membranes				
Dry axilla[5]	50	82	2.8	NS
Dry mucous membranes of mouth and nose[6]	85	58	NS	**0.3**
Longitudinal furrows on tongue[6]	85	58	NS	**0.3**
Sunken eyes[6]	62	82	NS	0.5
Neurologic findings				
Confusion[6]	57	73	NS	NS
Weakness[6]	43	82	NS	NS
Speech not clear or expressive[6]	56	82	NS	0.5

NS, not significant; Likelihood ratio (LR) if finding present = positive LR; LR if finding absent = negative LR.
*Diagnostic standard: For hypovolemia, elevated serum urea nitrogen-creatinine ratio, osmolarity, or sodium level.

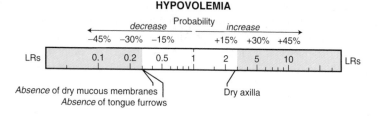

These studies show that only one finding, a dry axilla, argues somewhat *for* hypovolemia (likelihood ratio [LR] = 2.8, see EBM Box 9-1), and only two findings, the absence of tongue furrows and the presence of moist mucous membranes, argue *against* hypovolemia (LR = 0.3 for both findings). In these studies, the presence or absence of sunken eyes, confusion, weakness, or abnormal speech had little diagnostic value.

Another study confirms the association between dry axilla and hypovolemia.[7] Two studies have found poor skin turgor to have no diagnostic value in adults.[6,7] Although poor capillary refill time has been advanced as a reliable sign of hypovolemia, the only available studies either compare it to a questionable diagnostic standard (i.e., vital signs)[8] or find the sign has no diagnostic value.[6]

REFERENCES

1. Mange K, Matsuura D, Cizman B, et al. Language guiding therapy: The case of dehydration versus volume depletion. *Ann Intern Med.* 1997;127:848-853.
2. Osler W. *The principles and practice of medicine (facsimile by Classics of Medicine library).* New York: D. Appleton and Co; 1892.
3. Dorrington KL. Skin turgor: Do we understand the clinical sign? *Lancet.* 1981;1:264-265.
4. Aquilar OM, Albertal M. Images in clinical medicine. Poor skin turgor. *N Engl J Med.* 1998;338:25.
5. Eaton D, Bannister P, Mulley GP, Connolly MJ. Axillary sweating in clinical assessment of dehydration in ill elderly patients. *Br Med J.* 1994;308:1271.
6. Gross CR, Lindquist RD, Woolley AC, et al. Clinical indicators of dehydration severity in elderly patients. *J Emerg Med.* 1992;10:267-274.
7. Levitt MA, Lopez B, Lieberman ME, Sutton M. Evaluation of the tilt test in an adult emergency medicine population. *Ann Emerg Med.* 1992;21:713-718.
8. Schriger DL, Baraff LJ. Capillary refill: Is it a useful predictor of hypovolemic states? *Ann Emerg Med.* 1991;20:601-605.

10

Protein-Energy Malnutrition and Weight Loss

PROTEIN-ENERGY MALNUTRITION

I. INTRODUCTION

Protein energy malnutrition occurs when the supply of protein, calories, or both is inadequate. Decreased oral intake is the most common cause worldwide, although in industrialized countries, increased nutrient loss (e.g., malabsorption, diarrhea, nephrotic syndrome) and increased nutrient requirements (e.g., fever, cancer, infection, or surgery) play a more important role. Among patients admitted to surgical services in industrialized nations, 9% to 27% have signs of severe malnutrition.[1,2]

II. THE FINDINGS

Two distinct syndromes of protein-energy malnutrition have been described in children of developing nations: *marasmus* (predominant caloric deficiency), characterized by weight loss, muscle and fat wasting; and *kwashiorkor* (predominant protein deficiency), characterized by ascites and edema. In industrialized countries, however, most malnourished patients present less dramatically with features of both syndromes, including low body weight, atrophy of muscle and subcutaneous fat, weakness, and various laboratory abnormalities (e.g., low albumin or other serum proteins).

A. ARM MUSCLE CIRCUMFERENCE

Arm muscle circumference is a decades-old anthropometric measure designed to reflect the amount of muscle in the arm, which therefore provides an indirect measure of the total amount of muscle or protein in the body. After measuring the upper arm circumference with a flexible tape measure (C_a) and the triceps skinfold thickness with calipers (h), the clinician estimates arm muscle circumference (AMC) by using the following formula[*, 3]:

$$AMC = C_a - \pi h$$

Age- and sex-standardized values of the normal AMC have been published.[5] Similar measurements are made to calculate the forearm muscle circumference.

B. GRIP STRENGTH

Based on the hypothesis that skeletal muscle strength reflects total body protein stores and that protein-malnutrition becomes particularly important during periods of stress, such as surgery, Klidjian in 1980 investigated the grip strength of 102 patients and showed that weakness accurately predicted postoperative complications.[6] In his method, the patient squeezed a simple hand-held spring dynamometer three times, resting 10 seconds between each attempt, and the clinician recorded the highest value obtained. The presence of arthritis, stroke, or other obvious reasons for reduced grip strength makes the test uninterpretable.

   Age- and sex-standardized values of normal grip strength have been published.[7] Clinical studies of grip strength always test the nondominant arm, but this may be unnecessary because other studies show very little difference in strength between the two arms.[7]

---

*This formula assumes that the arm is a cylinder and ignores the contribution of the humerus[4]. To derive this formula, $AMC = \pi d_1$, where d_1 is the diameter of the muscle component of the arm; $d_1 = d_2 - h$, where d_2 is the diameter of the arm and h is the skinfold thickness (which includes a double layer of skin and subcutaneous tissue). Therefore $AMC = \pi d_1 = \pi(d_2 - h) = \pi d_2 - \pi h = C_a - \pi h$. If the clinician desires to directly enter the skinfold thickness in mm (as it is measured), 0.314 is substituted for π in the formula (i.e., AMC and C_a are measured in cm).

III. CLINICAL SIGNIFICANCE

EBM Box 10-1 applies the signs of weight loss, arm anthropometry, and grip strength to patients just before major surgery and addresses how accurately these signs predict significant postoperative complications, which are assumed in part to reflect the effects of malnutrition. "Significant complications" are those that prolong the hospital stay, threaten the patient's life, or cause death (e.g., sepsis, wound infections, myocardial infarction, stroke).

The findings of reduced arm or forearm muscle circumference [likelihood ratios (LRs) = 2.5–3.2], reduced grip strength (LR = 2.2), and low body weight (LR = 2.0) are all modest predictors of postoperative complications. Only one finding, a normal grip strength, argues *against* the development of complications (LR = 0.4). The presence of recent weight loss has little diagnostic value, presumably because this finding includes not only patients with significant ongoing weight loss but also obese patients who have lost weight (and thus reduced their complication rate)[12] and those who have lost weight but gained some of it back in the immediate preoperative period.

Another bedside tool, not reviewed in EBM Box 10-1, is the "subjective global assessment," which combines elements from the patient's history (weight change, dietary history, gastrointestinal symptoms, and functional capacity) and physical examination (absence of subcutaneous fat, muscle wasting, edema, and ascites) to accurately predict postsurgical complications.[1,15,16] The components of this scoring tool, however, are imprecisely defined,[2] making it difficult for clinicians to duplicate the accuracy of the original investigators.

WEIGHT LOSS

I. INTRODUCTION

Involuntary weight loss reflects diuresis, decreased caloric intake, or the increased caloric requirements of malabsorption, glucosuria, or a hypermetabolic state. In series of patients presenting with involuntary weight loss (exceeding 5% of their usual weight), organic disease is diagnosed in 65% of patients (most commonly cancer and gastrointestinal disorders, although virtually any chronic disease may cause weight loss) and a psychiatric disorder is diagnosed in 10% of patients (depression, anorexia nervosa, schizophrenia). In 25% of patients, the cause remains unknown despite at least 1-year follow-up.[17–20]

Box 10-1   Protein-Energy Malnutrition and Major Surgical Complications*

Finding (Ref)[†]	Sensitivity (%)	Specificity (%)	Likelihood Ratio if Finding Present	Absent
Body weight				
Weight loss >10% [6,8–11]	15–75	47–88	1.4	NS
Low body weight [6,9,10,12]	11–35	83–97	2.0	NS
Anthropometry				
Upper arm muscle circumference < 85% predicted [6,9,10]	26–38	83–91	2.5	0.8
Forearm muscle circumference < 85% predicted [6,9,10]	14–42	85–97	**3.2**	0.8
Muscle strength				
Reduced grip strength [6,7,9,10,13,14]	33–90	46–93	2.2	0.4

NS, not significant; likelihood ratio (LR) if finding present = positive LR; LR if finding absent = negative LR.

*Diagnostic standard: In each of these studies, disease is defined as a major postoperative complication, including those prolonging hospital stay, threatening the patient's life, or causing death.

[†]Definition of findings (all findings were assessed during the preoperative physical examination): for weight loss >10% (recalled usual weight − measured weight)/(recalled usual weight) × 100 >10); for low body weight, weight-for-height less than normal lower limit,[12] < 90% of predicted,[6] or < 85% of predicted[9,10]; for predicted arm muscle circumference, published standardized values[5]; for forearm muscle circumference <85%, <20 cm in men and < 16.3 cm in women,[6,10] and for reduced grip strength, specific thresholds differ but all correspond closely to published age- and sex-standardized abnormal values from reference 7.

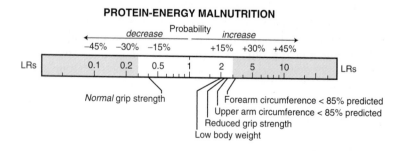

PROTEIN-ENERGY MALNUTRITION

II. CLINICAL SIGNIFICANCE

Weight loss is rarely due to occult disease and most diagnoses are made during the initial evaluation, including the patient interview, physical examination, and basic laboratory testing.[17,18,20]

In patients with involuntary weight loss, the presence of alcoholism (LR = 4.5) and cigarette smoking (LR = 2.2) increase the probability that an organic cause will be discovered during 6-months follow-up, whereas prior psychiatric disease (LR = 0.2) and a *normal* initial physical examination (LR = 0.4) decrease the probability of discovering organic disease.[21] Also, the patient's perceptions of the weight loss—whether he or she significantly underestimates or overestimates it—helps predict the final diagnosis. The patient is asked to estimate his or her weight before the illness (W) and the amount of weight lost (E). The observed weight loss (O) is the former weight (W) minus the current measured weight. Significant *underestimation* of weight loss, defined as (O − E) greater than 0.5 kg, predicts an *organic* cause of weight loss with a sensitivity of 40%, specificity of 92%, positive LR of 5.4, and negative LR of 0.6 [22]. Significant *overestimation* of weight loss, defined as (E − O) greater than 0.5 kg, predicts a *nonorganic* cause of weight loss with a sensitivity of 70%, specificity of 81%, positive LR of 3.6, and negative LR of 0.4.[22]

REFERENCES

1. Baker JP, Detsky AS, Wesson DE, et al. Nutritional assessment: A comparison of clinical judgment and objective measurements. *N Engl J Med.* 1982;306:969-972.
2. Detsky AS, McLaughlin JR, Baker JP, et al. What is subjective global assessment of nutritional status? *JPEN.* 1987;11:8-13.
3. Jelliffe DB. The assessment of the nutritional status of the community. *WHO Monograph Series.* 1966;53:1-271.
4. Hall JC, O'Quigley J, Giles GR, et al. Upper limb anthropometry: The value of measurement variance studies. *Am J Clin Nutr.* 1980;33:1846-1851.
5. Frisancho AR. New norms of upper limb fat and muscle areas for assessment of nutritional status. *Am J Clin Nutr.* 1981;34:2540-2545.
6. Klidjian AM, Foster KJ, Kammerling RM, et al. Relation of anthropometric and dynamometric variables to serious postoperative complications. *Br Med J.* 1980;281: 899-901.
7. Webb AR, Newman LA, Taylor M, Keogh JB. Hand grip dynamometry as a predictor of postoperative complications reappraisal using age standardized grip strengths. *JPEN.* 1989;13:30-33.
8. Windsor JA, Hill GL. Weight loss with physiologic impairment: A basic indicator of surgical risk. *Ann Surg.* 1988;207:290-296.

9. Klidjian AM, Archer TJ, Foster KJ, Karran SJ. Detection of dangerous malnutrition. *JPEN*. 1982;6:119-122.

10. Hunt DR, Rowlands BJ, Johnston D. Hand grip strength—A simple prognostic indicator in surgical patients. *JPEN*. 1985;9:701-704.

11. Katelaris PH, Bennett GB, Smith RC. Prediction of postoperative complications by clinical and nutritional assessment. *Aust N Z J Surg*. 1986;56:743-747.

12. Hickman DM, Miller RA, Rombeau JL, et al. Serum albumin and body weight as predictors of postoperative course in colorectal cancer. *JPEN*. 1980;4:314-316.

13. Davies CWT, Jones DM, Shearer JR. Hand grip—A simple test for morbidity after fracture of the neck of the femur. *J Roy Soc Med*. 1984;77:833-836.

14. Mahalakshmi VN, Ananthakrishnan N, Kate V, et al. Handgrip strength and endurance as a predictor of postoperative morbidity in surgical patients: Can it serve as a simple bedside test? *Int Surg*. 2004;89:115-121.

15. Detsky AS, Smalley PS, Chang J. Is this patient malnourished? *JAMA*. 1994;271:54-58.

16. Sungurtekin H, Sungurtekin U, Balci C, et al. The influence of nutritional status on complications after major intraabdominal surgery. *J Am Coll Nutr*. 2004;23:227-232.

17. Rabinovitz M, Pitlik SD, Leifer M, et al. Unintentional weight loss: A retrospective analysis of 154 cases. *Arch Intern Med*. 1986;146:186-187.

18. Marton KI, Sox HC, Krupp JR. Involuntary weight loss: Diagnostic and prognostic significance. *Ann Intern Med*. 1981;95:568-574.

19. Lankisch PG, Gerzmann M, Gerzmann JF, Lehnick D. Unintentional weight loss: Diagnosis and prognosis. The first prospective follow-up study from a secondary referral centre. *J Intern Med*. 2001;249:41-46.

20. Thompson MP, Morris LK. Unexplained weight loss in the ambulatory elderly. *J Am Geriatr Soc*. 1991;39:497-500.

21. Bilbao-Garay J, Barba R, Losa-Garcia JE, et al. Assessing clinical probability of organic disease in patients with involuntary weight loss: A simple score. *Eur J Intern Med*. 2002;13:240-245.

22. Ramboer C, Verhamme M, Vermeire L. Patients' perception of involuntary weight loss: Implications of underestimation and overestimation. *Br Med J*. 1985;291:1091.

Obesity

I. INTRODUCTION

Obesity increases the risk of coronary artery disease, diabetes, hypertension, osteoarthritis, cholelithiasis, certain cancers, and overall death.[1] Clinicians have recognized the hazards of obesity for thousands of years (according to one Hippocratic aphorism, "sudden death is more common in those who are naturally fat than in the lean").[2] At least one third of U.S. adults are overweight.[3]

II. THE FINDINGS AND THEIR SIGNIFICANCE

Several different anthropometric parameters have been used to identify those patients at greatest risk for the medical complications of obesity. The most important ones are body mass index, skinfold thickness, waist-to-hip ratio, waist circumference, and sagittal diameter.

A. BODY MASS INDEX (BMI)

1. The Finding

The BMI (or Quetelet index) is the patient's weight in kilograms divided by the square of his or her height in meters (kg/m^2). If pounds and inches are used, the quotient should be multiplied by 703.5 to convert the units to kg/m². An individual is overweight if the BMI exceeds 25 kg/m², and obese if the BMI exceeds 30 kg/m².[4,5]

The BMI was derived by a 17th century Belgian mathematician and astronomer, Lambert-Adolphe-Jacques Quetelet, who discovered that this ratio best expressed the natural relationship between weight and height.[6]

2. Clinical Significance

The BMI correlates well with precise measures of total body fat (r = 0.70–0.96),[7,8] much better that other formulas of weight (W) and height (H) (e.g., W/H, W/H³, W/H^0.3).[8] The BMI also correlates significantly with the patient's cholesterol level,[9] blood pressure,[9] incidence of coronary events,[10–13] and overall mortality.[12–15]

The arbitrary cutoff of 25 kg/m² was chosen in part because it reflects the level at which there is a significant increase in mortality, although increased rates of some complications such as diabetes appear at lower cutoffs.[1] Early studies of BMI and mortality revealed a J-shaped relationship (i.e., both lean and overweight patients had increased mortality),[15] but the increased risk for lean individuals disappears after controlling for the patient's age, cigarette use, and illness-related weight loss.[12,14,16]

B. SKINFOLD THICKNESS

Another measure of obesity is "total skinfold thickness," which is estimated by adding together the skinfold thickness (measured with calipers) of multiple sites (mid-biceps, mid-triceps, subscapular, and supra-iliac area).[8] This sum is then converted using a formula into an estimate of total body fat, which correlates well with more precise measures (r = 0.7–0.8).[8,17] Skinfold measurements rarely are used today to assess obesity, partly because they are too complex, but mostly because relatively few studies[10] show the number is clinically significant.

C. WAIST-TO-HIP RATIO

1. The Finding

The waist-to-hip ratio (WHR) is the circumference of the waist divided by that of the hips. It is based on the premise that the most important characteristic of obesity is its distribution, not its quantity. "Abdominal" obesity (also called "android," "upper body," or "apple-shaped" obesity, Fig. 11-1) has a much worse prognosis than "gluteal-femoral" obesity (also called "gynoid," "lower body," or "pear-shaped" obesity).

Although at least nine different methods of measuring WHR have been recommended,[9] most authorities measure the waist circumference at the midpoint between the lower costal margin and the iliac crest and the hip circumference at the widest part of the gluteal region.[19,20] Adverse health outcomes increase

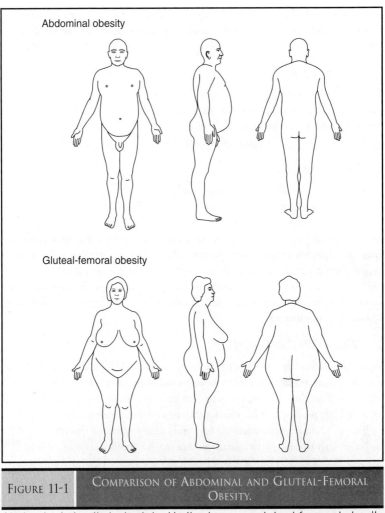

Abdominal obesity

Gluteal-femoral obesity

FIGURE 11-1	COMPARISON OF ABDOMINAL AND GLUTEAL-FEMORAL OBESITY.

Abdominal obesity is depicted in the top row; gluteal-femoral obesity in the bottom row. The drawings in this figure are adapted from photographs published by Jean Vague,[18] who is credited with first associating adverse health outcomes with abdominal obesity.

significantly when the WHR exceeds 1.0 in men and 0.85 in women,[19,21] values that are very close to the top quintiles in epidemiologic studies.[7,11,15,22]

The French diabetologist Jean Vague is usually credited with making the observation in the 1940s that abdominal obesity, common in men, is associated with worse health outcomes than obesity over the hips and thighs, more common in women (American life insurance companies, however, made the same

observation in the late 1800s).[23,24] Vague's original "index of masculine differentiation," a complicated index based on skinfolds and limb circumferences,[18] is no
longer used, having been replaced by the much simpler WHR in the 1980s.[25]

2. Clinical Significance

The WHR predicts health outcomes better than any other anthropometric
measure. Even after controlling for the effects of BMI, the WHR correlates significantly with blood pressure,[19,26] cholesterol level,[9,19,26] incidence of diabetes
mellitus,[19,26] stroke,[10,22,26] coronary events,[10,11,19,26] and overall mortality.[10,15]

3. Pathogenesis

The main contributor to abdominal obesity is visceral fat (i.e., omental, mesen-
teric, and retroperitoneal fat), not subcutaneous fat. Visceral fat is metabolically
very active, constantly releasing free fatty acids into the portal circulation,[23]
which probably contributes to hyperlipidemia, atherogenesis, and hyperinsu-
linemia.[23] Gluteal-femoral fat, on the other hand, is metabolically inactive
except during pregnancy and the postpartum period, which has led some to
suggest that the role of lower body fat is to help guarantee the survival of the
species, by providing a constant source of energy to the lactating female even
when external nutrients are unavailable.

D. WAIST CIRCUMFERENCE

Waist circumference is simply the numerator of the WHR calculation. It has
the advantages of being simpler to measure and of avoiding attention to the hips,
which, because they encompass bone and skeletal muscle as well as fat, should
have no biologically plausible relationship to diabetes, hypertension, and atherosclerosis.[21] Nonetheless, relatively few studies have validated this measure[9,27–29]
and some show the waist circumference to be inferior to the WHR.[10,22]
Recommended cutoffs for increased health risk are a waist circumference greater
than 102 cm (40 inches) for men and 88 cm (35 inches) for women.[4]

E. SAGITTAL DIAMETER

Because waist circumference encompasses both subcutaneous and visceral fat,
investigators have looked for anthropometric measures that reflect more precisely just visceral fat. One proposed measure is the sagittal diameter, which is
the total anterior-posterior distance between the anterior abdominal wall of the
supine patient and the surface of the examining table. Theoretically, visceral fat
maintains the abdominal depth in the supine patient, whereas subcutaneous fat
allows the abdominal depth to partially collapse from the force of gravity.[20]
Even so, there are few studies of this measure and most correlate it with variables of uncertain clinical significance, such as cardiovascular risk factors[30,31] or
the amount of visceral fat visualized on computed tomography.[7,32–34]

REFERENCES

1. Willett WC, Dietz WH, Colditz GA. Guidelines for healthy weight. *N Engl J Med*. 1999;341:427-434.
2. *Hippocratic writings*. Harmondsworth, Middlesex, England: Penguin Books; 1978.
3. Kuczmarski RJ, Flegal KM, Campbell SM, Johnson CL. Increasing prevalence of overweight among US adults: The National Health and Nutrition Examination Surveys 1960 to 1991. *JAMA*. 1994;272:205-211.
4. Executive summary of the clinical guidelines on the identification, evaluation, and treatment of overweight and obesity in adults. *Arch Intern Med*. 1998;158:1855-1867.
5. Bray GA, Dahms WT, Greenway FL, et al. Evaluation of the obese patient. II. Clinical findings. *JAMA*. 1976;235:2008-2010.
6. Jelliffe DB, Jeliffe EF. Underappreciated pioneers. Quetelet: Man and index. *Am J Clin Nutr*. 1979;32:2519-2521.
7. Pouliot M, Despres J, Lemieux S, et al. Waist circumference and abdominal sagittal diameter: Best simple anthropometric indexes of abdominal visceral adipose tissue accumulation and related cardiovascular risk in men and women. *Am J Card*. 1994;73:460-468.
8. Womersley J, Durnin JVGA. A comparison of the skinfold method with extent of "overweight" and various weight-height relationships in the assessment of obesity. *Br J Nutr*. 1977;38:271-284.
9. Seidell JC, Cigolini M, Charzewska J, Ellsinger B, Di Biase G. Fat distribution in European women: A comparison of anthropometric measurements in relation to cardiovascular risk factors. *Int J Epidemiol*. 1990;19:303-308.
10. Lapidus L, Bengtsson C, Larsson B, et al. Distribution of adipose tissue and risk of cardiovascular disease and death: A 12 year follow up of participants in the population study of women in Gothenburg, Sweden. *Br Med J*. 1984;289:1257-1261.
11. Rimm EB, Stampfer MJ, Giovannucci E, et al. Body size and fat distribution as predictors of coronary heart disease among middle-aged and older US men. *Am J Epidemiol*. 1995;141:1117-1127.
12. Manson JE, Willett WC, Stampfer MJ, et al. Body weight and mortality among women. *N Engl J Med*. 1995;333:677-685.
13. Stevens J, Cai J, Pamuk ER, Williamson DF, et al. The effect of age on the association between body-mass index and mortality. *N Engl J Med*. 1998;338:1-7.
14. Lee IM, Manson JE, Hennekens CH, Paffenbarger RS. Body weight and mortality: A 27-year follow-up of middle-aged men. *JAMA*. 1993;270:2823-2828.
15. Folsom AR, Kaye SA, Sellers TA, et al. Body fat distribution and 5-year risk of death in older women. *JAMA*. 1993;269:483-487.
16. Calle EE, Thun MJ, Petrelli JM, et al. Body-mass index and mortality in a prospective cohort of U. S. adults. *N Engl J Med*. 1999;341:1097-1105.
17. Jebb SA, Elia M. Techniques for the measurement of body composition: A practical guide. *Int J Obes Relat Metab Disord*. 1993;17:611-621.

18. Vague J. The degree of masculine differentiation of obesities: A factor determining predisposition to diabetes, atherosclerosis, gout, and uric calculous disease. *Am J Clin Nutr.* 1956;4:20-34.

19. Bjorntorp P. Obesity. *Lancet.* 1997;350:423-426.

20. van der Kooy K, Seidell JC. Techniques for the measurement of visceral fat: A practical guide. *Int J Obes Relat Metab Disord.* 1993;17:187-196.

21. Molarius A, Seidell JC. Selection of anthropometric indicators for classification of abdominal fatness: A critical review. *Int J Obes Relat Metab Disord.* 1998;22: 719-727.

22. Walker SP, Rimm EB, Ascherio A, et al. Body size and fat distribution as predictors of stroke among US men. *Am J Epidemiol.* 1996;144:1143-1150.

23. Kaplan NM. Obesity: Location matters. *Heart Dis Stroke.* 1992;1(3):148-150.

24. Kahn HS, Williamson DF. Abdominal obesity and mortality risk among men in nineteenth-century North America. *Int J Obes Relat Metab Disord.* 1994;18: 686-691.

25. Krotkeiwski M, Bjorntorp P, Sjostrom L, Smith U. Impact of obesity on metabolism in men and women. *J Clin Invest.* 1983;72:1150-1162.

26. Egger G. The case for using waist to hip ratio measurements in routine medical checks. *Med J Aust.* 1992;156:280-285.

27. Lemieux S, Prud'homme D, Bouchard C, et al. A single threshold value of waist girth identifies normal-weight and overweight subjects with excess visceral adipose tissue. *Am J Clin Nutr.* 1996;64:685-693.

28. Chan DC, Watts GF, Barrett PHR, Burke V. Waist circumference, waist-to-hip ratio and body mass index as predictors of adipose tissue compartments in men. *Q J Med.* 2003;96:441-447.

29. Janssen I, Katzmarzyk PT, Ross R. Body mass index, waist circumference, and health risk: Evidence in support of current National Institutes of Health guidelines. *Arch Intern Med.* 2002;162:2074-2079.

30. Ohrvall M, Berglund L, Vessby B. Sagittal abdominal diameter compared with other anthropometric measurements in relation to cardiovascular risk. *Int J Obes Relat Metab Disord.* 2000;24:497-501.

31. Turcato E, Bosello O, Francesco TB, et al. Waist circumference and abdominal sagittal diameter as surrogates of body fat distribution in the elderly: Their relation with cardiovascular risk factors. *Int J Obes Relat Metab Disord.* 2000;24: 1005-1010.

32. Seidell JC, Bouchard C. Visceral fat in relation to health: Is it a major culprit or simply an innocent bystander? *Int J Obesity.* 1997;21:626-631.

33. Harris TB, Visser M, Everhart J, et al. Waist circumference and sagittal diameter reflect total body fat better than visceral fat in older men and women: The health, aging, and body composition study. *Ann N Y Acad Sci.* 2000;904:462-473.

34. Zamboni M, Turcato E, Armellini F, et al. Sagittal abdominal diameter as a practical predictor of visceral fat. *Int J Obes Relat Metab Disord.* 1998;22:655-660.

Cushing's Syndrome

I. INTRODUCTION

"Cushing's syndrome" refers to various clinical findings—hypertension, central obesity, weakness, hirsutism (in women), depression, skin striae, and bruises— that are caused by excess circulating glucocorticoids. The most common cause is exogenous administration of corticosteroid hormones.[1,2] Endogenous Cushing's syndrome results from pituitary tumors producing adrenocorti- cotropic hormone (ACTH) (i.e., "Cushing's disease," 70% of all endogenous cases), ectopic production of ACTH (usually by small cell carcinoma of the lung or carcinoid tumors of the lung or mediastinum, 10% of cases), adrenal adenomas (15% of cases), or adrenal carcinoma (5% of cases).[2-7] Cushing's dis- ease and the ectopic ACTH syndrome are referred to as "ACTH-dependent," because the elevated cortisol levels are accompanied by inappropriately high ACTH levels. Adrenal tumors are "ACTH independent."

The bedside findings associated with Cushing's syndrome were originally described by Harvey Cushing in 1932.[8] Corticosteroid hormones were first used as therapeutic agents to treat patients with rheumatoid arthritis in 1949; within 2 years, clear descriptions of exogenous Cushing's syndrome appeared.[9]

II. THE FINDINGS AND THEIR PATHOGENESIS

Table 12-1 presents the physical signs found in 462 patients with Cushing's syndrome.

A. BODY HABITUS

Patients with Cushing's syndrome develop central obesity (or "truncal obesity," "centripedal obesity"), which means that fat accumulates centrally on the neck, chest, and abdomen, providing a striking visual contrast to the muscle atrophy that affects the extremities. The definitions of central obesity vary, depending on which clinical study is consulted: some define it subjectively as the appearance of obesity sparing the extremities.[10,15] Others define it more precisely using

Table 12-1	Cushing's Syndrome—Frequency of Individual Findings*

Physical Finding[†]	Frequency (%)[‡]
Vital signs	
Hypertension	64–88
Body habitus	
Moon facies	67–100
Central obesity	44–93
Buffalo hump	34–75
Skin findings	
Thin skin	24–84
Plethora	28–94
Hirsutism, women	48–81
Ecchymoses	24–77
Red or purple striae	64
Acne	21–52
Extremity findings	
Proximal muscle weakness	51
Edema	50
Other	
Significant depression	12–48

*Information is based on 462 patients from references 2, 5, 7, 10–16.
Diagnostic standard: For Cushing's syndrome, elevated daily cortisol or corticosteroid metabolites, or both, with loss of circadian rhythm and with abnormal dexamethasone suppression tests.
[†]Definition of finding: For hypertension, systolic blood pressure >140 mm Hg[15] or >150 mm Hg,[11] diastolic blood pressure >90 mm Hg,[5,11,15] or not defined.
[‡]Results are overall mean frequency or, if statistically heterogenous, the range of values.

the "central obesity index," which is the sum of three truncal circumferences—neck, chest, and abdomen—divided by the sum of six limb circumferences—bilateral arms, thighs, and lower legs. A central obesity index exceeding 1 is abnormal.[17] A third definition of central obesity—an abnormal waist-to-hip circumference ratio (>1.0 in men and >0.85 in women; see Chapter 11)[1]—is not recommended because of the high false-positive rate.[18]

Other characteristic features of the Cushing's body habitus are accumulation of fat in the bitemporal region ("moon facies"),[19] between the scapulae and behind the neck ("buffalo hump"), in the supraclavicular region (producing a "collar" around the base of the neck),[1] and in front of the sternum ("dewlap," named after its resemblance to the hanging fold of skin at the base of the bovine neck,[20] Fig. 12-1). Although many experts believe that the buffalo hump is not specific for Cushing's syndrome and may occur after weight gain from any cause,[4,21] this has not been formally tested. Morbid obesity (i.e., weight more than twice the ideal weight) is rare in Cushing's syndrome.[22]

The truncal obesity of Cushing's syndrome reflects an increase in intraabdominal visceral fat, not subcutaneous fat,[23] probably from glucocorticoid-induced reduction in lipolytic activity and activation of lipoprotein lipase, which allows tissues to accumulate triglyceride.[1,18]

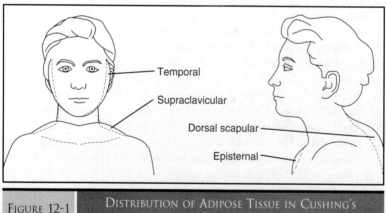

FIGURE 12-1	DISTRIBUTION OF ADIPOSE TISSUE IN CUSHING'S SYNDROME.

Rounding of cheeks and prominent bitemporal fat produces the characteristic "moon facies." Fat also may accumulate bilaterally above the clavicles ("supraclavicular collar"), in front of the sternum (episternal area, or "dewlap"), and over the back of the neck (dorsal cervical fat pad, or "buffalo hump"). In these drawings, the dotted line depicts normal contours of patients without Cushing's syndrome.

B. HYPERTENSION

Hypertension occurs in three of four patients with Cushing's syndrome. Proposed mechanisms are suppressed vasodepressor systems (prostaglandins, kallikrein-kinin), exaggerated pressor responses to vasoactive substances, and possible activation of the renin-angiotensin system.[24] Most patients do *not* have a positive salt and water balance.[1]

C. SKIN FINDINGS

The characteristic skin findings are thin skin, striae, plethora, hirsutism (in women), acne, and ecchymoses.

Significant thinning of the skin, which affects most patients,[25-28] probably arises from corticosteroid-induced inhibition of epidermal cell division and dermal collagen synthesis.[1] To assess skin thickness, many experts recommend using calipers (either skinfold calipers or electrocardiograph calipers) to measure skinfold thickness on the back of the patient's hand, an area lacking significant subcutaneous fat and thus representing just epidermis and dermis.[25,28] In women of reproductive age, this skinfold should be thicker than 1.8 mm.[25] Precise cutoffs have not been established for men, whose skin is normally thicker than women's, or for elderly patients, whose skin is normally thinner than younger patients.[28]

The striae of Cushing's syndrome are wide (>1 cm) and are colored deep red or purple, in contrast to the thinner and paler pink or white striae that sometimes occur in any individual after rapid weight gain.[10,29] Striae are usually found on the lower abdomen but may occur on the buttocks, hips, lower back, upper thighs, and arms. In one of Cushing's original patients, wide striae extended from the lower abdomen to the axillae.[8] Pathologically, striae are dermal scars, with collagen fibers all aligned in the direction of stress, covered by an abnormally thin epidermis.[30] The pathogenesis of striae is not understood, but they may represent actual rupture of the weakened connective tissue of the skin, under tension from central obesity, which leaves a thin translucent window to the red and purple colored dermal blood vessels. Striae are more common in younger patients with Cushing's syndrome than older patients.[11,29]

Plethora is an abnormal diffuse purple or reddish color of the face.[10] Hirsutism and acne occur because of increased adrenal androgens.[1,29,31] Ecchymoses probably appear because the blood vessels, lacking connective tissue support and protection, are more easily traumatized.

The severity of striae, acne, and hirsutism correlate poorly with cortisol levels, indicating that other factors—temporal, biochemical, or genetic—play a role in these physical signs.[29]

D. PROXIMAL WEAKNESS

Painless proximal weakness of the legs is common and prominent in Cushing's syndrome, especially elderly patients.[11,32-34] Because the weakness is a true myopathy, patients lack fasciculations, sensory changes, or reflex abnormalities.[32-34] Chapter 57 discusses how to assess proximal muscle strength.

E. DEPRESSION

Patients with Cushing's syndrome may have crying episodes, insomnia, impaired concentration, difficulty with memory, and suicide attempts.[14,35] The severity of depression correlates with the cortisol level,[35] and unless the depression antedates the endocrine symptoms by years, it usually improves dramatically after treatment.[14]

F. PSEUDOCUSHING'S SYNDROME

Several disorders, including chronic alcoholism, depression, and human immunodeficiency virus (HIV) infection, may mimic the physical findings and biochemical findings of Cushing's syndrome and are referred to as "pseudo-Cushing's syndrome." Patients with chronic alcoholism may develop the physical findings or the biochemical abnormalities, or both, probably because of overproduction of ACTH by the hypothalamic-pituitary axis, an abnormality that resolves after several weeks of abstinence.[36-39] Depressed patients may have the biochemical abnormalities of Cushing's syndrome, but they usually lack the physical findings.[40,41] Patients with HIV infection, particularly if they are receiving protease inhibitors, may develop some of the physical findings (especially the buffalo hump and truncal obesity) but rarely the biochemical abnormalities.[42-47]

III. CLINICAL SIGNIFICANCE

A. DIAGNOSTIC ACCURACY OF FINDING

EBM Box 12-1 presents the diagnostic accuracy of individual physical sign for Cushing's syndrome, as applied to 247 patients with suspected Cushing's syndrome.[10,15,17,25] According to these studies, the findings arguing the most *for* Cushing's syndrome are thin skinfold [likelihood ratio (LR) = 115.6], ecchymoses (LR = 4.5), central obesity (LR = 3.0), and plethora (LR = 2.7). (The astronomical LR for thin skinfold thickness (LR = 115.6) applies only to young women who have suspected disease because of hirsutism and menstrual irregularity.) The findings arguing the most *against* the diagnosis of Cushing's syndrome are the presence of generalized obesity (LR = 0.1), absence of moon facies (LR = 0.1), the absence of central obesity (LR = 0.2), and the presence of normal skinfold thickness (LR = 0.2).

In these same studies, one of the most powerful predictors of Cushing's syndrome is osteoporosis (sensitivity of 61%–63%, specificity of 94%–97%, positive LR = 17.6, and negative LR = 0.4).[10,15] Although osteoporosis was identified

Box
12-1

Cushing's Syndrome*

Finding (Ref)[†]	Sensitivity (%)	Specificity (%)	Likelihood Ratio if Finding	
			Present	Absent
Vital signs				
Hypertension[10,15]	25–38	83–94	2.3	0.8
Body habitus				
Moon facies[15]	98	41	1.6	**0.1**
Central obesity[10,15,17]	72–90	62–97	**3.0**	**0.2**
Generalized obesity[10]	4	38	**0.1**	2.5
Skin findings				
Thin skinfold[25]	78	99	**115.6**	**0.2**
Plethora[10]	83	69	2.7	**0.3**
Hirsutism, in women[10,15]	50–76	56–71	1.7	0.7
Ecchymoses[10,15]	54–71	69–94	**4.5**	0.5
Red or blue striae[10,15]	46–52	63–78	1.9	0.7
Acne[10]	52	76	2.2	0.6
Extremity findings				
Proximal muscle weakness[10,15]	62–63	69–93	NS	0.4
Edema[10,15]	38–57	56–83	1.8	0.7

NS, not significant; likelihood ratio (LR) if finding present = positive LR; LR if finding absent = negative LR.
*Diagnostic standard: For Cushing's syndrome, elevated daily cortisol or corticosteroid metabolites, or both, with loss of circadian rhythm and with abnormal dexamethasone suppression.
†Definition of findings: For hypertension, diastolic blood pressure >105 mm Hg; for central obesity, central obesity index exceeds 1[17] or subjective appearance of central obesity sparing the extremities[10,15]; for thin skinfold, skinfold thickness on back of hand <1.8 mm (women of reproductive age only).[25]

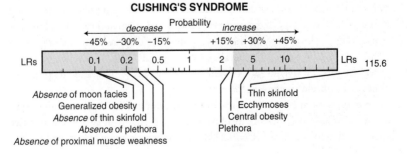

radiographically in these studies, it is often apparent at the bedside because of vertebral fractures, kyphosis, and loss of height. Presumably, these bedside findings also would accurately identify patients with Cushing's syndrome.

B. ETIOLOGY OF CUSHING'S SYNDROME AND BEDSIDE FINDINGS

Patients who take exogenous corticosteroids have the same frequency of central obesity, moon facies, and bruising as patients with endogenous Cushing's but a significantly lower incidence of hypertension, hirsutism, acne, striae, and buffalo humps.[2]

Patients with the ectopic ACTH syndrome from small cell carcinoma are more often male, have Cushing's syndrome of rapid onset (over months instead of years), and present with prominent weight loss, myopathy, hyperpigmentation, and edema.[4,40,41,48,49] The irregular hepatomegaly of metastatic disease also may suggest this diagnosis.[49] In studies of patients with ACTH-dependent Cushing's syndrome, two findings strongly argued for the ectopic ACTH syndrome and against Cushing's disease: weight loss (positive LR = 20.0) and symptom duration less than 18 months (positive LR = 15.0).[7,49]

Hirsutism and acne may occur in any woman with endogenous Cushing's syndrome, but the presence of virilization (i.e., male pattern baldness, deep voice, male musculature, clitoromegaly) argues strongly for adrenocortical carcinoma.[50–52]

REFERENCES

1. Yanovski JA, Cutler GB Jr. Glucocorticoid action and the clinical features of Cushing's syndrome. *Endocrinol Metab Clin North Am.* 1994;23:487-509.
2. Liou TC, Lam HC, Ho LT. Cushing's syndrome: Analysis of 188 cases. *J Formosan Med Assoc.* 1989;88:886-893.
3. Invitti C, Giraldi FP, de Martin M, Cavagnini F. Diagnosis and management of Cushing's syndrome: Results of an Italian multicentre study. Study Group of the Italian Society of Endocrinology on the Pathophysiology of the Hypothalamic-Pituitary-Adrenal Axis. *J Clin Endocrinol Metab.* 1999;84:440-448.
4. Newell-Price J, Trainer P, Besser M, Grossman A. The diagnosis and differential diagnosis of Cushing's syndrome and pseudo-Cushing's states. *Endocr Rev.* 1998;19:647-672.
5. Ross EJ, Linch DC. Cushing's syndrome—killing disease: Discriminatory value of signs and symptoms aiding early diagnosis. *Lancet.* 1982;2(8299):646-649.
6. Isidori AM, Kaltsas GA, Mohammed S, et al. Discriminatory value of the low-dose dexamethasone suppression test in establishing the diagnosis and differential diagnosis of Cushing's syndrome. *J Clin Endocrinol Metab.* 2003;88:5299-5306.

7. Su DH, Chang YC, Chang TC, et al. Characteristics of Cushing's syndrome in Taiwanese. *J Formos Med Assoc.* 2003;102:292-298.
8. Cushing H. The basophil adenomas of the pituitary body and their clinical manifestations (pituitary basophilism). *Bull Johns Hopkins Hosp.* 1932;50(3):137-195.
9. Freyberg RH, Traeger CH, Patterson M, et al. Problems of prolonged cortisone treatment for rheumatoid arthritis: Further investigation. *JAMA.* 1951;147:1538-1543.
10. Nugent CA, Warner HR, Dunn JT, Tyler FH. Probability theory in the diagnosis of Cushing's syndrome. *J Clin Endocrinol Metab.* 1964;24:621-630.
11. Urbanic RC, George JM. Cushing's disease—18 years' experience. *Medicine (Baltimore).* 1981;60:14-24.
12. Plotz CM, Knowlton AI, Ragan C. The natural history of Cushing's syndrome. *Am J Med.* 1952;13:597-614.
13. Soffer LJ, Iannoccone A, Gabrilove JL. Cushing's syndrome: A study of fifty patients. *Am J Med.* 1961;30:129-146.
14. Jeffcoate WJ, Silverstone JT, Edwards CR, Besser GM. Psychiatric manifestations of Cushing's syndrome: Response to lowering of plasma cortisol. *Q J Med.* 1979;48:465-472.
15. Streeten DHP, Stevenson CT, Dalakos TG, et al. The diagnosis of hypercortisolism. Biochemical criteria differentiating patients from lean and obese normal subjects and from females on oral contraceptives. *J Clin Endocrinol.* 1969;29:1191-1211.
16. Erem C, Algun E, Ozbey N, et al. Clinical laboratory findings and results of therapy in 55 patients with Cushing's syndrome. *J Endocrinol Invest.* 2003;26:65-72.
17. Hiramatsu R, Yoshida K, Sato T. A body measurement to evaluate the pattern of fat distribution in central obesity. A screening and monitoring technique for Cushing's syndrome. *JAMA.* 1983;250:3174-3178.
18. Rebuffe-Scrive M, Krotkiewski M, Elfversson J, Bjorntorp P. Muscle and adipose tissue morphology and metabolism in Cushing's syndrome. *J Clin Endocrinol Metab.* 1988;67:1122-1128.
19. Gottlieb NL. Temporal fat pad sign during corticosteroid treatment. *Arch Intern Med.* 1980;140:1507-1508.
20. Lucena GE, Bennett WM, Pierre RV. "Dewlap": A corticosteroid-induced episternal fatty tumor. *N Engl J Med.* 1966;275:834-835.
21. Orth DN. Cushing's syndrome. *N Engl J Med.* 1995;332:791-803.
22. Printen KJ, Blommers TJ. Morbid obesity in Cushing's syndrome: A nonentity? *Am J Surg.* 1977;134:579-580.
23. Mayo-Smith W, Hayes CW, Biller BM, et al. Body fat distribution measured with CT: Correlations in healthy subjects, patients with anorexia nervosa, and patients with Cushing syndrome. *Radiology.* 1989;170:515-518.
24. Saruto T, Suzuki H, Handa M, et al. Multiple factors contribute to the pathogenesis of hypertension in Cushing's syndrome. *J Clin Endocrinol Metab.* 1986;62:275-279.

25. Corenblum B, Kwan T, Gee S, Wong NCW. Bedside assessment of skin-fold thickness: A useful measurement for distinguishing Cushing's disease from other causes of hirsutism and oligomenorrhea. *Arch Intern Med.* 1994;154:777-781.

26. Ferguson JK, Donald RA, Weston TS, Espiner EA. Skin thickness in patients with acromegaly and Cushing's syndrome and response to treatment. *Clin Endocrinol (Oxf).* 1983;18:347-353.

27. Greenwood BM. Capillary resistance and skin-fold thickness in patients with rheumatoid arthritis. Effect of corticosteroid therapy. *Ann Rheum Dis.* 1966;25:272-277.

28. Wright AD, Joplin GF. Skin-fold thickness in normal subjects and in patients with acromegaly and Cushing's syndrome. *Acta Endocrinol (Copenh).* 1969;60:705-711.

29. Stratakis CA, Mastorakos G, Mitsiades NS, et al. Skin manifestations of Cushing disease in children and adolescents before and after the resolution of hypercortisolemia. *Pediatr Dermatol.* 1998;15:253-258.

30. Arem AJ, Kischer CW. Analysis of striae. *Plastic Reconstruct Surg.* 1980;65(1):22-29.

31. Smals AGH, Koppenborg PWC, Benraad TJ. Plasma testosterone profiles in Cushing's syndrome. *J Clin Endocrinol Metab.* 1977;45:240-245.

32. Mueller R, Kugelberg E. Myopathy in Cushing's syndrome. *J Neurol Neurosurg Psychiatry.* 1959;22:314-319.

33. Olafsson E, Jones HR, Jr., Guay AT, Thomas CB. Myopathy of endogenous Cushing's syndrome: A review of the clinical and electromyographic features in 8 patients. *Muscle Nerve.* 1994;17:692-693.

34. Pleasure DE, Walsh GO, Engel WK. Atrophy of skeletal muscle in patients with Cushing's syndrome. *Arch Neurol.* 1970;22:118-125.

35. Starkman MN, Schteingart DE. Neuropsychiatric manifestations of patients with Cushing's syndrome. Relationship to cortisol and adrenocorticotropic hormone levels. *Arch Intern Med.* 1981;141:215-219.

36. Elias AN, Meshkinpour H, Valenta LJ, Grossman MK. Pseudo-Cushing's syndrome: The role of alcohol. *J Clin Gastroenterol.* 1982;4:137-139.

37. Kirkman S, Nelson DH. Alcohol-induced pseudo-Cushing's disease: A study of prevalence with review of the literature. *Metabolism.* 1988;37:390-394.

38. Rees LH, Besser GM, Jeffcoate WJ, Goldie DJ, Marks V. Alcohol-induced pseudo-Cushing's syndrome. *Lancet.* 1977;1(8014):726-728.

39. Veldman RG, Meinders AE. On the mechanism of alcohol-induced pseudo-Cushing's syndrome. *Endocrine Rev.* 1996;17:262-268.

40. Trainer PJ, Grossman A. The diagnosis and differential diagnosis of Cushing's syndrome. *Clin Endocrinol (Oxf).* 1991;34:317-330.

41. Howlett TA, Rees LH, Besser G. Cushing's syndrome. *Clin Endocrinol Metab.* 1985;14:911-945.

42. Lo JC, Mulligan K, Tai VW, et al. "Buffalo hump" in men with HIV-1 infection. *Lancet.* 1998;351(9106):867-870.

43. Miller KD, Jones E, Yanovski JA, et al. Visceral abdominal-fat accumulation associated with use of indinavir. *Lancet.* 1998;351:871-875.

44. Aboulafia DM, Bundow D. Images in clinical medicine. Buffalo hump in a patient with the acquired immunodeficiency syndrome. *N Engl J Med.* 1998;339:1297.

45. Carr A, Cooper DA. Lipodystrophy associated with an HIV-protease inhibitor. *N Engl J Med.* 1998;339:1296.

46. De Luca A, Murri R, Damiano F, Ammassari A, Antinori A. "Buffalo hump" in HIV-1 infection. *Lancet.* 1998;352:320.

47. Miller KK, Daly PA, Sentochnik D, et al. Pseudo-Cushing's syndrome in human immunodeficiency virus-infected patients. *Clin Infect Dis.* 1998;27:68-72.

48. Sowers JR, Lippman HR. Cushing's syndrome due to ectopic ACTH production: Cutaneous manifestations. *Cutis.* 1985;36:351-353.

49. Blunt SB, Sandler LM, Burrin JM, Joplin GF. An evaluation of the distinction of ectopic and pituitary ACTH dependent Cushing's syndrome by clinical features, biochemical tests and radiological findings. *Q J Med.* 1990;77:1113-1133.

50. Bertagna C, Orth DN. Clinical and laboratory findings and results of therapy in 58 patients with adrenocortical tumors admitted to a single medical center (1951 to 1978). *Am J Med.* 1981;71:855-875.

51. Hutter AM, Kayhoe DE. Adrenal cortical carcinoma: Clinical features of 138 patients. *Am J Med.* 1966;41:572-580.

52. Luton JP, Cerdas S, Billaud L, et al. Clinical features of adrenocortical carcinoma, prognostic factors, and the effect of mitotane therapy. *N Engl J Med.* 1990;322:1195-1201.

3

VITAL SIGNS

13

Pulse Rate and Contour

PULSE RATE

I. INTRODUCTION

Taking the patient's pulse is one of the oldest physical examination techniques, practiced as long ago as 3500 BC by ancient Egyptian physicians, who believed a weakening pulse indicated advancing disease.[1] The pulse was one of Galen's (ca. 129–200 AD) favorite subjects, occupying several treatises, in which he instructed clinicians to observe the pulse's speed, force, and duration.[2,3] The first accurate observations of heart rate in disease were by John Foyer (1649–1734), who published his clinical observations in 1707 based on his invention, the "pulse-watch."[3] The first clinicians to establish the significance of bradycardia were Adams and Stokes, who, between 1827 and 1846, pointed out that not all seizures and fainting represented disease of the brain but instead could occur because of the slow pulse of heart block.[1]

II. TECHNIQUE

Most clinicians determine the pulse rate by palpating the radial pulse or, less often, by listening to the heart tones with the stethoscope (i.e. "apical rate"). Counting the pulse for 30 seconds and doubling the result is more accurate than 15 seconds of observation.[4] In patients with fast heart rates, especially if the patient has atrial fibrillation, counting the apical rate is more accurate than counting the radial pulse, and 60 seconds of observation is more accurate than shorter periods.[5]

A difference between the radial pulse rate and apical rate (the apical rate always being greater) is called the "pulse deficit." A pulse deficit has traditionally been associated with atrial fibrillation, although it is a common finding with extrasystoles and all fast heart rates and by itself has little diagnostic significance.[6]

III. THE FINDING

Many textbooks state that the normal sinus rate ranges from 60 to 100 beats/minute, but more recent information indicates that the heart rate of 95% of healthy persons instead ranges from 50 to 95 beats/minute.[7] **Bradycardia** is a pulse rate less than 50 beats/minute; **tachycardia** is a rate greater than 100 beats/minute.

IV. CLINICAL SIGNIFICANCE

An important role of any vital sign is to provide the clinician an early indication that trouble is afoot for the patient. EBM Box 13-1 shows that the finding of tachycardia serves this role well. In a wide variety of clinical disorders, including septic shock, pneumonia, myocardial infarction, gallstone pancreatitis, and pontine hemorrhage, the finding of tachycardia (variably defined as rate >90 beats/minute to >110 beats/minute) predicts both increased complications and worse survival [likelihood ratios (LRs) = 1.5 to 25.4]. In patients with myocardial infarction, the increased risk of adverse outcome is a continuum, being greater for patients with higher heart rates and persisting whether or not the patient has a low ejection fraction, takes beta-blocker medications, or receives thrombolytic therapy.[12,15–18] In patients with septic shock, the relationship between tachycardia and mortality is independent of whether the patient receives vasopressor medications,[9] and in patients with pontine hemorrhage, tachycardia is a better predictor of mortality than some other neurologic findings, such as extensor posturing or the absence of withdrawal to pain.[14] The

Box 13-1   Tachycardia

Finding (Ref)	Sensitivity (%)	Specificity (%)	Likelihood Ratio if Finding	
			Present	Absent
Heart rate >90 beats/min				
Predicting hospital mortality in trauma patients with hypotension[8]	94	38	1.5	**0.2**
Heart rate >95 beats/min				
Predicting hospital mortality in patients with septic shock[9]	97	53	2.0	**0.1**
Heart rate >100/min				
Predicting mortality in patients with pneumonia[10]	45	78	2.1	NS
Predicting hospital mortality in patients with myocardial infarction[11,12]	6–9	97–98	**3.0**	NS
Predicting complications in patients with gallstone pancreatitis[13]	86	87	**6.8**	NS
Heart rate >110 beats/min				
Predicting hospital mortality in patients with pontine hemorrhage[14]	70	97	**25.4**	0.3

NS, not significant; likelihood ratio (LR) if finding present = positive LR; LR if finding absent = negative LR.

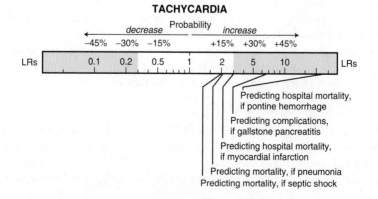

TACHYCARDIA

Predicting hospital mortality, if pontine hemorrhage

Predicting complications, if gallstone pancreatitis

Predicting hospital mortality, if myocardial infarction

Predicting mortality, if pneumonia

Predicting mortality, if septic shock

absence of tachycardia, on the other hand, decreases the probability of hospital mortality in patients with trauma, septic shock, and pontine hemorrhage (LRs = 0.1–0.3, see EBM Box 13-1)

Heart rates less than 50 beats/minute or greater than 120 beats/minute may also indicate heart rhythms other than sinus rhythm (e.g., complete heart block, atrial flutter), a subject discussed in Chapter 14.

ABNORMALITIES OF PULSE CONTOUR

I.   PULSUS ALTERNANS

A.   THE FINDING

Pulsus alternans describes a regular pulse that has alternating strong and weak beats (Fig. 13-1). The pulse must be absolutely regular to diagnose pulsus alternans and to distinguish it from the bigeminal pulse, which also has beats of alternating strength although the rhythm is irregular (see Chapter 14).[19] Rarely, in patients with pulsus alternans, the weak pulse is too small to feel and only half of the beats reach the radial artery ("total alternans").[20] Pulsus alternans is often accompanied by alternation of the intensity of heart sounds and murmurs ("auscultatory alternans").[19,21]

Traube first described pulsus alternans in 1872.[22]

B.   TECHNIQUE

Palpating the radial pulse or using the blood pressure cuff are the best ways to detect pulsus alternans. When using the blood pressure cuff, the clinician should stop deflating the cuff at the first appearance of Korotkoff sounds and hold the cuff pressure just below systolic level for several beats. In patients with pulsus alternans, only the Korotkoff sounds belonging to the strong beats are heard. After further deflation of the cuff, cuff pressure eventually falls below the systolic pressure of the weaker beats, causing the cadence of Korotkoff sounds to suddenly double. The usual difference in systolic pressure between the strong and weak beats is only 15 to 20 mm Hg.[20]

Pulsus alternans often is most prominent in the several beats immediately after a pause in the heart rhythm. Typically, the pause is caused by a premature beat or the abrupt termination of a paroxysmal tachycardia.[23]

C.   CLINICAL SIGNIFICANCE

In patients with normal heart rates, the finding of pulsus alternans indicates severe left ventricular dysfunction, caused by ischemic or valvular heart disease, long-standing hypertension, or idiopathic cardiomyopathy.[24–26] In one series of patients presenting for cardiac catheterization, investigators specifically looked for pulsus

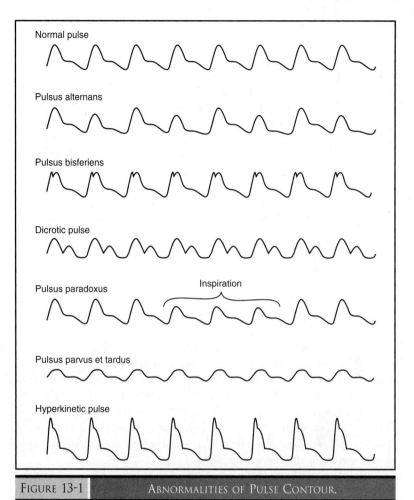

FIGURE 13-1 | ABNORMALITIES OF PULSE CONTOUR.

The normal pulse tracing (*top row*) is displayed with six tracings of abnormal pulse contours (*bottom rows*). **Pulsus alternans** (*second row*) is a *regular* pulse that has alternating strong and weak beats. Both **pulsus bisferiens** (*third row*) and the **dicrotic pulse** (*fourth row*) have two beats per cardiac cycle: in pulsus bisferiens both beats are systolic, whereas in the dicrotic pulse one is systolic and the other diastolic. **Pulsus paradoxus** (*fifth row*) is a pulse whose systolic blood pressure falls more than 10–12 mm Hg during inspiration. **Pulsus parvus et tardus** (*sixth row*) is a pulse that has a small volume and rises slowly. The **hyperkinetic pulse** (*last row*) is a pulse with unusually abrupt and strong force; it may have a normal diastolic blood pressure (e.g., severe mitral insufficiency) or low diastolic blood pressure (e.g., severe aortic regurgitation). These tracings are facsimiles of actual pulse tracings made more than 100 years ago. See text for pathogenesis and clinical significance.

alternans after premature beats or 10 seconds of pacemaker-induced atrial tachycardia: compared with patients without the finding, those with pulsus alternans had worse ejection fractions and higher left ventricular filling pressures.[23]

In patients with rapid heart rates, pulsus alternans has less significance because even patients with normal hearts sometimes develop the finding during paroxysmal tachycardia.[27] Also, pulsus alternans may rarely reflect an intermittent left bundle branch block that alternates with ventricular beats having normal conduction.[28]

D. PATHOGENESIS

There has been considerable debate over decades regarding whether the primary cause of pulsus alternans is alternation of intrinsic contractility of the heart ("contractility argument") or alternation of filling of the ventricles ("hemodynamic argument").

One version of the hemodynamic argument is particularly compelling.[22,29] In patients with a *regular* pulse, the sum of the length of systole and the length of the subsequent diastole must be constant. If systole lengthens for any reason, the subsequent diastole must be shorter; if systole shortens for any reason, the subsequent diastole must be longer. In patients with left ventricular dysfunction, a sudden increase in ventricular filling (such as that induced by a postextrasystolic pause) causes the subsequent systole to produce a strong beat, although it takes longer than normal for the weakened heart to eject this blood (i.e., thus lengthening systole). By prolonging systole, the strong beat thus shortens the next diastole, which reduces filling of the heart and causes the next beat to be weaker. The weaker beat is ejected more quickly, shortening systole and causing the next diastole to be longer, thus perpetuating the alternating pulse.

Nonetheless, the hemodynamic argument does not explain how pulsus alternans ever gets started when there is no pause in the rhythm from an extrasystole or termination of a tachycardia. Most experts now believe that alternation of intrinsic contractility is the fundamental problem in pulsus alternans, because alternation can even be demonstrated in vitro in isolated muscles at constant length and resting tension.[25,26] Once alternans begins, however, the hemodynamic effects probably contribute to the alternating amplitude of the pulse.

II.   PULSUS BISFERIENS

A. THE FINDING

Pulsus bisferiens (Latin *bis*, meaning "twice" and Latin *ferire*, meaning "to beat") has two beats per cardiac cycle, both of which occur in systole (the first beat is called the "percussion wave"; the second, the "tidal wave," see Fig. 13-1).[19] Descriptions of pulsus bisferiens appear in the writings of Galen.[30]

B. TECHNIQUE

Pulsus bisferiens is detected by palpating the brachial or carotid pulse with moderate compression of the vessel or by using the blood pressure cuff.[31] When using the blood pressure cuff, the clinician hears a quick double tapping sound instead of the typical single sound (the clinician can mimic the double sound by saying "pa-da . . . pa-da" as fast as possible).[32]

C. CLINICAL SIGNIFICANCE

Pulsus bisferiens is a finding in patients with moderate-to-severe aortic regurgitation.[30,32,33] Pulsus bisferiens also occurs in patients with combined aortic stenosis and regurgitation, although the principal lesion is usually the regurgitation and the stenosis is mild.[30,33,34] There are exceptional cases of the finding in severe aortic stenosis.[31]

Pulsus bisferiens is sometimes described in patients with hypertrophic cardiomyopathy,[35] although almost always as a finding seen on direct intraarterial pressure tracings, not as a finding palpated at the bedside.[36]

D. PATHOGENESIS

The bisferiens pulse probably results from rapid ejection of blood into a flexible aorta. Because of the Venturi effect, the rapidly moving blood stream temporarily draws the walls of the aorta together, reducing flow momentarily and producing a notch with two systolic peaks in the waveform (in hypertrophic cardiomyopathy, the Venturi effect draws the anterior leaflet of the mitral valve and the interventricular septum together).[31,37] Although this hypothesis was proposed over 35 years ago, direct evidence supporting it is difficult to find.

III. PULSUS PARADOXUS

A. THE FINDING

Pulsus paradoxus is an exaggerated decrease of systolic blood pressure during inspiration (see Figure 13-1).[19,38] Although the usual definition is an inspiratory fall in systolic blood pressure exceeding 10 mm Hg, a better threshold may be 12 mm Hg, which is the upper 95% confidence interval for inspiratory decline in normal persons (i.e., the average inspiratory decrease in systolic pressure of normal persons is 6 ± 3 mm Hg).[39] In patients with pulsus paradoxus, the systolic blood pressure and pulse pressure fall dramatically during inspiration, though the diastolic blood pressure changes little.[38,39]

In 1873, Kussmaul first described pulsus paradoxus in three patients with pericardial disease.[40,41] Kussmaul called the finding "paradoxical" because the pulse of his patients disappeared during inspiration even though the apical beat

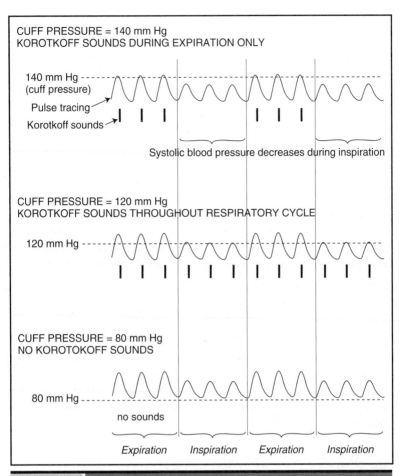

FIGURE 13-2   TECHNIQUE FOR MEASURING PULSUS PARADOXUS.

The figure simultaneously depicts the pressure in the blood pressure cuff (*dashed horizontal line*), the patient's pulse tracing (*solid line*), and Korotkoff sounds (*solid vertical bars* under pulse tracing) during two breaths (expiration and inspiration are separated by *vertical lines*). The pulse tracing shows the fall in systolic pressure during inspiration, which is characteristic of pulsus paradoxus. To detect and measure the paradoxical pulse, the clinician begins by checking the blood pressure in the usual way but slowly deflates the cuff to precisely identify the *cuff pressure* at three points: (1) the moment Korotkoff sounds first appear (*top tracing*). In patients with pulsus paradoxus, cuff pressure will fall below the systolic pressure of just the expiratory beats, and the Korotkoff sounds will repeatedly come and go during quiet respiration, disappearing with inspiration and reappearing with expiration; (2) the persisted throughout the respiratory cycle. The term is unfortunate, because the finding is nothing more than an exaggeration of normal physiologic change.

B. TECHNIQUE

When checking for pulsus paradoxus, the clinician should have the patient breathe quietly and regularly, because even normal persons can induce a pulsus paradoxus with vigorous respirations. Pulsus paradoxus is detected by palpating the pulse or using the blood pressure cuff, although only paradoxical pulses exceeding 15 to 20 mm Hg are palpable.[42,43] For this reason, most clinicians use the blood pressure cuff, which has the added advantage of quantifying the finding (Fig. 13-2).

Pulsus paradoxus also has been noted in pulse oximetry tracings, appearing as respiratory movement of the tracing's baseline.[44] The amplitude of this oscillation correlates with the severity of pulsus paradoxus[44] and, if a blood pressure cuff is used to quantify the pulsus paradoxus, the visual display of the pulse oximeter may substitute for actually listening to the Korotkoff sounds.[45]

C. CLINICAL SIGNIFICANCE

Pulsus paradoxus is a common finding in two conditions, cardiac tamponade and acute asthma.

1. Cardiac Tamponade

Pulsus paradoxus greater than 10 mm Hg occurs in 98% of patients with cardiac tamponade (i.e., a pericardial effusion under high pressure compressing the heart and compromising cardiac output; see Chapter 43). Because it is one of three key findings of tamponade—the others being elevated neck veins (sensitivity = 100%) and tachycardia (sensitivity = 81-100%)—the clinician should consider tamponade and check for pulsus paradoxus in any patient suspected of having pericardial disease, such as those with elevated neck veins, unexplained dyspnea, pericardial rub, or known pericardial effusion.[43]

---

moment when Korotkoff sounds persist throughout the respiratory cycle (*middle tracing*). At this point cuff pressure has fallen below systolic blood pressure of all beats; and (3) the moment when Korotkoff sounds disappear (i.e., the diastolic pressure, *bottom tracing*). In this patient, only expiratory Korotkoff sounds are heard between cuff pressures of 140 mm Hg and 120 mm Hg, but Korotkoff sounds are heard throughout the respiratory cycle between pressures of 120 mm Hg and 80 mm Hg. The patient's blood pressure is therefore "140/80 mm Hg with a paradox of 20 mm Hg" (i.e., 20 = 140 − 120).

In patients with pericardial effusions, the finding of pulsus paradoxus greater than 12 mm Hg discriminates patients with tamponade from those without tamponade with a sensitivity of 98%, specificity of 83%, positive LR of 5.9, and negative LR of 0.03.*[39]

2. Cardiac Tamponade Without Pulsus Paradoxus

In only 2% of patients with tamponade, pulsus paradoxus is absent. These patients usually have one of five associated disorders: (1) atrial septal defect, (2) severe left ventricular dysfunction (especially those with uremic pericarditis),[46] (3) regional tamponade (tamponade affecting only one or two heart chambers, a complication of cardiac surgery),[47] (4) severe hypotension,[48-50] or (5) aortic regurgitation. Knowing that aortic regurgitation may eliminate pulsus paradoxus is especially significant, because patients with proximal (type A) aortic dissection and hemopericardium usually lack the paradoxical pulse despite significant tamponade, and the unaware clinician may exclude the possibility of tamponade to the harm of the patient.

The section on pathogenesis explains why pulsus paradoxus is missing in each of these clinical disorders.

3. Asthma

EBM Box 13-2 shows that, in patients with acute asthma, pulsus paradoxus exceeding 20 mm Hg almost certainly indicates severe bronchospasm (LR = 8.2). Nonetheless, pulsus paradoxus has limited clinical utility in patients with acute asthma for two reasons: (1) Up to half of patients with severe bronchospasm lack a pulsus paradoxus of greater than 10 mm Hg (see EBM Box 13-2). The sensitivity is low because the pulsus paradoxus of asthma is notably dependent on respiratory rate and effort, even when the degree of airway obstruction remains constant.[52,54] (2) The best measure of bronchospasm (and the criterion standard in studies listed in EBM Box 13-2) is the peak expiratory flow rate. In a busy emergency department with an anxious and dyspneic patient, it is much more convenient to measure peak flow rates using hand-held flow-meters than trying to interpret the coming and going of Korotkoff sounds.

In patients being mechanically ventilated, the amount of pulsus paradoxus, as reflected in the changing baseline of the pulse oximeter tracing, correlates with the degree of the patient's auto-positive end-expiratory pressure (auto-PEEP) (a measure of expiratory difficulty in ventilated patients).[44]

---

*Tamponade was defined in this study as improvement in cardiac output of 20% or more following pericardiocentesis. See Chapter 43.

Box 13-2 Pulsus Paradoxus Predicting Severe Asthma*

Finding (Ref)	Sensitivity (%)	Specificity (%)	Likelihood Ratio if Finding	
			Present	Absent
Pulsus paradoxus >10 mm Hg[42,51-53]	52–68	69–92	2.7	0.5
Pulsus paradoxus >20 mm Hg[42,51,52]	19–39	91–100	**8.2**	0.8
Pulsus paradoxus >25 mm Hg[53]	16	99	**22.6**	0.8

FEV_1, forced expiratory volume in 1 second; FVC, forced vital capacity; likelihood ratio (LR) if finding present = positive LR; LR if finding absent = negative LR.
*Diagnostic standard: For severe asthma, a $FEV_1/FVC < 50\%$,[42] FEV1 < 1.0 L,[51] peak flow < 200 L/min,[53] and peak flow < 30% predicted.[52] All patients in these studies had acute asthma.

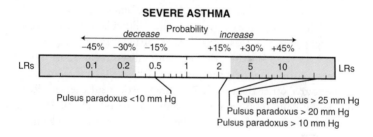

4. Pulsus Paradoxus in Other Conditions

Pulsus paradoxus has been described as an uncommon finding in constrictive pericarditis, right ventricular infarction, pulmonary embolism, and severe pectus excavatum (see Chapter 43).[38,55]

5. Reversed Pulsus Paradoxus[56]

Reversed pulsus paradoxus, which is a systolic blood pressure that falls greater than 10 mm Hg *during expiration*, occurs in three clinical disorders: (1) hypertrophic cardiomyopathy, (2) isorhythmic dissociation (i.e., inspiration accelerates the sinus rate, which temporarily positions the P waves before the QRS complex, thus coordinating the atrial and ventricular contractions and raising blood pressure; expiration slows the sinus rate, removes atrioventricular coordination, and lowers blood pressure), and (3) intermittent inspiratory positive-pressure breathing in the presence of left ventricular failure (this is a variation of the Valsalva square wave response in heart failure; see Chapter 44).

D. PATHOGENESIS

1. Cardiac Tamponade

Tamponade develops when the pressure of fluid inside the pericardial space exceeds the diastolic filling pressure of the heart chambers. Once this occurs, the diastolic pressure in the heart chambers, reflected in the neck veins, becomes a measurement of the force acting to compress the heart. The four chambers, now smaller in size, begin to compete for space, and an increase in the size of one comes at the expense of the size of another. Inspiration increases filling to the right side of the heart and shifts the interventricular septum to the left and posteriorly, thus obliterating the left ventricular chamber and causing the cardiac output to fall. During expiration, filling of the right side of the heart is less, which increases left ventricular size, and both cardiac output and blood pressure increase.[38,47,57-60]

This explains why pulsus paradoxus is absent in regional tamponade and tamponade associated with atrial septal defect, severe left ventricular dysfunction, and aortic insufficiency (see "Cardiac Tamponade Without Pulsus Paradoxus"). Inspiratory movement of the interventricular septum is prevented when the right ventricle does not fill more during inspiration (atrial septal defect, see Chapter 36), when the left ventricular pressures are very high (severe left ventricular dysfunction), or when the left ventricle fills from some source other than the left atrium (aortic insufficiency). Regional tamponade, by definition, compresses only one or two chambers, enough to impair cardiac output but too confined to cause the heart chambers to compete for space.

2. Asthma

The mechanism of pulsus paradoxus in asthma is complex and not fully understood. Difficulty breathing causes wide swings of intrapleural pressure, which then are transmitted directly to the aorta, contributing to the paradoxical pulse. This is not a complete explanation, however, because the amount of pulsus paradoxus in asthma often exceeds the pressure shifts of these respiratory excursions.[54] Furthermore, the pulse pressure also declines during inspiration of some asthma patients, which would not happen if transmission of pressures were the only cause. Other proposed mechanisms are an inspiratory reduction in pulmonary venous return to the left heart[38,54,61,62] and the compressive action of the hyperinflated chest, which, like tamponade, may reduce the size of the heart chambers and cause them to compete for space.[52,63]

IV.   PULSUS PARVUS ET TARDUS

A.   THE FINDING AND TECHNIQUE

Pulsus parvus et tardus describes a carotid pulse with a small volume ("pulsus parvus") that rises slowly and has a delayed systolic peak ("pulsus tardus", see Fig. 13-1).[19] It is routinely detected by palpation.

B.   CLINICAL SIGNIFICANCE

Pulsus parvus et tardus is a finding of aortic stenosis. Of its two components, pulsus tardus is the better discriminator, detecting severe aortic stenosis with a sensitivity of 31% to 90%, specificity of 68% to 93%, positive LR of 3.7, and negative LR of 0.4 (see Chapter 40).[64–67]

C.   PATHOGENESIS

Pulsus tardus depends on both obstruction to flow and the compliance of the vessel distal to the obstruction. The pulse waveform rises rapidly in stiff vessels, but slowly in more compliant vessels that act like low-pass filters and remove the high-frequency components of the waveform.[68] That the delay in the pulse reflects the severity of obstruction is a principle also used by Doppler sonography to gauge the severity of renal artery stenosis.[68]

V.   DICROTIC PULSE

A.   THE FINDING AND TECHNIQUE

The dicrotic pulse has two beats per cardiac cycle, but, unlike pulsus bisferiens, one peak is systolic and the other is diastolic (see Fig. 13-1).[19] It is usually detected by palpation of the carotid artery.[69]

The second wave of the dicrotic pulse is identical in timing to the small dicrotic wave of normal persons, obvious on arterial pressure tracings but never palpable. The dicrotic wave is felt to represent rebound of blood against the closed aortic valve.

B.   CLINICAL SIGNIFICANCE

The dicrotic pulse occurs in younger patients with severe myocardial dysfunction, low stroke volumes, and high systemic resistance.[69,70] In patients who have had valvular replacement surgery, the finding of a persistent dicrotic pulse is associated with a poor prognosis.[70]

C.   PATHOGENESIS

The dicrotic pulse has two components: (1) low stroke volume, which significantly lowers the height of the pulse's initial systolic wave, thus increasing the chances that the dicrotic wave will be palpable[71] and (2) a resilient arterial system, which amplifies the rebound of the pulse waveform during diastole. The importance of a resilient arterial system may explain why the dicrotic pulse usually occurs in young patients with cardiomyopathy, who have more compliant vessels than older patients.[69,70]

The importance of a low stroke volume to the dicrotic pulse is illustrated by the observation that the dicrotic pulse sometimes disappears with beats that have larger stroke volumes, such as the beat after a premature beat, the stronger beats of pulsus alternans, and the expiratory beats of pulsus paradoxus.[69,71] Vasodilators often cause the dicrotic pulse to disappear, perhaps because of better forward flow and a greater stroke volume.[69]

VI. HYPERKINETIC PULSE

A. THE FINDING
The hyperkinetic pulse strikes the examiner's fingers with unusually abrupt and strong force (see Fig. 13-1). Hyperkinetic pulses may have either a normal pulse pressure (e.g., severe mitral regurgitation, hypertrophic obstructive cardiomyopathy) or increased pulse pressure (e.g., aortic insufficiency and other disorders with abnormal aortic runoff).[19] In both severe mitral regurgitation and hypertrophic obstructive cardiomyopathy, the blood is ejected rapidly from the left ventricle but the integrity of the aortic valve preserves a normal arterial diastolic and pulse pressure.[72] In aortic regurgitation, the rapid ejection of blood is accompanied by an incompetent aortic valve, which causes a very low diastolic pressure in the aortic root, thus increasing the pulse pressure and causing the "Corrigan" or "water-hammer" pulse characteristic of this disorder (see Chapter 41).

B. CLINICAL SIGNIFICANCE
Chapter 41 discusses the significance of the water hammer pulse and large pulse pressure of aortic regurgitation.

In patients with mitral stenosis, the pulse is characteristically normal or diminished. If the clinician instead finds a hyperkinetic pulse in these patients, the probability is high that additional valvular disease is present, such as significant mitral regurgitation (sensitivity 71%, specificity 95%, positive LR = 14.2, negative LR = 0.3, see Chapter 42).[73]

VII. PULSES AND HYPOVOLEMIC SHOCK

In patients with hypovolemic shock, the peripheral pulses provide a rough guide to the patient's systolic blood pressure.[74] As blood pressure progressively

Box 13-3   Pulses and Hypovolemic Shock [74]

Finding	Sensitivity (%)	Specificity (%)	Likelihood Ratio if Finding Present	Absent
Detecting systolic blood pressure ≥ 60 mm Hg[*]				
Carotid pulse present	95	22	NS	NS
Femoral pulse present	95	67	2.9	**0.1**
Radial pulse present	52	89	NS	0.5

NS, not significant; likelihood ratio (LR) if finding present = positive LR; LR if finding absent = negative LR.

*Diagnostic standard: For systolic blood pressure, invasive arterial blood pressure measurements.

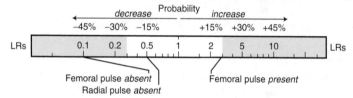

diminishes, the radial pulse generally disappears first, then the femoral pulse, and finally the carotid pulse. In one study of 20 patients with hypovolemic shock, summarized in EBM Box 13-3, the femoral pulse had the greatest diagnostic accuracy in determining severity of shock: the presence of a palpable femoral pulse argued modestly for a systolic blood pressure greater than 60 mm Hg (LR = 2.9), whereas its absence was a strong argument *against* a blood pressure this high (LR = 0.1).

REFERENCES

1. Schechter DC, Lillehei CW, Soffer A. History of sphygmology and of heart block. *Dis Chest.* 1969;55(Suppl 1):535-579.
2. Galen. On the pulse. In: Clendening L, ed. *Source book of medical history.* New York: Dover; 1960:42-47.
3. Geddes LA. Perspectives in physiological monitoring. *Med Instrument.* 1976;10(2): 91-97.

4. Hollerbach AD, Sneed NV. Accuracy of radial pulse assessment by length of counting interval. *Heart Lung.* 1990;19:258-264.

5. Sneed NV, Hollerbach AD. Accuracy of heart rate assessment in atrial fibrillation. *Heart Lung.* 1992;21:427-433.

6. Doyle MP, Jordan LE. A comparison of pulse deficit readings by serial and simultaneous measurement. *Nurs Res.* 1968;17:460-462.

7. Spodick DH. Normal sinus heart rate: Appropriate rate thresholds for sinus tachycardia and bradycardia. *South Med J.* 1996;89:666-667.

8. Victorino GP, Battistella FD, Wisner DH. Does tachycardia correlate with hypotension after trauma? *J Am Coll Surg.* 2003;196:679-684.

9. Parker MM, Shelhamer JH, Natanson C, Dalling DW, Parrillo JE. Serial cardiovascular variables in survivors and nonsurvivors of human septic shock: Heart rate as an early predictor of prognosis. *Crit Care Med.* 1987;15:923-929.

10. Starczewski AR, Allen SC, Vargas E, Lye M. Clinical prognostic indices of fatality in elderly patients admitted to hospital with acute pneumonia. *Age Ageing.* 1988;17:181-186.

11. Kovar D, Cannon CP, Bentley JH, et al. Does initial and delayed heart rate predict mortality in patients with acute coronary syndromes? *Clin Cardiol.* 2004;27:80-86.

12. Zuanetti G, Mantini L, Hernandez-Bernal F, et al. Relevance of heart rate as a prognostic factor in patients with acute myocardial infarction: Insights from the GISSI-2 study. *Eur Heart J.* 1998;19 (Suppl F):F19-F26.

13. Arnell TD, De Virgilio C, Chang L, et al. Admission factors can predict the need for ICU monitoring in gallstone pancreatitis. *Am Surg.* 1996;62:815-819.

14. Wijdicks EFM, St. Louis E. Clinical profiles predictive of outcome in pontine hemorrhage. *Neurol.* 1997;49:1342-1346.

15. Hjalmarson A, Gilpin EA, Kjekshus J, et al. Influence of heart rate on mortality after acute myocardial infarction. *Am J Cardiol.* 1990;65:547-553.

16. Disegni E, Goldbourt U, Reicher-Reiss H, et al. The predictive value of admission heart rate on mortality in patients with acute myocardial infarction. *J Clin Epidemiol.* 1995;48:1197-1205.

17. Hathaway WR, Peterson ED, Wagner GS, et al. Prognostic significance of the initial electrocardiogram in patients with acute myocardial infarction. *JAMA.* 1998;279:387-391.

18. Berton GS, Cordiano R, Palmieri R, et al. Heart rate during myocardial infarction: Relationship with one-year global mortality in men and women. *Can J Cardiol.* 2002;18:495-502.

19. Feinstein AR, Hochstein E, Luisada AA, et al. Glossary of cardiologic terms related to physical diagnosis: Part IV. Arterial pulses. *Am J Card.* 1971;27:708-709.

20. Liu CK, Luisada AA. Halving of the pulse due to severe alternans (pulsus bisectus). *Am Heart J.* 1955;50:927-932.

21. Tavel ME, Nasser WK. Murmur alternans in aortic stenosis. *Chest.* 1970;57:176-179.

22. Mitchell JH, Sarnoff SJ, Sonnenblick EH. The dynamics of pulsus alternans: Alternating end-diastolic fiber length as a causative factor. *J Clin Invest.* 1963;42: 55-63.
23. Schaefer S, Malloy CR, Schmitz JM, Dehmer GJ. Clinical and hemodynamic characteristics of patients with inducible pulsus alternans. *Am Heart J.* 1988;115: 1251-1257.
24. Swanton RH, Jenkins BS, Brooksby IAB, Webb-Peploe MM. An analysis of pulsus alternans in aortic stenosis. *Eur J Cardiol.* 1976;4:39-47.
25. Lab MJ, Seed WA. Pulsus alternans. *Cardiovasc Res.* 1993;27:1407-1412.
26. Surawicz B, Fisch C. Cardiac alternans: Diverse mechanisms and clinical manifestations. *J Am Coll Cardiol.* 1992;20:483-499.
27. Saunders DE, Ord JW. The hemodynamic effects of paroxysmal supraventricular tachycardia in patients with the Wolff-Parkinson-White syndrome. *Am J Card.* 1962;9:223-236.
28. Barold SS, Herweg B. Pulsus alternans caused by 2:1 left bundle branch block. *J Interv Card Electrophysiol.* 2005;12(3):221-222.
29. Gleason WL, Braunwald E. Studies on Starling's law of the heart: Relationships between left ventricular end-diastolic volume and stroke volume in man with observations on the mechanism of pulsus alternans. *Circulation.* 1962;25:841-848.
30. Fleming PR. The mechanism of the pulsus bisferiens. *Br Heart J.* 1957;19:519-524.
31. MacAlpin RN, Kattus AA. Brachial-artery bruits in aortic-valve disease and hypertrophic subaortic stenosis. *N Engl J Med.* 1965;273:1012-1018.
32. Ciesielski J, Rodbard S. Doubling of the arterial sounds in patients with pulsus bisferiens. *JAMA.* 1961;175:475-477.
33. Ikram H, Nixon PGF, Fox JA. The hemodynamic implications of the bisferiens pulse. *Br Heart J.* 1964;26:452-459.
34. Wood P. Aortic stenosis. *Am J Card.* 1958;1:553-571.
35. Frank S, Braunwald E. Idiopathic hypertrophic subaortic stenosis: Clinical analysis of 126 patients with emphasis on the natural history. *Circulation.* 1968;37: 759-788.
36. Perloff JK. Clinical recognition of aortic stenosis: The physical signs and differential diagnosis of the various forms of obstruction to left ventricular outflow. *Prog Cardiovasc Dis.* 1968;10:323-352.
37. Constant J. *Bedside cardiology.* Boston: Little, Brown and Company; 1985.
38. Shabetai R. *The pericardium.* New York: Grune and Stratton; 1981.
39. Curtiss EI, Reddy PS, Uretsky BF, Cecchetti AA. Pulsus paradoxus: Definition and relation to the severity of cardiac tamponade. *Am Heart J.* 1988;115:391-398.
40. Kussmaul A. Ueber schwielige Mediastino-Pericarditis und den paradoxen Puls. *Berl Klin Wochenschrift.* 1873;38:445-449.
41. Shapiro E, Salick AI. A clarification of the paradoxical pulse: Adolf Kussmaul's original description. *Am J Cardiol.* 1965;16:426-431.
42. Knowles GK, Clark TJH. Pulsus paradoxus as a valuable sign indicating severity of asthma. *Lancet.* 1973;2:1356-1359.

43. Fowler NO. Pulsus paradoxus. *Heart Dis Stroke.* 1994;3:68-69.

44. Hartert TV, Wheeler AP, Sheller JR. Use of pulse oximetry to recognize severity of airflow obstruction in obstructive airway disease: Correlation with pulsus paradoxus. *Chest.* 1999;115:475-481.

45. Clark JA, Lieh-Lai M, Thomas R, et al. Comparison of traditional and plethysmographic methods for measuring pulsus paradoxus. *Arch Pediatr Adolesc Med.* 2004;158:48-51.

46. Reddy PS, Curtiss EI, O'Toole JD, Shaver JA. Cardiac tamponade: Hemodynamic observations in man. *Circulation.* 1978;58:265-272.

47. Shabetai R. Changing concepts of cardiac tamponade. *J Am Coll Cardiol.* 1988;12:194-195.

48. Antman EM, Cargill V. Low-pressure tamponade. *Ann Intern Med.* 1979;91:403-406.

49. Himelman RB, Kircher B, Rockey DC, Schiller NB. Inferior vena cava plethora with blunted respiratory response: A sensitive echocardiographic sign of cardiac tamponade. *J Am Coll Cardiol.* 1988;12:1470-1477.

50. Hayes SN, Freeman WK, Gersh BJ. Low pressure cardiac tamponade: Diagnosis facilitated by Doppler echocardiography. *Br Heart J.* 1990;63:136-140.

51. Carden DL, Nowak RM, Sarkar D, Tomlanovich MC. Vital signs including pulsus paradoxus in the assessment of acute bronchial asthma. *Ann Emerg Med.* 1983;12:80-83.

52. Shim C, Williams MH. Pulsus paradoxus in asthma. *Lancet.* 1978;1:530-531.

53. Pearson MG, Spence DPS, Ryland I, Harrison BDW. Value of pulsus paradoxus in assessing acute severe asthma. *Br Med J.* 1993;307:659.

54. Martin J, Jardim J, Sampson M, Engel LE. Factors influencing pulsus paradoxus in asthma. *Chest.* 1981;80:543-549.

55. Yalamanchili K, Summer W, Valentine V. Pectus excavatum with inspiratory inferior vena cava compression: A new presentation of pulsus paradoxus. *Am J Med Sci.* 2005;329:45-47.

56. Massumi RA, Mason DT, Vera Z, et al. Reversed pulsus paradoxus. *N Engl J Med.* 1973;289:1272-1275.

57. Savitt MA, Tyson GS, Elbeery JR, et al. Physiology of cardiac tamponade and paradoxical pulse in conscious dogs. *Am J Physiol.* 1993;265(6 Pt 2):H1996-2008.

58. Settle HP, Adolph RJ, Fowler NO, et al. Echocardiographic study of cardiac tamponade. *Circulation.* 1977;56:951-959.

59. Yeh E. Varying ejection fractions of both ventricles in paradoxical pulses: Demonstration by radionuclide study. *Chest.* 1978;74:687-689.

60. Santoro IH, Neumann A, Carroll JD, et al. Pulsus paradoxus: A definition revisited. *J Am Soc Echocardiography.* 1991;4:409-412.

61. Squara P, Dhainaut JF, Schremmer B, et al. Decreased paradoxic pulse from increased venous return in severe asthma. *Chest.* 1990;97:377-383.

62. Settle HP, Engel PJ, Fowler NO, et al. Echocardiographic study of the paradoxical arterial pulse in chronic obstructive lung disease. *Circulation.* 1980;62:1297-1307.

63. Rebuck AS, Pengelly LD. Development of pulsus paradoxus in the presence of airways obstruction. *N Engl J Med.* 1973;288:66-69.

64. Aronow WS, Kronzon I. Prevalence and severity of valvular aortic stenosis determined by Doppler echocardiography and its association with echocardiographic and electrocardiographic left ventricular hypertrophy and physical signs of aortic stenosis in elderly patients. *Am J Cardiol.* 1991;67:776-777.

65. Forssell G, Jonasson R, Orinius E. Identifying severe aortic valvular stenosis by bedside examination. *Acta Med Scand.* 1985;218:397-400.

66. Hoagland PM, Cook EF, Wynne J, Goldman L. Value of noninvasive testing in adults with suspected aortic stenosis. *Am J Med.* 1986;80:1041-1050.

67. Aronow WS, Kronzon I. Correlation of prevalence and severity of valvular aortic stenosis determined by continuous-wave Doppler echocardiography with physical signs of aortic stenosis in patients aged 62 to 100 years with aortic systolic ejection murmurs. *Am J Cardiol.* 1987;60:399-401.

68. Bude RO, Rubin JM, Platt JF, et al. Pulsus tardus: Its cause and potential limitations in detection of arterial stenosis. *Radiology.* 1994;190:779-784.

69. Ewy GA, Rios JC, Marcus FI. The dicrotic arterial pulse. *Circulation.* 1969;39:655-661.

70. Orchard RC, Craige E. Dicrotic pulse after open heart surgery. *Circulation.* 1980;62:1107-1114.

71. Smith D, Craige E. Mechanisms of the dicrotic pulse. *Br Heart J.* 1986;56:531-534.

72. Perloff JK. The physiologic mechanisms of cardiac and vascular physical signs. *J Am Coll Cardiol.* 1983;1:184-198.

73. Wood P. An appreciation of mitral stenosis: Part 1. Clinical features. Part 2. Investigations and results. *Br Med J.* 1954;1:1051-1063, 1113-1024.

74. Deakin CD, Low JL. Accuracy of the advanced trauma life support guidelines for predicting systolic blood pressure using carotid, femoral, and radial pulses: Observation study. *BMJ.* 2000;321:673-674.

14

Abnormalities of Pulse Rhythm

I. INTRODUCTION

In the late 19th and early 20th centuries, before the introduction of electrocardiography, clinicians could examine the patient's arterial pulse, heart tones, and jugular venous waveforms, and, from these observations alone, diagnose atrial and ventricular premature contractions, atrial flutter, atrial fibrillation, complete heart block, Mobitz 1 and 2 atrioventricular block, and sinoatrial block.[1-3] In fact, clinicians were familiar enough with the bedside findings of these arrhythmias that early textbooks of electrocardiography included tracings of the arterial and venous pulse to help explain the electrocardiogram (ECG, Fig. 14-1).[4]

The bedside diagnosis of arrhythmias today is probably little more than an intellectual game, because all significant arrhythmias require electrocardiography for confirmation and monitoring. Nonetheless, bedside diagnosis of arrhythmias is still possible, using the principles discovered 100 years ago by Mackenzie, Wenckebach, and Lewis. These principles, based on extensive investigation and many polygraph recordings of the arterial and venous pulse,[1-4] allow diagnosis of simple arrhythmias when the electrocardiograph is not nearby.

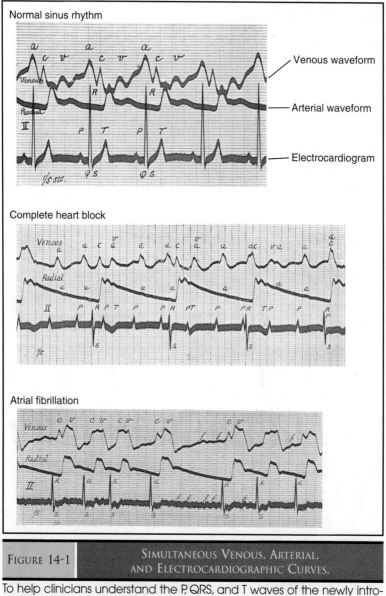

FIGURE 14-1	SIMULTANEOUS VENOUS, ARTERIAL, AND ELECTROCARDIOGRAPHIC CURVES.

To help clinicians understand the P, QRS, and T waves of the newly introduced electrocardiogram, early textbooks displayed simultaneous venous and arterial waveforms with the electrocardiogram. These examples, reproduced from Sir Thomas Lewis's 1925 *Mechanism and graphic registration of the heart beat,*[4] depict normal sinus rhythm (*top*), complete heart block (*middle*), and atrial fibrillation (*bottom*). See text.

II. TECHNIQUE

The first step in diagnosing arrhythmias is to determine the basic rhythm of the patient's radial pulse. Most arrhythmias can be classified into one of five basic abnormalities: (1) the pause, (2) regular bradycardia, (3) regular tachycardia, (4) irregular rhythm that varies with respiration, and (5) irregularly irregular (or "chaotic") rhythm (Fig. 14-2).

The radial pulse may not correspond to the ventricular pulse (or "apical pulse"), as determined by auscultation of the heart tones or palpation of the cardiac impulse, because some ventricular contractions are too weak to propel blood to the radial artery. Although the clinician must compare the radial pulse with the ventricular pulse to diagnose arrhythmias, the difference in *rate* between the two by itself indicates no particular diagnosis.

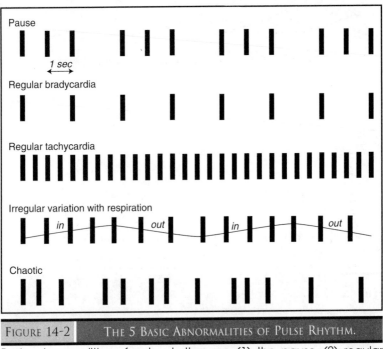

FIGURE 14-2	THE 5 BASIC ABNORMALITIES OF PULSE RHYTHM.

Basic abnormalities of pulse rhythm are (1) the pause, (2) regular bradycardia, (3) regular tachycardia, (4) irregular rhythm that varies with respiration ("in" depicts inspiration and "out" depicts expiration), and (5) irregularly irregular (or "chaotic") rhythm. See text.

After the basic rhythm of the radial pulse is identified, analysis of the jugular venous waveforms, heart tones, and response of the heart rhythm to vagal maneuvers may further distinguish the various causes.

III. THE FINDINGS AND THEIR CLINICAL SIGNIFICANCE

A. THE PAUSE

The pause has two important causes, premature contractions (common) and heart block (uncommon).

1. Terminology

When the radial pulse consists of the regular repetition of two beats followed by a pause, the term "bigeminal pulse" or "bigeminal rhythm" is used. When there are three radial pulse beats between each pause, the appropriate term is "trigeminal" pulse or rhythm. The finding of several beats between each pause is usually called "group beating," and much longer periods of regular rhythm interrupted by the rare pause is sometimes referred to as "pulse intermissions." The basic mechanism for all of these rhythm disturbances is the same, only the frequency of premature beats or heart block differs among them.

Because the cadence of these rhythms becomes predictable after short periods of observation, the term "regularly irregular" is sometimes used. This term, however, inaccurately conveys to others what actually is going on, and it is best discarded.

2. Basic Mechanism of the Pause

The pause has three basic mechanisms, illustrated in Fig. 14-3. The two most important questions that distinguish these mechanisms are (1) Is there a premature radial pulse immediately preceding the pause? and (2) Do additional ventricular beats (identified by listening to the heart tones or palpating the apical pulse) occur during the pause?

a. Premature Beat

Patients with premature contractions (the first two examples in Fig. 14-3) have evidence of a premature ventricular beat during or immediately preceding the pause in the radial pulse. This early beat is always evident in the form of a palpable apical impulse or additional heart tones, although it may not be felt in the radial artery.

Some premature contractions are strong enough to open the aortic valve (first example in Fig. 14-3). If so, the clinician will feel a quick beat in the radial pulse just preceding the pause, although the quick beat is usually not as strong as a normal

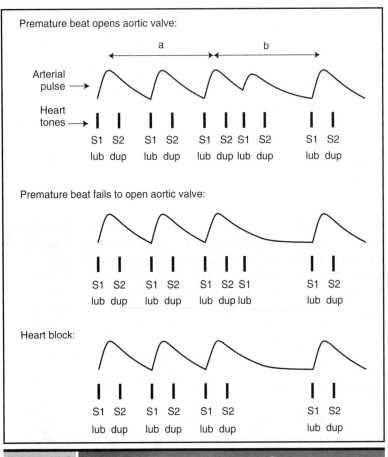

Premature beat opens aortic valve:

Arterial pulse →

Heart tones →

S1	S2	S1	S2	S1	S2	S1	S2	S1	S2
lub	dup	lub	dup	lub	dup	lub	dup	lub	dup

Premature beat fails to open aortic valve:

S1	S2	S1	S2	S1	S2	S1		S1	S2
lub	dup	lub	dup	lub	dup	lub		lub	dup

Heart block:

S1	S2	S1	S2	S1	S2		S1	S2
lub	dup	lub	dup	lub	dup		lub	dup

FIGURE 14-3	MECHANISM OF THE PAUSE.

The radial pulse tracing and heart tones are presented, illustrating the three mechanisms for the pause: (1) premature contraction that opens the aortic valve, (2) premature contraction that fails to open the aortic valve, and (3) heart block. Onomatopoeia of the heart tones appears below each tracing ("lub" is the first heart sound, "dup" is the second heart sound). See text.

sinus beat. When listening to the heart tones, the clinician will hear both the first and second heart sounds of the early beat, which produces the following characteristic cadence:

lub dup   lub dup   lub dup lub dup   lub dup

(In this and the following two examples, "*lub*" is the first heart sound and "*dup*" is the second sound; each rhythm begins with three normal beats, i.e., three "*lub dups*").

If the premature contraction is too weak to open the aortic valve (second example in Fig. 14-3), the clinician palpating the pulse will not detect the quick beat but will only feel the pause. Listening to the heart, he or she will hear only the first sound of the premature beat (S_2 is absent because the aortic valve never opens):

lub dup   lub dup   lub dup lub   lub dup

b. Heart Block

Patients with heart block (third example in Fig. 14-3), whether sinoatrial or atrioventricular, have no palpable apical impulse or extra heart tones during the pause. The cadence of heart tones contrasts with those of the premature beat:

lub dup   lub dup   lub dup   lub dup

3. Bigeminal and Trigeminal Rhythms, and Grouped Beating

Based on the mechanisms previously discussed, there are three causes of the bigeminal rhythm: (1) alternating normal and premature contractions. In this case, the second beat of the couplet is weaker; (2) premature contractions occurring every third beat, although the premature contraction is too weak to open the aortic valve; and, (3) 3:2 heart block (atrioventricular or sinoatrial). In causes 2 and 3, both beats of the couplet are strong, but cause 2 has evidence of a ventricular contraction during the pause whereas cause 3 does not.

The same analysis is used for trigeminal rhythms (i.e., possible causes are premature contractions after every two or three normal beats or 4:3 heart block) and grouped beating.

4. Atrial Versus Ventricular Premature Contractions

Two helpful bedside findings distinguish atrial premature contractions from ventricular ones.

a. Compensatory Pause

Beats that originate in the ventricle usually do not upset the underlying sinus rhythm, causing the beat immediately following the pause to fall exactly where the clinician anticipates it would. Tapping the foot during the normal regular rhythm helps determine this. In Fig. 14-3, the distance b equals a, meaning there is a "complete compensatory pause."

Beats that originate in the atria, in contrast, often reset the sinus node, causing the next beat to appear early. In Fig. 14-3, b would be less than a, and the clinician tapping the foot would find that the basic meter of rhythm changes.

This rule is much more helpful when the pause is not compensatory (i.e. b < a, indicating the beat is atrial), because many atrial premature contractions also seem to have a complete compensatory pause at the bedside.

b. Cannon A Waves

The appearance of a sudden prominent venous wave in the neck (cannon A wave) *during the pause* indicates that the premature beat was ventricular (see also Chapter 32). This occurs because the right atrium, still beating under the direction of the uninterrupted sinus impulses, contracts after the ventricular premature contraction has closed the tricuspid valve. Rarely, a very early atrial premature beat may also have a cannon A wave, but this wave precedes the first heart sound of the premature contraction, whereas cannon A waves from ventricular premature contractions always follow the first heart sound of the premature beat.

B. REGULAR BRADYCARDIA (RATE < 50 BEATS/MINUTE)

There are three causes of regular bradycardia that are recognizable at the bedside: sinus bradycardia, complete heart block, and "halved pulse."

1. Sinus Bradycardia

This arrhythmia resembles the normal rhythm in every way except for the abnormally slow rate: The venous waveforms in the neck are normal, the intensity of the first heart sound is the same with each beat, and there is no evidence of ventricular contractions between radial pulsations (as determined by palpation of apical impulse or auscultation of the heart tones).

2. Complete Heart Block

In complete heart block, the atria and ventricles beat independently of each other (i.e., atrioventricular dissociation). Sometimes the atrial and ventricular contractions are contiguous and sometimes they are far apart. Atrioventricular dissociation causes two important bedside findings: changing intensity of the first heart sound and intermittent cannon A waves in the venous pulse.

a. Changing Intensity of the First Heart Sound

In complete heart block, the first heart sound of most beats is faint. Intermittently, however, the atrium contracts just before the ventricle contracts, which results in a first heart of booming intensity (named "bruit de canon" for its explosive quality; see Chapter 36 for pathophysiology of S_1 intensity).[5]

The finding of a changing first heart sound is only significant when the pulse is regular, because in irregular rhythms its intensity varies with the length of the previous diastole (i.e., long diastoles cause next first heart sound to be loud; short ones cause it to be soft). If the ventricular pulse is regular, however, a changing first heart sound (or intermittent "booming" of the first heart sound) indicates only one diagnosis, atrioventricular dissociation.

b. Intermittent Appearance of Cannon A Waves in the Venous Pulse

When the atrial contraction falls intermittently just after a ventricular contraction in complete heart block, the right atrium is contracting against a closed tricuspid valve, causing an abrupt systolic outward wave in the jugular venous pulse (i.e., cannon A wave; see also Chapter 32).

Cannon A waves appearing with every arterial pulse occur in many different arrhythmias. If the cannon A wave appears *intermittently*, however, in a patient whose ventricular pulse is regular, the only diagnosis is atrioventricular dissociation.

c. Other Evidence of Atrioventricular Dissociation

Other uncommon signs of atrioventricular dissociation are regular small A waves in the venous pulse; regular muffled fourth heart sounds at the apex; or, in patients with mitral stenosis, regular short murmurs from the atrium pushing blood across the stenotic valve. All of these findings represent regular atrial contractions that continue during the long ventricular diastoles.

A rare sign of complete heart block is an intermittently audible summation gallop (or third heart sound; see Chapter 37).[6]

3. Halved Pulse

Halved pulse refers to the finding of twice as many ventricular beats as radial pulse beats. This is almost always due to premature contractions, which appear every other beat but are too weak to open the aortic valve and reach the radial pulse. Rarely, pulsus alternans may be the cause ("total alternans"),[7] although in these patients the heart tones at the apex are regular, whereas in premature contractions they are bigeminal.

C. REGULAR TACHYCARDIA

The regular tachycardias that *sometimes* are recognizable at the bedside include sinus tachycardia, atrial flutter, paroxysmal supraventricular tachycardia, and ventricular tachycardia. The bedside observations that distinguish these arrhythmias are response to vagal maneuvers, signs of atrioventricular dissociation, and abnormalities of the neck veins. Even so, bedside examination is diagnostic in only the minority of patients with rapid rates, and the careful clinician always relies on electrocardiography for diagnosis.

1. Vagal Maneuvers

The usual maneuvers are the Valsalva maneuver and carotid artery massage.

a. Technique

Both maneuvers are performed when the patient is supine. To perform the Valsalva maneuver, the clinician asks the patient to bear down and strain against a closed glottis as if "having a bowel movement." Patients who have difficulty following this instruction sometimes respond better when asked to put the tip of their own thumb in their mouth and pretend it is a balloon to blow up. In patients with supraventricular tachycardia, 15 seconds of straining is as effective as 30 seconds.[8] The maneuver increases vagal tone and has its maximal effect on tachycardias *after* the release of the Valsalva, not while the patient is straining.[8]

In carotid artery massage, the clinician finds the bifurcation of one carotid artery, located just below the angle of the jaw, and massages or presses on it for 5 seconds.[8,9]

The Valsalva maneuver is preferred for two reasons: (1) it tends to be more efficacious, terminating supraventricular tachycardia 20% to 50% of the time, compared with only a 10% efficacy with carotid massage,[8,10] and (2) in elderly patients with carotid artery disease, carotid artery massage risks causing strokes.[9,11–13]

b. Response of Regular Tachycardias to Vagal Maneuvers[9]

Transient slowing of the pulse during a vagal maneuver indicates sinus tachycardia. **Abrupt termination** of the tachycardia indicates paroxysmal supraventricular tachycardia (this occurs with both nodal re-entry tachycardias and reciprocating tachycardias using an accessory pathway). **Abrupt halving** of the rate may occur in atrial flutter. **No response** is unhelpful, being characteristic of ventricular tachycardia[14] but also occurring with every other regular tachycardia.[8,10]

2. Atrioventricular Dissociation

Any finding of atrioventricular dissociation in patients with regular tachycardia indicates the rhythm is ventricular tachycardia. These findings include the *intermittent* appearance of cannon A waves in the neck veins, changing intensity of the first heart sound, and changing systolic blood pressure (usually detected with the blood pressure cuff).[15] In one study of patients with ventricular tachycardia, in which atrioventricular association or dissociation was determined by pacing (EBM Box 14-1), the finding of a changing S_1 argued strongly *for* atrioventricular dissociation [likelihood ratio (LR) = 24.4] and the *absence* of

Box 14-1   Atrioventricular Dissociation and Ventricular Tachycardia*

Finding (Ref)†	Sensitivity (%)	Specificity (%)	Likelihood Ratio if Finding	
			Present	Absent
Varying arterial pulse[16]	63	70	NS	NS
Intermittent cannon A waves, neck veins [16]	96	75	**3.8**	**0.1**
Changing intensity S_1[16]	58	98	**24.4**	0.4

NS, not significant; likelihood ratio (LR) if finding present = positive LR; LR if finding absent = negative LR.
*Diagnostic standards: For atrioventricular dissociation, ventricular-paced rhythm at a rate independent of the atrial rate.
†Definition of findings: For varying arterial pulse, varying amplitude of radial or carotid pulse by palpation.

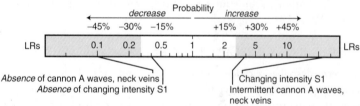

ATRIOVENTRICULAR DISSOCIATION (IF TACHYCARDIA)

intermittent cannon A waves argued convincingly *against* atrioventricular dissociation (LR = 0.1).

Even so, these LRs are somewhat misleading because some patients with ventricular tachycardia lack atrioventricular dissociation and instead have 1:1 retrograde conduction or atrial fibrillation.[14] Given the serious consequences of misdiagnosing this arrhythmia, an ECG should always be obtained.

3. Flutter Waves in the Venous Pulse

In elderly patients with a ventricular pulse of 130 to 160 beats/minute, the clinician should suspect atrial flutter with 2:1 conduction. In addition to performing vagal maneuvers, the clinician may see rapid, small undulations (with a rate about 300/minute) in the venous pulse, which are called flutter waves (or f waves) and which correspond to the wave of the same name on the ECG.[17]

4. Sensation of Pounding in the Neck

In one study of 244 consecutive patients referred for electrophysiologic testing, all of whom had intermittent rapid palpitations, the history of feeling rapid and regular pounding in the neck during the palpitations discriminated atrioventricular nodal reentrant tachycardia from other causes of tachycardia, with a sensitivity of 92%, specificity of 100%, positive LR of 350.7, and negative LR of 0.1.[18] The pounding occurs because both the carotid pulsation and cannon A waves arrive in the neck simultaneously (atrial and ventricular pulsations practically coincide in these patients). Patients with reciprocating tachycardias using an accessory pathway, another common supraventricular tachycardia, lack these pounding sensations, because the atrial contraction is delayed until well after the ventricular contraction.

D.   IRREGULAR RHYTHM THAT VARIES WITH RESPIRATION

This rhythm is sinus arrhythmia, an especially common and prominent arrhythmia of younger patients. The pulse characteristically quickens during inspiration and slows during exhalation (see Fig. 14-2).[19] The slowing during expiration is sometimes so conspicuous it mimics the finding of a pause.

E.   IRREGULARLY IRREGULAR RHYTHM ("CHAOTIC" RHYTHM)

This term describes a cadence of ventricular and radial beats that is completely irregular and unpredictable. The diagnosis is usually atrial fibrillation. Frequent premature contractions may sometimes seem chaotic at the bedside, but two findings distinguish this rhythm from atrial fibrillation: (1) **Venous pulse.** In atrial fibrillation, the venous pulse is simple and consists of only one wave per cardiac cycle (i.e., there is no A wave and the x′ descent is diminished; see Chapter 32). In frequent premature contractions, in contrast, the venous pulse is complex and consists of intermittent cannon A waves superimposed on two venous movements per cardiac cycle. (2) **Rhythm of ventricular pulse** (Fig. 14-4). In atrial fibrillation, the interval between ventricular beats is random, and it is quite common to have one pause followed by an even longer pause. In frequent premature contractions, this is impossible because the pause must be followed by another quick beat or the normal sinus interval. This difference in rhythm, which again focuses on the ventricular rhythm at the apex, not the radial pulse, is quite conspicuous once the clinician is aware of it.

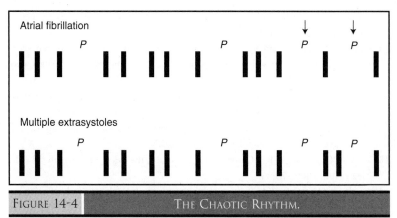

FIGURE 14-4	THE CHAOTIC RHYTHM.

The irregularly irregular or "chaotic" rhythm may represent atrial fibrillation (*top*) or sinus rhythm with multiple extrasystoles (*bottom*). "P" marks conspicuous pauses that appear in the cadence of *apical* heart tones (each bar depicts one cardiac cycle, or one "lub dup"). In this example, the cadence of the two arrhythmias is identical until the end of the tracing: In atrial fibrillation, two pauses occur in a row (*arrows*), thus distinguishing it from the pauses of multiple extrasystoles that are flanked by quick beats or beats of normal cadence. See text.

REFERENCES

1. Mackenzie J. *The study of the pulse: Arterial, venous, and hepatic and of the movements of the heart* (facsimile by the Classics of Cardiology Library). Edinburgh: Young J. Pentland; 1902.

2. Wenckebach KF. *Arrhythmia of the heart: A physiological and clinical study* (facsimile by the Classics of Cardiology Library). Edinburgh: William Green and Sons; 1904.

3. Lewis T. *Clinical disorders of the heart beat*, 4th ed. London: Shaw and Sons; 1918.

4. Lewis T. *The mechanism and graphic registration of the heart beat*, 3rd ed. London: Shaw and Sons Ltd.; 1925.

5. Burggraf GW, Craige E. The first heart sound in complete heart block: Phono-echocardiographic correlations. *Circulation.* 1974;50:17-24.

6. Iga K, Konishi T. Intermittently audible "third heart sound" as a sign of complete atrioventricular block in patients with a VVI pacemaker. *Int J Cardiol.* 1999;71:135-139.

7. Liu CK, Luisada AA. Halving of the pulse due to severe alternans (pulsus bisectus). *Am Heart J.* 1955;50:927-932.

8. Mehta D, Wafa S, Ward DE, Camm AJ. Relative efficacy of various physical manoeuvres in the termination of junctional tachycardia. *Lancet.* 1988;1:1181-1185.

9. Schweitzer P, Teichholz LE. Carotid sinus massage: Its diagnostic and therapeutic value in arrhythmias. *Am J Med.* 1985;78:645-654.

10. Lim SH, Anantharaman V, Teo WS, et al. Comparison of treatment of supraventricular tachycardia by Valsalva maneuver and carotid sinus massage. *Ann Emerg Med.* 1998;31:30-35.

11. Richardson DA, Bexton R, Shaw FE, et al. Complications of carotid sinus massage—A prospective series of older patients. *Age Ageing.* 2000;29:412-417.

12. Davies AJ, Kenny RA. Frequency of neurologic complications following carotid sinus massage. *Am J Cardiol.* 1998;81:1256-1257.

13. Veitch PC, Montague RE. Carotid sinus massage in the elderly: Is it worth the risk? *Med J Aust.* 2000;173:83.

14. Armbrust CA, Levine SA. Paroxysmal ventricular tachycardia: A study of one hundred and seven cases. *Circulation.* 1950;1:28-40.

15. Wilson WS, Judge RD, Siegel JH. A simple diagnostic sign in ventricular tachycardia. *N Engl J Med.* 1964;270:446-448.

16. Garratt CJ, Griffith MJ, Young G, et al. Value of physical signs in the diagnosis of ventricular tachycardia. *Circulation.* 1994;90:3103-3107.

17. Hartman H. The jugular venous tracing. *Am Heart J.* 1960;59:698-717.

18. Gursoy S, Steurer G, Brugada J, et al. The hemodynamic mechanism of pounding in the neck in atrioventricular nodal reentrant tachycardia. *N Engl J Med.* 1992;327:772-774.

19. van Ravenswaaij-Arts CMA, Kollee LAA, Hopman JCW, et al. Heart rate variability. *Ann Intern Med.* 1993;118:436-447.

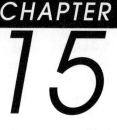

Blood Pressure

I. INTRODUCTION

Systolic blood pressure is the maximal pressure within the artery during ventricular systole, **diastolic blood pressure** is the lowest pressure in the vessel just before the next systole, and **pulse pressure** is the difference between them. Pulse pressure may be normal, abnormally small ("narrow"), or abnormally large ("wide"; see "Abnormal Pulse Pressure" later). The mean arterial pressure can be estimated by $(S+2D)/3$, where S is systolic blood pressure and D is diastolic blood pressure.[1]

The first person to measure blood pressure was Stephen Hales, an English clergyman of creative genius, who in 1708 directly connected the left crural artery of a horse to a 9-feet tall glass manometer using brass tubes and a trachea of goose.[2,3] Vierordt of Germany introduced the indirect method of measuring blood pressure in 1855, based on the principle that blood pressure is equal to the amount of external pressure necessary to obliterate the distal pulse. Indirect measurements required cumbersome mechanical devices and were not widely accepted until 1896, when the Italian Riva-Rocci invented the blood pressure cuff.[2,3]

Blood pressure was the last of the four traditional vital signs to be routinely monitored in hospitalized patients. In 1901, after Harvey Cushing first brought the blood pressure cuff to America and encouraged its use in neurosurgical patients, most clinicians resisted using it because they believed palpation of pulse revealed much more information, characterized by the pulse's "fullness," "tension," "rate," "rhythm," "size," "force," and "duration."[4,5] Two events were responsible for clinicians eventually accepting the blood pressure cuff: (1) Korotkoff described his sounds in 1905, which allowed clinicians to easily measure systolic and diastolic blood pressure and (2) Janeway published his book *Clinical Study of Blood Pressure* in 1907, which proved that monitoring blood pressure was clinically useful (e.g., Janeway showed that the first sign of intestinal perforation or hemorrhage in typhoid fever was a falling blood pressure).[6] By the First World War, blood pressure was routinely recorded by most clinicians along with the patient's pulse, respirations, and temperature.[5,7,8]

II. TECHNIQUE

A. RECOMMENDED METHOD OF MEASURING BLOOD PRESSURE[9,10]

Published recommendations for measuring blood pressure are based on the consensus opinion of expert committees who have reviewed all available scientific evidence. These recommendations, however, are designed to avoid misdiagnosis of hypertension and may not be as relevant to clinicians using the blood pressure cuff to diagnose other abnormalities, such as hypotension or abnormalities of pulse contour (see later and Chapter 13).

The important elements of the correct technique are as follows: (1) the patient should sit in a chair with his or her back supported and should rest for at least 5 minutes before the blood pressure is measured; (2) the patient's arm should be at the heart level; (3) the length of the blood pressure cuff's bladder should encircle at least 80% of the arm's circumference; (4) the clinician should inflate the cuff to a pressure 20 to 30 mm Hg above systolic pressure, as first identified by palpation of the distal pulse (i.e., the pulse disappears when cuff pressure exceeds systolic pressure); (5) the pressure in the cuff should be released at a rate of 2 mm Hg per second; (6) the clinician should obtain at least two readings separated by at least 30 seconds and average them; if these differ by more than 5 mm Hg, additional readings are necessary; and (7) the readings should be rounded off to the nearest 2 mm Hg.

These recommendations sometimes state that the bell of the stethoscope should be used, because Korotkoff sounds contain primarily low-frequency sound, although this technique is often inconvenient and one study showed that measurements made by the bell and diaphragm were the same.[11]

In some clinical scenarios, described in "The Findings and Their Clinical Significance," additional measurements are necessary, including those of the legs or opposite arm or measurements taken with the patient in different positions.

B. KOROTKOFF SOUNDS

1. Definition of Systolic and Diastolic Blood Pressure

As the cuff is slowly deflated from a point above systolic pressure, the first appearance of sound (Korotkoff phase 1) indicates systolic blood pressure.* Clinicians have debated for decades whether the muffling of sound (Korotkoff phase 4) or disappearance of sound (Korotkoff phase 5) better indicates diastolic blood pressure, although now all experts favor using phase 5 for the following reasons: (1) in most studies, phase 5 sounds correlate better with intra-arterial measurements of diastolic blood pressure;[15,16] (2) many persons lack phase 4 sounds;[15,17] (3) interobserver agreement is better for phase 5 sounds than phase 4 sounds;[15,17] and, most importantly, (4) long-term studies showing that hypertension increases the risk of cardiovascular events and that treatment reduces this risk have used phase 5 sounds as the definition of diastolic blood pressure.[18–20]

2. Pathogenesis

Korotkoff sounds are produced underneath the *distal* half of the blood pressure cuff.[21] The sounds occur with cuff pressures between the systolic and diastolic blood pressure, because the underlying artery is collapsing completely and then reopening with each heart beat. The artery collapses because cuff pressure exceeds diastolic pressure; it opens again with each beat because cuff pressure is less than systolic pressure. The sound represents the sudden deceleration of the rapidly opening arterial walls, which causes a snapping or tapping sound just like the sail of a boat that snaps when it suddenly tenses after tacking in the wind or like a handkerchief that snaps when its ends are suddenly drawn taut.[21–25] Once cuff pressure falls below the diastolic blood pressure, the sound disappears, because the vessel wall no longer collapses but instead gently ebbs and expands with each beat, being held open by diastolic pressure.

The genesis of the Korotkoff sounds, therefore, is similar to the genesis of other snapping or tapping sounds produced by the sudden deceleration of other biologic membranes, such as the normal first and second heart sounds or the femoral pistol shot sounds of aortic regurgitation (see Chapters 36 and 41).

---

*There are five Korotkoff phases, numbered in order as they appear during deflation of the cuff. The initial tapping sound at systolic blood pressure is phase 1, a swishing murmur is phase 2, the reappearance of a softer tapping sound is phase 3, the disappearance of the tapping and appearance of a much softer murmur ("muffling") is phase 4, and the disappearance of all sound is phase 5.[2] Korotkoff described only four of these sounds (phases 1, 2, 3, and 5). Ettinger added the muffling point (phase 4) in 1907.[7,12,13] All five phases are audible with electronic stethoscopes in 40% of adults.[14]

C. MEASUREMENT USING PALPATION

Even before the discovery of Korotkoff sounds, clinicians used the blood pressure cuff to measure both systolic and diastolic blood pressure.[6] Systolic blood pressure was simply the amount of cuff pressure necessary to obliterate the pulse. Clinicians still use this technique to measure the pressure of patients with hypotension, when Korotkoff sounds are faint, or to determine whether the patient has an auscultatory gap (see later).

To identify diastolic pressure, clinicians can use one of two methods. In the first method, the clinician applies light pressure to palpate the brachial artery just below the blood pressure cuff. As the cuff is deflated, the first appearance of a pulse indicates systolic blood pressure. As the cuff pressure falls more and approaches diastolic pressure, the pulsatile forces distending the artery distal to the cuff progressively grow, eventually causing a sudden shock to strike the clinician's fingers as the artery abruptly opens and then completely collapses with each beat (this abrupt tapping sensation is similar to the "water-hammer pulse" of aortic regurgitation).[22] At the moment the cuff pressure falls below diastolic blood pressure, the shocking sensations disappear, being replaced by a much gentler pulse, because the underlying artery no longer collapses completely between beats. The cuff pressure at this "lower limit of maximal pulsation" indicates the diastolic blood pressure.[6]

A second method requires a rigid and tightly applied cuff, so that the arterial pulsations under the cuff are actually transmitted to the manometer. As the cuff pressure decreases, the mercury column of a mercury manometer or the indicator needle of an aneroid manometer starts to bob with increasing amplitude, until the bobbing suddenly disappears at the moment cuff pressure falls below diastolic pressure.[6] Many patients with tightly applied cuffs also experience a similar pounding sensation in their arm near the diastolic pressure, which abruptly disappears the moment cuff pressure falls below diastolic blood pressure.

Measurements of systolic and diastolic blood pressure by palpation differ from readings by auscultation by only 6 to 8 mm Hg or less.[26,27]

D. POSTURAL VITAL SIGNS[28]

When obtaining postural vital signs (i.e., comparison of measurements when the patient is supine with those when the patient is upright), clinicians should wait 2 minutes before measuring the supine vital signs and 1 minute after standing before measuring the upright vital signs. These recommendations are based on the following observations: (1) shorter periods of supine rest significantly reduce the sensitivity of postural vital signs for detecting blood loss and (2) after normal persons stand, the pulse change stabilizes after 45 to 60 seconds and the blood pressure stabilizes after 1 to 2 minutes. Counting the heart rate first, beginning at 1 minute, allows more time for the blood pressure to stabilize.

Supine vital signs should always be compared with standing vital signs, because sitting instead of standing significantly reduces the clinician's ability to detect postural changes after blood loss.[29,30]

E. COMMON ERRORS

Biologic variation of blood pressure is common, and many studies show that blood pressure measurements vary with physical activity, smoking, caffeine ingestion, emotional state, temperature of the room, and season.[20,31,32] In addition, the blood pressure measurement may be inaccurate because of inappropriate technique, improper equipment, or other biases related to the observer.[13,32]

1. Wrong Cuff Size

In 1901, von Recklinghausen discovered that Riva-Rocci's original blood pressure cuff, whose bladder was about the size of a bicycle tire, was too narrow and often overestimated the true blood pressure, especially in larger arms.[7,33,34] Subsequent investigations have shown that both the bladder width and length affect the measurement, although if the bladder encircles at least 80% of the arm's circumference, the effect of width is minimized.[16,33,35] The bladder of the standard cuff measures 12 × 23 cm and thus is appropriate only for arm circumferences up to 28 cm, which includes only 60% to 70% of the European adult population.[33]

Cuffs that are too short overestimate blood pressure because they transmit cuff pressure inefficiently to the underlying soft tissues. Much higher cuff pressures are then necessary to cause collapse of the artery, leading the clinician to misdiagnose hypertension when it is not present.[35] This error is greater the farther the *center* of the bladder is positioned from the brachial artery.[16]

The significance of the opposite error—underestimation of true blood pressure by using too large a cuff—is controversial, although most studies show that such an error is small. Table 15-1 presents the mean errors resulting from using cuffs too small or too large. These data are based on measurements of blood pressure in the same individual with three cuffs of different sizes, assuming that the most accurate measurement is the one made with the smallest cuff encircling 80% of the arm. The greatest errors, according to these data, occur from using too small of a cuff; the risk of underestimating true pressure with too large a cuff is relatively small.

2. Auscultatory Gap

Up to 20% of elderly patients with hypertension have an auscultatory gap, which means that the phase 1 Korotkoff sounds normally appear at systolic pressure but then disappear for varying lengths of time before they reappear above the diastolic pressure.[37] This "auscultatory gap" is important because

| Table 15-1 | Blood Pressure Cuff Size and Error in Measurement* |

Cuff Bladder Size	Arm Circumference		
	28 cm or Less	29 to 42 cm	43 cm or More
Regular (12 × 23 cm)	Accurate	Overestimates SBP by 4–8 mm Hg DBP by 3–6 mm Hg	Overestimates SBP by 16–17 mm Hg DBP by 10–11 mm Hg
Large (15 × 33 cm)	Underestimates SBP by 2–3 mm Hg DBP by 1–2 mm Hg	Accurate	Overestimates SBP by 5–7 mm Hg DBP by 2–4 mm Hg
Thigh (18 × 36 cm)	Underestimates SBP by 5–7 mm Hg DBP by 1–3 mm Hg	Underestimates SBP by 5–7 mm Hg DBP by 2–4 mm Hg	Accurate

DBP, diastolic blood pressure reading; SBP, systolic blood pressure reading.
*Overestimation means that hypertension may be diagnosed in someone with normal blood pressure; underestimation means that the blood pressure reading may be normal in someone who actually has high blood pressure. See text for further discussion. Data from reference 36.

inflation of the cuff only to the initial disappearance of sounds (i.e., auscultatory gap) significantly underestimates the true systolic blood pressure. Because the distal pulse persists during the auscultatory gap, however, clinicians can avoid this mistake by palpating the systolic pressure before using the stethoscope.

The cause of the auscultatory gap remains a mystery. Patients with auscultatory gaps have twice as much arterial atherosclerotic plaque as those without a gap, suggesting perhaps that the gap is somehow related to arterial stiffness.[37] Venous congestion also seems to promote auscultatory gaps, because slow cuff inflation (which increases venous congestion) sometimes makes auscultatory gaps appear and elevation of the arm before inflating the cuff makes them disappear.[34]

The auscultatory gap was discovered by Krylov in 1906, 1 year after Korotkoff's discovery.[12] In part, the discovery of the auscultatory gap was responsible for the initial reluctance of clinicians to adopt Korotkoff's method of indirect blood pressure measurement.[7]

3.   Stethoscope Pressure Too Firm

Excessive pressure with the stethoscope artificially lowers the diastolic reading, sometimes by 10 mm Hg or more, although the systolic reading is usually unaffected.[38] This error occurs because the stethoscope pressure then contributes to the collapse of the underlying artery (i.e., the total tissue pressure around the artery represents the sum of both cuff and stethoscope pressure). If the clinician applies 10 mm Hg of stethoscope pressure to the arm of a patient whose intra-arterial diastolic pressure is 80 mm Hg, the diastolic reading will be 70 mm Hg (i.e., Korotkoff sounds disappear at a tissue pressure of 80 mm Hg = 70 mm Hg cuff pressure, the basis for the reading, and 10 mm Hg of stethoscope pressure).

4.   Inappropriate Level of the Arm

The recommended position of the patient's elbow is the "level of the heart," which is usually regarded to be the fourth intercostal space at the sternum. If the patient's arm is instead 6 to 7 cm higher (e.g., level of the sternomanubrial junction), both the systolic and diastolic readings will be about 5 mm Hg lower. If the arm is 7 to 8 cm lower (e.g. level of the xiphosternal junction), the pressures will be about 6 mm Hg higher.[39]

These errors are completely explained by the hydrostatic effect. When the arm is at the lower position, for example, the measured pressure is the sum of the blood pressure in the artery plus the weight of a column of blood 8 cm high (i.e., 8 cm blood = $(8 \div 13.6) \times 1.06 = 0.6$ cm or 6 mm Hg; 13.6 = density of mercury; 1.06 = density of blood).

5.   Terminal Digit Preference[31,32]

Clinicians often tend to round off blood pressure readings to the nearest 0, 5, or other preferred number, a bias called terminal digit preference. Clinical studies minimize this and other observer biases by using oscillometric devices, which measure oscillations of pressure instead of Korotkoff sounds and use computer programs to digitally display the blood pressure reading,[10] or by using a random zero sphygmomanometer, which blinds the clinician to the true reading.[20,40]

III.   THE FINDINGS AND THEIR CLINICAL SIGNIFICANCE

A.   HYPERTENSION
1.   Essential Hypertension

Essential hypertension is defined as three or more blood pressure readings taken over three visits separated by weeks whose average exceeds 140/90 (i.e., systolic blood pressure of 140 mm Hg and diastolic blood pressure of 90 mm Hg).[9] The threshold is lower for patients with diabetes or chronic kidney disease (i.e., hypertension=readings>130/80 mm Hg). Detecting essential hypertension is the reason blood pressure should be measured in every person, even when asymptomatic, because the disorder is common and treatable and because treatment reduces cardiovascular morbidity and overall mortality.

2. Pseudohypertension and Osler's Sign

"Pseudohypertension" describes the finding of elevated indirect measurements in persons who have normal intra-arterial pressure. The traditional explanation for pseudohypertension is that the artery under the cuff is so stiff and calcified it remains open long after the cuff pressure exceeds systolic blood pressure, continuing to produce Korotkoff sounds.

The diagnosis of pseudohypertension requires direct cannulation of the patient's artery, which is of course inappropriate and impractical during daily routine. A single study from 1985 proposed that a simple physical finding, Osler's sign, accurately identifies patients with pseudohypertension.[41] This sign is positive if the patient's radial or brachial artery distal to the cuff remains palpable after inflation of the cuff above systolic blood pressure.

Osler's sign, however, has limited clinical value. It occurs commonly in elderly individuals, whether or not they have hypertension (11% older than the age of 75 years and 44% older than 85 years have a positive Osler's sign).[42] Other investigators have shown that almost all patients with Osler's sign do not have pseudohypertension but instead actually have direct measurements that exceed the indirect ones.[43,44]

Although pseudohypertension remains an important problem in blood pressure measurements of the legs, especially in diabetic patients with intermittent claudication (see Chapter 50), undue emphasis on pseudohypertension in the brachial artery misses the point that all clinical studies demonstrating the benefits of treating essential hypertension used the blood pressure cuff and indirect measurements, not intra-arterial measurements.

B. HYPOTENSION

In patients with acute illness, hypotension is ominous. It predicts death in patients hospitalized in the intensive care unit (likelihood ratio [LR] = 4.0, EBM Box 15-1) and in patients with bacteremia (LR = 4.9), pneumonia (LR = 10.0), and myocardial infarction (LR = 15.5). Presumably, it predicts mortality in many other acute disorders as well. The Acute Physiology and Chronic Health Evaluation (APACHE) scoring system, which predicts the risk of hospital mortality among patients in the intensive care unit, assigns more

Box
15-1

Hypotension and Prognosis

Finding (Ref)	Sensitivity (%)	Specificity (%)	Likelihood Ratio if Finding	
			Present	Absent
Systolic blood pressure <90 mm Hg				
Predicting mortality in intensive care unit[45]	21	95	**4.0**	0.8
Predicting mortality in patients with bacteremia[46,47]	13–71	85–91	**4.9**	NS
Predicting mortality in patients with pneumonia[48–50]	11–35	97–99	**10.0**	NS
Systolic blood pressure ≤80 mm Hg				
Predicting mortality in patients with acute myocardial infarction[51]	32	98	**15.5**	0.7

NS, not significant; likelihood ratio (LR) if finding present = positive LR; LR if finding absent = negative LR.

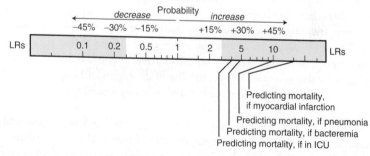

HYPOTENSION

decrease Probability increase

−45% −30% −15%   +15% +30% +45%

LRs   0.1   0.2   0.5   1   2   5   10   LRs

Predicting mortality, if myocardial infarction
Predicting mortality, if pneumonia
Predicting mortality, if bacteremia
Predicting mortality, if in ICU

points (and thus a higher risk) to severe hypotension than to any other physiologic variable.[52] In patients with myocardial infarction, a systolic blood pressure less than 80 mm Hg also predicts a much higher incidence of congestive heart failure, ventricular tachycardia and fibrillation, and complete heart block.[51]

C. DIFFERENCES IN PRESSURE BETWEEN THE ARMS

The average difference in systolic blood pressure between the two arms is 6 to 10 mm Hg.[53,54] Differences of 20 mm Hg or more are uncommon and usually indicate obstructed flow in the subclavian artery leading to the arm with the lower pressure. This is a significant finding in the following two clinical settings:

1. Subclavian Steal Syndrome

The finding of one weak radial pulse in a patient with symptoms of vertebral-basilar ischemia (episodic vertigo, visual complaints, hemiparesis, ataxia, or diplopia) suggests the subclavian steal syndrome. In this syndrome, stenosis or occlusion of one subclavian artery proximal to the origin of the vertebral artery reduces the pressure distal to the obstruction, which causes the flow in the vertebral artery to reverse directions: instead of traveling normally up the vertebral artery to perfuse the brain, blood flow courses downward to perfuse the arm (i.e., the arm "steals" blood from the posterior circulation).[55] Ninety-four percent of patients with subclavian steal have a systolic blood pressure that is 20 mm Hg or more lower on the affected side compared to the opposite arm (the mean difference between the arms is 45 mm Hg in affected patients).[56] Most patients have an ipsilateral radial pulse that is diminished or absent and a systolic bruit over the ipsilateral subclavian artery.[56] The left side is affected in 70% and the right side in 30%.[56]

2. Aortic Dissection

The finding of a difference in blood pressure between the two arms in a patient with acute chest pain suggests aortic dissection. EBM Box 15-2 presents the accuracy of physical examination in more than 400 patients presenting to emergency departments with acute chest or upper back pain suspicious for aortic dissection. In these studies, two findings were compelling arguments for aortic dissection: focal neurologic signs (from obstruction of cranial or spinal arteries, LR = 33.4), and the presence of a pulse deficit (i.e., absent extremity or carotid pulse, LR = 6.0). Mediastinal or aortic widening on chest radiography also increased the probability of dissection, although only modestly (LR = 2.0); the *absence* of mediastinal widening argued *against* dissection (LR = 0.3).[57,59,60]

In these studies, the murmur of aortic regurgitation was diagnostically unhelpful, possibly because of the highly selected nature of enrolled patients: these patients represented only 0.3% of patients with chest or back pain evaluated in these centers[59]; one third had the murmur of aortic regurgitation, and one half had the diagnosis of dissection eventually confirmed.

Von Kodolitsch et al.[59] have identified three independent predictors of aortic dissection in patients with acute chest pain: (1) pain that is tearing or ripping; (2) pulse deficits, blood pressure differentials (>20 mm Hg), or both (see

Box 15-2   Aortic Dissection *

Finding (Ref)[†]	Sensitivity (%)	Specificity (%)	Likelihood Ratio if Finding	
			Present	Absent
Individual findings				
Pulse deficit[57-59]	12–49	82–99	**6.0**	NS
Aortic regurgitation murmur[57-60]	15–49	45–95	NS	NS
Focal neurologic signs[59]	14	100	**33.4**	NS
Combined findings[59]				
0 predictors	4	47	**0.1**	...
1 predictor	20	...	0.5	...
2 predictors	49	...	**5.3**	...
3 predictors	27	100	**65.8**	...

NS, not significant; likelihood ratio (LR) if finding present = positive LR; LR if finding absent = negative LR.

*Diagnostic standard: For aortic dissection, transesophageal echocardiography,[57,60] aortography,[58] or any of a variety of tests (i.e., computed tomography, magnetic resonance imaging, transesophageal echocardiography, or digital angiography).[59]

[†]Definition of findings: For pulse deficit, absent extremity or carotid pulse[57,58] or 20 mm Hg difference in blood pressure in the arms, absent extremity or carotid pulse, or both[59]; for combined findings, see text.

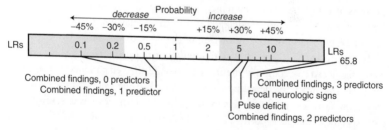

AORTIC DISSECTION

footnote to EBM Box 15-2 for definition); and (3) mediastinal or aortic widening on chest radiography. The absence of all three predictors argues *against* the diagnosis of dissection (LR = 0.1, see EBM Box 15-2); two predictors argues *for* dissection (LR = 5.3), and the presence of all three predictors is pathognomonic for dissection (LR = 65.8).

Rare patients with aortic dissection present with the physical findings of pulsatile sternoclavicular joints[61] or unilateral femoral pistol shot sounds (see Chapter 41).[62]

In patients with established aortic dissection, three findings increase the probability that the dissection involves the proximal aorta (i.e., it is a type A dissection, not a type B dissection): systolic blood pressure less than 100 mm Hg (LR = 5.0), murmur of aortic regurgitation (LR = 5.0), and a pulse deficit (LR = 2.3).[57,58,61,63,64] In patients with acute type A dissection, pulse deficits are associated with increased hospital mortality.[65]

D. DIFFERENCES IN PRESSURE BETWEEN ARMS AND LEGS

This finding is valuable in two clinical settings.

1. Chronic Ischemia of the Lower Extremities

Chapter 50 describes calculation of the ankle-arm index, which is the principal bedside tool used in patients with intermittent claudication.

2. Coarctation of the Aorta

In young patients with hypertension, the finding of an unobtainable blood pressure in the legs or a blood pressure that is much lower in the legs than arms suggests the diagnosis of coarctation of the aorta.[66,67] These patients also have hypertension of the arms (96% have a blood pressure >140/90 mm Hg), femoral pulses that are absent or diminished and delayed (100%), augmented carotid pulsations, various murmurs (usually a systolic murmur at the sternal border and a continuous murmur posteriorly over the upper spine), and visible collateral arteries (usually around the scapula, intercostal spaces, or axilla).[66,67]

During simultaneous palpation of the femoral and radial arteries of healthy persons, it is impossible to tell which comes first. In patients with coarctation, however, the femoral pulse is delayed, due both to delay in arrival at the legs and to more rapid than normal conduction of the wave to the arms.[68]

In one study of 1206 children with unexplained heart murmurs, clinicians correctly diagnosed coarctation of the aorta in 18 of 22 affected patients (in this study, the overall accuracy for detecting coarctation by bedside examination—presumably using arm-to-leg blood pressure or pulse discrepancies—was sensitivity of 82%, specificity of 100%, positive LR = 242.2, and negative LR = 0.2).[69]

E. ABNORMAL PULSE CONTOUR

The three abnormalities of pulse contour—pulsus paradoxus, pulsus alternans, and pulsus bisferiens—are easily detectable using the blood pressure cuff (see Chapter 13).

F. ABNORMAL PULSE PRESSURE

1. Abnormally Small Pulse Pressure

Because the pulse pressure depends on stroke volume, clinicians have tried for decades to use it as a way to quantify cardiac output. This relationship has been validated in only one setting, in patients with known left ventricular dysfunction: In these patients, the finding of a proportional pulse pressure (i.e., the pulse pressure divided by the systolic pressure) less than 0.25 detects a cardiac index less than 2.2 L/min/m² with a sensitivity of 70% to 91%, specificity of 83% to 93%, positive LR = 6.9, and negative LR = 0.2.[70,71]

In contrast to conventional teachings, many patients with significant aortic stenosis have a normal pulse pressure (see Chapter 40).[72]

2. Abnormally Large Pulse Pressure

In patients with the murmur of aortic insufficiency, a pulse pressure of 80 mm Hg or greater argues that the regurgitation is moderate or severe, with a sensitivity of 57%, specificity of 95%, and positive LR = 10.9.[73]

G. ORTHOSTATIC HYPOTENSION

When a person stands, 350 to 600 mL of blood shifts to the lower body. Normally, the blood pressure remains relatively stable during this shift because of compensatory increases in cardiac output, heart rate, and systemic vascular resistance, and transfer of blood from the pulmonary circulation to the systemic side.[28] Orthostatic hypotension, usually defined as a fall in systolic blood pressure of 20 mm Hg or greater when the patient stands from the supine position, may occur if: (1) compensatory mechanisms fail (i.e., "autonomic insufficiency") or (2) the patient has lost excessive amounts of fluid from the vascular space (e.g., acute blood loss).

1. Postural Vital Signs in Healthy Persons

As normovolemic persons stand up from the supine position, the pulse increases on average by 10.9 beats/minute, systolic blood pressure decreases by 3.5 mm Hg, and diastolic blood pressure increases by 5.2 mm Hg.[28] Postural hypotension, defined as a decrement in systolic blood pressure of 20 mm Hg or greater, occurs in 10% of normovolemic individuals younger than 65 years and in 11% to 30% older than 65 years.[28] As persons age, the postural pulse increment diminishes (r = −0.50, p<.02); this phenomenon and the observation that older persons have more postural hypotension suggests that autonomic reflexes decline as persons age.

2. Vital Signs and Hypovolemia

Table 15-2 presents the vital signs from normal persons before and after phlebotomy of 450 to 630 mL (moderate blood loss) or 630 to 1150 mL (large blood loss).* Chapter 9 reviews the other physical findings of hypovolemia.

a. Postural Change in Pulse

Table 15-2 shows that the most valuable observation is *either* a postural pulse increment of 30/minute or more *or* the inability of the patient to stand long enough for vital signs because of severe dizziness. Most persons have one or both of these findings after large amounts of blood loss (sensitivity = 98%), but only one of five persons develop either of them after moderate blood loss (sensitivity ranges from 7% to 57%, see Table 15-2).[28] These findings are durable after hemorrhage, lasting at least 12 to 72 hours if intravenous fluids are withheld.[30,82,83]

b. Postural Change in Blood Pressure

After excluding those patients unable to stand for vital signs (which includes almost all patients after large amounts of blood loss), the finding of postural hypotension (≥ 20 mm Hg postural decrement in systolic blood pressure) has no proven value, being found just as often in patients before blood loss as after it. For example, in persons younger than 65 years, postural hypotension is found in 8% before moderate blood loss and 9% after blood loss. For those 65 years or older, postural hypotension is detected in 11% to 30% before blood loss and about 25% after blood loss.[28,75]

Obviously, because severe dizziness with standing is a valuable finding, but postural hypotension of 20 mm Hg is not, there must be an intermediate level of postural fall (e.g., 30 mm Hg, 40 mm Hg, or another value), not yet identified, that better discriminates between patients with and without blood loss.

c. Supine Pulse and Supine Blood Pressure

In patients with suspected blood loss, both supine tachycardia and supine hypotension are specific indicators of significant blood loss, although both are infrequent. After moderate blood loss, 0% have tachycardia in the supine position and only 13% have supine hypotension; after large blood loss, only 10% have tachycardia and 31% have hypotension.

---

*Calculating LRs for these data is not appropriate because "acute blood loss" has endless gradations of severity, many of which are important to the clinician. For example, the LR of physical signs for moderate blood loss are of little use to the clinician who, when taking care of the patient with melena, regards blood loss of 400 mL ("disease-negative" according to the LR) to be as significant as a loss of 500 mL ("disease-positive"). Table 15-2 instead just illustrates the general trends of vital signs with increasing amounts of blood loss.

Table 15-2	Vital Signs and Acute Blood Loss*		
Physical Finding (Ref)[†]	Moderate Blood Loss, Sensitivity (%)	Large Blood Loss, Sensitivity (%)	Specificity (%)
Postural pulse increment ≥30/min or severe postural dizziness[29,74-76]	7–57	98	99
Postural hypotension (≥20 mm Hg decrease in SBP)[74,75]	9	...	90–98
Supine tachycardia (pulse>100/min)[30,76-79]	1	10	99
Supine hypotension (SBP<95 mm Hg)[30,77,78,80,81]	13	31	98

SBP, systolic blood pressure.
*Data obtained from 568 normal persons, mostly young and healthy, after "moderate" blood loss (phlebotomy of 450–630 mL) or "large" blood loss (phlebotomy of 630–1150 mL). "Specificity" from same patients when euvolemic, before blood loss. Results are overall mean frequency or, if statistically heterogenous, the range of values. Adapted from reference 28.
†Definition of finding: For postural, the difference between supine and standing measurements; for postural hypotension (≥20 mm Hg decrease in SBP), the finding applies only to patients able to stand without severe dizziness.

Sinus bradycardia, in contrast, is a common arrhythmia after blood loss and often precedes the drop in blood pressure that causes patients to faint.[28]

H. BLOOD PRESSURE AND IMPAIRED CONSCIOUSNESS

Patients with impaired consciousness may have either a structural intracranial lesion (e.g., stroke or brain tumors) or metabolic encephalopathy (e.g., hepatic encephalopathy, diabetic coma, drug intoxication, or sepsis). Patients with structural lesions tend to have higher blood pressures (from reflex responses to increases in intracranial pressure—the Cushing reflex—or from the etiologic association of hypertension and stroke) than patients with metabolic encephalopathy (whose severe comorbidities often are associated with lower blood pressure). In one study of 529 consecutive patients with impaired consciousness (i.e., Glasgow coma scale <15) but no head trauma, a systolic blood pressure of 160 mm Hg or greater argued significantly *for* a structural lesion (LR = 10.4, EBM Box 15-3), whereas readings less than 120 mm Hg argued against structural disorders (LR = 0.1) and thus *for* metabolic encephalopathy.[84]

I. CAPILLARY FRAGILITY TEST (RUMPEL-LEEDE TEST)

Traditionally, the blood pressure cuff also was used to test capillary fragility, although measurements of blood pressure were not part of the test. Capillary fragility tests were designed to detect abnormally weakened capillary walls in the skin that would burst more easily when distended, resulting in appearance of high numbers of petechiae. The diseases associated with capillary fragility were legion, ranging from coagulopathies, vitamin deficiencies (e.g., scurvy), infectious diseases (e.g., scarlet fever), and endocrine disorders (e.g. hyperthyroidism), to dermatologic disorders (e.g., Osler-Weber-Rendu syndrome).[85] Both negative and positive pressure methods were used. The negative pressure technique applied suction to a defined area of the skin, a technique whose undoing was the eventual

 Box 15-3 Systolic Blood Pressure and Impaired Consciousness[84]

Finding	Sensitivity (%)	Specificity (%)	Likelihood Ratio if Finding Present
Detecting structural brain lesion			
Systolic blood pressure <120 mm Hg	7	35	**0.1**
Systolic blood pressure 120-159 mm Hg	35	...	NS
Systolic blood pressure ≥160 mm Hg	58	94	**10.4**

NS, not significant; likelihood ratio (LR) if finding present = positive LR.

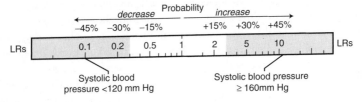

STRUCTURAL BRAIN LESION (IF COMA)

demonstration that the number of resulting petechiae depended not only on the age of patient but also on the time of day, season, and psychic influences.[86] Positive pressure methods, introduced at the turn of the century by Drs. Rumpel and Leede, consisted of raising the venous pressure by a tourniquet or blood pressure cuff around the arm and counting petechiae that subsequently developed in a defined area distally. This test was eventually standardized,[86] but interest fell after the introduction of better diagnostic tests for coagulation and the other associated disorders. More recently, increased capillary fragility was believed to represent a sign of diabetic retinopathy,[87] but this was soon disproven.[88]

REFERENCES

1. Thulin T, Andersson G, Schersten B. Measurement of blood pressure: A routine test in need of standardization. *Postgrad Med J.* 1975;51:390-395.
2. Burch GE, DePasquale NP. *Primer of clinical measurement of blood pressure.* St. Louis: CV Mosby Co; 1962.
3. Major RH. The history of taking the blood pressure. *Ann Med Hist.* 1930;2:47-55.
4. Gibson GA, Russell W. *Physical diagnosis: A guide to methods of clinical investigation,* 2nd ed. New York: D. Appleton and Co.; 1893.
5. Crenner CW. Introduction of the blood pressure cuff into U. S. medical practice: Technology and skilled practice. *Ann Intern Med.* 1998;128:488-493.
6. Janeway TC. *The clinical study of blood-pressure: A guide to the use of the sphygomomanometer.* New York: Appleton and Co; 1907.
7. Geddes LA, Hoff HE, Badger AS. Introduction of the auscultatory method of measuring blood pressure: Including a translation of Korotkoff's original paper. *Cardiovasc Res Center Bull.* 1966;5:57-74.
8. Geddes LA. Perspectives in physiological monitoring. *Med Instrument.* 1976;10: 91-97.
9. Chobanian AV, Bakris GL, Black HR, et al. The Seventh report of the Joint National Committee on prevention, detection, evaluation, and treatment of high blood pressure. The JNC 7 report. *JAMA.* 2003;289:2560-2572.
10. Pickering TG, Hall JE, Appel LJ, et al. Recommendations for blood pressure measurement in humans and experimental animals. Part 1: Blood pressure measurement in humans: A statement for professionals from the subcommittee of professional and public education of the American Heart Association Council on high blood pressure research. *Circulation.* 2005;111:697-716.
11. Cushman WC, Cooper KM, Horne RA, Meydrech EF. Effect of back support and stethoscope head on seated blood pressure determination. *Am J Hypertension.* 1990;3:240-241.
12. Askey JM. The auscultatory gap in sphygmomanometry. *Ann Intern Med.* 1974;80: 94-97.

13. Perloff D, Grim C, Flack J, et al. Human blood pressure determination by sphygmomanometry. *Circulation*. 1993;88(5 Pt 1):2460-2470.
14. O'Sullivan J, Allen J, Murray A. The forgotten Korotkoff phases: How often are phases II and III present, and how do they relate to the other Korotkoff phases? *Am J Hypertens*. 2002;15:264-268.
15. London SB, London RE. Critique of indirect diastolic end point. *Arch Intern Med*. 1967;119:39-49.
16. Karvonen MJ, Telivuo LJ, Jarvinen EJK. Sphygmomanometer cuff size and the accuracy of indirect measurement of blood pressure. *Am J Card*. 1964;13:688-693.
17. Penny J, Shennan A, De Swiet M. The reproducibility of Korotkoff 4 and 5. *Am J Hypertension*. 1996;9:839.
18. Medical Research Council Working Party. MRC trial of treatment of mild hypertension: Principal results. *Br Med J*. 1985;291:97-104.
19. Hypertension Detection and Follow-up Program Cooperative Group. Five-year findings of the hypertension detection and follow-up program. I. Reduction in mortality of persons with high blood pressure, including mild hypertension. *JAMA*. 1979;242:2562-2571.
20. Bailey RH, Bauer JH. A review of common errors in the indirect measurement of blood pressure (sphygmomanometry). *Arch Intern Med*. 1993;153:2741-2748.
21. Tavel ME, Faris J, Nasser WK, Feigenbaum H, Fisch C. Korotkoff sounds: Observations on pressure-pulse changes underlying their formation. *Circulation*. 1969;39:465-474.
22. Enselberg CD. Measurement of diastolic blood pressure by palpation. *N Engl J Med*. 1961;265:272-274.
23. Dock W. Korotkoff's sounds. *N Engl J Med*. 1980;302:1264-1267.
24. Ur A, Gordon M. Origin of Korotkoff sounds. *Am J Physiol*. 1970;218:524-529.
25. McCutcheon EP, Rushmer RF. Korotkoff sounds: An experimental critique. *Circ Res*. 1967;20:149-161.
26. Segall HN. A note on the measurement of diastolic and systolic blood pressure by the palpation of arterial vibrations (sounds) over the brachial artery. *Can Med Assoc J*. 1940;42:311-313.
27. Putt AM. A comparison of blood pressure readings by auscultation and palpation. *Nurs Res*. 1966;15:311-316.
28. McGee S, Abernethy WB, Simel DL. Is this patient hypovolemic? *JAMA*. 1999;281:1022-1029.
29. Knopp R, Claypool R, Leonardi D. Use of the tilt test in measuring acute blood loss. *Ann Emerg Med*. 1980;9:72-75.
30. Wallace J, Sharpey-Schafer EP. Blood changes following controlled haemorrhage in man. *Lancet*. 1941;241:393-395.
31. Rose GA, Holland WW, Crowley EA. A sphygmomanometer for epidemiologists. *Lancet*. 1964;1:296-300.
32. Reeves RA. Does this patient have hypertension? How to measure blood pressure. *JAMA*. 1995;273:1211-1218.

33. O'Brien E. Review: A century of confusion; which bladder for accurate blood pressure measurement? *J Human Hypertension*. 1996;10:565-572.
34. Ragan C, Bordley J. The accuracy of clinical measurements of arterial blood pressure. *Bull Johns Hopkins Hosp*. 1941;69:504-528.
35. King GE. Errors in clinical measurement of blood pressure in obesity. *Clin Sci*. 1967;32:223-237.
36. Maxwell MH, Waks AU, Schroth PC, Karam M, Dornfeld LP. Error in blood-pressure measurement due to incorrect cuff size in obese patients. *Lancet*. 1982;2: 33-35.
37. Cavallini MC, Roman MJ, Blank SG, Pini R, Pickering TG, Devereux RB. Association of the auscultatory gap with vascular disease in hypertensive patients. *Ann Intern Med*. 1996;124:877-883.
38. Londe S, Klitzner TS. Auscultatory blood pressure measurement: Effect of pressure on the head of the stethoscope. *West J Med*. 1984;141:193-195.
39. Mitchell PL, Parlin RW, Blackburn H. Effect of vertical displacement of the arm on indirect blood-pressure measurement. *N Engl J Med*. 1964;271:72-74.
40. Wright BM, Dore CF. A random-zero sphygmomanometer. *Lancet*. 1970;1:337-338.
41. Messerli FH, Ventura HO, Amodeo C. Osler's maneuver and pseudohypertension. *N Engl J Med*. 1985;312:1548-1551.
42. Tsapatsaris NP, Napolitana BT, Rothchild J. Osler's maneuver in an outpatient clinic setting. *Arch Intern Med*. 1991;151:2209-2211.
43. Kuwajima I, Hoh E, Suzuki Y, et al. Pseudohypertension in the elderly. *J Hypertension*. 1990;8:429-432.
44. Belmin J, Visintin JM, Salvatore R, et al. Osler's maneuver: Absence of usefulness for the detection of pseudohypertension in an elderly population. *Am J Med*. 1995; 98:42-49.
45. Lemeshow S, Teres D, Klar J, et al. Mortality probability models (MPM II) based on an international cohort of intensive care unit patients. *JAMA*. 1993;270:2478-2486.
46. Shapiro NI, Wolfe RE, Moore RB, et al. Mortality in emergency department sepsis (MEDS) score: A prospectively derived and validated clinical prediction rule. *Crit Care Med*. 2003;31:670-675.
47. Vales EC, Abraira V, Sanchez JCC, et al. A predictive model for mortality of blood stream infections: Bedside analysis with the Weibull function. *J Clin Epidemiol*. 2002;55:563-572.
48. Allen SC. Lobar pneumonia in Northern Zambia: Clinical study of 502 adult patients. *Thorax*. 1984;39:612-616.
49. Conte HA, Chen YT, Mehal W, et al. A prognostic rule for elderly patients admitted with community-acquired pneumonia. *Am J Med*. 1999;106:20-28.
50. Fedullo AJ, Swinburne AJ. Relationship of patient age to clinical features and outcome for in-hospital treatment of pneumonia. *J Gerontol*. 1985;40:29-33.
51. Goldberg RJ, Gore JM, Alpert JS, et al. Cardiogenic shock after acute myocardial infarction: Incidence and mortality from a community-wide perspective, 1975 to 1988. *N Engl J Med*. 1991;325:1117-1122.

52. Knaus WA, Wagner DP, Draper EA, et al. The APACHE III prognostic system: Risk prediction of hospital mortality for critically ill hospitalized adults. *Chest.* 1991;100:1619-1636.
53. Lane D, Beevers M, Barnes N, et al. Inter-arm differences in blood pressure: When are they clinical significant? *J Hypertens.* 2002;20:1089-1095.
54. Singer AJ, Hollander JE. Blood pressure: Assessment of interarm differences. *Arch Intern Med.* 1996;156:2005-2008.
55. Fisher CM. A new vascular syndrome: "The subclavian steal". *N Engl J Med.* 1961;265:912-913.
56. Fields WS, Lemak NA. Joint study of extracranial arterial occlusion. VII. Subclavian steal: A review of 168 cases. *JAMA.* 1972;222:1139-1143.
57. Armstrong WF, Bach DS, Carey LM, et al. Clinical and echocardiographic findings in patients with suspected acute aortic dissection. *Am Heart J.* 1998;136:1051-1060.
58. Enia F, Ledda G, Mauro RL, et al. Utility of echocardiography in the diagnosis of aortic dissection involving the ascending aorta. *Chest.* 1989;95:124-129.
59. von Kodolitsch Y, Schwartz AG, Nienaber CA. Clinical prediction of acute aortic dissection. *Arch Intern Med.* 2000;160:2977-2982.
60. Chan KL. Usefulness of transesophageal echocardiography in the diagnosis of conditions mimicking aortic dissection. *Am Heart J.* 1991;122:495-504.
61. Slater EE, DeSanctis RW. The clinical recognition of dissecting aortic aneurysm. *Am J Med.* 1976;60:625-633.
62. McGee SR, Adcox M. Unilateral femoral pistol-shot sounds: A clue to aortic dissection. *West J Med.* 1995;162:547-548.
63. Hagan PG, Nienaber CA, Isselbacher EM, et al. The international registry of acute aortic dissection (IRAD): New insights into an old disease. *JAMA.* 2000;283:897-903.
64. Spittell PC, Spittell JA, Joyce JW, et al. Clinical features and differential diagnosis of aortic dissection: Experience with 236 cases (1980 through 1990). *Mayo Clin Proc.* 1993;68:642-651.
65. Bossone E, Rampoldi V, Nienaber CA, et al. Usefulness of pulse deficit to predict in-hospital complications and mortality in patients with acute type A aortic dissection. *Am J Cardiol.* 2002;89:851-855.
66. Ostermiller WE, Somerndike JM, Hunter JA, et al. Coarctation of the aorta in adult patients. *J Thor Cardiovasc Surg.* 1971;61:125-130.
67. Cleland WP, Counihan TB, Goodwin JF, Steiner RE. Coarctation of the aorta. *Br Med J.* 1956;2:379-390.
68. Lewis T. Material relating to coarctation of the aorta of the adult type. *Heart.* 1933;16:205-261.
69. Danford DA, Fletcher SE, Martin AB, Gumbiner CH. Accuracy of clinical diagnosis of left heart valvular or obstructive lesions in pediatric outpatients with heart murmur. *Am J Cardiol.* 2002;89:878-884.
70. Stevenson LW, Perloff JK. The limited reliability of physical signs for estimating hemodynamics in chronic heart failure. *JAMA.* 1989;261:884-888.

71. Rohde LE, Beck-da-Silva L, Goldraich L, et al. Reliability and prognostic value of traditional signs and symptoms in outpatients with congestive heart failure. *Can J Cardiol*. 2004;20:697-702.

72. Hancock EW, Abelmann WH. A clinical study of the brachial arterial pulse form: With special reference to the diagnosis of aortic valvular disease. *Circulation*. 1957;16:572-581.

73. Frank MJ, Casanegra P, Migliori AJ, Levinson GE. The clinical evaluation of aortic regurgitation. *Arch Intern Med*. 1965;116:357-365.

74. Baraff LJ, Schriger DL. Orthostatic vital signs: Variation with age, specificity, and sensitivity in detecting a 450-mL blood loss. *Am J Emerg Med*. 1992;10:99-103.

75. Witting MD, Wears RL, Li S. Defining the positive tilt test. *Ann Emerg Med*. 1994;23:1320-1323.

76. Kosowsky JM, Han JH, Collins SP, et al. Assessment of stroke index using impedance cardiography: Comparison with traditional vital signs for detection of moderate acute blood loss in health volunteers. *Acad Emerg Med*. 2002;9:775-780.

77. Skillman JJ, Olson JE, Lyons JH, Moore FD. The hemodynamic effect of acute blood loss in normal man, with observations on the effect of the Valsalva maneuver and breath holding. *Ann Surg*. 1967;166:713-738.

78. Shenkin HA, Cheney RH, Govons SR, et al. On the diagnosis of hemorrhage in man. *Am J Med Sci*. 1944;208:421-436.

79. Ralston LA, Cobb LA, Bruce RA. Acute circulatory effects of arterial bleeding as determined by indicator-dilution curves in normal human subjects. *Am Heart J*. 1961;61:770-776.

80. Bergenwald L, Freyschuss U, Sjostrand T. The mechanism of orthostatic and haemorrhage fainting. *Scand J Clin Lab Invest*. 1977;37:209-216.

81. Warren JV, Brannon ES, Stead EA, Merrill AJ. The effect of venesection and the pooling of blood in the extremities on the atrial pressure and cardiac output in normal subjects with observations on acute circulatory collapse in three instances. *J Clin Invest*. 1945;24:337-344.

82. Green DM, Metheny D. The estimation of acute blood loss by the tilt test. *Surg Gynecol Obstet*. 1947;84:1045-1050.

83. Ebert RV, Stead EA, Gibson JG. Response of normal subjects to acute blood loss. *Arch Intern Med*. 1941;68:578-590.

84. Ikeda M, Matsunaga T, Irabu N, Yoshida S. Using vital signs to diagnose impaired consciousness: Cross sectional observation study. *BMJ*. 2002;325:800-802.

85. Peck SM, Copley AL. Diagnosis and treatment of skin manifestations of capillary fragility. *N Engl J Med*. 1946;235:900-906.

86. Beaser SB, Rudy A, Seligman AM. Capillary fragility in relation to diabetes mellitus, hypertension, and age. *Arch Intern Med*. 1944;73:18-22.

87. Reynolds WA. Identification of diabetic retinopathy (letter). *JAMA*. 1983;249:1267.

88. Williams R, Jones L. The tourniquet test and screening for diabetic retinopathy (letter). *JAMA*. 1985;254:235.

16

Temperature

I. INTRODUCTION

Fever is a fundamental sign of almost all infectious diseases and many noninfectious disorders. Clinicians began to monitor the temperature of febrile patients in the 1850s and 1860s, after Traube introduced the thermometer to hospital wards and Wunderlich published an analysis based on observation of an estimated 20,000 subjects that convinced clinicians of the value of graphing temperature over time.[1-3] These temperature charts, the first vital sign to be routinely recorded in hospitalized patients, were originally named "Wunderlich curves."[4]

II. TECHNIQUE

A. SITE OF MEASUREMENT

Thermometers are used to measure the temperature of the patient's oral cavity, rectum, axilla, or, using infrared technology, tympanic membrane. Rectal temperatures are on average 0.4° to 0.5°C (0.7°–1.0°F) higher than oral temperatures,[5-8] which in turn are 0.4° to 0.7°C (0.7°–1.3°F) higher than axillary measurements[9,10] and 0.4°C (0.7°F) higher than tympanic membrane measurements.[7,11,12] These differences, however, are only average values; the difference between rectal and oral measurements in one person on successive days may vary from −0.4° to 1.3°C (−0.8° to 2.4°F).[8]

Tympanic measurements are potentially ideal because they are rapid, convenient, and theoretically best reflect core temperature (i.e., the core temperature is the temperature of the hypothalamus, which is supplied by the same artery as the tympanic membrane).[13] Nonetheless, tympanic measurements of a single person vary over time much more than do oral or rectal measurements,[7,9,11–14] and some studies question their precision, demonstrating that the correlation between the right and left tympanic temperatures in the same person, measured only minutes apart, is poor (r=0.57).[14]

B.   VARIABLES AFFECTING THE TEMPERATURE MEASUREMENT

1.   Eating and Smoking[7,15,16]

The *oral* temperature measurement increases about 0.3°C after sustained chewing and stays elevated for up to 20 minutes, probably because of increased blood flow to the muscles of mastication. Drinking hot liquids also increases oral readings about 0.9°C for up to 15 minutes, and smoking a cigarette increases oral readings about 0.2°C for 30 minutes. Drinking ice water causes the oral reading to fall 0.3° to 1.2°C, a reduction lasting about 10 to 15 minutes.

2.   Tachypnea

Tachypnea reduces the *oral* temperature reading about 0.5°C for every 10 breaths/minute increase in the respiratory rate.[5,6] This phenomenon probably explains why marathon runners, at the end of their race, often have a large discrepancy between normal oral temperatures and high rectal temperatures.[17]

In contrast, administration of oxygen by nasal canula does not affect oral temperature.[18]

3.   Cerumen

Cerumen lowers *tympanic* temperature readings, simply because it obstructs radiation of heat from the tympanic membrane.[7]

4.   Hemiparesis

In patients with hemiparesis, *axillary* temperature readings are about 0.5°C lower on the weak side compared with the healthy side. The discrepancy between the two sides correlates poorly with the severity of the patient's weakness, suggesting that it is not due to difficulty holding the thermometer under the arm, but instead to other factors, such as differences in cutaneous blood flow between the two sides.[19]

III. THE FINDING

A. NORMAL TEMPERATURE AND FEVER

In healthy persons, the mean oral temperature is 36.8°C (98.2°F),[20] a value slightly lower than Wunderlich's original estimate of 37°C (98.6°F), which in turn had been established using foot-long axillary thermometers that may have been calibrated higher than the thermometers used today.[1] The temperature is usually lowest at 6 AM and highest at 4 to 6 PM (a variation called "diurnal variation").[20] Fever is defined as the 99th percentile of maximum temperatures in healthy persons, which is an oral temperature greater than 37.7°C (99.9°F).[20]

B. FEVER PATTERNS

In the early days of clinical thermometry, clinicians observed that prolonged fevers could be categorized into one of four fever patterns—sustained, intermittent, remittent, and relapsing (Fig. 16-1).[3,21-23] **(1) Sustained fever.** In this pattern the fever varies little from day to day (the modern definition is variation ≤0.3°C (≤0.5°F) each day); **(2) Intermittent fever.** In this pattern the temperature returns to normal between exacerbations. If the exacerbations occur daily, the fever is "quotidian"; if they occur every 48 hours, it is "tertian" (i.e., they appear again on the third day); and if they occur every 72 hours, it is "quartan" (i.e., they appear again on the fourth day). **(3) Remittent.** Remittent fevers vary at least 0.3°C (0.5°F) each day but do not return to normal. **Hectic fevers** are intermittent or remittent fevers with wide swings in temperature, usually greater than 1.4°C (2.5°F) each day. **(4) Relapsing fevers.** These fevers are characterized by periods of fever lasting days interspersed by equally long afebrile periods.

Each of these patterns was associated with prototypic diseases: for sustained fever—lobar pneumonia (lasting 7 days until it disappeared abruptly by "crisis" or gradually by "lysis"), for intermittent fever—malarial infection, for remittent fever—typhoid fever (causing several days of ascending remittent fever, whose curve resemble climbing steps, before becoming sustained), for hectic fever—chronic tuberculosis or pyogenic abscesses, and for relapsing fever—relapse of a previous infection (e.g., typhoid fever). Other causes of relapsing fever are the Pel-Ebstein fever of Hodgkin's disease,[24] rat-bite fever (*Spirillum minus* or *Streptobacillus moniliformis*),[25] and *Borrelia* infections.[26]

Despite these etiologic associations, early clinicians recognized that the diagnostic significance of fever patterns was limited.[27] Instead, they used these labels more often to communicate a specific observation at the bedside rather than imply a specific diagnosis, much like we use the words "systolic murmur" or "lung crackle" today.

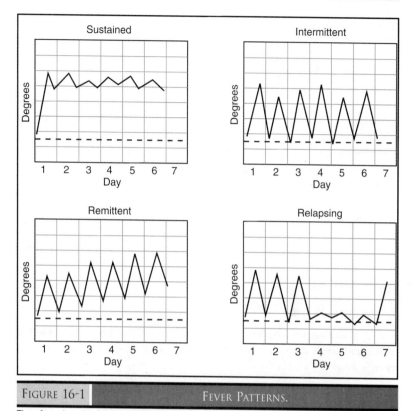

FIGURE 16-1   FEVER PATTERNS.

The four basic fever patterns are sustained, intermittent, remittent, and relapsing fever. The dashed line in each chart depicts normal temperature. See text for definitions and clinical significance.

C. ASSOCIATED FINDINGS

1. Focal Findings

More than 80% of patients with bacterial infections have specific focal signs or symptoms that point the clinician to the correct diagnosis.[28] There are countless focal signs associated with febrile illness (e.g., the tender swelling of an abscess or the diastolic murmur of endocarditis), which are reviewed in detail in infectious diseases textbooks. One potentially misleading focal sign, however, is jaundice. Although fever and jaundice are often due to hepatitis or cholangitis, jaundice is also a nonspecific complication of bacterial infection distant to the liver, occurring in 1% of all bacteremias.[29,30] This "reactive hepatopathy of bacteremia" was recognized over a century ago by Osler, who wrote that jaundice appeared in pneumococcal pneumonia with curious irregularity in different outbreaks.[27]

2. Relative Bradycardia

Relative bradycardia, a traditional sign of intracellular bacterial infections (e.g., typhoid fever), refers to a pulse rate that is inappropriately slow for the patient's temperature. The best definition is a pulse rate that is lower than the 95% confidence limit for the patient's temperature, which can be estimated by multiplying the patient temperature in degrees Celsius times 10 and then subtracting 323.[31] For example, if the patient's temperature is 39°C, relative bradycardia would refer to pulse rates below 67/minute (i.e., 390−323).*

3. Anhidrosis

Classically, patients with heat stroke have "bone-dry skin," but most modern studies show that anhidrosis appears very late in the course and has a sensitivity of only 3% to 60%.[32-34] In contrast, 91% of patients with heat stroke have significant pyrexia (exceeding 40°C), and 100% have abnormal mental status.

4. Muscle Rigidity

Muscle rigidity suggests the diagnosis of neuroleptic malignant syndrome (a febrile complication from dopamine antagonists) or serotonin syndrome (from proserotonergic drugs).[35,36]

IV. CLINICAL SIGNIFICANCE

A. DETECTION OF FEVER

Two findings modestly increase the probability of fever: the patient's subjective report of fever and the clinician's perception that the patient's skin is abnormally warm [both likelihood ratios (LRs) = 2.9, EBM Box 16-1]. When either of these findings is absent, the probability of fever decreases (LR = 0.3).

B. PREDICTORS OF BACTEREMIA IN FEBRILE PATIENTS

In patients hospitalized with fever, 8% to 21% will have documented bacteremia,[40-48] a finding associated with an increased hospital mortality.[49] Of all the bedside findings that help diagnose bacteremia, the most important are the

---

*This formula combines separate formulae for women (<11 × T °C − 359) and men (<10.2 × T °C − 333) provided in reference 31, which in turn were based on observations of 700 febrile patients.

Box 16-1 Detection of Fever*

Finding (Ref)	Sensitivity (%)	Specificity (%)	Likelihood Ratio if Finding	
			Present	Absent
Patient's report of fever[37,38]	80–83	55–83	2.9	**0.3**
Patient's forehead abnormally warm[38,39]	71–85	72	2.9	**0.3**

*Diagnostic standard: For fever, measured axillary temperature >37.5°C,[38] oral temperature >38°C,[37] or rectal temperature >38.1°C.[39]

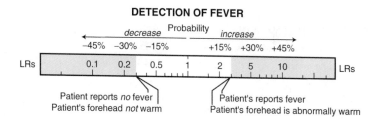

patient's underlying disorders, in particular the presence of renal failure (LR = 4.6, EBM Box 16-2), hospitalization for trauma (LR = 3.0), and poor functional status (i.e., bedridden or requiring attendance, LR = 3.6).* A few physical findings also modestly increase the probability of bacteremia: hypotension (LR = 2.6), presence of an indwelling urinary catheter (LR = 2.4), and presence of a central venous catheter (LR = 2.0). The only finding arguing significantly against the diagnosis of bacteremia is age younger than 50 years (LR = 0.3).

The presence of "shaking chills" discriminates only weakly between bacteremia and other causes of fever (sensitivity 24%–67%; specificity 64%–88%; positive LR = 1.8, negative LR = 0.8).[42,44,45,47,48,51] The "toxic appearance" fails to discriminate serious infection from trivial illness.[28,53]

---

*For comparison, the LRs of these findings are superior to those for traditional laboratory signs of bacteremia, such as leukocytosis and bandemia. In detecting bacteremia, a WBC >15,000 has a LR of only 1.6,[28,41,48,52] whereas a band count >1,500 has an LR of 2.6.[28,41,44]

Box 16-2

Detection of Bacteremia in Febrile Patients*

Finding (Ref)[†]	Sensitivity (%)	Specificity (%)	Likelihood Ratio if Finding Present	Absent
RISK FACTORS				
Age 50 years or more[28,41]	89–95	32–33	1.4	**0.3**
Renal failure[42]	19–28	95	**4.6**	0.8
Hospitalization for trauma[40,50]	12–63	79–98	**3.0**	NS
Intravenous drug use[45]	7	98	2.9	NS
Previous stroke[42]	17	94	2.8	NS
Diabetes mellitus[28,41,42,44,48]	17–38	82–89	1.5	NS
Poor functional performance[42]	48–61	83–87	**3.6**	0.6
Rapidly fatal disease (<1 mo)[45,47]	2–30	88–99	2.7	NS
PHYSICAL EXAMINATION				
Indwelling lines and catheters				
Indwelling urinary catheter present[41,42,44,48]	22–38	83–95	2.4	NS
Central intravenous line present[40,51]	16–24	90–91	2.0	NS
Vital signs				
Temperature ≥ 38.5°C[44]	87	27	1.2	NS
Tachycardia[40,48]	61–73	42–48	1.2	0.7
Respiratory rate >20/min[48]	65	30	NS	NS
Hypotension[44,45,48]	7–20	93–99	2.6	NS
Other findings				
Acute abdomen[45,47,51]	2–20	90–100	1.7	NS
Confusion or depressed sensorium[40,44,48,51]	10–52	68–95	1.5	NS

NS, not significant; likelihood ratio (LR) if finding present = positive LR; LR if finding absent = negative LR.

*Diagnostic standard: For bacteremia, true bacteremia (not contamination), as determined by number of positive cultures, organism type, and results of other cultures.

†Definition of findings: For renal failure, serum creatinine >2.0 mg/dL; for rapidly fatal disease, >50% probability of fatality within 1 month (e.g., relapsed leukemia without treatment, hepatorenal syndrome); for poor functional status, see text; for tachycardia, pulse rate >90 beats/min[40] or >100 beats/min[48]; for hypotension, systolic blood pressure <100 mm Hg,[48] <90 mm Hg,[45] or "shock."[44]

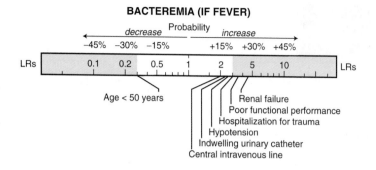

C. EXTREME PYREXIA AND HYPOTHERMIA

Extreme pyrexia (i.e., temperature exceeding 41.1 °C or 106 °F) has diagnostic significance because the cause is usually gram-negative bacteremia or problems with temperature regulation (heat stroke, intracranial hemorrhage, severe burns).[34]

In a wide variety of disorders, the finding of a very high or low temperature indicates a worse prognosis.[54,55] For example, temperatures greater than 39 °C are associated with an increased risk of death in patients with pontine hemorrhage (LR = 23.7, EBM Box 16-3). Very low temperatures are associated with an increased risk of death in patients hospitalized with congestive heart failure (LR = 6.7), pneumonia (LR = 3.5), and bacteremia (LR = 3.3).

D. FEVER PATTERNS

Most fevers today, whether infectious or noninfectious in origin, are intermittent or remittent and lack any other characteristic feature.[61,62] Antibiotic medications have changed many traditional fever patterns. For example, the fever of lobar pneumonia, which in the preantibiotic era was sustained and lasted 7 days, now lasts only 2 to 3 days.[63,64] The double quotidian fever pattern (i.e., two daily fever spikes), a feature of gonococcal endocarditis present in 50% of cases during the preantibiotic era, is consistently absent in reported cases from the modern era.[65] The characteristic tertian or quartan intermittent fever of malaria infection also is uncommon today, because most patients are treated before the characteristic synchronization of the malaria cycle.[66]

Nonetheless, although traditional fever patterns may be less common, they still have significance. In tropical countries, the presence of the "stepladder" remittent pattern of fever is highly specific for the diagnosis of typhoid fever (LR = 177.4).[67] Also, among travelers with malarial infection who reported a tertian pattern, most were infected with *Plasmodium vivax* (traditionally the most common cause of this pattern).[68]

Moreover, the antibiotic era has given fever patterns a new significance, because once antibiotics have been started, the finding of an unusually prolonged

**Box
16-3** Extremes of Temperature and Prognosis

Finding (Ref)	Sensitivity (%)	Specificity (%)	Likelihood Ratio if Finding	
			Present	Absent
Temperature >39°C				
Predicting hospital mortality in patients with pontine hemorrhage[56]	66	97	**23.7**	0.4
Hypothermia*				
Predicting hospital mortality from pump failure in patients with congestive heart failure[57]	29	96	**6.7**	NS
Predicting hospital mortality in patients with pneumonia[58,59]	14–43	93	**3.5**	NS
Predicting hospital mortality in patients with bacteremia[60]	13	96	**3.3**	NS

NS, not significant; likelihood ratio (LR) if finding present = positive LR; LR if finding absent = negative LR.
*Definition of findings: For hypothermia, temperature <35.2°C,[57] <36.1°C,[59] <36.5°C,[60] or <37.0°C.[58]

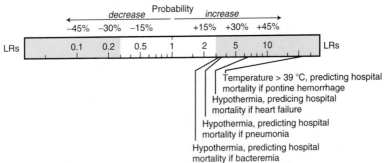

EXTREMES OF TEMPERATURE

Temperature > 39 °C, predicting hospital mortality if pontine hemorrhage
Hypothermia, predicting hospital mortality if heart failure
Hypothermia, predicting hospital mortality if pneumonia
Hypothermia, predicting hospital mortality if bacteremia

fever is an important sign indicating either that the diagnosis of infection was incorrect (e.g., the patient instead has a connective tissue disorder or neoplasm) or that the patient has one of several complications, such as resistant organisms, superinfection, drug fever, or an abscess requiring surgical drainage.

E. RELATIVE BRADYCARDIA

Clinical studies demonstrate that some infections, such as intracellular bacterial infections (e.g., typhoid fever and Legionnaire's disease) and arboviral infections (e.g., sandfly fever and dengue fever), do produce less tachycardia than other infections, but, because very few patients with these infections actually have a relative bradycardia (as previously defined), the clinical utility of this observation is limited.[31,69]

REFERENCES

1. Mackowiak PA, Worden G. Carl Reinhold August Wunderlich and the evolution of clinical thermometry. *Clin Inf Dis*. 1994;18:458-467.
2. Wright-St. Clair RE. Go to the bedside. *J Roy Coll Gen Pract*. 1971;21:442-452.
3. Guttman P. *A handbook of physical diagnosis: Comprising the throat, thorax, and abdomen*. New York: William Wood and Co; 1880.
4. Geddes LA. Perspectives in physiological monitoring. *Med Instrument*. 1976;10:91-97.
5. Tandberg D, Sklar D. Effect of tachypnea on the estimation of body temperature by an oral thermometer. *N Engl J Med*. 1983;308:945-946.
6. Durham ML, Swanson B, Paulford N. Effect of tachypnea on oral temperature estimation: A replication. *Nurs Res*. 1986;35:211-214.
7. Rabinowitz RP, Cookson ST, Wasserman SS, Mackowiak PA. Effects of anatomic site, oral stimulation, and body position on estimates of body temperature. *Arch Intern Med*. 1996;156:777-780.
8. Horvath SM, Menduke H, Piersol GM. Oral and rectal temperatures of man. *JAMA*. 1950;144:1562-1565.
9. Nichols GA, Ruskin MM, Glor BAK, Kelly WH. Oral, axillary, and rectal temperature determinations and relationships. *Nurs Res*. 1966;15:307-310.
10. Erickson RS, Kirklin SK. Comparison of ear-based, bladder, oral, and axillary methods for core temperature measurement. *Crit Care Med*. 1993;21:1528-1534.
11. Abolnik IZ, Kithas PA, McDonnald JJ, et al. Comparison of oral and tympanic temperatures in a Veterans Administration outpatient clinic. *Am J Med Sci*. 1999;317:301-303.
12. Giuliano KK, Giuliano AJ, Scott SS, et al. Temperature measurement in critically ill adults: A comparison of tympanic and oral methods. *Am J Crit Care*. 2000;9: 254-261.

13. Klein DG, Mitchell C, Petrinec A, et al. A comparison of pulmonary artery, rectal, and tympanic membrane temperature measurement in the ICU. *Heart Lung.* 1993; 22:435-441.

14. Chu A, Burnham RS. Reliability and validity of tympanic temperature measurement in persons with high spinal cord injuries. *Paraplegia.* 1995;33:476-479.

15. Terndrup TE, Allegra JR, Kealy JA. A comparison of oral, rectal, and tympanic membrane-derived temperature changes after ingestion of liquids and smoking. *Am J Emerg Med.* 1989;7:150-154.

16. Newman BH, Martin CA. The effect of hot beverages, cold beverages, and chewing gum on oral temperature. *Transfusion.* 2001;41:1241-1243.

17. Maron MB. Effect of tachypnea on estimation of body temperature (letter). *N Engl J Med.* 1983;309:612-613.

18. Lim-Levy F. The effect of oxygen inhalation on oral temperature. *Nurs Res.* 1982; 31:150-152.

19. Mulley G. Axillary temperature differences in hemiplegia. *Postgrad Med J.* 1980;56: 248-249.

20. Mackowiak PA, Wasserman SS, Levine MM. A critical appraisal of 98.6 degrees F, the upper limit of the normal body temperature, and other legacies of Carl Reinhold August Wunderlich. *JAMA.* 1992;268:1578-1580.

21. Sahli H. *A treatise on diagnostic methods of examination.* Philadelphia: W.B. Saunders; 1911.

22. Gibson GA, Russell W. *Physical diagnosis: A guide to methods of clinical investigation,* 2nd ed. New York: D. Appleton and Co; 1893.

23. Brown JG. *Medical diagnosis: A manual of clinical methods.* New York: Bermingham and Co; 1884.

24. Reimann HA. Periodic (Pel-Ebstein) fever of lymphomas. *Ann Clin Lab Sci.* 1977;7:1-5.

25. Beeson PB. The problem of the etiology of rat bite fever: Report of 2 cases due to spirillum minus. *JAMA.* 1943;123:332-334.

26. Bennett IL. The significance of fever in infections. *Yale J Biol Med.* 1954;26:491-505.

27. Osler W. *The principles and practice of medicine* (facsimile by Classics of Medicine library). New York: D. Appleton and Co; 1892.

28. Mellors JW, Horwitz RI, Harvey MR, Horwitz SM. A simple index to identify occult bacterial infection in adults with acute unexplained fever. *Arch Intern Med.* 1987;147:666-671.

29. Franson TR, Hierholzer WJ, LaBrecque DR. Frequency and characteristics of hyperbilirubinemia associated with bacteremia. *Rev Infect Dis.* 1985;7:1-9.

30. Vermillion SE, Gregg JA, Baggenstoss AH, Bartholomew LG. Jaundice associated with bacteremia. *Arch Intern Med.* 1969;124:611-618.

31. Ostergaard L, Huniche B, Andersen PL. Relative bradycardia in infectious diseases. *J Infect.* 1996;33:185-191.

32. Costrini AM, Pitt HA, Gustafson AB, Uddin DE. Cardiovascular and metabolic manifestations of heat stroke and severe heat exhaustion. *Am J Med*. 1979;66:296-302.

33. Shibolet S, Coll R, Gilat T, Sohar E. Heatstroke: Its clinical picture and mechanism in 36 cases. *Q J Med*. 1967;36:525-548.

34. Simon HB. Extreme pyrexia. *JAMA*. 1976;236:2419-2421.

35. Kurlan R, Hamill R, Shoulson I. Neuroleptic malignant syndrome. *Clin Neuropharmacol*. 1984;7:109-120.

36. Boyer EW, Shannon M. The serotonin syndrome. *N Engl J Med*. 2005;352:1112-1120.

37. Buckley RG, Conine M. Reliability of subjective fever in triage of adult patients. *Ann Emerg Med*. 1996;27:693-695.

38. Singh M, Pai M, Kalantri SP. Accuracy of perception and touch for detecting fever in adults: A hospital-based study from a rural, tertiary hospital in Central India. *Trop Med Int Health*. 2003;8:408-414.

39. Hung OL, Kwon NS, Cole AE, et al. Evaluation of the physician's ability to recognize the presence or absence of anemia, fever, and jaundice. *Acad Emerg Med*. 2000;7:146-156.

40. Jaimes F, Arango C, Ruiz G, et al. Predicting bacteremia at the bedside. *Clin Infect Dis*. 2004;38:357-362.

41. Leibovici L, Cohen O, Wysenbeek AJ. Occult bacterial infection in adults with unexplained fever: Validation of a diagnostic index. *Arch Intern Med*. 1990;150: 1270-1272.

42. Leibovici L, Greenshtain S, Cohen O, et al. Bacteremia in febrile patients: A clinical model for diagnosis. *Arch Intern Med*. 1991;151:1801-1806.

43. Mozes B, Milatiner D, Block C, et al. Inconsistency of a model aimed at predicting bacteremia in hospitalized patients. *J Clin Epidemiol*. 1993;46:1035-1040.

44. Pfitzenmeyer P, Decrey H, Auckenthaler R, Michel JP. Predicting bacteremia in older patients. *J Am Geriatr Soc*. 1995;43:230-235.

45. Bates DW, Cook EF, Goldman L, Lee TH. Predicting bacteremia in hospitalized patients: A prospectively validated model. *Ann Intern Med*. 1990;113:495-500.

46. Mylotte JM, Pisano MA, Ram S, et al. Validation of a bacteremia prediction model. *Infect Control Hosp Epidemiol*. 1995;16:203-209.

47. Yehezkelli Y, Subah S, Elhanan G, et al. Two rules for early prediction of bacteremia: Testing in a University and a community hospital. *J Gen Intern Med*. 1996; 11:98-103.

48. Fontanarosa PB, Kaeberlein FJ, Gerson LW, Thomson RB. Difficulty in predicting bacteremia in elderly emergency patients. *Ann Emerg Med*. 1992;21:842-848.

49. Bates DW, Pruess KE, Lee TH. How bad are bacteremia and sepsis? Outcomes in a cohort with suspected bacteremia. *Arch Intern Med*. 1995;155:593-598.

50. Mellors JW, Kelly JJ, Gusberg RJ, Horwitz SM, Horwitz RI. A simple index to estimate the likelihood of bacterial infection in patients developing fever after abdominal surgery. *Am Surg*. 1988;54:558-564.

51. Bates DW, Sands K, Miller E, et al. Predicting bacteremia in patients with sepsis syndrome. *J Infect Dis*. 1997;176:1538-1551.

52. Wolfe RE, Bates DW, Spear J, et al. Age has little effect on the predictive value of the CBC for bacteremia. *Acad Emerg Med.* 2004;11:473.

53. Marantz PR, Linzer M, Feiner CJ, et al. Inability to predict diagnosis in febrile intravenous drug abusers. *Ann Intern Med.* 1987;106:823-828.

54. Fine MJ, Orloff JJ, Arisumi D, et al. Prognosis of patients hospitalized with community-acquired pneumonia. *Am J Med.* 1990;88:5-1N-8N.

55. Knaus WA, Wagner DP, Draper EA, et al. The APACHE III prognostic system: Risk prediction of hospital mortality for critically ill hospitalized adults. *Chest.* 1991;100:1619-1636.

56. Wijdicks EFM, St. Louis E. Clinical profiles predictive of outcome in pontine hemorrhage. *Neurology.* 1997;49:1342-1346.

57. Casscells W, Vasseghi MF, Siadaty MS, et al. Hypothermia is a bedside predictor of imminent death in patients with congestive heart failure. *Am Heart J.* 2005;149: 927-933.

58. Allen SC. Lobar pneumonia in Northern Zambia: Clinical study of 502 adult patients. *Thorax.* 1984;39:612-616.

59. Conte HA, Chen YT, Mehal W, et al. A prognostic rule for elderly patients admitted with community-acquired pneumonia. *Am J Med.* 1999;106:20-28.

60. Pittet D, Thievent B, Wenzel RP, et al. Bedside prediction of mortality from bacteremic sepsis: A dynamic analysis of ICU patients. *Am J Respir Crit Care Med.* 1996;153:684-693.

61. Mackowiak PA, LeMaistre CF. Drug fever: A critical appraisal of conventional concepts. *Ann Intern Med.* 1987;106:728-733.

62. Musher DM, Fainstein V, Young EJ, Pruett TL. Fever patterns: Their lack of clinical significance. *Arch Intern Med.* 1979;139:1225-1228.

63. Halm EA, Fine MJ, Marrie TJ, et al. Time to clinical stability in patients hospitalized with community-acquired pneumonia: Implications for practice guidelines. *JAMA.* 1998;279:1452-1457.

64. van Metre TE. Pneumococcal pneumonia treated with antibiotics: The prognostic significance of certain clinical findings. *N Engl J Med.* 1954;251:1048-1052.

65. Fernandez GC, Chapman AJ, Bolli R, et al. Gonococcal endocarditis: A case series demonstrating modern presentation of an old disease. *Am Heart J.* 1984;108: 1326-1334.

66. Stanley J. Malaria. *Emerg Med Clin North Am.* 1997;15:113-155.

67. Haq SA, Alam MN, Hossain SM, et al. Value of clinical features in the diagnosis of enteric fever. *Bangladesh Med Res Counc Bull.* 1997;23:42-46.

68. Svenson JE, MacLean JD, Gyorkos TW, Keyston J. Imported malaria: Clinical presentation and examination of symptomatic travelers. *Arch Intern Med.* 1995;155: 861-868.

69. Wittesjo B, Bjornham A, Eitrem R. Relative bradycardia in infectious diseases. *J Infect.* 1999;39:246-247.

Respiratory Rate and Abnormal Breathing Patterns

RESPIRATORY RATE

I. INTRODUCTION

The respiratory rate (i.e., number of breaths per minute) is one of the four traditional vital signs, the others being heart rate, blood pressure, and temperature.

One of the first clinicians to recommend routine measurement of the respiratory rate was Stokes in 1825,[1] although routine charting of this vital sign was infrequent until the late 19th century.[2,3]

II. TECHNIQUE

The respiratory rate is usually measured while the clinician is holding the patient's wrist and ostensibly measuring the pulse, primarily because the respiratory rate may change if attention is drawn to it. This practice seems reasonable, because the respiratory rate is the only vital sign that is under voluntary control.

As routinely recorded in the patient's hospital record, the respiratory rate is often inaccurate.[4,5] In one study of patients whose actual respiratory rates ranged from 11 to 33 breaths/minute, the recorded rate 98% of the time was from 18 to 22 breaths/minute.[5] Some of these errors represent too short a period of observation (i.e., the clinician counting the number of breaths in 10 seconds multiplying the result times 6). Consequently, it is probably good practice to observe respirations for at least 30 to 60 seconds, which not only may make the measured rate more accurate but also allows detection of unusual breathing patterns, such as Cheyne-Stokes respirations (see later).

III. FINDING

A. THE NORMAL RESPIRATORY RATE

The normal respiratory rate averages 20 breaths/minute (range 16–25 breaths/minute), based on careful measurement in persons without fever, heart disease, or lung disease.[6,7] This estimate is identical to that made more than 150 years ago by Lambert Quetelet, who was the first to compile and analyze vital and social statistics.*[8] For unclear reasons, many textbooks, citing no data, mistakenly record the normal rate as 12 to 18 breaths/minute.[6]

B. TACHYPNEA

Definitions of tachypnea vary, but the most reasonable one, based on the normal range and clinical studies, is a respiratory rate ≥25 breaths/minute.

C. BRADYPNEA

Bradypnea is defined as a respiratory rate less than 8 breaths/minute, a threshold derived from studies of patients taking opioid medications, because this rate best predicts respiratory depression and correlates well with level of sedation.[9]

IV. CLINICAL SIGNIFICANCE

A. TACHYPNEA

The finding of tachypnea has both diagnostic and prognostic value. As a diagnostic sign, it argues modestly for the diagnosis of pneumonia in outpatients

---

*Quetelet's 1835 monumental treatise also provided our current formula for body mass index, known as the Quetelet index (see Chapter 11).

with cough and fever [likelihood ratio (LR) = 2.0, EBM Box 17-1]. Tachypnea also argues for pneumonia in hospitalized patients, the abnormal sign sometimes appearing as early as 1 to 2 days before the diagnosis is apparent by other means.[7, 18]

One characteristic of a vital sign is that it accurately predicts the patient's prognosis, and EBM Box 17-1 shows that tachypnea predicts subsequent cardiopulmonary arrest in hospitalized patients (LR = 3.1), much better than does tachycardia or abnormal blood pressure.[11] During trials of weaning from a ventilator, tachypnea also is a significant although modest predictor of weaning failure (LR = 2.9).[10,19] In patients hospitalized with pneumonia, severe tachypnea (i.e., rate >30 breaths/minute) predicts subsequent hospital death (LR = 2.1).

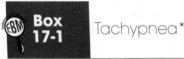

Box 17-1   Tachypnea*

Finding (Ref)	Sensitivity (%)	Specificity (%)	Likelihood Ratio if Finding Present	Likelihood Ratio if Finding Absent
Rate >24/min				
Predicting failure of weaning from the ventilator, in intubated patients[10]	94	68	2.9	NS
Rate >27/min				
Predicting cardiopulmonary arrest, in medical inpatients[11]	54	82	**3.1**	0.6
Rate >28/min				
Detecting pneumonia, in outpatients with cough and fever[12]	36	82	2.0	0.8
Rate >30/min				
Predicting hospital mortality, in patients with pneumonia[13–17]	41–85	63–87	2.1	0.6

NS, not significant; likelihood ratio (LR) if finding present = positive LR; LR if finding absent = negative LR.
*Diagnostic standard: For failure of weaning, progressive hypoxemia or respiratory acidosis; for pneumonia, infiltrate on chest radiograph.

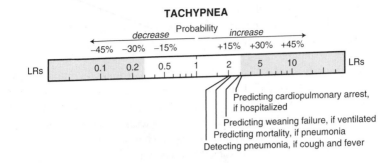

B. TACHYPNEA AND OXYGEN SATURATION

The respiratory rate correlates poorly with the patient's level of oxygen desaturation ($r = 0.16$).[20] Although this at first seems surprising (i.e., the lower the oxygen level, the more rapid a patient should breathe), this actually is expected because some hypoxemic patients, by breathing rapidly, are able to bring their oxygen level back up to normal (i.e., hyperventilation raises arterial oxygen levels) and because other patients are hypoxemic simply because they have a primary hypoventilatory disorder. Consequently, the respiratory rate and oxygen saturation are both valuable to the clinician, each providing information independent from the other.

ABNORMAL BREATHING PATTERNS

I. CHEYNE-STOKES BREATHING ("PERIODIC BREATHING")

A. INTRODUCTION

Cheyne-Stokes breathing consists of alternating periods of apnea and hyperpnea (Fig. 17-1). Some authors equate the term "periodic breathing" with Cheyne-Stokes breathing,[21,22] whereas others reserve "periodic breathing" for oscillations of tidal volume that lack intervening periods of apnea.[23]

Cheyne-Stokes breathing was described by John Cheyne in 1818 and William Stokes in 1854.[24]

B. THE FINDING

1. The Breathing Pattern

At the end of each apneic period, breathing commences with excursions of the chest that initially are small but gradually increase for several breaths and then diminish until apnea returns. The respiratory rate is constant during the hypernea phase and does not gradually increase and then decrease as often surmised.[25]

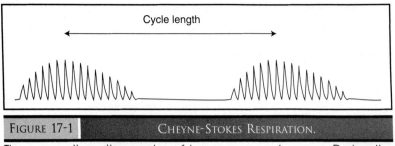

| FIGURE 17-1 | CHEYNE-STOKES RESPIRATION. |

There are alternating cycles of hyperpnea and apnea. During the hyperpnea phase only the tidal volume oscillates; the respiratory frequency is constant.

Cheyne-Stokes breathing often first appears when the patient lies down, probably because this position reduces the patient's functional residual capacity, thus diminishing the lung's ability to buffer changes in carbon dioxide (see "Pathogenesis" later).[22,26]

The time between two consecutive peaks of hyperpnea is called the "cycle length" or "period." Each cycle length is divided into a hyperpnea phase (lasting about 30 seconds on average in patients with congestive heart failure) and an apnea phase (lasting about 25 seconds on average).[27]

2. Associated Bedside Observations

Several additional findings appear in patients with Cheyne-Stokes breathing. During the hyperpnea phase, the patient is alert and sometimes agitated, with dilated pupils, hyperactive muscle stretch reflexes, and increased muscle tone. During the apnea phase, the patient appears motionless and asleep with constricted pupils, hypoactive reflexes, and reduced muscle tone.[28,29] The agitation of the hyperpnea phase can easily startle a patient out of sleep, a nocturnal symptom that clinicians can mistake for the paroxysmal nocturnal dyspnea of heart failure caused by transient pulmonary edema.[30,31]

C. CLINICAL SIGNIFICANCE
1. Associated Conditions

Cheyne-Stokes breathing affects 30% of patients with stable congestive heart failure.[23] The breathing pattern also appears in many neurologic disorders, including hemorrhage, infarction, tumors, meningitis, and head trauma involving the brainstem or higher levels of the central nervous system.[28,29,32,33] Normal persons often develop Cheyne-Stokes breathing during sleep[21] or at high altitudes.[28]

2. Prognostic Importance

Modern studies confirm Dr. Stokes' original impression that, in patients with heart disease, this breathing pattern carries a poor prognosis. Compared with heart failure patients with normal breathing, patients with Cheyne-Stokes breathing have lower cardiac outputs, higher pulmonary capillary wedge pressures, and shorter survival.[23,34–37]

D. PATHOGENESIS

The fundamental problem causing Cheyne-Stokes breathing is enhanced sensitivity to carbon dioxide. The circulatory delay between the lungs and systemic arteries, caused by poor cardiac output, also contributes to the waxing and waning of breaths. Cerebral blood flow increases during hyperpnea and decreases during apnea, perhaps explaining the fluctuations of mental status.[27,38]

1. Enhanced Sensitivity to Carbon Dioxide

Whether because of congestive heart failure or neurologic disease, patients with Cheyne-Stokes breathing have two to three times the normal sensitivity to carbon dioxide.[28,38–40] This causes patients to hyperventilate excessively, eventually driving the carbon dioxide level so low that central apnea results. After they stop breathing, carbon dioxide levels again rise, eliciting another hyperventilatory response and thus perpetuating the alternating cycles of apnea and hyperpnea.

Mountain climbers develop Cheyne-Stokes breathing because hypoxia induces hypersensitivity to carbon dioxide. In contrast, their native Sherpa guides, who are acclimated to hypoxia, lack an exaggerated ventilatory response and do not develop Cheyne-Stokes breathing.[28]

2. Circulatory Delay Between Lungs and Arteries

Ventilation is normally controlled by the medullary respiratory center, which monitors arterial carbon dioxide levels and directs the lungs to ventilate more if carbon dioxide levels are too high and less if levels are too low. The medulla signals the lungs almost immediately, the message traveling via the nervous system. The feedback to the medulla, however, is much slower because it requires circulation of blood from lungs back to systemic arteries.

In Cheyne-Stokes breathing, the carbon dioxide levels in the alveoli and those of the systemic arteries are precisely out of sync. During peak hyperpnea, carbon dioxide levels in the alveoli are very low, yet the medulla is just beginning to sample blood containing high carbon dioxide levels from the previous apnea phase and thus still directs the lungs to continue breathing deeply.[28] The delay in feedback to the medulla contributes to the gradual waxing and waning of tidal volume.

The length of circulatory delay also governs the cycle length of Cheyne-Stokes breathing, the two correlating closely (r = 0.8 between cycle length and circulation time from lung to arteries, $p<0.05$).[27,38] The cycle length is about two times the circulation time, just as would be expected from the observation that carbon dioxide levels in the lungs and arteries are precisely out of sync. This suggests that the clinician should be able to take a stopwatch to the bedside and time the patient's cycle length, using this number as a rough guide to the patient's cardiac output. This idea, however, has never been formally tested.

II. KUSSMAUL'S RESPIRATION

Kussmaul's respirations are rapid and deep and appear in patients with metabolic acidosis.[41] The unusually deep respirations are distinctive, because other causes of tachypnea, such as heart and lung disease, reduce vital capacity and thus cause rapid, *shallow* respirations.

III. GRUNTING RESPIRATIONS

A. DEFINITION

Grunting respirations are short, explosive sounds of low-to-medium pitch produced by vocal cord closure during expiration. The actual sound is the rush of air that occurs when the glottis opens and suddenly allows air to escape. Grunting respirations are more common in children,[42] although the finding also has been described in adults as a sign of respiratory muscle fatigue[43] and, in the preantibiotic era, as a cardinal sign of lobar pneumonia, usually appearing after 4 to 6 days of illness.[3,44]

B. PATHOGENESIS

Grunting respirations slow down expiration and allow more time for maximal gas exchange.[43] In animal experiments, artificial mimicking of grunting respirations causes the PO_2 to increase by 10% and the PCO_2 to fall by 11%, whether or not the animal has pneumonia.[45] Grunting respirations also produce positive pressure exhalation that may reduce exudation of fluid into the alveoli, based on an old observation that administration of morphine to patients with pneumonia often reduced the grunting respirations but was sometimes followed immediately by fatal pulmonary edema.[44]

IV. ABNORMAL ABDOMINAL MOVEMENTS

A. NORMAL ABDOMINAL MOVEMENTS

In the absence of massive gaseous distension, the abdominal viscera are non-compressible and act like hydraulic coupling fluid that directly transmits movements of the diaphragm to the anterior abdominal wall.[46] Abdominal respiratory movements, therefore, indicate indirectly how the diaphragm is moving. During normal respiration, the chest and abdomen move synchronously: both out during inspiration and both in during expiration (Fig. 17-2). The chest wall moves more when the person is upright, and the abdomen moves more when the person is supine.[47,48]

B.   ABNORMAL ABDOMINAL MOVEMENTS

Three abnormal abdominal movements are all signs of chronic airflow obstruction or respiratory muscle weakness: asynchronous breathing, respiratory alternans, and paradoxical abdominal movements.

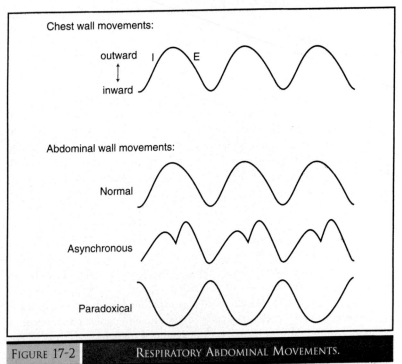

FIGURE 17-2	RESPIRATORY ABDOMINAL MOVEMENTS.

Chest movements are depicted in the first row. I, inspiration; E, expiration. Upward sloping lines on the drawing indicate outward body wall movements; downward sloping lines, inward movements. In normal persons, the abdominal and chest wall movements are completely in sync. In asynchronous breathing, only expiratory abdominal movements are abnormal. In paradoxical abdominal movements, both inspiratory and expiratory abdominal movements are abnormal. See text.

1. Asynchronous Breathing
a. Findings

Asynchronous breathing is an abnormal *expiratory* movement that sometimes develops in patients with chronic airflow obstruction. In these patients, the normal smooth inward abdominal movement during expiration is replaced by an abrupt inward and then outward movement (see Fig. 17-2).[49,50]

b. Clinical Significance

In patients with chronic airflow obstruction, asynchronous breathing correlates with lower forced expiratory volumes and a much poorer prognosis.[50] Among patients with chronic airflow obstruction who develop acute respiratory symptoms, the presence of an asynchronous breathing pattern predicts subsequent hospital death or the need for artificial ventilation with a sensitivity of 64%, specificity of 80%, and positive LR of 3.2 (negative LR not significant).[49]

c. Pathogenesis

The outward abdominal movement during expiration probably reflects the strong action of chest wall accessory muscles during expiration, which push the flattened diaphragm temporarily downward and thus the abdomen abruptly outward.[47,49]

2. Respiratory Alternans

Respiratory alternans describes a breathing pattern that alternates between inspiratory movements that are mostly abdominal and inspiratory movements that are mostly thoracic.[19]

3. Paradoxical Abdominal Movements
a. Finding

Paradoxical abdominal movements are completely out of sync with those of the chest wall. During inspiration the abdomen moves in as the chest wall moves out; during expiration, the abdomen moves out as chest moves in.[46,51-53]

b. Clinical Significance

The finding of paradoxical abdominal movements is a sign of bilateral diaphragm weakness. Most of these patients also complain of severe orthopnea. In one study of patients with dyspnea and neuromuscular disease, the finding of paradoxical abdominal movements detected diaphragm weakness with a sensitivity of 95%, specificity of 70%, and positive LR of 3.2 (in this study, the definition of paradoxical movements was any inspiratory inward abdominal movement, and the definition of diaphragm weakness was a maximal transdiaphragmatic pressure ≤ 30 cm H_2O; the normal sniff transdiaphragmatic pressure is > 98 cm H_2O).[51]

c. Pathogenesis

If the diaphragm is totally paralyzed, the inspiratory outward movement of the chest wall will draw the diaphragm upward and thus the abdomen inward. The weight of the abdominal viscera probably also plays a role, because paradoxical movements are most obvious in affected patients who are positioned supine and are often absent when the patient is upright.[51]

V.   ORTHOPNEA, TREPOPNEA, AND PLATYPNEA

These terms describe tachypnea (and dyspnea) that appears abruptly in particular positions: when the patient is supine (orthopnea), lying on a side (trepopnea), or upright (platypnea). These findings are often first diagnosed during observation of the patient's respirations at the bedside.

A.   ORTHOPNEA

1.   Finding

Orthopnea describes dyspnea that appears when the patient lies down but is relieved when the patient sits up (from the Greek words *ortho* meaning straight or vertical, and *pnea* meaning to breathe).

2.   Clinical Significance

Orthopnea occurs in a variety of disorders, including massive ascites, bilateral diaphragm paralysis, pleural effusion, morbid obesity, and severe pneumonia, although its most important clinical association is congestive heart failure.[51,52,54] In one study of patients with known chronic obstructive pulmonary disease, the finding of orthopnea distinguished between those patients with abnormally low ejection fraction (<0.50) and those with normal ejection fraction with a sensitivity of 97%, specificity of 64%, positive LR of 2.7, and negative LR of 0.04.[55] This suggests that, in patients with lung disease, the *presence* of orthopnea has limited value (i.e., occurs in both lung and heart disease), but the *absence* of orthopnea is more compelling, arguing *against* the presence of associated left ventricular dysfunction (LR = 0.04).

3.   Pathogenesis

In patients with orthopnea, lung compliance and vital capacity fall significantly after moving from the upright to supine position. This explains in part why dyspnea worsens in the supine position and why orthopnea is a finding common to so many different clinical conditions.[54,56,57] However, orthopnea cannot be entirely caused by postural changes in lung mechanics, for several reasons. First, orthopnea is uncommon in other disorders with similar reductions of vital capacity and compliance (e.g., interstitial fibrosis). Second, in patients with congestive heart failure, orthopnea correlates poorly with the pulmonary artery wedge pressure, which should have some relation to interstitial edema and pulmonary mechanics.[58] Finally, elevation of the head alone brings prompt relief to some orthopneic patients. It was once believed that elevation of the head relieved dyspnea because it reduced intracranial venous pressure and thus improved cerebral perfusion, although this hypothesis has been experimentally disproved.[54]

B. TREPOPNEA

1. Finding

Trepopnea* (from Greek *trepo* meaning twist or turn) describes dyspnea that is worse in one lateral decubitus position and relieved in the other.

2. Clinical Significance

There are three primary causes of trepopnea.

a. Unilateral Lung Disease[61,62]

Affected patients usually prefer to position their healthy lung down, which improves oxygenation because blood preferentially flows to the lower lung.

b. Congestive Heart Failure from Dilated Cardiomyopathy[59,60,63]

Patients usually prefer to have their right side down. Whether this is due to positional changes in lung mechanics (e.g., left lung atelectasis from cardiomegaly), right ventricular preload, or airway compression is unclear.

c. Mediastinal or Endobronchial Tumor

Tumors may compress the airways or central blood vessels in one position but not the other.[64–66] A clue to this diagnosis is a localized wheeze that appears in the position causing symptoms.[64]

---

*In 1937, Drs. Wood and Wolferth first described trepopnea in patients with congestive heart failure.[59] In searching for a name for the finding, a patent lawyer suggested to them "rolling relief," which they translated into "rotopnea," until a Dr. Kern pointed out that "roto" was a Latin root and the pure Greek term "trepopnea" would be better.[60]

C. PLATYPNEA

1. Finding

Platypnea (from the Greek *platus*, meaning "flat") is the opposite of orthopnea: patients experience worse dyspnea when they sit up and relief when they lie down (a related term, "orthodeoxia," described a similar deterioration of oxygen saturation in the upright position). This rare syndrome was first described in 1949, and the term "platypnea" was first coined in 1969.[67,68]

2. Clinical Significance

Platypnea occurs in patients with right-to-left shunting of blood through intracardiac or intrapulmonary shunts.

a. Right-to-Left Shunting of Blood Through a Patent Foramen Ovale or Atrial Septal Defect

These patients often first develop the finding after undergoing pneumonectomy or developing a pulmonary embolus or pericardial effusion, which for unclear reasons promotes right-to-left shunting in the upright position.[69–74]

b. Right-to-Left Shunting of Blood Through Intrapulmonary Shunts

Shunting through intrapulmonary shunts located in the bases of the lungs occurs in the hepatopulmonary syndrome, a complication of chronic liver disease.[75] In these patients, the upright position causes more blood to flow to the bases, thus aggravating the right-to-left shunting of blood and the patient's hypoxemia.

REFERENCES

1. Stokes W. *An introduction to the use of the stethoscope* (facsimile edition by the Classics of Cardiology Library). Edinburgh: Maclachlin and Stewart; 1825.
2. Geddes LA. Perspectives in physiological monitoring. *Med Instrument.* 1976;10: 91-97.
3. Osler W. *The principles and practice of medicine* (facsimile by Classics of Medicine library). New York: D. Appleton and Co; 1892.
4. Krieger B, Feinerman D, Zaron A, Bizousky F. Continuous noninvasive monitoring of respiratory rate in critically ill patients. *Chest.* 1986;90:632-634.
5. Kory RC. Routine measurement of respiratory rate: An expensive tribute to tradition. *JAMA.* 1957;165:448-450.
6. Hooker EA, O'Brien DJ, Danzl DF, et al. Respiratory rates in emergency department patients. *J Emerg Med.* 1989;7:129-132.

7. McFadden JP, Price RC, Eastwood HD, Briggs RS. Raised respiratory rate in elderly patients: A valuable physical sign. *Br Med J.* 1982;284:626-627.

8. Quetelet LAJ. *A treatise on man and the development of his faculties* (1969 facsimile by Scholars facsimiles and reprints). Edinburgh: William and Robert Chambers; 1842.

9. Mulroy MF. Monitoring opioids. *Reg Anesthesia.* 1996;21:89-93.

10. Tobin MJ, Perez W, Guenther SM, et al. The pattern of breathing during successful and unsuccessful trials of weaning from mechanical ventilation. *Am Rev Respir Dis.* 1986;134:1111-1118.

11. Fieselmann JF, Hendryx MS, Helms CM, Wakefield DS. Respiratory rate predicts cardiopulmonary arrest for internal medicine inpatients. *J Gen Intern Med.* 1993;8: 354-360.

12. Heckerling PS. The need for chest roentgenograms in adults with acute respiratory illness: Clinical predictors. *Arch Intern Med.* 1986;146:1321-1324.

13. Research Committee of the British Thoracic Society. Community-acquired pneumonia in adults in British hospitals in 1982-1983: A survey of aetiology, mortality, prognostic factors and outcome. *Q J Med.* 1987;62239:195-220.

14. Conte HA, Chen YT, Mehal W, et al. A prognostic rule for elderly patients admitted with community-acquired pneumonia. *Am J Med.* 1999;106:20-28.

15. Farr BM, Sloman AJ, Fisch MJ. Predicting death in patients hospitalized for community-acquired pneumonia. *Ann Intern Med.* 1991;115:428-436.

16. Brancati FL, Chow JW, Wagener MM, et al. Is pneumonia really the old man's friend? Two-year prognosis after community-acquired pneumonia. *Lancet.* 1993; 342:30-33.

17. Ewig S, Kleinfeld T, Seifert K, et al. Comparative validation of prognostic rules for community-acquired pneumonia in an elderly population. *Eur Respir J.* 1999;14: 370-375.

18. Gravelyn TR, Weg JG. Respiratory rate as an indicator of acute respiratory dysfunction. *JAMA.* 1980;244:1123-1125.

19. Cohen CA, Zagelbaum G, Gross D, et al. Clinical manifestations of inspiratory muscle fatigue. *Am J Med.* 1982;73:308-316.

20. Mower WR, Sachs C, Nicklin EL, et al. A comparison of pulse oximetry and respiratory rate in patient screening. *Resp Med.* 1996;90:593-599.

21. Webb P. Periodic breathing during sleep. *J Appl Physiol.* 1974;37:899-903.

22. Altschule MD, Iglauer A. The effect of position on periodic breathing in chronic cardiac decompensation. *N Engl J Med.* 1958;259:1064-1066.

23. Mortara A, Sleight P, Pinna GD, et al. Association between hemodynamic impairment and Cheyne-Stokes respiration and periodic breathing in chronic stable congestive heart failure secondary to ischemic or idiopathic dilated cardiomyopathy. *Am J Cardiol.* 1999;84:900-904.

24. Sternbach GL. John Cheyne and William Stokes: Periodic respiration. *J Emerg Med.* 1985;3:233-236.

25. Morse SR, Chandrasekhar AJ, Cugell DW. Cheyne-Stokes respiration redefined. *Chest.* 1974;66:345-346.

26. Lange RL, Hecht HH. The mechanism of Cheyne-Stokes respiration. *J Clin Invest.* 1962;41(1):42-52.

27. Franklin KA, Sandstrom E, Johansson G, Balsfors EM. Hemodynamics, cerebral circulation, and oxygen saturation in Cheyne-Stokes respiration. *J Appl Physiol.* 1997;83:1184-1191.

28. Tobin MJ, Snyder JV. Cheyne-Stokes respiration revisited: Controversies and implications. *Crit Care Med.* 1984;12:882-887.

29. Dowell AR, Buckley E, Cohen R, et al. Cheyne-Stokes respiration: A review of clinical manifestations and critique of physiological mechanisms. *Arch Intern Med.* 1971;127:712-726.

30. Harrison TR, King CE, Calhoun JA, Harrison WG. Congestive heart failure: XX. Cheyne-Stokes respiration as the cause of paroxysmal dyspnea at the onset of sleep. *Arch Intern Med.* 1934;53:891-910.

31. Rees PJ, Clark TJH. Paroxysmal nocturnal dyspnea and periodic respiration. *Lancet.* 1979;2:1315-1317.

32. Lee MC, Klassen AC, Heaney LM, Resch JA. Respiratory rate and pattern disturbances in acute brainstem infarction. *Stroke.* 1976;7:382-385.

33. Brown HW, Plum F. The neurologic basis of Cheyne-Stokes respiration. *Am J Med.* 1961;30:849-860.

34. Andreas S, Hagenah G, Moeller C, et al. Cheyne-Stokes respiration and prognosis in congestive heart failure. *Am J Cardiol.* 1996;78:1260-1264.

35. Hanly PJ, Zuberi-Khokhar NS. Increased mortality associated with Cheyne-Stokes respiration in patients with congestive heart failure. *Am J Respir Crit Care Med.* 1996;153:272-276.

36. Findley LJ, Zwillich CW, Ancoli-Israel S, et al. Cheyne-Stokes breathing during sleep in patients with left ventricular heart failure. *South Med J.* 1985;78:11-15.

37. Lanfranchi PA, Braghiroli A, Bosimini E, et al. Prognostic value of nocturnal Cheyne-Stokes respiration in chronic heart failure. *Circulation.* 1999;99:1435-1440.

38. Karp HR, Sieker HO, Heyman A. Cerebral circulation and function in Cheyne-Stokes respiration. *Am J Med.* 1961;30:861-870.

39. Javaheri S. A mechanism of central sleep apnea in patients with heart failure. *N Engl J Med.* 1999;341:949-954.

40. Naughton MT. Pathophysiology and treatment of Cheyne-Stokes respiration. *Thorax.* 1998;53:514-518.

41. Minagar A, Weiner WJ. Adolf Kussmaul and his respiratory sign. *J Med Biograph.* 2001;9:181-183.

42. Poole SR, Chetham M, Anderson M. Grunting respirations in infants and children. *Pediatr Emerg Care.* 1995;11:158-161.

43. Grinman S, Whitelaw WA. Pattern of breathing in a case of generalized respiratory muscle weakness. *Chest.* 1983;84:770-772.

44. Barach AL. Physiologic advantages of grunting, groaning, and pursed-lip breathing: Adaptive symptoms related to the development of continuous positive pressure breathing. *Bull N Y Acad Med.* 1973;49:666-673.

45. Knelson JH, Howatt WF, DeMutyh GR. The physiologic significance of grunting respiration. *Pediatrics.* 1969;44:393-400.

46. Loh L, Goldman M, Newsome Davis J. The assessment of diaphragm function. *Medicine.* 1977;56:165-169.

47. Goldman MD, Williams AJ, Soo Hoo G, Trang TTH. Asynchronous thoracoabdominal movements in chronic airflow obstruction (CAO). *Adv Exp Med Biol.* 1995;393:95-100.

48. Sharp JT, Goldberg NB, Druz WS, Danon J. Relative contributions of rib cage and abdomen to breathing in normal subjects. *J Appl Physiol.* 1975;39:608-618.

49. Gilbert R, Ashtosh K, Auchinocloss JH, et al. Prospective study of controlled oxygen therapy: Poor prognosis of patients with asynchronous breathing. *Chest.* 1977;71:456-462.

50. Ashutosh K, Gilbert R, Auchincloss JH, Peppi D. Asynchronous breathing movements in patients with chronic obstructive pulmonary disease. *Chest.* 1975; 67:553-557.

51. Mier-Jedrzejowicz A, Brophy C, Moxham J, Green M. Assessment of diaphragm weakness. *Am Rev Respir Dis.* 1988;137:877-883.

52. Chan CK, Loke J, Virgulto JA, Mohsenin V, et al. Bilateral diaphragmatic paralysis: Clinical spectrum, prognosis, and diagnostic approach. *Arch Phys Med Rehabil.* 1988;69:976-979.

53. Newsom Davis J, Goldman M, Loh L, Casson M. Diaphragm function and alveolar hypoventilation. *Q J Med.* 1976;45:87-100.

54. Calhoun JA, Cullen GE, Harrison TR, et al. Studies in congestive heart failure. XIV. Orthopnea: Its relation to ventilation, vital capacity, oxygen saturation and acid-base condition of arterial and jugular blood. *J Clin Invest.* 1931;10:833-855.

55. Zema MJ, Masters AP, Margouleff D. Dyspnea: The heart or the lungs? Differentiation at bedside by use of the simple Valsalva maneuver. *Chest.* 1984;85:59-64.

56. Sharp JT, Rakowski D, Keefer D. The effect of body position change on lung compliance in normal subjects and in patients with congestive heart failure. *J Clin Invest.* 1959;38:659-667.

57. Nava S, Larovere MT, Fanfulla F, et al. Orthopnea and inspiratory effort in chronic heart failure patients. *Resp Med.* 2003;97:647-653.

58. Chakko S, Woska D, Martinez H, et al. Clinical, radiographic, and hemodynamic correlations in chronic congestive heart failure: Conflicting results may lead to inappropriate care. *Am J Med.* 1991;90:353-359.

59. Wood FC, Wolferth CC. The tolerance of certain cardiac patients for various recumbent positions (trepopnea). *Am J Med Sci.* 1937;193:354-378.

60. Wood FC. Trepopnea. *Arch Int Med.* 1959;104:966-973.

61. Zack MB, Pontoppidan H, Kazemi H. The effect of lateral positions on gas exchange in pulmonary disease: A prospective evaluation. *Am Rev Resp Dis.* 1974; 110:49-55.

62. Remolina C, Khan AU, Santiago TV, Edelman NH. Positional hypoxemia in unilateral lung disease. *N Engl J Med.* 1981;304:523-525.

63. Fujita M, Miyamoto S, Tambara K, Budgell B. Trepopnea in patients with chronic heart failure. *Int J Cardiol.* 2002;84:115-118.

64. Acosta J, Khan F, Chitkara R. Trepopnea resulting from large aneurysm of sinus of Valsalva and descending aorta. *Heart Lung.* 1982;11:342-344.

65. Mahler DA, Snyder PE, Virgulto JA, Loke J. Positional dyspnea and oxygen desaturation related to carcinoma of the lung: Up with the good lung. *Chest.* 1983;83: 826-827.

66. Tsunezuka Y, Sato H, Tsukioka T, Shimizu H. Trepopnea due to recurrent lung cancer. *Respiration.* 2000;67:98-100.

67. Altman M, Robin ED. Platypnea (diffuse zone 1 phenomenon?). *N Engl J Med.* 1969;281:1347-1348.

68. Robin ED, McCauley RF. An analysis of platypnea-orthodeoxia syndrome, including a "new" therapeutic approach. *Chest.* 1997;112:1449-1451.

69. LaBresh KA, Pietro DA, Coates EO, et al. Platypnea syndrome after left pneumonectomy. *Chest.* 1981;79:605-607.

70. Seward JB, Hayes DL, Smith HC, et al. Platypnea-orthodeoxia: Clinical profile, diagnostic workup, management, and report of seven cases. *Mayo Clin Proc.* 1984;59:221-231.

71. Wright RS, Simari RD, Orszulak TA, et al. Eosinophilic endomyocardial disease presenting as cyanosis, platypnea, and orthodeoxia. *Ann Intern Med.* 1992;117: 482-483.

72. Adolph EA, Lacy WO, Hermoni YI, et al. Reversible orthodeoxia and platypnea due to right-to-left intracardiac shunting related to pericardial effusion. *Ann Intern Med.* 1992;116:138-139.

73. Begin R. Platypnea after pneumonectomy. *N Engl J Med.* 1975;293:342-343.

74. Hussain SF, Mekan SF. Platypnea-orthodeoxia: Report of two cases and review of the literature. *South Med J.* 2004;97:657-662.

75. Robin ED, Laman D, Horn BR, Theodore J. Platypnea related to orthodeoxia caused by true vascular lung shunts. *N Engl J Med.* 1976;294:941-943.

18

Pulse Oximetry

I. INTRODUCTION

Pulse oximetry measures the arterial oxygen saturation rapidly and conveniently. It is now regarded as the fifth vital sign[1,2] although some clinicians argue that pulse oximetry is a diagnostic test, not a physical sign, because it requires special equipment. Measurement of oxygen saturation, however, is no different from the other vital signs whose measurement requires a thermometer, sphygmomanometer, or stopwatch.

Takuo Aoyagi of Japan discovered the basic principle of pulse oximetry—pulsatile transmission of light through tissue depends on the patient's arterial saturation—in the mid-1970s.[3] The first pulse oximeters were successfully marketed in the 1980s.[4]

II. THE FINDING

Measurements are obtained by using a self-adhesive or clip-type probe attached to the patient's finger or ear. The oximeter makes several hundred measurements each second and then displays an average value based on the previous 3 to 6 seconds, which is updated about every second.[5] Although the digital display of pulse oximeters creates a sense of precision, studies show that, between oxygen saturation levels of 70% and 100%, pulse oximeters are only accurate within 5% (i.e., ±2 standard deviations) of measurements made by in vitro arterial blood gas analysis using co-oximetry.[4,6,7]

The most common causes of inadequate oximeter signals are poor perfusion (resulting from cold or hypotension), excessive ambient light, and motion artifact. The clinician can sometimes correct these problems and thus improve the signal by warming or rubbing the patient's hand, repositioning the probe, or resting the patient's hand on a soft surface.[5] If inadequate signals persist, the clinician should try obtaining measurements with the clip probe attached to the lobule or pinna of the patient's ear.

In patients with hemiparesis, the results of pulse oximetry on the right and left sides of the body are the same.[8]

III.   CLINICAL SIGNIFICANCE

A.   ADVANTAGES OF PULSE OXIMETRY

As a sign of low oxygen levels, pulse oximetry is superior to the physical sign of cyanosis, because oximetry is more sensitive and because readings do not depend on the patient's hemoglobin level (see Chapter 7). Consequently, pulse oximetry has become indispensable in the monitoring of patients in emergency departments, recovery and operating rooms, pulmonary clinics, and intensive care units, where measurements often reveal unsuspected oxygen desaturation, leading to changes in diagnosis and treatment.[9] Oxygen therapy prolongs survival of some hypoxemic patients, such as patients chronically hypoxemic from lung disease.[10,11] Presumably, oxygen therapy benefits patients with acute hypoxemia as well.

B.   LIMITATIONS OF PULSE OXIMETRY[4,6,12,13]

Because pulse oximetry readings indicate only the degree of oxygen saturation of hemoglobin, they fail to detect problems of poor oxygen delivery (e.g., anemia, poor cardiac output), hyperoxia, and hypercapnia. Other limitations of pulse oximetry measurements are discussed in the following sections.

1.   Dyshemoglobinemias

The pulse oximeter interprets carboxyhemoglobin to be oxyhemoglobin and therefore seriously underestimates the degree of oxygen desaturation in patients with carbon monoxide poisoning. In patients with methemoglobinemia, the pulse oximetry readings decrease initially but eventually plateau at around 85%, despite true oxyhemoglobin levels that continue to decrease to much lower levels.

2. Dyes

Methylene blue causes a spurious decrease in oxygen saturation readings. Some colors of nail polish and finger pigments also interfere with oximetry and should be removed before pulse oximetry monitoring.[14-16] Hyperbilirubinemia and jaundice, however, do not affect the pulse oximeter's accuracy.

3. Low Perfusion Pressure

In patients with hypotension or peripheral vascular disease, the arterial pulse may be so weak that the pulse oximeter is unable to pick up the arterial signal, thus making measurements difficult or impossible.

4. Exaggerated Venous Pulsations

In patients with right-sided heart failure or tricuspid regurgitation, the oximeter may mistake the venous waveform for the arterial one, leading to spuriously low oxygen saturation readings.

5. Excessive Ambient Light

Excessive ambient light (or malposition of the probe allowing ambient light to reach the sensor) also may interfere with the oximeter's accuracy, falsely lowering the value in patients with normal oxygen saturation and, more importantly, overestimating it in patients with significant hypoxemia.

REFERENCES

1. Tierney LM, Whooley MA, Saint S. Oxygen saturation: A fifth vital sign? *West J Med.* 1997;166:285-286.
2. Neff TA. Routine oximetry: A fifth vital sign? *Chest.* 1988;94:227.
3. Aoyagi T. Pulse oximetry: Its invention, theory, and future. *J Anesth.* 2003;17:259-266.
4. Tremper KK, Barker SJ. Pulse oximetry. *Anesthesiology.* 1989;70:98-108.
5. Hanning CD, Alexander-Williams JM. Pulse oximetry: A practical review. *Br Med J.* 1995;311:367-370.
6. Sinex JE. Pulse oximetry: Principles and limitations. *Am J Emerg Med.* 1999;17:59-66.
7. Jensen LA, Onyskiw JE, Prasad NGN. Meta-analysis of arterial oxygen saturation monitoring by pulse oximetry in adults. *Heart Lung.* 1998;27:387-408.
8. Roffe C, Sills S, Wilde K, Crome P. Effect of hemiparetic stroke on pulse oximetry readings on the affected side. *Stroke.* 2001;32:1808-1810.
9. Mower WR, Myers G, Nicklin EL, et al. Pulse oximetry as a fifth vital sign in emergency geriatric assessment. *Acad Emerg Med.* 1998;5:858-865.

10. Medical Research Council Working Party. Long term domiciliary oxygen therapy in chronic hypoxic cor pulmonale complicating chronic bronchitis and emphysema. *Lancet*. 1981;1:681-686.

11. Nocturnal Oxygen Therapy Trial Group. Continuous or nocturnal oxygen therapy in hypoxemic chronic obstructive lung disease: A clinical trial. *Ann Intern Med*. 1980;93:391-398.

12. Schnapp LM, Cohen NH. Pulse oximetry: Uses and abuses. *Chest*. 1990;98:1244-1250.

13. Soubani AO. Noninvasive monitoring of oxygen and carbon dioxide. *Am J Emerg Med*. 2001;19:141-146.

14. Cote CJ, Goldstein A, Fuchsman WH, Hoaglin DC. The effect of nail polish on pulse oximetry. *Anesth Analg*. 1988;67:683-686.

15. Battito MF. The effect of fingerprinting ink on pulse oximetry. *Anesth Analg*. 1989;69:265.

16. Goucke R. Hazards of henna. *Anesth Analg*. 1989;69:416.

HEAD AND NECK

19

The Pupils

NORMAL PUPIL

I. INTRODUCTION

The integrity of the pupil depends on the iris, cranial nerves II and III, and the sympathetic nerves innervating the eye.

II. SIZE

The size of the normal pupil decreases as persons grow older ($r = -0.75$, $p < 0.001$): At 10 years of age the mean diameter is 7 mm, at 30 years it is 6 mm, and at 80 years it is 4 mm.[1,2] Throughout human history, large pupils have been associated with youth, beauty, and vigor, explaining why the plant yielding the pupillary dilator atropine was named *belladonna*, which literally means "beautiful lady."

III. HIPPUS

Under steady illumination the normal pupil is in continual motion, repeatedly dilating and contracting small amounts. This restless undulation, called "hippus" or "pupillary unrest," is more prominent in younger patients and during exposure to bright light. Clinicians of the 19th century associated hippus with all sorts of diseases, from myasthenia gravis to brain tumors, but hippus is now known to be a normal phenomenon.[3] The oscillations of the right and left pupil are synchronous, which suggests hippus is under central control.

IV. SIMPLE ANISOCORIA

Simple anisocoria, a normal finding, is defined as a 0.4 mm or more difference in size of the right and left pupil that cannot be attributed to any of the abnormal pupils discussed later, intraocular drugs, ocular injury, or ocular inflammation.[2] Simple anisocoria occurs in up to 38% of healthy persons (only half of these patients have anisocoria at any given moment) and affects 3% of persons all of the time. When simple anisocoria waxes and wanes, the same eye usually displays the larger pupil.[2]

The difference in pupil size in simple anisocoria rarely exceeds 1 mm.[2] Other features distinguishing it from pathologic anisocoria are described later, under "abnormal pupils."

V. NORMAL LIGHT REFLEX

A. ANATOMY

Figure 19-1 illustrates the nerves responsible for the normal light reflex. Because both pupillary constrictor muscles normally receive identical signals from the midbrain, they constrict the same amount, which may be small or large depending on the *summation* of light intensity coming into *both* eyes. For example, both pupils dilate the same amount in darkness, constrict an identical small amount when a dim light is held in front of one eye, and constrict an identical larger amount when a bright light is held in front of one eye.

With a light held in front of one eye, ipsilateral pupillary constriction is called "direct reaction" to light and contralateral constriction is called "consensual reaction."

B. CLINICAL SIGNIFICANCE

The anatomy of the normal light reflex has two important clinical implications.

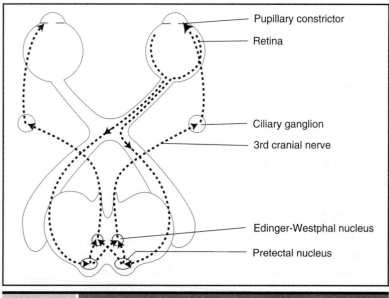

Pupillary constrictor

Retina

Ciliary ganglion

3rd cranial nerve

Edinger-Westphal nucleus

Pretectal nucleus

FIGURE 19-1	ANATOMY OF THE PUPILLARY LIGHT REFLEX.

The dotted lines show how nerve impulses from the retina and optic nerve on one side (right eye in this example) contribute to the nerve impulses of both third nerves, via the crossing of the nerve impulses from the nasal retina in the optic chiasm and the abundant inter-connections between both pretectal nuclei and both Edinger-Westphal nuclei. Unless there is asymmetric disease of the efferent pathway (i.e., third nerve, ciliary ganglion and postganglionic fibers, iris), the pupils are thus symmetric.

1.   Anisocoria Is Absent in Disorders of the Optic Nerve or Retina (i.e., the Afferent Connections)

Because the signal in both outgoing third nerves is identical in these disorders, representing the summation of light intensity from both eyes, the pupils are the same size. Unilateral afferent disease is similar to the experiment previously described of holding a bright light in front of one eye (i.e., the eye not being illuminated is similar to an eye with an afferent defect: despite receiving less light on one side, the pupils are the same).

2.   Anisocoria Indicates Asymmetric Disease of the Iris, Third Nerve, or Sympathetic Nerves (i.e., Efferent Connections and Iris)

Asymmetric disease of the efferent connections guarantees that the signals arriving at the pupil are different and that the pupil size, therefore, will be different.

VI. NEAR SYNKINESIS REACTION

The near synkinesis reaction occurs when a person focuses on a near object. The reaction has three parts: (1) constriction of the pupils (pupilloconstrictor muscle), (2) convergence of eyes (medial rectus muscles), and (3) accommodation of the lenses (ciliary body).

ABNORMAL PUPILS

I. RELATIVE AFFERENT PUPILLARY DEFECT (MARCUS GUNN PUPIL)

A. INTRODUCTION
The relative afferent pupillary defect is the most common abnormal pupillary finding, more common than all other pupillary defects combined.[4]

Although the relative afferent pupillary defect was described by R. Marcus Gunn in 1904, it is clear from his report that the sign was generally known to clinicians of his time. Kestenbaum named the finding in 1946 after Marcus Gunn,[4] and in 1959, Levatin[5] introduced the "swinging flashlight test," which is how most clinicians now elicit the finding.

B. THE FINDING
Because the pupils are equal in patients with disorders of the retina and optic nerves (see "Normal Pupils" and Fig. 19-1), the swinging flashlight test is necessary to uncover disorders of the afferent half of the light reflex. This test compares the amount of pupilloconstriction produced by illuminating one eye with that produced by illuminating the other.

To perform the test, the clinician swings the flashlight back and forth from eye to eye, holding it over each pupil 1 to 2 seconds at a time before immediately shifting it to the other (Fig. 19-2). Both pupils constrict strongly when the light is shining into the normal eye, but, as the light moves to illuminate the abnormal eye, both pupils dilate (dilation occurs because the pupils respond as if the light were much dimmer, producing a smaller bilateral constriction—or net dilation—compared with when the light is shining in the normal eye).[4,6] As long as the clinician swings the light back and forth, the reaction persists— pupils constrict with light into the normal eye and dilate with light into the abnormal eye. Because the clinician usually just focuses on the illuminated pupil, the one that dilates is labeled as having a "relative afferent pupillary defect" or the "Marcus Gunn pupil."

There has been some debate whether eyes with afferent defects also display abnormal pupillary release (pupillary release occurs during steady illumination

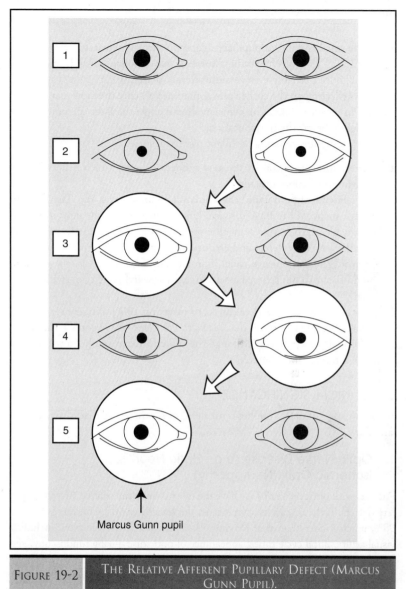

| FIGURE 19-2 | THE RELATIVE AFFERENT PUPILLARY DEFECT (MARCUS GUNN PUPIL). |

The figure depicts a patient with an abnormal *right* optic nerve. Under normal room light illumination (*row 1*), the pupils are symmetric. During the swinging flashlight test, the pupils constrict when the normal eye is illuminated (*rows 2 and 4*) but dilate when the abnormal eye is illuminated (*rows 3 and 5*). Although both pupils constrict or dilate simultaneously, the clinician is usually focused on just the illuminated pupil. The pupil that dilates during the swinging flashlight test has the "relative afferent pupillary defect" and is labeled the "Marcus Gunn pupil." See text.

and is the small amount of pupillary dilatation that immediately follows initial constriction).[7] Two careful studies, however, have shown that only the swinging flashlight test reliably uncovers the afferent defect.[8,9]

Light reflecting off the cornea may sometimes obscure the movements of the pupils. To overcome this, the clinician should angle the light to come from a point slightly below the horizontal axis.

Interpreting the swinging flashlight test has three caveats[6,10]:

1. **Correct interpretation of the test ignores hippus,** which otherwise can make interpretation difficult.
2. **The clinician should avoid the tendency to linger with the flashlight on the eye suspected to have disease.** Uneven swinging of the light may temporarily bleach the retina being illuminated more, thus eventually producing a relative pupillary defect and erroneously confirming the initial suspicion. To avoid this and ensure equal illumination of both retinas, the clinician should count to himself or herself: "one, two, switch, one two, switch," and so on.
3. **Only one working iris is required to interpret this pupillary sign.** If the patient has only one pupil that reacts to light (see "Anisocoria"), the test is performed the same way, although the clinician focuses only on the normal iris to interpret the results.

C. CLINICAL SIGNIFICANCE

A relative afferent defect implies optic nerve or severe retinal disease of the ipsilateral eye.

1. Optic Nerve Disease (e.g., Optic Neuritis, Ischemic Optic Neuropathy)

Patients with optic nerve disease have the most prominent relative afferent pupillary defects. If the disease is asymmetric, the sensitivity of the finding is 92% to 98%, much higher than that for any other test of afferent function, including visual acuity, pupil cycle times, appearance of optic disc during funduscopy, and visual evoked potentials.[11,12] The finding depends, however, on *asymmetric* optic nerve function (hence the word "relative" in its label); consequently, in patients with suspected unilateral disease but without the afferent pupillary finding, bilateral optic nerve disease is eventually found two thirds of the time.[12]

2. Retinal Disease

Severe retinal disease may cause a relative afferent pupillary defect, although the retinal disease must be markedly asymmetric to produce the finding and, once the finding appears, it is subtle compared with that seen in optic nerve disease.[13,14]

3. Cataracts Do Not Cause the Relative Afferent Pupillary Defect[13,15]

Although this seems surprising, it is because the retina, if healthy, compensates over minutes for any diminished brightness, just as it does when as person walks into a dark movie theater. In fact, in Galen's time it was known that an intact pupillary light reaction was a good prognostic sign for vision if cataract couching was being considered (i.e., the retina and optic nerve behind the cataract are intact).[4,16]

II. ARGYLL ROBERTSON PUPILS

A. THE FINDING[17,18]

Argyll Robertson pupils have four characteristic findings: (1) bilateral involvement, (2) small pupils that fail to dilate fully in dim light, (3) no light reaction, and (4) brisk constriction to near vision and brisk redilation to far vision.

Originally described by Douglas Moray Cooper Lamb Argyll Robertson in 1868, this finding had great significance a century ago because it settled a long-standing debate whether general paresis and tabes dorsalis were the same disease. The pupillary abnormality was found in a high proportion of patients with both diseases and was limited to these diseases, arguing for a common syphilitic origin of both. The introduction of Wassermann's serologic test for syphilis in 1906 confirmed that the two diseases had the same cause.

B. CLINICAL SIGNIFICANCE

1. Associated Disorders

In addition to neurosyphilis, there are rare, scattered reports of Argyll Robertson pupils in patients with various other disorders, including diabetes mellitus, neurosarcoidosis, and Lyme disease (see "Diabetic Pupil").[17] The responsible lesion is probably located in the dorsal midbrain, where damage would interrupt the light reflex fibers but spare the more ventrally located fibers innervating the Edinger-Westphal nuclei that control the near reaction.[19]

2. Differential Diagnosis of Light-Near Dissociation

Argyll Robertson pupils display light-near dissociation, that is, they fail to react to light but constrict during near vision. Several other causes of light-near dissociation include the following.

a. Adie's Tonic Pupil (See Later)

b. Optic Nerve or Severe Retinal Disease

Either of these disorders may eliminate the light reaction when light is directed into the abnormal eye, although the pupils still constrict with the near synkinesis.

In contrast to other causes of light-near dissociation, however, optic nerve and retinal disease severely impair vision.

c. Dorsal Midbrain Syndrome (Also Known as "Parinaud's Syndrome," "Sylvian Aqueduct Syndrome," or "Pretectal Syndrome")

Characteristic findings of dorsal midbrain syndrome are light-near dissociation, vertical gaze palsy, lid retraction, and convergence-retraction nystagmus (a rhythmic inward movement of both eyes from co-contraction of the extraocular muscles, usually elicited during convergence or upward gaze; most neuro-ophthalmologists use a optokinetic drum rotating downward to elicit the finding). Common causes of the dorsal midbrain syndrome are pinealoma in younger patients and multiple sclerosis and basilar artery strokes in older patients.[20]

d. Aberrant Regeneration of the Third Nerve

After damage to the third nerve (from trauma, aneurysms, or tumors but *not* ischemia), regenerating fibers originally destined for the medial rectus muscle may instead reinnervate the pupillary constrictor, thus causing pupillary constriction during convergence but no reaction to light. Unlike Argyll Robertson pupils, however, this finding is unilateral, and most patients also have anisocoria, ptosis, and diplopia.[21,22]

3. "Near-Light Dissociation"

The phenomenon opposite to light-near dissociation, near-light dissociation describes pupils that react to light but not during the near synkinesis. Near-light dissociation was historically described as a finding of von Economo's encephalitis lethargica, although now it usually means the patient is not trying hard enough to focus on a near object.[17] For this reason, many neuro-ophthalmologists save time during their examination and skip testing the near response unless the patient demonstrates no pupillary light reaction.

III. OVAL PUPIL

There are three causes of the oval pupil.

A. Evolving Third Nerve Palsy from Brain Herniation

These patients are invariably comatose from cerebral catastrophes causing elevated intracranial pressure.[23,24] As the pupil marches on to become fully round, dilated, and fixed, it may appear oval for a short time.

B. ADIE'S TONIC PUPIL (SEE LATER)

Adie's tonic pupil may sometimes appear oval from segmental iris palsy.[25] These patients are alert and, if complaining of anything, describe only blurring of vision in the involved eye (from paralysis of accommodation).

C. PREVIOUS SURGERY OR TRAUMA TO THE IRIS

IV. ANISOCORIA

A. DEFINITION

Anisocoria is defined as a difference ≥0.4 mm in the diameter of the pupils. It represents either a problem with the pupillary constrictor muscle (parasympathetic denervation, iris disorder, pharmacologic pupil) or the pupillary dilator muscle (sympathetic denervation, simple anisocoria).

B. TECHNIQUE

Figures 19-3 and 19-4 summarize the initial approach to anisocoria. The most important initial questions follow:

1. **Is the anisocoria old or new?** Examination of driver's license photograph or other facial photograph, magnified with the direct ophthalmoscope (using the +10 lens), may reveal a preexisting pupillary inequality.[28]
2. **Do both pupils constrict normally during the light reflex?** If there is a poor light reaction in the eye with the larger pupil, the pupillary constrictor of that eye is abnormal. If there is a good light reaction in both eyes, the pupillary dilator of the eye with the smaller pupil is abnormal.
3. **Is the anisocoria worse in bright light or dim light/darkness?** If anisocoria is worse in light than darkness, the pupillary constrictor of the eye with the larger pupil is abnormal. If anisocoria is worse in darkness than light, the pupillary dilator of the eye with the smaller pupil is abnormal (see Fig. 19-4).*[29]

C. ABNORMAL PUPILLARY CONSTRICTOR (THE "FIXED, DILATED PUPIL," RESULTING FROM PARASYMPATHETIC DEFECT, IRIS DISORDER, OR PHARMACOLOGIC BLOCKADE)

The most important questions in these patients are (1) Is there a full third nerve palsy or are the findings confined to the pupillary constrictor? (Fig. 19-5) and (2) Is there altered mental status or other neurologic findings?

---

*To determine the amount of anisocoria in darkness, neuro-ophthalmologists often take a flash picture of the patient in darkness. Because there is a delay of about 1.5 seconds between the flash of light and subsequent pupillary constriction, such a picture actually reflects pupil size in darkness (this delay explains why cameras designed to reduce "red eye" actually flash repeatedly *before* the picture is taken).[4]

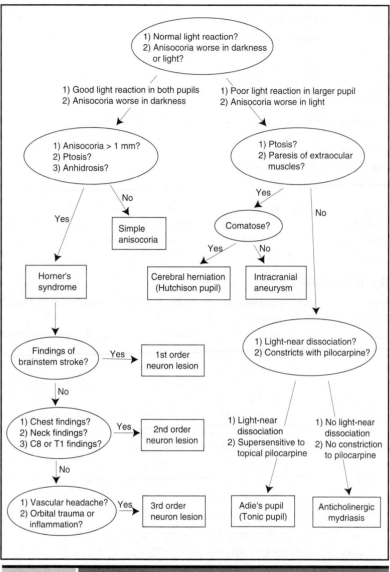

FIGURE 19-3   SUMMARY OF APPROACH TO ANISOCORIA.

The first two questions (Is there a normal light reaction? and Is aniso-coria worse in darkness or light?, see also Fig. 19-4) distinguish problems with the pupillary dilator muscle (i.e., Horner's syndrome, simple anisocoria; *left side* of figure) from problems with the pupillary constrictor muscle (i.e., third cranial nerve, iris; *right side* of figure). Two other tests distinguish Horner's syndrome from simple anisocoria: the cocaine test (see Fig. 19-8) and pupillary dilator lag (i.e., the pupil dilates slowly in darkness, as documented by photographs, see text). Based on references 26 and 27.

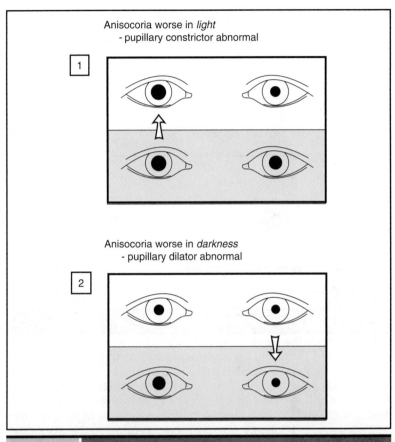

Anisocoria worse in *light*
- pupillary constrictor abnormal

Anisocoria worse in *darkness*
- pupillary dilator abnormal

FIGURE 19-4   COMPARING ANISOCORIA IN LIGHT AND DARKNESS.

Patient 1 (*top*) has more prominent anisocoria in light than darkness, indicating that the pupillary *constrictor* of the *larger* pupil is abnormal (i.e., it fails to constrict in light, *arrow*). Patient 2 has more prominent anisocoria in darkness than light, indicating that the pupillary *dilator* of the *smaller* pupil is abnormal (i.e., it fails to dilate in darkness, *arrow*). The diagnosis in patient 1 (abnormal pupillary constrictor) could be a third nerve palsy, tonic pupil, pharmacologic mydriasis, or a disorder of the iris (right side of Fig. 19-3). The diagnosis in patient 2 (abnormal pupillary dilator, left side of Fig. 19-3) could be Horner's syndrome or simple anisocoria. In patient 2, both pupils will react to light, whereas the larger pupil of patient 1 will not react well to light.

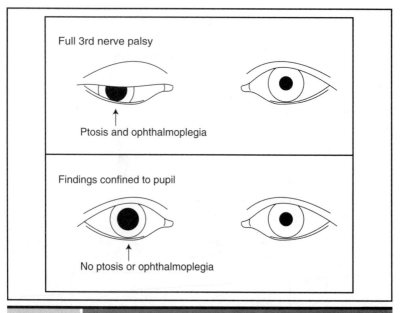

Full 3rd nerve palsy

↑
Ptosis and ophthalmoplegia

Findings confined to pupil

↑
No ptosis or ophthalmoplegia

| FIGURE 19-5 | TYPES OF ABNORMAL PUPILLARY CONSTRICTOR. |

Both patients in this figure have a paralyzed right pupillary constrictor (i.e., a dilated pupil that fails to react well to light; see Fig. 19-4). The patient in the top row also has ptosis and ophthalmoplegia (i.e., eyes not aligned), indicating a full third nerve palsy: Possible diagnoses are transtentorial herniation (if comatose) or intracranial aneurysm (if mentally alert). The patient in the bottom row lacks ptosis and ophthalmoplegia, indicating the findings are confined to the pupil itself: possible diagnoses are the tonic pupil, pharmacologic mydriasis, or a disorder of the iris. See text.

1. Full Third Nerve Palsy: Associated Ptosis and Paralysis of Ocular Movements

Because the third cranial nerve controls the levator palpebrae (which lifts the eyelid) and four of the six eye muscles (medial, inferior, and superior recti, and inferior oblique), a full third nerve palsy causes a dilated pupil, ptosis, ophthalmoplegia, and an eye that is deviated outward and downward (see Fig. 19-5, *top row*). In patients with anisocoria, this has two important causes.

a. Ipsilateral Brain Herniation (Hutchinson Pupil)[30,31]

These patients are in the midst of a neurologic catastrophe from an expanding unilateral cerebral mass that causes coma, damage to the ipsilateral third nerve (dilated pupil, ptosis, and ophthalmoplegia), and, eventually, damage to the contralateral cerebral peduncle (which may lead to the false localizing sign of hemiplegia on the *same* side of the lesion). Although the involvement of the ocular muscles may be difficult to recognize, most patients have a narrowed palpebral fissure and an eye that, if not dysconjugate, moves poorly during the vestibulo-ocular reflex. The expanding mass is on the same side as the dilated pupil 77% to 96% of the time.[32-34]

In patients with coma, examination of the pupils is one of the key physical findings distinguishing intracranial structural disorders (e.g., expanding hemispheric or posterior fossa masses; 33% to 59% of patients with coma) from metabolic encephalopathy (e.g., drug overdose, hypoglycemia, sepsis, uremia, or other metabolic disorder; 41% to 67% of patients with coma).[35-37] Abnormal pupils support a structural cause; normal pupils argue for metabolic encephalopathy. In one study of 115 adults with coma (i.e., Glasgow Coma Scale $\leq$7),[37] anisocoria greater than 1 mm significantly increased the probability of an intracranial structural disorder [likelihood ratio (LR) = 9.0, EBM Box 19-1], whereas preservation of light reactions in both pupils argued against a structural disorder (LR = 0.2) and thus *for* metabolic encephalopathy.

b. Posterior Communicating Artery Aneurysm

Posterior communicating artery aneurysms are the most common of all intracranial aneurysms. Twenty percent to 61% of patients present with an ipsilateral third nerve palsy, which dilates the pupil. It is essential to recognize this disorder promptly because of the risk of subsequent, devastating subarachnoid hemorrhage. Importantly, the abnormal pupil is almost always accompanied by ptosis and ophthalmoplegia (i.e., full third nerve palsy, see Fig. 19-5): In reports of 332 aneurysms that give details of the third nerve paresis, 71% had dilated pupil and complete ophthalmoplegia, 25% had dilated pupil and partial ophthalmoplegia, 4% had sparing of the pupil with partial ophthalmoplegia, and only 1 patient had isolated involvement of the pupil.[43-51]

2. The Tonic Pupil
a. The Finding

The tonic pupil has five important features (Fig. 19-6): (1) unilateral dilation of a pupil; (2) poor or absent response to light; (3) extensive, slow (over seconds), and long-lasting constriction during near vision (this is why the pupil is "tonic"; i.e., it is analogous to "myotonia"); (4) disturbances of accommodation (which causes the main concern for many patients, i.e., an inability to focus vision in the involved eye); and (5) supersensitivity of pupillary constriction to pilocarpine.[25,52,53]

Although both the Argyll Robertson pupil and the tonic pupil display light-near dissociation, they are easily distinguished by the characteristics in Table 19-1.

Box 19-1 Pupils*

Finding (Ref)	Sensitivity (%)	Specificity (%)	Likelihood Ratio if Finding	
			Present	Absent
Detecting intracranial structural lesion in patients with coma[37]				
Anisocoria >1 mm	39	96	**9.0**	0.6
Absent light reflex in at least one eye	83	77	**3.6**	**0.2**
Detecting Horner's syndrome[38,39]				
Post-topical cocaine anisocoria ≥1mm	95	99	**96.8**	**0.1**
Detecting first or second order neuron lesion in Horner's syndrome[40,41]				
Dilation with topical hydroxyamphetamine (Paredrine)	83-92	79-96	**9.2**	**0.2**
Detecting serious eye disease in patients with unilaterally red eye[42]				
Anisocoria ≥1 mm	19	97	**6.5**	0.8

Likelihood ratio (LR) if finding present = positive LR; LR if finding absent = negative LR.
*Diagnostic standard: For structural lesion, supratentorial and subtentorial lesions with gross anatomical abnormality, including cerebrovascular disease, intracranial hematoma, tumor, and contusion; for serious eye disease, corneal foreign body or abrasion, keratitis, or uveitis.

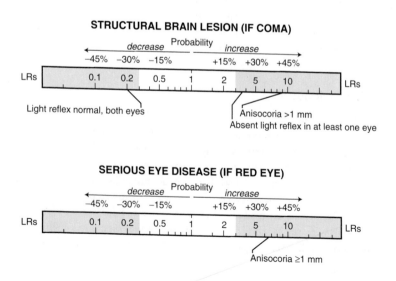

STRUCTURAL BRAIN LESION (IF COMA)

SERIOUS EYE DISEASE (IF RED EYE)

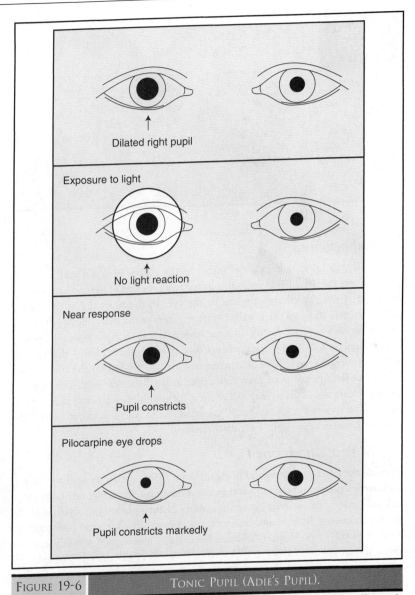

Dilated right pupil

Exposure to light

No light reaction

Near response

Pupil constricts

Pilocarpine eye drops

Pupil constricts markedly

FIGURE 19-6   TONIC PUPIL (ADIE'S PUPIL).

The patient in this figure has a *right* tonic pupil. At baseline, there is anisocoria with the right pupil larger than the left (*first row*). The dilated pupil fails to react to light (*second row*) but constricts slowly (i.e., "tonic" contraction) when the patient focuses on a near object (*third row*). After instillation of dilute pilocarpine eye drops (*fourth row*), the pupil constricts markedly.

Table 19-1	Comparison of Tonic Pupil and Argyll Robertson Pupil*	
Finding	Tonic Pupil	Argyll Robertson Pupils
Pupil size	Large	Small
Laterality	Mostly unilateral	Mostly bilateral
Reaction to near vision	Extremely slow and prolonged with slow redilation	Normal with brisk redilation

*Based on reference 52.

b. Pathogenesis

The tonic pupil occurs because of injury to the ciliary ganglion and postganglionic fibers (see Fig. 19-1) and subsequent misdirection of nerve fibers as they regenerate from the ciliary ganglion to the eye. In the normal eye, the ciliary ganglion sends 30 times the number of nerve fibers to the ciliary body (the muscle that focuses the lens during the near synkinesis) as to the iris (i.e., the pupillary constrictor).[54] Once these fibers are disrupted, odds are 30 to 1 that the iris will receive regenerating fibers that were originally intended for the ciliary body instead of the normal ones that participate in the light reaction. The pupil of these patients thus fails to respond to light, although during near vision, which normally activates the ciliary body, the misdirected fibers to the iris cause the pupil to constrict (i.e., light-near dissociation).

c. Clinical Significance

Because the ciliary ganglion and postganglionic fibers are contiguous to the eyeball, any of various injuries may cause the tonic pupil, including orbital trauma, orbital tumors, or varicella-zoster infections of the ophthalmic division of the trigeminal nerve. Most cases, however, are idiopathic, which has been dubbed "Adie's pupil" (named after William John Adie, although the syndrome was more thoroughly and accurately described by others before his 1931 paper).[52]

3. Disorders of the Iris

a. Pharmacologic Blockade of the Pupil with Topical Anticholinergic Drugs

Pharmacologic blockade causes an isolated fixed, dilated pupil without paralysis of eye movements. Not all patients with this problem are surreptitiously instilling mydriatic drops. Causes include unintended exposure of the eye to anticholinergic nebulizer treatments,[55] scopolamine patches,[56] and plants containing anticholinergic substances (blue nightshade, angel's trumpet, jimsonweed, moonflower).[57-60] Nebulizer treatments are an important cause to recognize in the intensive care unit, where metabolic encephalopathy is also common, leading clinicians to misdiagnose the Hutchison pupil in patients with pharmacologic anisocoria and unresponsiveness.

The pharmacologic pupil characteristically fails to constrict to topical pilocarpine (see later).

4. The Poorly Reactive Pupil—Response to Pilocarpine

In difficult diagnostic problems, especially when pharmacologic blockade is a consideration, the pupil's response to topical pilocarpine solution is helpful. Pilocarpine constricts Adie's pupil and the dilated pupil from parasympathetic denervation (Hutchinson pupil or intracranial aneurysm) but not the dilated pupil from pharmacologic blockade.[61]

D. ABNORMAL PUPILLARY DILATOR

1. Definition

The most important cause of an abnormal pupillary dilator muscle is sympathetic denervation of the pupil, or **Horner's syndrome**, which has three characteristics: (1) ipsilateral miosis (paralyzed pupillodilator muscle), (2) ipsilateral ptosis (paralyzed superior tarsal muscle), and (3) ipsilateral anhidrosis of the face (from damage to sudomotor fibers). Figure 19-7 describes the neuroanatomy of the sympathetic pathways innervating the eye.

Horner's syndrome is named after the Swiss ophthalmologist Johann Horner, who published a description of the syndrome in 1869. Like other eponymous pupillary findings (Adie's pupil and Marcus Gunn pupil), other clinicians had published earlier descriptions of the same finding.[62,63]

2. Horner's Syndrome Versus Simple Anisocoria

When evaluating a pupil that dilates abnormally (see left half of Fig. 19-3; patient 2 in Fig. 19-4), the findings of anisocoria greater than 1 mm, associated ptosis, or asymmetric facial sweating all indicate Horner's syndrome.

In difficult cases, the definitive test of sympathetic denervation is the cocaine test (cocaine drops diminish the anisocoria of simple anisocoria but aggravate that of Horner's syndrome. Fig. 19-8). In one study of 169 persons, the presence of post-cocaine anisocoria ≥ 1 mm was pathognomonic for Horner's syndrome (LR = 96.8, see EBM Box 19-1); the absence of this finding was a strong argument against the diagnosis (LR = 0.1). Nonetheless, topical cocaine has the disadvantage of being a controlled narcotic that must be prepared by local pharmacies. In addition, testing renders the patient's urine test positive for cocaine up to 48 hours.[64,65] The topical glaucoma

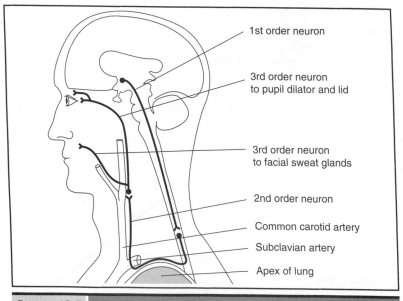

1st order neuron

3rd order neuron
to pupil dilator and lid

3rd order neuron
to facial sweat glands

2nd order neuron

Common carotid artery

Subclavian artery

Apex of lung

FIGURE 19-7   ANATOMY OF SYMPATHETIC PATHWAYS TO THE EYE.

The sympathetic innervation of the eye consists of three neurons connected in series: first order neurons, second order neurons, and third order neurons. The first order neurons ("central" neurons) extend from the posterior hypothalamus to the C8-T2 level of the spinal cord. The second order neurons ("preganglionic" neurons) leave the spinal cord and travel over the lung apex, around the subclavian artery, and along the carotid artery to the superior cervical ganglion. The third order neurons ("postganglionic neurons") diverge and take two paths: those to the pupil and lid muscles travel along the internal carotid artery through the cavernous sinus to reach the orbit; those to the facial sweat glands travel with the external carotid artery to the face. Lesions in any of these neurons causes Horner's syndrome and distinct associated physical signs (see Fig. 19-3 and text).

medication, apraclonidine, may replace topical cocaine when testing for Horner's syndrome in the future.[65-69]

3. Clinical Significance of Horner's Syndrome

a. Etiology

Which etiologies of Horner's syndrome a clinician is likely to see depends on the clinician's specialty. On a neurologic service, 70% of patients with Horner's

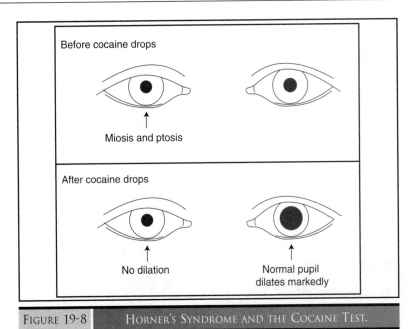

Before cocaine drops

Miosis and ptosis

After cocaine drops

No dilation   Normal pupil
                     dilates markedly

FIGURE 19-8   HORNER'S SYNDROME AND THE COCAINE TEST.

Both pictures are of the same patient, before (*top*) and 45 minutes after (*bottom*) installation of cocaine drops into each eye. At baseline, there is a mild right ptosis and miosis, which suggests the diagnosis of Horner's syndrome of the right pupil. After installation of the cocaine eyedrops into both eyes, the right pupil fails to dilate, markedly aggravating the anisocoria and confirming the diagnosis of Horner's syndrome. Cocaine eye drops block the reuptake of norepinephrine at the myoneural junction of the iris dilator, causing the pupil to dilate unless norepinephrine is absent because of sympathetic denervation.

syndrome have lesions in the first order neuron, usually strokes in the brainstem (see Table 58-2 in Chapter 58).[70] On a medical service, 70% of patients have a lesion in the second order neuron, usually from tumors (e.g., lung and thyroid) or trauma (e.g., to the neck, chest, spinal nerves, subclavian or carotid arteries).[62] Ophthalmologists tend to see second and third order neuron lesions (causes of lesions in the third order neuron are vascular headache, skull fracture, and cavernous sinus syndrome).[40,41,71]

b. Localizing the Lesion

(1) Associated Findings Helpful features are (1) findings from the ipsilateral brainstem (e.g., lateral medullary syndrome), pointing to a first order

neuron lesion (see Table 58-2 in Chapter 58); (2) abnormal chest or neck findings, a supraclavicular mass, or motor, reflex, or sensory findings of the ipsilateral C8T1 spinal roots, all pointing to the second order neuron lesion; and (3) orbital trauma, orbital inflammation, migraine or neck pain, pointing to a third order neuron lesion.

(2) Facial Sweating The sudomotor sympathetic fibers to the face diverge from the sympathetic pathway at the bifurcation of the carotid artery and therefore do not accompany the sympathetic nerves to the pupil and lid. Theoretically, therefore, Horner's syndrome from a third order neuron lesions would preserve facial sweating, whereas Horner's syndrome from a first and second order neurons would cause asymmetric facial sweating. In one study, however, this finding lacked diagnostic value: the finding of asymmetric facial sweating argued *for* a first or second order lesion and *against* a third order lesion with a sensitivity of only 53%, a specificity of 78%, and a positive LR that was not significant.[72]

(3) Paredrine Test In patients whose Horner's syndrome remains unexplained, the Paredrine test was historically used to identify the site of the lesion. In first and second order neuron lesions, but not third order neuron lesions, topical hydroxyamphetamine (Paredrine) causes pupillary dilation (positive LR = 9.2, negative LR = 0.2, see EBM Box 19-1). Unfortunately, hydroxyamphetamine is no longer being manufactured, although it is possible the homologous compound hydroxymethylamphetamine (Pholedrine) may serve as a substitute.[73,74]

E. INTRAOCULAR INFLAMMATION

As part of the eye's response to intraocular inflammation, the ipsilateral pupil often constricts. In one study of 317 patients with the unilaterally red eye, anisocoria ≥ 1 mm with the small pupil in the red eye significantly increased the probability of serious eye disease (i.e., corneal foreign body or abrasion, keratitis, and uveitis, LR = 6.5, EBM Box 19-1) and argued against more benign problems (i.e., subconjunctival hemorrhage, conjunctivitis). The absence of anisocoria was unhelpful in this study (LR = 0.8).

V. DIABETES AND THE PUPIL

The pupils of patients with long-standing diabetes show signs of sympathetic denervation (small size and poor dilation in darkness)[1,75–80] and parasympathetic denervation (sluggish light reaction).[1,75,78,79,81] Diabetes also reduces the amplitude of hippus.[1,82] Denervation alone, however, does not explain all of the diabetic pupillary abnormalities, because the pupils of many patients also respond poorly to dilating and constricting eye drops, which suggests an additional disorder of the iris itself (i.e., denervated pupils are classically supersensitive to eye drops).[77] Some reviews state that diabetes causes the Argyll Robertson pupil, but the data for this are meager and what exists suggests that the finding is very rare.[17,83,84]

REFERENCES

1. Smith SE, Smith SA, Brown PM, et al. Pupillary signs in diabetic autonomic neuropathy. *Br Med J.* 1978;2:924-927.
2. Lam BL, Thompson HS, Corbett JJ. The prevalence of simple anisocoria. *Am J Ophthalmol.* 1987;104:69-73.
3. Thompson HS, Franceschetti AT, Thompson PM. Hippus: Semantic and historic considerations of the word. *Am J Ophthalmol.* 1971;71:1116-1120.
4. Thompson HS. Afferent pupillary defects: Pupillary findings associated with defects of the afferent arm of the pupillary light reflex arc. *Am J Ophthalmol.* 1966; 62:861-871.
5. Levatin P. Pupillary escape in disease of the retina or optic nerve. *Arch Ophthalmol.* 1959;62:768-779.
6. Thompson HS, Corbett JJ, Cox TA. How to measure the relative afferent pupillary defect. *Surv Ophthalmol.* 1981;26:39-42.
7. Landau WM. The Marcus Gunn phenomenon: Loose canon of neuro-ophthalmology. *Neurology.* 1988;38:1141-1142.
8. Cox TA. Pupillary escape. *Neurology.* 1992;42:1271-1273.
9. Enyedi LB, Dev S, Cox TA. A comparison of the Marcus Gunn and alternating light tests for afferent pupillary defects. *Ophthalmology.* 1998;105:871-873.
10. Thompson HS, Corbett JJ. Swinging flashlight test. *Neurology.* 1989;38:154-156.
11. Cox TA, Thompson HS, Hayreh SS, Snyder JE. Visual evoked potential and pupillary signs: A comparison in optic nerve disease. *Arch Ophthalmol.* 1982;100: 1603-1606.
12. Cox TA, Thompson HS, Corbett JJ. Relative afferent pupillary defects in optic neuritis. *Am J Ophthalmol.* 1981;92:685-690.
13. Newsome DA, Milton RC. Afferent pupillary defect in macular degeneration. *Am J Ophthalmol.* 1981;92:396-402.
14. Girkin CA. Evaluation of the pupillary light response as an objective measure of visual function. *Ophthalmol Clin North Am.* 2003;16:143-153.
15. Sadun AA, Bassi CJ, Lessell S. Why cataracts do not produce afferent pupillary defects. *Am J Ophthalmol.* 1990;110:712-714.
16. Thompson HS. The vitality of the pupil: A history of the clinical use of the pupil as an indicator of visual potential. *J Neuro-Ophthalmol.* 2003;23:213-224.

17. Loewenfeld IE. The Argyll Robertson pupil, 1869-1969: A critical survey of the literature. *Surv Ophthalmol.* 1969;14:199-299.

18. Dacso CC. Significance of the Argyll Robertson pupil in clinical medicine. *Am J Med.* 1989;86:199-202.

19. Poole CJM. Argyll Robertson pupils due to neurosarcoidosis: Evidence for site of lesion. *Br Med J.* 1984;289:356.

20. David NJ. Optokinetic nystagmus: A clinical review. *J Clin Neuro-ophthalmol.* 1989;9:258-266.

21. Ford FR, Walsh FB, King A. Clinical observations on the pupillary phenomena resulting from regeneration of the third nerve with especial reference to the Argyll Robertson pupil. *Bull Johns Hopkins Hosp.* 1941;68:309-318.

22. Spector RH, Faria MA. Aberrant regeneration of the inferior division of the oculomotor nerve. *Arch Neurol.* 1981;38:460-461.

23. Marshall LF, Barba D, Toole BM, Bowers SA. The oval pupil: Clinical significance and relationship to intracranial hypertension. *J Neurosurg.* 1983;58:566-568.

24. Fisher CM. Oval pupils. *Arch Neurol.* 1980;37:502-503.

25. Thompson HS. Segmental palsy of the iris sphincter in Adie's syndrome. *Arch Ophthalmol.* 1978;96:1615-1620.

26. Czarnecki JSC, Pilley SFJ, Thompson HS. The analysis of anisocoria: The use of photography in the clinical evaluation of unequal pupils. *Can J Ophthalmol.* 1979; 14:297-302.

27. Thompson HS, Pilley SFJ. Unequal pupils: A flow chart for sorting out the anisocorias. *Surv Ophthalmol.* 1976;21:45-48.

28. Zito G, Gennaro P. Clinical evaluation of anisocoria (letter). *Arch Neurol.* 1982;39:604.

29. Lam BL, Thompson HS, Walls RC. Effect of light on the prevalence of simple anisocoria. *Ophthalmology.* 1996;103:790-793.

30. Sunderland S, Bradley KC. Disturbances of oculomotor function accompanying extradural haemorrhage. *J Neurol Neurosurg Psychiatry.* 1953;16:35-46.

31. Ropper AH. The opposite pupil in herniation. *Neurology.* 1990;40:1707-1709.

32. Mitsumoto H, Conomy JP, Regula G. Ophthalmologic aspects of subdural hematoma. *Cleve Clin Q.* 1977;44:101-105.

33. Stone JL, Rifai MHS, Sugar O, et al. Subdural hematomas I. Acute subdural hematoma: Progress in definition, clinical pathology, and therapy. *Surg Neurol.* 1983;19:216-231.

34. Talalla A, Morin MA. Acute traumatic subdural hematoma: A review of one hundred consecutive cases. *J Trauma.* 1971;11:771-777.

35. Ikeda M, Matsunaga T, Irabu N, Yoshida S. Using vital signs to diagnose impaired consciousness: Cross sectional observation study. *BMJ.* 2002;325:800-802.

36. Plum F, Posner JB. *The diagnosis of stupor and coma,* 3rd ed. Philadelphia: F.A. Davis; 1980.

37. Tokuda Y, Nakazato N, Stein GH. Pupillary evaluation for differential diagnosis of coma. *Postgrad Med.* 2003;79:49-51.

38. Kardon RH, Denison CE, Brown CK, Thompson HS. Critical evaluation of the cocaine test in the diagnosis of Horner's syndrome. *Arch Ophthalmol.* 1990;108: 384-387.

39. Kardon RH, Denison CE, Brown CK, Thompson HS. The cocaine test and Horner's syndrome. *Arch Ophthalmol.* 1990;108:1667-1668.

40. Cremer SA, Thompson HS, Digre KB, Kardon RH. Hydroxyamphetamine mydriasis in Horner's syndrome. *Am J Ophthalmol.* 1990;110:71-76.

41. Maloney WF, Younge BR, Moyer NJ. Evaluation of the causes and accuracy of pharmacologic localization in Horner's syndrome. *Am J Ophthalmol.* 1980;90: 394-402.

42. Rose GE, Pearson RV. Unequal pupil size in patients with unilateral red eye. *Br Med J.* 1991;302:571-572.

43. Fujiwara S, Fujii K, Nishio S, et al. Oculomotor nerve palsy in patients with cerebral aneurysms. *Neurosurg Rev.* 1989;12:123-132.

44. Kissel JT, Burde RM, Klingele TG, Zeiger HE. Pupil-sparing oculomotor palsies with internal carotid-posterior communicating artery aneurysms. *Ann Neurol.* 1983;13:149-154.

45. Capo H, Warren F, Kupersmith MJ. Evolution of oculomotor nerve palsies. *J Clin Neuro-ophthalmol.* 1992;12:12-15.

46. Cogan DG, Mount HTJ. Intracranial aneurysms causing ophthalmoplegia. *Arch Ophthalmol.* 1963;70:757-771.

47. Green WR, Hackett ER, Schlezinger NS. Neuro-ophthalmologic evaluation of oculomotor nerve paralysis. *Arch Ophthalmol.* 1964;72:154-167.

48. Rucker CW. The causes of paralysis of the third, fourth and sixth cranial nerves. *Am J Ophthalmol.* 1966;61:1293-1298.

49. Keane JR. Aneurysms and third nerve palsies. *Ann Neurol.* 1983;14:696-697.

50. Raja IA. Aneurysm-induced third nerve palsy. *J Neurosurg.* 1972;36:548-551.

51. Botterell EH, Lloyd LA, Hoffman HJ. Oculomotor palsy due to supraclinoid internal carotid artery berry aneurysm. *Am J Ophthalmol.* 1962;54:609-616.

52. Loewenstein O, Loewenfeld IR. Pupillotonic pseudotabes (syndrome of Markus-Weill and Reys-Holmes-Adie): A critical review of the literature. *Surv Ophthalmol.* 1967;10:129-185.

53. Loewenfeld IR, Thompson HS. The tonic pupil: A re-evaluation. *Am J Ophthalmol.* 1967;63:46-87.

54. Warwick R. The ocular parasympathetic nerve supply and its mesencephalic sources. *J Anat.* 1954;88:71-93.

55. Helprin GA, Clarke GM. Unilateral fixed dilated pupil associated with nebulised ipratropium bromide. *Lancet.* 1986;2:1469.

56. Riddick FA, Jordan JD. Cruise ship anisocoria. *Ann Intern Med.* 1992;117:95.

57. Rubinfeld RS, Currie JN. Accidental mydriasis from blue nightshade "lipstick". *J Clin Neuro-ophthalmol.* 1987;7:34-37.

58. Savitt DL, Roberts JR, Siegel EG. Anisocoria from jimsonweed. *JAMA.* 1986;255:1439-1440.

59. Voltz R, Hohlfeld R, Liebler M, Hertel H. Gardener's mydriasis. *Lancet.* 1992; 339:752.

60. Meng K, Graetz DK. Moonflower-induced anisocoria. *Ann Emerg Med.* 2004;44:665-666.

61. Thompson HS, Newsome DA, Loewenfeld IE. The fixed dilated pupil: Sudden iridoplegia or mydriatic drops? A simple diagnostic test. *Arch Ophthalmol.* 1971;86:21-27.

62. Giles CL, Henderson JW. Horner's syndrome: An analysis of 216 cases. *Am J Ophthalmol.* 1958;46:289-296.

63. Ross IB. The role of Claude Bernard and others in the discovery of Horner's syndrome. *J Am Coll Surg.* 2004;199:976-980.

64. Jacobson DM, Berg R, Grinstead GF, Kruse JR. Duration of positive urine for cocaine metabolite after ophthalmic administration: Implications for testing patients with suspected Horner syndrome using ophthalmic cocaine. *Am J Ophthalmol.* 2001; 131:742-747.

65. Bacal DA, Levy SR. The use of apraclonidine in the diagnosis of Horner syndrome in pediatric patients. *Arch Ophthalmol.* 2004;122:276-279.

66. Brown SM, Aouchiche R, Freedman KA. The utility of 0.5% apraclonidine in the diagnosis of Horner syndrome. *Arch Ophthalmol.* 2003;121:1201-1203.

67. Freedman KA, Brown SM. Topical apraclonidine in the diagnosis of suspected Horner syndrome. *J Neuro-Ophthalmol.* 2005;25:83-85.

68. Morales J, Brown SM, Abdul-Rahim AS, Crosson CE. Ocular effects of apraclonidine in Horner syndrome. *Arch Ophthalmol.* 2000;118:951-954.

69. Kardon R. Are we ready to replace cocaine with apraclonidine in the pharmacologic diagnosis of Horner syndrome? *J Neuro-Ophthalmol.* 2005;25:69-70.

70. Keane JR. Oculosympathetic paresis: Analysis of 100 hospitalized patients. *Arch Neurol.* 1979;36:13-16.

71. Van der Wiel HL, Van Gijn J. Localization of Horner's syndrome: Use and limitations of the hydroxyamphetamine test. *J Neurol Sci.* 1983;59:229-235.

72. Rosenberg ML. The friction sweat test as a new method for detecting facial anhidrosis in patients with Horner's syndrome. *Am J Ophthalmol.* 1989;108:443-447.

73. Bates AT, Chamberlain S, Champion M, et al. Pholedrine: A substitute for hydroxyamphetamine as a diagnostic eyedrop test in Horner's syndrome. *J Neurol Neurosurg Psychiatry.* 1995;58:215-217.

74. Burde RM, Thompson HS. Hydroxyamphetamine. A good drug lost? *Am J Ophthalmol.* 1991;111:100-102.

75. Hreidarsson AB, Gundersen HJG. The pupillary response to light in type 1 (insulin-dependent) diabetes. *Diabetologia.* 1985;28:815-821.

76. Hreidarsson AB. Pupil size in insulin-dependent diabetes: Relationship to duration, metabolic control, and long-term manifestations. *Diabetes.* 1982;31:442-448.

77. Alio J, Hernandez I, Millan A, Sanchez J. Pupil responsiveness in diabetes mellitus. *Ann Ophthalmol.* 1989;21:132-137.

78. Smith SA, Smith SE. Reduced pupillary light reflexes in diabetic autonomic neuropathy. *Diabetologia*. 1983;24:330-332.

79. Lanting P, Bos JE, Aartsen J, et al. Assessment of pupillary light reflex latency and darkness adapted pupil size in control subjects and in diabetic patients with and without cardiovascular autonomic neuropathy. *J Neurol Neurosurg Psychiatry*. 1990;53:912-914.

80. Smith SA, Smith SE. Evidence for a neuropathic aetiology in the small pupil of diabetes mellitus. *Br J Ophthalmol*. 1983;67:89-93.

81. Friedman SA, Feinberg R, Podolak E, Bedell RHS. Pupillary abnormalities in diabetic neuropathy. *Ann Intern Med*. 1967;67:977-983.

82. Hreidarsson AB, Gundersen HJG. Reduced pupillary unrest: Autonomic nervous system abnormality in diabetes mellitus. *Diabetes*. 1988;37:446-451.

83. Waite JH, Beetham WP. The visual mechanism in diabetes mellitus (A comparative study of 2002 diabetics and 457 non-diabetics for control). *N Engl J Med*. 1935;212:367-379.

84. Martin MM. Diabetic neuropathy: A clinical study of 150 cases. *Brain*. 1953;76:594-624.

20

Diabetic Retinopathy

I.   INTRODUCTION

Diabetic retinopathy is the leading cause of blindness in adults between the ages of 25 and 74.[1] Whether a patient develops retinopathy depends to a large extent on the type and duration of diabetes: Patients with type 1 diabetes have a 0% risk of proliferative retinopathy at 5 years after diagnosis, 4% at 10 years and 50% at 20 years, whereas those with type 2 diabetes, especially if taking insulin, the risk is 3% to 4% at the time of diagnosis, 10% at 10 years, and 20% at 15 years.[2] Once retinopathy develops, however, one of the best predictors of progression to sight-threatening retinopathy is the extent of retinopathy during the baseline examination: The higher the grade of retinopathy during the initial examination, the greater the risk of progression (Table 20-1). In type 1 diabetics, pregnancy increases the risk of progression 2.3-fold.[2]

In large cross-sectional surveys of diabetic patients seen by general practitioners, sight-threatening retinopathy (i.e., proliferative retinopathy and more severe forms of nonproliferative retinopathy) is found in 5% to 15% of patients.[7-11]

| Table 20-1 | Progression to High-Risk Proliferative Diabetic Retinopathy* | | |

Grade of Baseline Retinopathy	Principal Clinical Findings	Cumulative Risk (%) of High-Risk Proliferative Retinopathy	
		1 Year	5 Years
Nonproliferative retinopathy			
Mild	Microaneurysms Dot and blot hemorrhages Soft exudates	1	16
Moderate	Extensive microaneurysms and hemorrhages IRMA Venous beading	3–8	27–39
Severe	Same as moderate[†]	15	56
Very severe	Same as moderate[†]	45	71
Proliferative retinopathy[‡]			
	Neovascularization Preretinal/vitreous hemorrhages Fibrovascular proliferation	22–46	64–75

IRMA, intraretinal microvascular abnormalities; NVD, neovascularization within one disc diameter of the optic disc; NVE, neovascularization elsewhere, i.e., beyond one disc diameter of the optic disc (see text).
*High-risk proliferative retinopathy is NVD >1/4 disc area in size, NVD <1/4 disc area and vitreous or preretinal hemorrhage, OR NVE >1/2 disc area and vitreous or preretinal hemorrhage.[3] These figures, based on references 4 and 5, assume that the patient is untreated.
[†]Moderate, severe, and very severe nonproliferative retinopathy share the same funduscopic findings, although they differ in severity (based on standardized photographs)[6] and the number of retinal quadrants involved.[5]
[‡]Percentages are for patients whose baseline evaluation reveals proliferative retinopathy with less than high-risk characteristics.

II. THE FINDINGS

The findings of diabetic retinopathy are divided into nonproliferative changes, which occur *within* the retina, and proliferative changes, which are located on the inner surface of the retina or in the vitreous.[12] The terms "background retinopathy" and "preproliferative retinopathy" are outdated and no longer recommended,

having been replaced by the grades of retinopathy shown in Table 20-1.[13] Diabetic retinopathy progresses in an orderly fashion through these grades.

A. NONPROLIFERATIVE CHANGES (FIG. 20-1)

The earliest changes to appear in diabetic retinopathy are **microaneurysms,** which are distinct red, round spots that are less than one-twelfth the diameter of an average optic disc, or 125 μm in its longest dimension (a long-standing convention assumes the average optic disc is 1500 μm in diameter; 125 μm is approximately the width of an average major vein at the disc margin).[6] **Dot hemorrhages** are larger red dots with sharp borders; red spots with indistinct borders are **blot hemorrhages.** Both dot and blot hemorrhages are located in the inner retinal layers. **Hard exudates** (deposition of lipid in the inner retina) are small, white or yellowish-white deposits with sharp margins that often have a waxy or glistening appearance.[6] **Soft exudates** (or "cotton wool" exudates) are ischemic swellings of the superficial nerve fiber layer, which appear as white, round, or oval patches with ill-defined (feathery) edges.[6] As retinal ischemia progresses, two other abnormalities appear: venous beading (veins sometimes resemble a string of beads) and intraretinal microvascular abnormalities (IRMA—extra tortuous vessels *within* the retina, which may be either new vessels or dilated preexisting capillaries).[6,14]

B. PROLIFERATIVE RETINOPATHY

Proliferative retinopathy is new vessel formation (i.e., **neovascularization**) on the inner surface of the retina or vitreous, which subsequently can threaten vision by causing retinal detachment or vitreous hemorrhage. These new vessels often resemble a small wagon wheel, with individual vessels radiating like spokes to a circumferential vessel forming the rim.[12] New vessel formation is subdivided into neovascularization of the disc (NVD; within one disc diameter of the optic disc) and neovascularization elsewhere (NVE). Of the two, NVD has a much worse visual prognosis.[5]

C. MACULAR EDEMA

Macular edema may accompany any stage of nonproliferative or proliferative retinopathy. It is very difficult to visualize using the direct ophthalmoscope, although important clues are rings of hard exudates (often surrounding the edematous area) and diminished visual acuity.[12]

III. CLINICAL SIGNIFICANCE

In patients with high-risk proliferative retinopathy or those with clinically significant macular edema, laser photocoagulation reduces the risk of subsequent

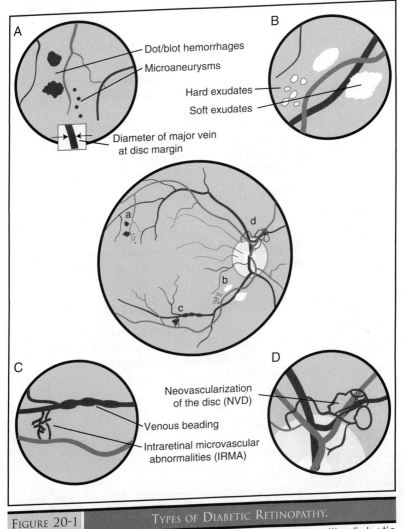

FIGURE 20-1   TYPES OF DIABETIC RETINOPATHY.

The center figure depicting the fundus of a patient with diabetic retinopathy is surrounded by four enlarged views, each labeled with a letter (*a–d*) that corresponds to a specific location on the center figure: *a*, microaneurysms and dot/blot hemorrhages. The diameter of microaneurysms is less than the width of a major vein at the disc margin (reproduced in square inset). *b*, Hard and soft exudates. *c*, venous beading and intraretinal microvascular abnormalities (IRMA). *d*, Neovascularization, which may be located within one disc diameter of the optic disc (NVD) or elsewhere (NVE). Although both IRMA and neovascularization represent the formation of new blood vessels, IRMA is confined to the layers of the retina, whereas neovascularization is on the inner surface of the retina or vitreous. See text.

visual loss by at least 50% (the footnote to Table 20-1 defines high-risk proliferative retinopathy).[3] Retinal examination is the only way to detect these lesions, thereby making diabetic retinopathy one of the best examples of a disorder in which careful, attentive physical examination has profound positive effects on a patient's health.

The findings that best predict subsequent proliferative retinopathy are venous beading, intraretinal microvascular abnormalities, and the extent of microaneurysms and hemorrhages. Soft exudates are less predictive, and the extent of hard exudates correlates poorly with subsequent proliferative retinopathy.[5]

A. VISUAL ACUITY AND DIABETIC RETINOPATHY

Diminished visual acuity per se is a poor screening test for diabetic retinopathy. In one community survey of more than 3500 patients, the presence or absence of reading acuity of 20/60 or worse failed to distinguish patients with diabetic retinopathy from those without it [both positive and negative likelihood ratios (LRs) not significant].[15]

B. DIAGNOSTIC ACCURACY OF OPHTHALMOSCOPY

EBM Box 20-1 presents the accuracy of direct ophthalmoscopy for sight-threatening retinopathy (i.e., proliferative changes and macular edema), using retinal photographs through dilated pupils or slit-lamp biomicroscopy as the diagnostic standard. Not surprisingly, specialists perform better than general

Box 20-1   Ophthalmoscopy and Diabetic Retinopathy*

Finding (Ref)†	Sensitivity (%)	Specificity (%)	Likelihood Ratio if Finding	
			Present	Absent
Detecting sight-threatening retinopathy, using the following technique:				
Nondilated pupils[16]	50	92	**6.2**	0.5
Dilated pupils, general providers[8,10,11,17]	53–69	91–96	**10.2**	0.4
Dilated pupils, specialists[9–11,18]	48–82	90–99	**18.6**	**0.3**

Likelihood ratio (LR) if finding present = positive LR; LR if finding absent = negative LR.
*Diagnostic standard: For sight-threatening retinopathy, retinal photographs through dilated pupils or slit-lamp biomicroscopy reveal proliferative retinopathy, macular edema, or both.
†Definition of findings: For sight-threatening retinopathy, direct ophthalmoscopy reveals proliferative retinopathy, macular edema, or both.

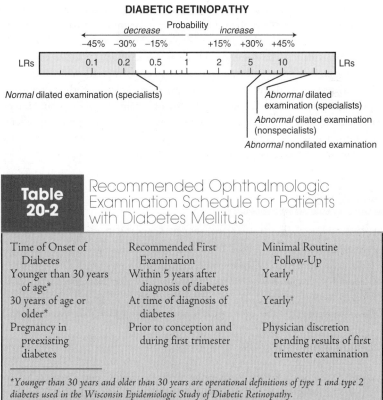

DIABETIC RETINOPATHY

Normal dilated examination (specialists)

Abnormal dilated examination (specialists)

Abnormal dilated examination (nonspecialists)

Abnormal nondilated examination

Table 20-2	Recommended Ophthalmologic Examination Schedule for Patients with Diabetes Mellitus	
Time of Onset of Diabetes	Recommended First Examination	Minimal Routine Follow-Up
Younger than 30 years of age*	Within 5 years after diagnosis of diabetes	Yearly†
30 years of age or older*	At time of diagnosis of diabetes	Yearly†
Pregnancy in preexisting diabetes	Prior to conception and during first trimester	Physician discretion pending results of first trimester examination

*Younger than 30 years and older than 30 years are operational definitions of type 1 and type 2 diabetes used in the Wisconsin Epidemiologic Study of Diabetic Retinopathy.
†In some patients with normal eye examinations, eye specialists may advise less frequent examinations (every 2–3 years).[20,21]

clinicians, and dilated examinations are superior to nondilated ones. If general providers examine with ophthalmoscopy and also review retinal photographs of the patient, sensitivity improves to greater than 80%, suggesting that this approach may become the most effective screening strategy when access to specialists is limited.[8,10,17]

Macular edema is rarely detected by general providers using direct ophthalmoscopy (sensitivity is close to 0%).[19] Because many patients with macular edema have normal visual acuity (i.e., the sensitivity of "visual acuity worse than 20/30" for macular edema is only 38%),[19] clinicians who exclude the diagnosis of macular edema because the patient's visual acuity is normal are missing many patients who would benefit from laser photocoagulation.

C.   SCREENING RECOMMENDATIONS

Diabetic retinopathy is a common and treatable problem that is detectable during a long asymptomatic period using simple tools. Consequently, it meets every criteria for a disease that benefits from screening. Screening programs are cost-saving, being less expensive than the disability payments that otherwise would go to people who develop blindness.[1,2] Table 20-2 reviews the screening schedule recommended by the American Diabetes Association.[20,22] Given the stakes of missing serious retinopathy and the less than optimal performance of general clinicians using just direct ophthalmoscopy, only clinicians with training and experience—in most cases, optometrists and ophthalmologists—should screen patients. Any patient with macular edema, more than moderate nonproliferative retinopathy, or proliferative retinopathy should be seen by eye care providers with experience in the management of diabetic retinopathy.[1]

REFERENCES

1. Diabetic retinopathy. *Diabetes Care*. 1998;21(Suppl 1):S47-49.
2. Singer DE, Nathan DM, Fogel HA, Schachat AP. Screening for diabetic retinopathy. *Ann Intern Med*. 1992;116:660-671.
3. Aiello LM, Cavallerano J. Diabetic retinopathy. *Curr Ther Endocrinol Metab*. 1997; 6:475-485.
4. Early Treatment Diabetic Retinopathy Study Research Group. Early photocoagulation for diabetic retinopathy. *Ophthalmology*. 1991;98:766-785.
5. Early Treatment Diabetic Retinopathy Study Research Group. Fundus photographic risk factors for progression of diabetic retinopathy. *Ophthalmology*. 1991;98:823-833.
6. Early Treatment Diabetic Retinopathy Study Research Group. Grading diabetic retinopathy from stereoscopic color fundus photographs: An extension of the modified Airlie House Classification. ETDRS report number 10. *Ophthalmology*. 1991;98:786-806.
7. Lee VS, Kingsley RM, Lee ET, et al. The diagnosis of diabetic retinopathy: Ophthalmoscopy versus fundus photography. *Ophthalmology*. 1993;100:1504-1512.
8. O'Hare JP, Hopper A, Madhaven C, et al. Adding retinal photography to screening for diabetic retinopathy: A prospective study in primary care. *Br Med J*. 1996;312:679-682.
9. Harding SP, Broadbent DM, Neoh C, et al. Sensitivity and specificity of photography and direct ophthalmoscopy in screening for sight threatening eye disease: The Liverpool Diabetic Eye Study. *BMJ*. 1995;311:1131-1135.
10. Gibbons RL, Owens DR, Allen JC, Eastman L. Practical application of the European Field Guide in screening for diabetic retinopathy by using ophthalmoscopy and 35 mm slides. *Diabetologia*. 1998;41:59-64.
11. Buxton MJ, Sculpher MJ, Ferguson BA, et al. Screening for treatable diabetic retinopathy: A comparison of different methods. *Diabet Med*. 1991;8:371-377.
12. Fonseca V, Munshi M, Merin LM, Bradrord JD. Diabetic retinopathy: A review for the primary care physician. *South Med J*. 1996;89:839-846.

13. Aiello LP, Gardner TW, King GL, et al. Diabetic retinopathy. *Diabetes Care.* 1998;21:143-156.
14. Ferris FL, Davis MD, Aiello LM. Treatment of diabetic retinopathy. *N Engl J Med.* 1999;341:667-667.
15. Ivers RQ, Macaskill P, Cumming RG, Mitchell P. Sensitivity and specificity of tests to detect eye disease in an older population. *Ophthalmology.* 2001;108:968-975.
16. Klein R, Klein BEK, Neider MW, et al. Diabetic retinopathy as detected using ophthalmoscopy, a nonmydriatic camera and a standard fundus camera. *Ophthalmology.* 1985;92:485-491.
17. Owens DR, Gibbins RL, Lewis PA, et al. Screening for diabetic retinopathy by general practitioners: Ophthalmoscopy or retinal photography as 35 mm colour transparencies? *Diabet Med.* 1998;15:170-175.
18. Moss SE, Klein R, Kessler SD, Richie KA. Comparison between ophthalmoscopy and fundus photography in determining severity of diabetic retinopathy. *Ophthalmology.* 1985;92:62-67.
19. Nathan DM, Fogel HA, Godine JE, et al. Role of diabetologist in evaluating diabetic retinopathy. *Diabetes Care.* 1991;14:26-33.
20. Association AD. Standards of medical care in diabetes. *Diabetes Care.* 2005; 28(Suppl 1):S1-S36.
21. Vijan S, Hofer TP, Hayward RA. Cost-utility analysis of screening intervals for diabetic retinopathy in patients with type 2 diabetes mellitus. *JAMA.* 2000;283: 889-896.
22. Fong DS, Aiello L, Gardner TW, et al. Retinopathy in diabetes. *Diabetes Care.* 2004;27(Suppl 1):S84-S87.

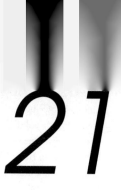

Hearing

I. INTRODUCTION

Hearing loss, which affects 25% to 40% of individuals older than the age of 65 years, is associated with depression, difficulty communicating, and reduced mobility.[1,2] Clinicians using casual assessment in the office overlook significant hearing loss about half the time.[3] The causes of hearing loss are either "neurosensory" (i.e., damage to the auditory nerve) or "conductive" (i.e., damage to the parts of the ear that conduct sound from air to the cochlea). Most neurosensory hearing loss is due to presbyacusis (the degenerative hearing loss of aging).[4] Less common causes are Ménière's disease and acoustic neuroma. The most common causes of conductive loss are impacted cerumen, otitis media, perforated eardrum, and otosclerosis.[2,5,6]

II. TECHNIQUE

A. WHISPERED VOICE TEST

Many tests of hearing are available to general clinicians, some more formal (hand-held audiometer) than others (listening to whisper, watch, or tuning fork).[1,7] The best validated test not requiring special tools is the "whispered voice test." In this test, the clinician whispers a combination of three letters or numbers (e.g., 5, B, 6) while standing arm's length (i.e., about 2 feet) behind the patient and then asks the patient to repeat the sequence. If the patient answers correctly, hearing is considered normal and testing is stopped. If the patient misidentifies any of the three items, the clinician repeats different triplets of numbers or letters one or two more times. If 50% or more of the items in the two or three triplets are incorrect, the test is abnormal.[3,8,9]

The clinician stands behind the patient to prevent lip-reading. Only one ear is tested at a time, the other being masked by the examiner's finger occluding the external auditory canal and making a continuous circular rubbing motion (occlusion without rubbing is insufficient masking). The clinician should quietly exhale before whispering to produce the quietest whisper possible.[8]

B.   TUNING FORK TESTS

1.   Introduction

Once hearing loss is identified, tuning forks tests distinguish neurosensory from conductive loss. All tuning fork tests are based on the fundamental principle, discovered almost 500 years ago,* that sound conducts through bone preferentially to an ear with conductive hearing loss. Tuning fork tests were introduced into clinical otology in the early 1800s, and at one time were the otologist's favorite tool consisting of more than 15 distinct tests.[11] After introduction of audiometry, however, enthusiasm for these tests waned, and only two are commonly used today, the Weber and Rinne test.[12]

2.   The Frequency of the Tuning Fork

Most authorities recommend using the 512 Hz tuning fork for tuning fork tests,[13] because frequencies above 512 Hz detect conductive hearing loss less well[6,14–16] and because frequencies of 128 Hz or lower generate so many vibrations that even patients without hearing can sense them.[6] The 512-Hz fork is preferred to the 256-Hz fork because the 256-Hz fork, in some studies of tuning fork tests, is less specific.[17,18]

3.   Method of Striking the Fork

Most authorities recommend striking the fork against a soft surface, such as a rubber pad or the muscles of the forearm.[13] The principal tone produced is the

---

*The Italian physician Capivacci made this fundamental observation after connecting his subject's teeth to a zither and then plucking the zither's strings.[10]

same whether the tines are struck on a soft or harder surface, but the harder surface generates multiple overtones that may confound interpretation of the test.[11] Weights, sometimes added to the tines to minimize overtones, also shorten the time of vibration and are not recommended.[11]

4. Weber Test

In this test, the clinician strikes the fork, places it in the middle of the patient's vertex, forehead, or bridge of nose, and asks the patient "Where do you hear the sound?" (Fig. 21-1). In patients *with unilateral hearing loss,* the sound is heard preferentially in the *good* ear if the loss is neurosensory and in the *bad* ear if the loss is conductive.[13,19] Weber himself recommended placing the vibrating fork on the incisors[20] and subsequent studies do show this is the most sensitive technique,[21] although concerns of transmitting infectious diseases prohibit using this method now.

According to traditional teachings, persons with normal hearing perceive the sound in the midline or inside their head, but studies show that up to 40% of normal-hearing persons also lateralize the Weber test.[16] Therefore, the Weber test should be interpreted only in patients with hearing loss.

5. Rinne Test (Pronounced "RIN-neh")

In this test, the clinician tests each ear individually to determine whether that ear detects sound better through air or bone (see Fig. 21-1). Air conduction (AC) is tested by holding the vibrating fork about 2.5 cm away from the ear, with the axis joining the tips of the tines in line with the axis through both external auditory canals.* Bone conduction (BC) is tested by holding the stem of the vibrating fork against the mastoid (excessive force should not be used because it causes sounds to be heard longer and diminishes the test's specificity).[22] The clinician compares air and bone conduction by either the (1) loudness comparison technique, in which the fork is held about 2 seconds in each position and the patient indicates which position is louder or the (2) threshold technique, in which the clinician uses a stopwatch to time how long the patient hears the sound, from the moment the fork is struck to when the sound disappears, first for AC and then BC.[13,19,21]

---

*During air conduction, the orientation of the tines of the fork is important because the sound waves emanate in two directions from the fork: one direction is parallel to the axis of the tines and the other is perpendicular to it. If the tines are held at an oblique angle, these sound waves may actually cancel each other out and diminish the sound.[11] Clinicians can easily convince themselves of this by rotating the stem of a vibrating fork near their own ear, noting that the sound intermittently disappears.

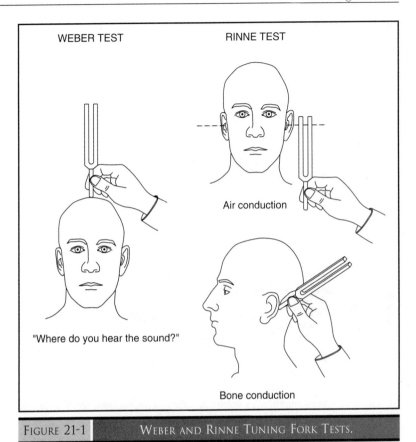

FIGURE 21-1	WEBER AND RINNE TUNING FORK TESTS.

In the Weber test (*left*), the clinician holds the vibrating tuning fork in the midline against the patient's vertex, forehead, or bridge of nose and asks "Where do you hear the sound?" In the Rinne test (*right*), the clinician tests one ear at a time, comparing perception of sound conducted through air (*top right*) to perception of sound conducted through bone (*bottom right*). When testing air conduction, the tuning fork is held so that an axis through both external auditory canals (dashed line) passes through both tines of the fork. When testing bone conduction, the stem of the vibrating fork is held against the mastoid.

Patients with normal hearing or neurosensory hearing loss perceive the sound better through AC than through BC. Patients with conductive hearing loss, in contrast, perceive the sound better (i.e., louder or longer) through BC: According to a confusing tradition, this result is recorded "Rinne negative," although it is more explicit to record "BC > AC" for the abnormal result.

Table 21-1	Tuning Fork Tests—Traditional Interpretation*	

Weber test	Rinne test	Possible Interpretations
Midline	AC > BC, bilateral	1. Normal hearing, bilateral 2. Neurosensory loss, bilateral
Louder in left	BC > AC, left AC > BC, right	1. Conductive loss, left
Louder in left	AC > BC, bilateral	1. Normal hearing, bilateral 2. Neurosensory loss, worse on right
Louder in right	BC > AC, bilateral	1. Conductive loss, bilateral but worse on right 2. Conductive loss on right and severe neurosensory loss on left[†]

AC, air conduction; BC, bone conduction.
*From reference 13.
[†]Some patients with severe neurosensory loss have the finding BC > AC because the BC stimulus is cross-heard by the better cochlea on the nontest side.

Table 21-1 presents some examples of different results from the Weber and Rinne test and their possible interpretations.

III.   CLINICAL SIGNIFICANCE

A.   WHISPERED VOICE TEST

EBM Box 21-1 reveals that the whispered voice test is an accurate test, arguing for significant hearing loss (i.e., >30 dB) when it is positive [likelihood ratio (LR) = 6.0] and practically excluding significant hearing loss when it is negative (LR = 0.03).

B.   TUNING FORK TESTS

EBM Box 21-1 shows that the Rinne test (by the loudness comparison technique) is an accurate test of conductive hearing loss. The finding of "BC > AC" argues strongly for an air-bone gap greater than 20 dB on audiometry (LR = 16.8); the finding of "AC > BC" argues against an air-bone gap this large (LR = 0.2). The larger the patient's air-bone gap on audiometry, the more likely the

Box 21-1   Hearing Tests*

Finding (Ref)[†]	Sensitivity (%)	Specificity (%)	Likelihood Ratio if Finding	
			Present	Absent
Hearing Tests				
Abnormal whispered voice test[3,8,9]	90–99	80–87	**6.0**	**0.03**
Tuning Fork Tests (Patients With Unilateral Hearing Loss)				
Rinne test, detecting conductive hearing loss[5,18]	60–90	95–98	**16.8**	**0.2**
Weber test lateralizes to good ear, detecting neurosensory loss[16]	58	79	2.7	NS
Weber test lateralizes to bad ear, detecting conductive loss[16]	54	92	NS	0.5

NS, not significant; likelihood ratio (LR) if finding present = positive LR; LR if finding absent = negative LR.

*Diagnostic standard: For hearing loss (whispered voice test), mean pure tone threshold >30 dB on audiometry; for conductive hearing loss (Rinne test), air-bone gap on audiometry ≥ 20 dB.

†Definition of findings: For abnormal whispered voice test, see text; for Rinne test, bone conduction (BC) greater than air conduction (AC), using the loudness comparison technique; all tuning fork tests used 512-Hz tuning fork.

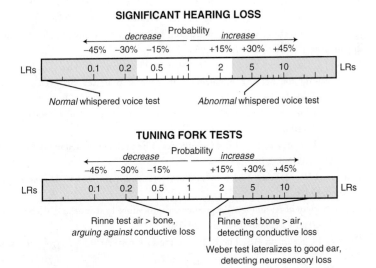

Rinne test will reveal "BC > AC" (for comparison, the mean air-bone gap in otosclerosis and otitis media is 21–27 dB).[5,18,23]

The Weber test, on the other hand, is less accurate, arguing only somewhat for neurosensory hearing loss when it lateralizes to the good ear (LR = 2.7). The Weber test performs poorly because many patients with unilateral hearing loss, whether neurosensory or conductive, hear the tuning fork in the midline.[16]

Tuning fork tests cannot distinguish normal hearing from bilateral neurosensory losses (see Table 21-1), and therefore, they should always follow hearing tests. Moreover, tuning fork tests cannot distinguish a pure conductive loss from a mixed conductive and neurosensory defect (see Table 21-1).[24]

REFERENCES

1. Lichtenstein MJ, Bess FH, Logan SA. Validation of screening tools for identifying hearing-impaired elderly in primary care. *JAMA*. 1988;259:2875-2878.
2. Yueh B, Shapiro N, MacLean CH, Shekelle PG. Screening and management of adult hearing loss in primary care: Scientific review. *JAMA*. 2003;289:1976-1985.
3. Macphee GJA, Crowther JA, McAlpine CH. A simple screening test for hearing impairment in elderly patients. *Age Ageing*. 1988;17:347-351.
4. Nadol JB. Hearing loss. *N Engl J Med*. 1993;329:1092-1102.
5. Burkey JM, Lippy WH, Schuring AG, Rizer FM. Clinical utility of the 512-Hz Rinne tuning fork test. *Am J Otol*. 1998;19:59-62.
6. Gelfand SA. Clinical precision of the Rinne test. *Acta Otolaryngol*. 1977;83:480-487.
7. Arbit E. A sensitive bedside hearing test. *Ann Neurol*. 1977;2:250-251.
8. Swan IRC, Browning GB. The whispered voice as a screening test for hearing impairment. *J Roy Coll Gen Pract*. 1985;35:197.
9. Eekhof JAH, de Bock GH, de Laat JAPM, et al. The whispered voice: The best test for screening for hearing impairment in general practice? *Br J Gen Pract*. 1996;46:473-474.
10. Ng M, Jackler RK. Early history of tuning-fork tests. *Am J Otolaryngol*. 1993;14:100-105.
11. Samuel J, Eitelberg E, Habil I. Tuning forks: The problem of striking. *J Laryngol Otol*. 1989;103:1-6.
12. Johnson EW. Tuning forks to audiometers and back again. *Laryngoscope*. 1970;80:49-68.
13. British Society of Audiology. Recommended procedure for Rinne and Weber tuning-fork tests. *Br J Audiol*. 1987;21:229-230.
14. Crowley H, Kaufman RS. The Rinne tuning fork test. *Arch Otolarygol*. 1966;84: 70-72.

15. Jacob V, Alexander P, Nalinesha KM, Nayar RC. Can Rinne's test quantify hearing loss? *ENT J.* 1993;72(2):152-153.
16. Stankiewicz JA, Mowry HJ. Clinical accuracy of tuning fork tests. *Laryngoscope.* 1979;89:1956-1973.
17. Browning GG, Swan IRC. Sensitivity and specificity of Rinne tuning fork test. *Br Med J.* 1988;297:1381-1382.
18. Chole RA, Cook GB. The Rinne test for conductive deafness: A critical reappraisal. *Arch Otolaryngol Head Neck Surg.* 1988;114:399-403.
19. Sheehy JL, Gardner G, Hambley WM. Tuning fork tests in modern otology. *Arch Otolaryngol.* 1971;94:132-138.
20. Huizing EH. The early description of the so-called tuning fork tests of Weber and Rinne I. the `Weber test" and its first description by Schmalz. *ORL.* 1973;35:278-282.
21. Golabek W, Stephens SDG. Some tuning fork tests revisited. *Clin Otolaryngol.* 1979;4:421-430.
22. Johnston DF. A new modification of the Rinne test. *Clin Otolaryngol.* 1992;17:322-326.
23. Wilson WR, Woods LA. Accuracy of the Bing and Rinne tuning fork tests. *Arch Otolaryngol.* 1975;101:81-85.
24. Doyle PJ, Anderson DW, Pijl S. The tuning fork: An essential instrument in otologic practice. *J Otolaryngol.* 1984;13(2):83-86.

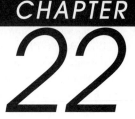
The Thyroid and Its Disorders

GOITER

I. INTRODUCTION

In industrialized areas of the world, goiter (i.e., enlarged thyroid) occurs in up to 10% of women and 2% of men, the usual causes being multinodular goiter, Hashimoto's thyroiditis, or Graves' disease (the most common cause worldwide is endemic goiter, largely from inadequate iodine intake).[1] About 80% of patients with goiter are clinically euthyroid, 10% are hypothyroid, and 10% are hyperthyroid.[1,2] Most patients are asymptomatic or present for evaluation of a neck mass. A few, especially those with substernal goiters, present with dyspnea, stridor, hoarseness, or dysphagia.[3,4]

Endemic goiter has been described for millennia, although it is unclear whether early clinicians distinguished goiter from other causes of neck swelling such as tuberculous lymphadenitis. The first person to clearly differentiate cystic goiter from cervical lymphadenopathy was Celsus, the Roman physician, writing in AD 30.[5]

II. TECHNIQUE

A. NORMAL THYROID

The important landmarks for locating the thyroid gland are the "V" at the top of the thyroid cartilage (the *laryngeal prominence* of the thyroid cartilage) and the cricoid cartilage (Fig. 22-1). These two structures, which are usually 3 cm apart, are the most conspicuous structures in the midline of the neck. The isthmus of the normal thyroid lies just below the cricoid cartilage and is usually 1.5 cm wide, covering the second, third, and fourth tracheal rings.[6,7] Each lateral lobe of the thyroid is 4 to 5 cm long and hugs the trachea tightly, extending from the middle of the thyroid cartilage down to the fifth or sixth tracheal rings.[7] A pyramidal lobe is found in up to 50% of anatomic dissections, usually on the left side, and is palpable in 10% of nontoxic goiters but seldom in normal-sized glands.[7,8]

The thyroid has a constant relationship with the laryngeal prominence (which is about 4 cm above the thyroid isthmus) and the cricoid cartilage (which is just above the isthmus), but the position of these structures in the neck (and thus of the thyroid in the neck) varies considerably among patients (see Fig. 22-1).[9] If the laryngeal prominence and suprasternal notch of the manubrium are far apart (e.g., 10–12 cm), the patient has a "high-lying" thyroid,

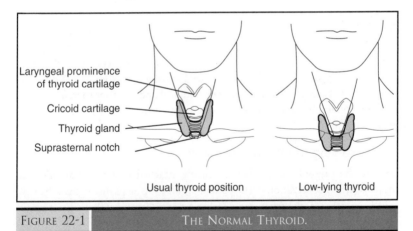

Laryngeal prominence of thyroid cartilage
Cricoid cartilage
Thyroid gland
Suprasternal notch

Usual thyroid position   Low-lying thyroid

FIGURE 22-1 | THE NORMAL THYROID.

The thyroid gland has a constant relationship with the two most prominent landmarks of the middle of the neck—the laryngeal prominence of the thyroid cartilage and the cricoid cartilage. On the left is the usual position of the thyroid gland. On the right is a "low-lying" thyroid, most of which is hidden behind the clavicles and sternum, inaccessible to palpation.

which is sometimes so conspicuous it suggests goiter even though it is normal-sized (see "Pseudogoiter"). If the laryngeal prominence is close to the suprasternal notch (e.g., 5 cm or less apart), the patient has a "low-lying" thyroid, which may be concealed behind the sternocleidomastoid muscles and clavicles, making complete palpation of the gland impossible.[9-11] Low-lying thyroids are more common in elderly patients.[11]

In areas of the world with iodine-replete diets, the normal thyroid is less than 20 mL in volume.[12,13]

B. EXAMINATION FOR GOITER

1. Inspection

Two maneuvers make the thyroid more conspicuous: (1) extending the patient's neck, which lifts the trachea (and thyroid) about 3 cm away from the suprasternal notch and stretches the skin against the thyroid and (2) inspecting the patient's neck from the side. In patients with normal- or high-lying thyroids, the line between the cricoid prominence and suprasternal notch, when viewed from the side, should be straight. Anterior bowing of this line suggests a goiter (Fig. 22-2).[14]

2. Palpation

The clinician may stand in front or behind the patient when palpating the thyroid, whichever position is most comfortable and effective, because no study has shown the superiority of either method.[13] Most authorities recommend palpating the thyroid with the patient's neck slightly flexed, to relax the sternocleidomastoid and sternohyoid muscles. A firm technique should be used. Special features to note during palpation are thyroid size, consistency (whether it is soft, firm, or hard; a "soft" thyroid has the consistency of the surrounding tissue in the neck), and texture (diffuse or nodular) and whether there is thyroid tenderness, tracheal deviation (a clue to asymmetric goiter), or cervical lymphadenopathy.

3. Observing the Patient Swallow.

Because the thyroid and trachea are firmly attached by ligaments and must move together, observation of the patient swallowing helps distinguish the thyroid from other neck structures. During a normal swallow, both the thyroid and trachea make an initial upward movement of 1.5 to 3.5 cm; the larger the oral bolus, the greater the movement.[15] The thyroid and trachea then hesitate 0.2 to 0.7 seconds before returning to their original position.

Therefore, a neck mass is probably *not* in the thyroid, if (1) the mass does not move during a swallow, or it moves less than the thyroid cartilage; (2) the mass does not hesitate before descending to its original position; or (3) the mass returns to its original position before complete descent of the thyroid cartilage.[15]

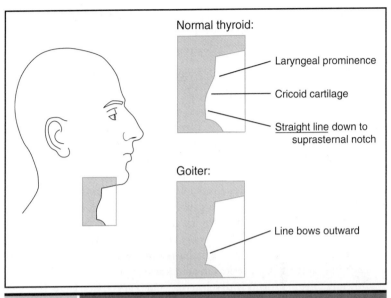

Normal thyroid:

— Laryngeal prominence

— Cricoid cartilage

— <u>Straight line</u> down to suprasternal notch

Goiter:

— Line bows outward

| FIGURE 22-2 | NECK CONTOUR AND GOITER. |

The shaded profile of the neck (*left*) is enlarged on the right, to contrast the normal thyroid contour with that of a goiter. Below the cricoid cartilage, the contour of the normal neck in the midline (*top right*) is a straight line downward to the suprasternal notch. In patients with goiter, this line bows outward (*bottom right*) because of enlargement of the thyroid isthmus. This line is visible only in patients with normal-lying and high-lying thyroids, not low-lying thyroids (see Fig. 22-1).

III. THE FINDINGS

A. CERVICAL GOITER

Some of the more common definitions of goiter include the following: (**1**) **The "rule of thumb,"** which states that a lateral lobe is enlarged if it is larger than the distal phalanx of the patient's thumb. (**2**) **Estimates of thyroid volume from palpation.** For example, a thyroid whose lateral lobes each measure 3 cm wide, 2 cm deep, and 5 cm long would have an estimated volume of 60 mL (i.e., $2 \times 3 \times 2 \times 5 = 60$). Any estimate greater than 20 mL is classified as a goiter (i.e., each lateral lobe is normally <10 mL). (**3**) **Epidemiologic definitions of goiter.** These definitions are designed for clinicians who rapidly survey large numbers of persons in areas of endemic goiter (these clinicians sometimes perform as many as 150–200 examinations per hour).[16] The World Health Organization has recently simplified their epidemiologic classification from five categories to only three: grade 0—no palpable or visible goiter, grade 1—a goiter that is palpable *but not visible* with the head in the normal position, and grade 2—a goiter that is clearly visible when the neck is in a normal position.[17]

B. SUBSTERNAL AND RETROCLAVICULAR GOITERS[18-23]

Large goiters may extend from the neck to the superior mediastinum, passing through the inflexible thoracic inlet (i.e., the bony ring formed by the upper sternum, first ribs, and first thoracic vertebral body). At the thoracic inlet, a goiter may compress the trachea, esophagus, or neck veins and cause dyspnea, dysphagia, facial plethora, cough, and hoarseness. Sometimes, when these patients flex or elevate the arms, the thoracic inlet is pulled up into the cervical goiter, just as if the thyroid were a cork and the thoracic inlet were the neck of a bottle. This causes a characteristic sign, **Pemberton's sign,** which is congestion of the face, cyanosis, and eventual distress induced by arm elevation (Fig. 22-3).[21,24–26] The exact frequency of Pemberton's sign is unknown. In two small series of patients with substernal goiter, it was positive in every patient[20,21]; two other larger series did not mention it at all.[22, 23]

Other findings in patients with substernal goiters are cervical goiter (i.e., palpable goiter above the thoracic inlet, 86% of patients), tracheal deviation (33%), distention of neck veins (22%), and stridor (10%) (for comparison, 75% have tracheal deviation on the chest radiograph).

C. THYROGLOSSAL CYST[27-31]

Thyroglossal cysts are cystic swellings of the thyroglossal duct, an epithelium-lined remnant marking the embryologic descent of thyroid tissue from the base of the tongue to its final location anterior to the larynx. Thyroglossal cysts present at any age, appearing as tense, nontender (unless infected or after acute hemorrhage into the capsule), mobile, nonlobulated round tumors, usually at the level of the hyoid bone or just below it (the hyoid bone is *above* the thyroid cartilage). They are in the midline in the neck, unless they are so low they lie to one side of the thyroid cartilage. Despite their cystic structure, they do not usually transilluminate. If the cyst remains attached to the base of the tongue or hyoid bone, a characteristic physical sign of thyroglossal cysts is upward movement when the patient protrudes the tongue, just as if the two structures were connected by a string. Thyroglossal cysts account for three-quarters of congenital neck masses, the other one quarter being branchial cleft cysts, which are located more laterally, usually anterior to the sternocleidomastoid muscle at the level of the hyoid bone.[32,33]

D. PSEUDOGOITER

Pseudogoiter refers to thyroid glands that appear enlarged even though they are normal-sized. There are three causes: **(1) High-lying thyroid gland,** which,

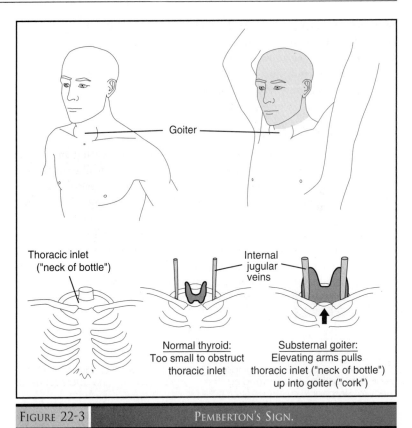

Goiter

Thoracic inlet
("neck of bottle")

Internal
jugular
veins

Normal thyroid:
Too small to obstruct
thoracic inlet

Substernal goiter:
Elevating arms pulls
thoracic inlet ("neck of bottle")
up into goiter ("cork")

FIGURE 22-3   PEMBERTON'S SIGN.

If a patient with retrosternal goiter elevates the arms (*top row*), dramatic facial congestion may occur (i.e., Pemberton's sign). This occurs because the thoracic inlet ("neck of bottle," *bottom left*) is an inflexible bony ring formed by the first thoracic vertebra, first ribs, and upper sternum (its outline is about the same size and shape as the patient's kidney). A normal-sized thyroid (*bottom middle*) is too small to obstruct the thoracic inlet. In contrast, a goiter of sufficient size (*bottom right*) may obstruct the thoracic inlet, especially if the goiter extends below the sternum and the patient elevates his arms (which pulls the thoracic inlet, or "neck of bottle" up into the goiter, or "cork," *arrow*).

although normal-sized, lies so high in the neck it is unusually conspicuous after neck extension. This diagnosis is suggested when the patient's laryngeal prominence is more than 10 cm above the suprasternal notch and both thyroid lobes are smaller than the distal phalanx of the patient's thumb. In one study, high-lying but normal-sized thyroids accounted for 8% of suspected goiters referred to an endocrinology service.[9] (**2**) **Other cervical masses,** such as adipose tissue, cervical lymphadenopathy, branchial cleft cysts, and pharyngeal diverticula (see Chapter 24). Observation during swallowing helps identify these lesions. (**3**) **Modigliani syndrome,** which describes a normal-sized thyroid lying in front of an exaggerated cervical spine lordosis,[34] named after the painter Amedeo Modigliani, whose portraits had subjects with long, curved necks.

E. THE DELPHIAN NODE

The Delphian node, a lymph node that drains the thyroid gland and larynx, lies directly anterior to the cricothyroid ligament (just cephalad to the thyroid isthmus, Fig. 22-4).[35,36] When enlarged, the node is readily palpable because of its superficial location and the fact that it lies against the unyielding trachea. The node is called "Delphian" because it is the first one exposed during surgery, and its appearance often foretells what the surgeon will find in the thyroid (e.g., carcinoma), just as the oracle at Delphi foretold the future.*[37] The Delphian node enlarges in some patients with thyroid cancer, Hashimoto's thyroiditis, and laryngeal cancer.[35] Its involvement in laryngeal cancer carries an ominous prognosis,[36,38,39] but no studies of its significance in thyroid cancer could be found.

---

*The word "Delphian" was originally suggested by Raymond Randall, a fourth-year medical student attending the thyroid clinic at The Massachusetts General Hospital.[37]

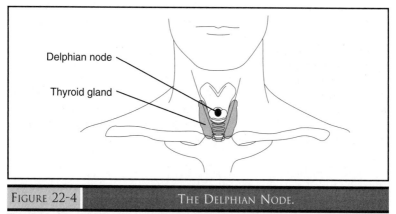

FIGURE 22-4   THE DELPHIAN NODE.

The Delphian node lies in midline of the neck, just above the thyroid isthmus and in front of the cricothyroid ligament, where it can easily be palpated against the unyielding cricoid cartilage.

IV. CLINICAL SIGNIFICANCE

A. DETECTING GOITER

The findings listed in EBM Box 22-1 are categorized into three levels: (1) no goiter by palpation or inspection (including inspection of the extended neck); (2) goiter by palpation, although the gland is visible only after extending the neck; and (3) goiter by palpation and inspection of the neck in the normal position. The first finding, absence of goiter by inspection and palpation, argues somewhat *against* the presence of an enlarged thyroid [likelihood ratio (LR) = 0.4, EBM Box 22-1; enlarged thyroid is defined as thyroid volume >20–25 mL]. Up to half of patients with an enlarged gland by ultrasonography have this finding, but presumably these goiters are small. The intermediate finding (i.e., goiter by palpation but visible only after neck extension) fails to distinguish goiter from normal-sized glands (LR not significant). Although this finding was tested in only one study, it suggests that subtle enlargement by palpation, not confirmed by inspection of the neck in the normal position, is an unreliable sign

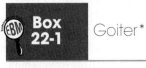 **Box 22-1** Goiter*

Finding (Ref)	Sensitivity (%)	Specificity (%)	Likelihood Ratio if Finding Present
No goiter by palpation or inspection[14,40–44]	5–57	0–26	0.4
Goiter by palpation, visible only after neck extension[40]	13	...	NS
Goiter by palpation and inspection with neck in normal position[40–42,44]	43–82	88–100	**26.3**

NS, not significant; likelihood ratio (LR) if finding present = positive LR.
*Diagnostic standard: For goiter, ultrasound volume >20 mL,[40–42,44] ultrasound volume >18 mL (women) or >25 mL (men),[43] or surgical weight >23 g.[14]

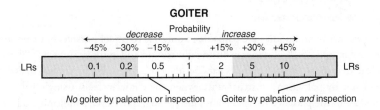

GOITER

of goiter. The most compelling finding arguing for an enlarged thyroid is a gland that is both enlarged by palpation and visible with the neck in the normal position (LR = 26.3).

B. ETIOLOGY OF GOITER

In a clinically euthyroid patient with goiter, the most common causes are multinodular goiter or Hashimoto's thyroiditis. In the hypothyroid patient it is Hashimoto's thyroiditis, and in the hyperthyroid patient it is Graves' disease or multinodular goiter. The associated finding of ophthalmopathy (tearing, diplopia, proptosis) or dermopathy (pretibial myxedema) indicates Graves' disease (see later).

Although thyroid cancer can also cause a goiter, cancer usually presents instead as a thyroid nodule (see "Thyroid Nodule").[45,46] Three findings argue strongly that a goiter contains carcinoma: vocal cord paralysis (LR = 45.2, EBM Box 22-2), cervical adenopathy (LR = 13.4), and fixation of the goiter to surrounding tissues (LR = 9.7).

Silent and postpartum thyroiditis also cause goiter, but goiter is present in only 50% or less of patients and it is rarely prominent, the clinician's attention instead directed toward the findings of hyperthyroidism.[49] The finding of a painful or tender thyroid gland, sometimes mimicking pharyngitis, suggests subacute thyroiditis[50-52] or hemorrhage into a cyst or nodule (although most thyroid hemorrhage is painless).[53] In subacute thyroiditis, the thyroid is modestly enlarged, usually 1.5 to 3 times the normal size.

THYROID NODULES

I. INTRODUCTION

Palpable thyroid nodules occur in about 5% of women and 1% of men, most of whom are clinically euthyroid.[54-56] Although thyroid nodules raise concerns about thyroid cancer, more than 95% of nodules reflect benign disorders, such as colloid cysts, adenomas, or dominant nodules of a multinodular gland.[57]

II. OCCULT NODULES

Because thyroid nodules are palpable in only 1% to 5% of persons but they are found in up to 50% of patients during ultrasound and autopsy surveys,[58-61] it is clear that most thyroid nodules are "occult" (i.e., detectable by clinical imaging but not by palpation). Furthermore, when the clinician feels a single *palpable* nodule in the patient's thyroid gland, ultrasonography reveals multiple nodules half the time.[62,63] Occult nodules are not palpable either because the patient's

Box 22-2 Goiter and Thyroid Nodules—Findings Predicting Carcinoma*

Finding (Ref)[†]	Sensitivity (%)	Specificity (%)	Likelihood Ratio if Finding	
			Present	Absent
GOITER				
Vocal cord paralysis[8]	24	99	**45.2**	0.8
Cervical adenopathy[8]	45	97	**13.4**	0.6
Fixation to surrounding tissues[8]	60	94	**9.7**	0.4
Goiter nodular (vs. diffuse)[8]	78	49	1.5	0.5
Pyramidal lobe present[8]	3	90	NS	NS
THYROID NODULE				
Vocal cord paralysis[47]	14	99	**12.0**	NS
Fixation to surrounding tissues[47,48]	13–37	95–98	**7.8**	NS
Cervical adenopathy[47]	31	96	**7.4**	0.7
Diameter ≥4 cm[48]	66	66	1.9	0.5
Very firm nodule[47]	4	99	NS	NS

NS, not significant; likelihood ratio (LR) if finding present = positive LR; LR if finding absent = negative LR.

*Diagnostic standard: For carcinoma, pathologic examination of tissue.[8,47,48]

[†]Definition of findings: For vocal cord paralysis, direct visualization of vocal cords.

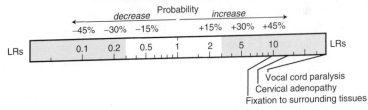

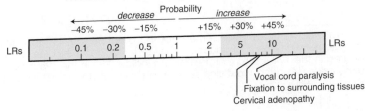

neck is too short or thick,[64] the nodules are buried in the posterior parts of the gland,[65] or the nodules are too small. (The mean diameter of a *palpable* nodule is 3 cm; palpation fails to detect 50% of nodules less than 2 cm in diameter and more than 90% of nodules less than 1 cm in diameter.)[58,62,64]

Although the large number of occult nodules raises the concern that palpation of the thyroid misses many thyroid cancers, it is important to emphasize that occult nodules rarely contain clinically important carcinoma[54,60,61,64] and that the most common presentation for thyroid carcinoma remains the *palpable* thyroid nodule.[45,46,66,67]

III. CLINICAL SIGNIFICANCE

The most important diagnostic test for thyroid nodules is fine needle aspiration. Nonetheless, a few physical signs, if present, argue strongly that the thyroid nodule contains carcinoma (see EBM Box 22-2): vocal cord paralysis (LR = 12.0), fixation of the nodule to surrounding tissues (LR = 7.8), and cervical adenopathy (LR = 7.4). Fewer than one of three patients with thyroid carcinoma, however, has any of these findings.

HYPOTHYROIDISM (MYXEDEMA)

I. INTRODUCTION

Hypothyroidism is a clinical syndrome that results from diminished levels of thyroid hormone, which slows the patient's metabolic rate and neuromuscular reactions and causes accumulation of mucopolysaccharides in the skin and other tissues throughout the body. In areas of the industrialized world with iodine-replete diets, hypothyroidism affects 9% of women and 1% of men[1]. The usual cause is disease in the thyroid gland itself (primary hypothyroidism), usually from Hashimoto's thyroiditis (60%–70% of cases) or previous radioiodine treatment for Grave's disease (20%–30% of cases).[1]

The diagnosis of hypothyroidism relies on laboratory tests, which have been available for more than 100 years.* Nonetheless, bedside diagnosis still has two important roles: (1) it estimates the likelihood of thyroid disease, which then

---

*The first thyroid test was measurements of the basal metabolic rate (BMR) (i.e., oxygen consumption), introduced in the 1890s. Radioactive iodine uptake appeared in the 1940s, serum protein-bound iodide (PBI) in the 1950s, serum total thyroxine (T4) in the 1960s, and sensitive assays for thyroid stimulating hormone in the 1980s.[68,69]

can be used to identify subgroups of patients with high or low probability of abnormal thyroid function, thus increasing the yield of laboratory testing[70] and (2) it is essential to the diagnosis of subclinical hypothyroidism or sick euthyroid syndrome, conditions that, by definition, describe patients with abnormal laboratory tests but without bedside findings of thyroid disease.

All of the classic bedside findings of hypothyroidism—the puffy skin, slow reflexes, thick speech, and sluggish thinking—were first described by William Gull and William Ord in the 1870s.[71–73]

II. FINDINGS AND THEIR PATHOGENESIS

A. SKIN AND SOFT TISSUE

The nonpitting puffiness of hypothyroidism results from dermal accumulation of mucopolysaccharides (mostly hyaluronic acid and chondroitin sulfate), which freely bind water.[29] These changes cause a "jelly-like swelling (and) overgrowth of mucus-yielding cement," which led Ord to coin the term "myxedema" in 1877.[73] Even after effective thyroid replacement, these changes may persist for months or longer.[74]

Some myxedematous patients also have a yellow tint to their skin, which occurs because of hypercarotenemia from diminished conversion of carotenoids to retinol.[75,76] The apparent coolness of the skin is attributed to diminished dermal blood flow,[77] and dryness results in part from decreased sebum production.[78] The loss of hair from the lateral eyebrows occurs in about a third of hypothyroid patients and is one of the least specific signs, commonly found in euthyroid patients.[79]

B. THE ACHILLES REFLEX

The ankle jerk has been investigated more extensively than any other physical finding of thyroid disease. By the 1970s, at least nine different instruments had been designed to precisely measure the duration of reflex to the nearest millisecond (msec).[80,81]

Both the contraction and relaxation phase of the ankle jerk are prolonged in hypothyroidism,[81–84] although prolonged relaxation seems most prominent to the human eye (and on many of the tracings of the reflex). In one study, the mean half-relaxation time (i.e., the time from the hammer tap to the moment the Achilles tendon has returned half-way to its original position) for hypothyroid patients was 460 msec [standard deviation (SD) 40 msec], compared with 310 msec (SD 30 msec) for euthyroid patients.[84] Experiments in hypothyroid rats suggest that the prolongation results from diminished calcium transport by the sarcoplasmic reticulum and subsequent slowing of the interaction between actin and myosin.[85]

When testing for hypothyroidism, clinicians usually elicit the ankle jerk by tapping on the Achilles tendon with the patient kneeling on a chair.[82,84,86] The force of the tap does not affect the duration of the reflex, although slightly more force is necessary in hypothyroid patients to generate a reflex than in hyperthyroid patients.[82]

C. HYPOTHYROID SPEECH

Hypothyroid speech, seen in about one third of patients with hypothyroidism,[87,88] has a slow rate and rhythm and is characteristically deep, low-pitched, and hyponasal (i.e., as if the patient has a cold).[89–91] Some patients even slur their words slightly, leading one clinician to describe the hypothyroid voice as "a bad gramophone record of a drowsy, slightly intoxicated person with a bad cold and a plum in the mouth."[92] Biopsies of vocal cords have revealed deposition of mucinous material.[93]

D. OBESITY IS NO MORE COMMON IN HYPOTHYROID PATIENTS THAN IN EUTHYROID PATIENTS[94]

III. CLINICAL SIGNIFICANCE

EBM Box 22-3 summarizes the diagnostic accuracy of physical signs associated with hypothyroidism, as applied to more than 1500 patients with suspected thyroid disease. The Billewicz scoring scheme, which appears on the bottom of EBM Box 22-3, is fully described in Table 22-1.

In patients with suspected thyroid disease, the findings arguing the most *for* hypothyroidism are hypothyroid speech (LR = 5.4, EBM Box 22-3), cool *and* dry skin (LR = 4.7), slow pulse rate (LR = 4.1), coarse skin (LR = 3.4), and delayed ankle reflexes (LR = 3.4).[*] Hair loss of the eyebrows was one of the least compelling diagnostic signs (LR = 1.9), and the finding of *isolated* coolness or dryness of the palms is unhelpful (LR not significant). No single finding, when absent, argues convincingly *against* hypothyroidism (i.e., no LR has a value <0.6).

A Billewicz score of +30 points or more argues convincingly *for* hypothyroidism (LR = 18.8), whereas a score less than −15 points argues convincingly *against* hypothyroidism (LR = 0.1). The mean ages of the patients in these studies is unknown[†]; the Billewicz score may perform less well in elderly patients, who, as a rule, have fewer findings than younger patients.[100]

---

*For comparison, precise measurements of the ankle jerk using special instruments discriminate well between patients with and without hypothyroidism: the finding of a half-relaxation time >370–380 msec detects hypothyroidism with a sensitivity 91%–99%, specificity 94%–97%, positive LR = 18.7, and negative LR = 0.1[84,86,95]

†One study[98] presented the range of ages (17–73 years), but the other study[97] presented no information about age.

Box 22-3 Hypothyroidism*

Finding (Ref)[†]	Sensitivity (%)	Specificity (%)	Likelihood Ratio if Finding Present	Likelihood Ratio if Finding Absent
Skin				
Cool and dry skin[95]	16	97	**4.7**	0.9
Coarse skin[87,96]	29–61	74–95	**3.4**	0.7
Cold palms[87]	37	77	NS	NS
Dry palms[87]	42	73	NS	NS
Periorbital puffiness[87,96]	53–91	21–81	NS	0.6
Puffiness of wrists[87]	39	86	2.9	0.7
Hair loss of eyebrows[87]	29	85	1.9	NS
Pretibial edema[96]	78	31	NS	NS
Speech				
Hypothyroid speech[87]	37	93	**5.4**	0.7
Pulse				
Slow pulse rate[95,96]	29–43	89–93	**4.1**	0.8
Thyroid				
Enlarged thyroid[95]	46	84	2.8	0.6
Neurologic				
Delayed ankle reflexes[96]	48	86	**3.4**	0.6
Slow movements[96]	87	13	NS	NS
Billewicz score[97,98]				
Less than −15 points	3–4	28–68	**0.1**	...
−15 to +29 points	35–39	...	NS	...
+30 points or more	57–61	90–99	**18.8**	...

NS, not significant; likelihood ratio (LR) if finding present = positive LR; LR if finding absent = negative LR.

*Diagnostic standard: For hypothyroidism, low free T_4 level and high thyroid stimulating hormone (TSH),[96,98] or low protein-bound iodide (PBI) level.[87,95,97] The PBI level and total T_4 level correlate closely, except in patients with thyroiditis and those who ingest exogenous iodides (e.g., radiocontrast dye, cough suppressants), diagnoses in which the PBI level may be falsely high.[99] These diagnoses, however, were largely excluded from the studies reviewed here.

[†]Definition of findings: For slow pulse rate, <60 beats/min[96] or <70 beats/min[95]; for delayed ankle reflexes, assessment of contraction and relaxation of calf muscle by naked eye[96]; for slow movements, patients required more than 1 minute to fold a 2-m-long bed sheet.[96]

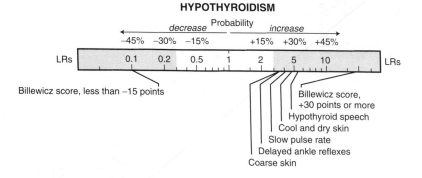

HYPOTHYROIDISM

Billewicz score, less than −15 points

Billewicz score, +30 points or more
Hypothyroid speech
Cool and dry skin
Slow pulse rate
Delayed ankle reflexes
Coarse skin

Table 22-1	Billewicz Diagnostic Index for Hypothyroidism*		
Finding†	**Points Scored if Finding**		
		Present	**Absent**
SYMPTOMS			
Diminished sweating		+6	−2
Dry skin		+3	−6
Cold intolerance		+4	−5
Weight increase		+1	−1
Constipation		+2	−1
Hoarseness		+5	−6
Paresthesiae		+5	−4
Deafness		+2	0
PHYSICAL SIGNS			
Slow movements		+11	−3
Coarse skin		+7	−7
Cold skin		+3	−2
Periorbital puffiness		+4	−6
Pulse rate < 75/min		+4	−4
Slow ankle jerk		+15	−6

*Source: Reference 97.
†Definition of findings: For weight increase, recorded increase in weight or tightness in clothing; for slow movements, observations while patient removing and replacing a buttoned garment; for coarse skin, roughness and thickening of skin of hands, forearms, and elbows; for slow ankle jerk, reflex appears slow with patient kneeling on a chair, grasping its back.

HYPERTHYROIDISM

I. INTRODUCTION

Hyperthyroidism is a clinical syndrome resulting from increased production or release of thyroid hormone, which elevates the metabolic rate and causes characteristic findings of the skin, thyroid, eyes, and neuromuscular system. The most common causes of hyperthyroidism are Graves' disease (60%–90% of cases), toxic nodular goiter, thyroiditis (subacute, silent, or postpartum), and iatrogenic overtreatment with thyroid replacement.[101] Hyperthyroidism affects women (4% prevalence) more than men (0.2% prevalence).

Three clinicians—Caleb Parry, Robert Graves, and Adolf von Basedow—all writing between 1825 and 1840, independently described the classic physical signs associated with thyrotoxicosis. All three were especially impressed with the triad of goiter, prominent eyes, and forceful tachycardia.[102]

II. FINDINGS AND THEIR PATHOGENESIS

A. THE THYROID

A goiter is present in 70%–93% of patients with hyperthyroidism.[103–105] The goiter is diffuse and symmetric in patients with Graves' disease and thyroiditis but nodular in those with toxic nodular goiter.[49,105]

A thyroid bruit is a common feature of Graves' disease (73% of patients in one study).[106] Nonetheless, the finding also was noted in 30% of elderly patients with toxic nodular goiter,[107] suggesting that the finding is not as specific for Graves' disease as is classically taught. Bruits often radiate far from their source, and perhaps the "thyroid bruit" in the elderly with toxic nodular goiter is actually a carotid bruit made prominent by the increased cardiac output of hyperthyroidism.*

B. EYE FINDINGS

Three distinct eye findings are associated with hyperthyroidism: lid lag (von Graefe's sign, 1864), lid retraction (Dalrymple's sign, 1849),† and Graves'

---

*The opposite phenomenon—a "carotid bruit" actually emanating from a superior thyroid artery—has also been described.[108.]
†The British eye surgeon John Dalrymple (1803-1852) apparently thought so little of his sign that he never published a description of it. Writing in 1849, W. White Cooper attributed the sign to his friend Dalrymple.[109] Albrecht von Graefe (1828-1870) described his sign in 1864.[102] Ruedemann coined the term "lid lag" in 1932.[110]

ophthalmopathy. Graves' ophthalmopathy afflicts exclusively patients with Graves' disease, whereas lid lag and lid retraction may occur in hyperthyroidism from any etiology.[52,111]

1. Lid Lag

This sign describes the appearance of white sclera between the margin of the upper eyelid and corneal limbus as the patient looks downward. In von Graefe's words, " . . . as the cornea looks down, the upper eyelid does not follow."[102]

2. Lid Retraction

This sign describes a peculiar staring appearance of the eyes, caused by a widened palpebral fissure. As the patient looks straight ahead, the upper eyelid is positioned abnormally high, revealing white sclera between the lid margin and superior limbus. Normally the margin of the upper eyelid rests just below the edge of the corneal limbus and covers about 1 mm of the iris.[112,113]

Both lid lag and lid retraction are attributed to the sympathetic hyperactivity of hyperthyroidism, which causes excess contraction of Mueller's muscle (the involuntary lid elevator whose paralysis causes the ptosis of Horner's syndrome). Although the findings improve after treatment with β-blocking medications,[114] mechanisms other than sympathetic hyperactivity must contribute to the lid findings of patients with Graves' disease (even those without exophthalmos or obvious ophthalmopathy, see below), because the lid findings of Graves' disease are often unilateral and persist after the patient becomes euthyroid, and because the pupils of patients with lid findings are usually normal-sized (instead of the dilated pupils of sympathetic hyperactivity).[115–118]

Other common causes of lid retraction are unilateral ptosis, facial muscle weakness, previous eyelid surgery, or the irritation of wearing contact lenses.[119] Ptosis causes contralateral lid retraction because attempts to elevate the weakened lid generate excessive neural signals to the motor neuron of the healthy lid, thus elevating it.[120] A simple test confirming ptosis as the cause is to occlude the eye that has ptosis, which then causes the lid retraction in the opposite eye to resolve. Facial weakness causes retraction of the ipsilateral eyelid because the lid elevators are no longer opposed by the orbicularis oculi muscle.[121]

3. Graves' Ophthalmopathy

Graves' ophthalmopathy is a constellation of findings, apparent in 25%–50% of patients with Graves' disease[116,122] that results from edema and lymphocytic infiltration of orbital fat, connective tissue, and eye muscles.[123] Characteristic physical findings are lid edema, limitation of eye movements, conjunctival chemosis and injection, and exophthalmos (as measured with an exophthalmometer).[113] Clinicians should suspect Graves' ophthalmopathy when patients complain of gritty sensation in the eyes, tearing, eye discomfort, or diplopia.

The orbital swelling of Graves' ophthalmopathy may threaten the optic nerve and vision. The bedside findings best predicting incipient optic neuropathy are lid edema and limitation of eye movements—not, surprisingly, the degree of proptosis (proptosis does not predict incipient optic neuropathy perhaps because intraocular pressure is relieved by the outward protrusion).[118,124]

C. CARDIOVASCULAR FINDINGS

Hyperthyroidism may cause a fast heart rate, loud snapping first heart sounds, midsystolic flow murmurs, and supraventricular arrhythmias.[106,125–128] Rare patients with severe hyperthyroidism may develop the Means-Lerman scratch,[129] a systolic rub or murmur with a prominent rough or grating character that appears near the left second intercostals space. Its pathogenesis is unknown.

D. SKIN FINDINGS

The skin of hyperthyroid patients is warm, moist, and smooth,[29] probably because of increased sympathetic tone to sweat glands and increased dermal blood flow. These skin findings often resolve after treatment with β-blocker medications.[77,106,125]

Up to 4% of patients with Graves' disease develop a skin lesion with the confusing name "pretibial myxedema," characterized by bilateral, asymmetric raised, firm plaques or nodules, which are pink to purple-brown in color and usually distributed over the anterior shins.[29,130]

E. NEUROMUSCULAR FINDINGS

The neuromuscular findings of hyperthyroidism are weakness and diminished exercise tolerance, tremor, and brisk ankle jerks. The diminished exercise tolerance (affecting 67% of patients) is due to an inability to increase cardiac output appropriately with exercise and to proximal muscle wasting and weakness from accelerated protein catabolism.[105,128,131–133] The fine tremor of hyperthyroidism occurs because of increased sympathetic tone and resolves with β-blocking medications.[106,125] Brisk reflexes are noted at the bedside in only 25% of patients or less,[79] and even precise measurements of the half-relaxation time (see "Hypothyroidism" for definition) reveal considerable overlap between normal values (range 230–420 msec) and hyperthyroid values (range 200–300 msec).[84]

III. CLINICAL SIGNIFICANCE

EBM Box 22-4 presents the diagnostic accuracy of physical signs for hyperthyroidism, as applied to more than 1700 patients with suspected thyroid disease. At the bottom of EBM Box 22-4 is the accuracy of the Wayne index, a diagnostic scoring scheme described in Table 22-2.

**Box
22-4**   Hyperthyroidism*

Finding (Ref)	Sensitivity (%)	Specificity (%)	Likelihood Ratio if Finding	
			Present	Absent
Pulse				
Pulse ≥90 beats/min[105]	80	82	**4.4**	**0.2**
Skin				
Skin moist and warm[105]	34	95	**6.7**	0.7
Thyroid				
Enlarged thyroid[105]	93	59	2.3	**0.1**
Eyes				
Eyelid retraction[105]	34	99	**31.5**	0.7
Eyelid lag[105]	19	99	**17.6**	0.8
Neurologic				
Fine finger tremor[105]	69	94	**11.4**	**0.3**
Wayne index[134,135]				
< 11 points	1–6	13–32	**0.04**	...
11–19 points	12–30	...	NS	...
≥ 20 points	66–88	92–99	**18.2**	...

NS, not significant; likelihood ratio (LR) if finding present = positive LR; LR if finding absent = negative LR.
*Diagnostic standards: For hyperthyroidism, high levels of PBI for patients evaluated in the 1960s, total T_4 for those in the 1970s, and total T_4 and TSH for those in the 1980s and 1990s (see footnote to Table 22-3 for discussion of PBI).

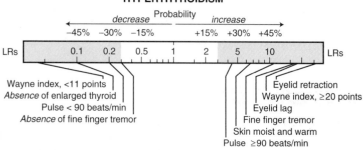

HYPERTHYROIDISM

Table 22-2	Wayne Diagnostic Index for Hyperthyroidism*			
Symptoms of Recent Onset or Increased Severity	Present	Signs	Present	Absent
Dyspnea on effort	+1	Palpable thyroid	+3	−3
Palpitations	+2	Bruit over thyroid	+2	−2
Tiredness	+2	Exophthalmos	+2	
Preference for heat (irrespective of duration)	−5	Lid retraction	+2	
Preference for cold	+5	Lid lag	+1	
Excessive sweating	+3	Hyperkinetic movements	+4	−2
Nervousness	+2	Fine finger tremor	+1	
Appetite increased	+3	Hands:		
Appetite decreased	−3	Hot	+2	−2
Weight increased	−3	Moist	+1	−1
Weight decreased	+3	Casual pulse rate:		
		Atrial fibrillation	+4	
		<80, regular	−3	
		80–90, regular	0	
		>90, regular	+3	

*From reference 134.

The findings that argue *for* the diagnosis of hyperthyroidism, in descending order of their LRs, are lid retraction (LR = 31.5, see EBM Box 22-4), lid lag (LR = 17.6), fine finger tremor (LR = 11.4), moist and warm skin (LR = 6.7), and pulse ≥90 beats/minute (LR = 4.4). Those findings arguing convincingly *against* hyperthyroidism are normal thyroid size (LR = 0.1), pulse less than 90 beats/minute (LR = 0.2), and absence of finger tremor (LR = 0.3).

A Wayne index score of 20 or more points argues *for* hyperthyroidism (LR = 18.2) and one of 10 or fewer points argues *against* hyperthyroidism (LR = 0.04). This index, however, may be less useful in elderly patients,[136] who, as a rule, have less goiter and tachycardia than younger patients.[137-139] In one study, 36% of elderly hyperthyroid patients had scores less than 11.[107] Elderly patients also have more weight loss and atrial fibrillation than younger patients,[105,107,140,141] but the frequency of lid retraction and lid lag is the same.[105,107]

REFERENCES

1. Vanderpump MPJ, Tunbridge WMG, French JM, et al. The incidence of thyroid disorders in the community: A twenty-year follow-up of the Whickham Survey. *Clin Endocrinol.* 1995;43:55-68.

2. Hurley DL, Gharib H. Evaluation and management of multinodular goiter. *Otolaryngol Clin North Am.* 1996;29:527-540.

3. Zorrilla L, Tsai J, Freedman M. Airway obstruction due to goiter in older patients. *J Am Geriatr Soc.* 1989;37:1153-1156.

4. Close LG, Costin BS, Kim EE. Acute symptoms of the aerodigestive tract caused by rapidly enlarging thyroid neoplasms. *Otolaryngology.* 1983;91:441-445.

5. Celsus. De Medicina. Spencer WG, trans. *De Medicina (English translation of Latin edition written between A.D. 25 and 35, printed in 1478).* Cambridge: Harvard University Press; 1953:140-141, 374-145.

6. Calhoun KH, Weiss RL, Scott B, et al. Management of the thyroid isthmus in tracheostomy: A prospective and retrospective study. *Otolaryngol Head Neck Surg.* 1994;111:450-452.

7. Hansen JT. Embryology and surgical anatomy of the lower neck and superior mediastinum. In: Falk SA, ed. *Thyroid disease: Endocrinology, surgery, nuclear medicine, and radiotherapy,* 2nd ed. Philadelphia: Lippincott-Raven; 1997:15-27.

8. Boyle JA, Greig WR, Franklin DA, et al. Construction of a model for computer-assisted diagnosis: Application to the problem of non-toxic goitre. *Q J Med.* 1966;35:565-588.

9. Gwinup G, Morton ME. The high lying thyroid: A cause of pseudogoiter. *J Clin Endocrinol Metab.* 1975;40:37-42.

10. Dobyns BM. Goiter. *Curr Prob Surg.* 1969:2-60.

11. Slater S. Cricoid cartilage and suprasternal notch: The "low-lying thyroid". *South Med J.* 1979;72:1621-1622.

12. Hegedus L, Perrild H, Poulsen LR, et al. The determination of thyroid volume by ultrasound and its relationship to body weight, age, and sex in normal subjects. *J Clin Endocrinol Metab.* 1983;56:260-263.

13. Siminoski K. The rational clinical examination: Does this patient have a goiter? *JAMA.* 1995;273:813-817.

14. Silink K, Reisenauer R. Geographical spread of endemic goitre and problems of its mapping. In: Silink K, Cerny K, eds. *Endemic goitre and allied diseases.* Bratislava: Publishing House of the Slovak Academy of Sciences; 1966:33-47.

15. Siminoski K. Differential movement during swallowing as an aid in the detection of thyroid pseudonodules. *Head Neck.* 1994;16:21-24.

16. Perez D, Scrimshaw NS, Munoz JA. Classification of goitre and technique of endemic goitre surveys. *Bull World Health Org.* 1958;18:217-232.

17. *Assessment of iodine deficiency disorders and monitoring their elimination: A guide for programme managers. WHO/NHD/01.1,* 2nd ed. World Health Organization; 2001.

18. Sherman PH, Shahbahrami F. Mediastinal goiter: Review of ten cases. *Am Surg.* 1966;32:137-142.
19. Singh B, Lucente FE, Shaha AR. Substernal goiter: A clinical review. *Am J Otolaryngol.* 1994;15:409-416.
20. Klassen-Udding LM, van Lijf JH, Napel HHT. Substernal goitre, deep venous thrombosis of the arm, and Pemberton's sign. *Neth J Med.* 1983;26:228-231.
21. Blum M, Biller BJ, Bergman DA. The thyroid cork: Obstruction of the thoracic inlet due to retroclavicular goiter. *JAMA.* 1974;227:189-191.
22. Katlic MR, Grillo HC, Wang C. Substernal goiter: Analysis of 80 patients from Massachusetts General Hospital. *Am J Surg.* 1985;149:283-287.
23. Reeve TS, Rundle FF, Hales IB, et al. The investigation and management of intrathoracic goiter. *Surg Gynecol Obstet.* 1962;115:223-229.
24. Wallace C, Siminoski K. The Pemberton sign. *Ann Intern Med.* 1996;125:568-569.
25. Pemberton HS. Sign of submerged goitre. *Lancet.* 1946;251:509.
26. Basaria S, Salvatori R. Pemberton's sign. *N Engl J Med.* 2004;350:1338.
27. Pounds LA. Neck masses of congenital origin. *Pediatr Clin North Am.* 1981;28:841-844.
28. Girard M, Deluca SA. Thyroglossal duct cyst. *Am Fam Phys.* 1990;42:665-668.
29. Heymann WR. Cutaneous manifestations of thyroid disease. *J Am Acad Dermatol.* 1992;26:885-902.
30. Marshall SF, Becker WF. Thyroglossal cysts and sinuses. *Ann Surg.* 1949;129:642-651.
31. Dedivitis RA, Camargo DL, Peixoto GL, et al. Thyroglossal duct: A review of 55 cases. *J Am Coll Surg.* 2002;194:274-277.
32. Liston SL, Siegel LG. Branchial cysts, sinuses, and fistulas. *ENT J.* 1979;58:504-509.
33. Himalstein MR. Branchial cysts and fistulas. *ENT J.* 1980;59:23-29.
34. Mercer RD. Pseudo-goiter: The Modigliani syndrome. *Cleve Clin J Med.* 1975;42:319-326.
35. Cope O, Dobyns BM, Hamlin E, Hopkirk J. What thyroid nodules are to be feared? *J Clin Endocrinol Metab.* 1949;9:1012-1022.
36. Olsen KD, DeSanto LW, Pearson BW. Positive Delphian lymph node: Clinical significance in laryngeal cancer. *Laryngoscope.* 1987;97:1033-1037.
37. Cope O. The surgery of the thyroid. In: Means JH, ed. *The thyroid and its diseases,* 2nd ed. Philadelphia: J.B. Lippincott Co.
38. Foote RL, Buskirk SJ, Stanley RJ, et al. Patterns of failure after total laryngectomy for glottic carcinoma. *Cancer.* 1989;64:143-149.
39. Thaler ER, Montone K, Tucker J, Weinstein GS. Delphian lymph node in laryngeal carcinoma: A whole organ study. *Laryngoscope.* 1997;107:332-334.
40. Berghout A, Wiersinga WM, Smits NJ, Touber JL. The value of thyroid volume measured by ultrasonography in the diagnosis of goitre. *Clin Endocrinol.* 1988;28:409-414.
41. Hegedus L, Karstrup S, Veiergang D, et al. High frequency of goitre in cigarette smokers. *Clin Endocrinol.* 1985;22:287-292.

42. Hegedus L, Hansen JM, Luehdorf K, et al. Increased frequency of goitre in epileptic patients on long-term phenytoin or carbamazepine treatment. *Clin Endocrinol.* 1985;23:423-429.

43. Hintze G, Windeler J, Baumert J, et al. Thyroid volume and goitre prevalence in the elderly as determined by ultrasound and their relationships to laboratory indices. *Acta Endocrinol (Copenh).* 1991;124:12-18.

44. Perrild H, Hegedus L, Baastrup PC, et al. Thyroid function and ultrasonically determined thyroid size in patients receiving long-term lithium treatment. *Am J Psychiatry.* 1990;147:1518-1521.

45. Christensen SB, Ljungberg O, Tibblin S. Thyroid carcinoma in Malmo, 1960-1977: Epidemiologic, clinical, and prognostic findings in a defined urban population. *Cancer.* 1984;53:1625-1633.

46. Mazzaferri EL, Young RL, Oertel JE, et al. Papillary thyroid carcinoma: The impact of therapy in 576 patients. *Medicine.* 1977;56:171-196.

47. Hamming JF, Goslings BM, van Steenis GJ, et al. The value of fine-needle aspiration biopsy in patients with nodular thyroid disease divided into groups of suspicion of malignant neoplasms on clinical grounds. *Arch Intern Med.* 1990;150:113-116.

48. Carrillo JF, Frias-Mendivil M, Ochoa-Carrillo FJ, Ibarra M. Accuracy of fine-needle aspiration biopsy of the thyroid combined with an evaluation of clinical and radiologic factors. *Otolaryngol Head Neck Surg.* 2000;122:917-921.

49. Woolf PD. Transient painless thyroiditis with hyperthyroidism: A variant of lymphocytic thyroiditis? *Endocrinol Rev.* 1980;1:411-420.

50. Greene JN. Subacute thyroiditis. *Am J Med.* 1971;51:97-108.

51. Murray IPC, Stewart RDH, Indyk JS. The diagnosis of the painful thyroid. *Med J Austral.* 1970;2:1055-1061.

52. Volpe R, Johnston MW. Subacute thyroiditis: A disease commonly mistaken for pharyngitis. *Can Med Assoc J.* 1957;77:297-307.

53. Mizokami T, Okamura K, Hirata T, et al. Acute spontaneous hemorrhagic degeneration of the thyroid nodule with subacute thyroiditis-like symptoms and laboratory findings. *Endocrine J.* 1995;42:683-689.

54. Vander JB, Gaston EA, Dawber TR. The significance of nontoxic thyroid nodules: Final report of a 15-year study of the incidence of thyroid malignancy. *Ann Intern Med.* 1968;69:537-540.

55. Tunbridge WMG, Evered DC, Hall R, et al. The spectrum of thyroid disease in a community: The Whickham survey. *Clin Endocrinol.* 1977;7:481-493.

56. Wang C, Crapo LM. The epidemiology of thyroid disease and implications for screening. *Endocrinol Metab Clin North Am.* 1997;26:189-218.

57. Hermus AR, Huysmans DA. Treatment of benign nodular thyroid disease. *N Engl J Med.* 1998;338:1438-1446.

58. Tomimori E, Pedrinola F, Cavaliere H, et al. Prevalence of incidental thyroid disease in a relatively low iodine intake area. *Thyroid.* 1995;5:273-276.

59. Ridgeway EC. Clinical review 30: Clinician's evaluation of a solitary thyroid nodule. *J Endocrinol Clin Metab.* 1992;74:231-235.

60. Ezzat S, Sarti DA, Cain DR, Braunstein GD. Thyroid incidentalomas: Prevalence by palpation and ultrasonography. *Arch Intern Med.* 1994;154:1838-1840.

61. Burguera B, Gharib H. Thyroid incidentalomas: Prevalence, diagnosis, significance, and management. *Endocrinol Metab Clin North Am.* 2000;29:187-203.

62. Brander A, Viiginkoski P, Tuuhea J, et al. Clinical versus ultrasound examination of the thyroid gland in common clinical practice. *J Clin Ultrasound.* 1992;20:37-42.

63. Tan GH, Gharib H, Reading CC. Solitary thyroid nodule: Comparison between palpation and ultrasonography. *Arch Intern Med.* 1995;155:2418-2423.

64. Witterick IJ, Abel SM, Hartwick W, et al. Incidence and types of non-palpable thyroid nodules in thyroids removed for palpable disease. *J Otolaryngol.* 1993;22:294-300.

65. Schneider AB, Bekerman C, Leland J, et al. Thyroid nodules in the follow-up of irradiated individuals: Comparison of thyroid ultrasound with scanning and palpation. *J Clin Endocrinol Metab.* 1997;82:4020-4027.

66. Brennan MD, Bergstralh EJ, van Heerden JA, McConahey WM. Follicular thyroid cancer treated at the Mayo Clinic, 1946 through 1970: Initial manifestations, pathologic findings, therapy, and outcome. *Mayo Clin Proc.* 1991;66:11-22.

67. McConahey WM, Hay ID, Woolner LB, et al. Papillary thyroid cancer treated at the Mayo Clinic, 1946 through 1970: Initial manifestations, pathologic findings, therapy, and outcome. *Mayo Clin Proc.* 1986;61:978-996.

68. Gruhn JG, Barsano CP, Kumar Y. The development of tests of thyroid function. *Arch Pathol Lab Med.* 1987;111:84-100.

69. Dubois EF. *Basal metabolism in health and disease.* Philadelphia: Lea & Febiger; 1927.

70. White GH. Can the initial clinical assessment of thyroid function be improved? *Lancet.* 1978;2:933-935.

71. Beahrs OH. American Association of Endocrine Surgeons. Presidential address: Lest we forget. *Surgery.* 1987;102:893-897.

72. Hoffenberg R. The thyroid and Osler. *J Coll Physicians Lond.* 1985;19(2):80-84.

73. Rolleston HD. *The endocrine organs in health and disease with an historical review.* London: Oxford University Press; 1936.

74. Gabrilove JL, Ludwig AW. The histogenesis of myxedema. *J Clin Endocrinol Metab.* 1957;17:925-932.

75. Al-Jubouri MA, Coombes EJ, Young RM, McLaughlin NP. Xanthoderma: An unusual presentation of hypothyroidism. *J Clin Pathol.* 1994;47:850-851.

76. Escamilla RF. Carotinemia in myxedema: Explanation of the typical slightly icteric tint. *J Clin Metab Endocrinol.* 1942;2:33-35.

77. Thomson JA. Alterations in capillary fragility in thyroid disease. *Clin Sci.* 1964;26:55-60.

78. Goolamali SK, Evered D, Shuster S. Thyroid disease and sebaceous function. *Br Med J.* 1976;1:432-433.

79. Danowski TS. *Clinical endocrinology*. Baltimore: Wm. Wilkins; 1962.

80. Chaney WC. Tendon reflexes in myxedema: A valuable aid in diagnosis. *JAMA*. 1924;82:2013-2016.

81. Rives KL, Furth ED, Becker DV. Limitations of the ankle jerk test: Intercomparison with other tests of thyroid function. *Ann Intern Med*. 1965;62: 1139-1146.

82. Lawson JD. The free Achilles reflex in hypothyroidism and hyperthyroidism. *N Engl J Med*. 1958;259:761-764.

83. Sherman L. The Achilles reflex (letter). *Lancet*. 1963;2:942-943.

84. Sherman M, Larson FC. The Achilles reflex: A diagnostic test of thyroid function. *Lancet*. 1963;1:243-245.

85. Fanburg BL. Calcium transport by skeletal muscle sarcoplasmic reticulum in the hypothyroid rat. *J Clin Invest*. 1968;47:2499-2506.

86. Reinfrank RF, Kaufman RP, Wetstone HJ, Glennon JA. Observations of the Achilles reflex test. *JAMA*. 1967;199:59-62.

87. Barker DJ, Bishop JM. Computer-based screening system for patients at risk of hypothyroidism. *Lancet*. 1969;2:835-838.

88. Cassidy CE, Eddy RL. Hypothyroidism in patients with goiter. *Metabolism*. 1970;19:751-759.

89. Lloyd WH. Value of the voice in diagnosis of myxoedema in the elderly. *Br Med J*. 1959;1:1208-1211.

90. Maragos NE. Vocal abnormalities: What listening can tell you. *Postgrad Med*. 1984;76:25-34.

91. Wolf S. Hypothyroidism (letter). *J Fam Pract*. 1993;37:225.

92. Asher R. Myxoedematous madness. *Br Med J*. 1949;2:555-562.

93. Bicknell PG. Mild hypothyroidism and its effects on the larynx. *J Laryngol Otol*. 1973;87:123-127.

94. Plummer WA. Body weight and spontaneous myxedema. *West J Surg*. 1942;50:85-92.

95. Nordyke RA, Kulikowski CA, Kulikowski CW. A comparison of methods for the automated diagnosis of thyroid dysfunction. *Comput Biomed Res*. 1971;4: 374-389.

96. Indra R, Patil SS, Joshi R, et al. Accuracy of physical examination in the diagnosis of hypothyroidism: A cross-sectional, double-blind study. *J Postgrad Med*. 2004;50:7-11.

97. Billewicz WZ, Chapman RS, Crooks J, et al. Statistical methods applied to the diagnosis of hypothyroidism. *Q J Med*. 1969;38:255-266.

98. Seshadri MS, Samuel BU, Kanagasabapathy AS, Cherian AM. Clinical scoring system for hypothyroidism: Is it useful? *J Gen Intern Med*. 1989;4: 490-492.

99. Sisson JC. Principles of, and pitfalls in, thyroid function tests. *J Nuc Med*. 1965;6:853-901.

100. Doucet J, Trivalle C, Chassagne P, et al. Does age play a role in clinical presentation of hypothyroidism? *J Am Geriatr Soc*. 1994;42:984-986.

101. Franklyn JA. The management of hyperthyroidism. *N Engl J Med*. 1994;330: 1731-1738.

102. Major RH. *Classic descriptions of disease: With biographical sketches of the authors.* Springfield: Charles C. Thomas; 1932.

103. Hegedus L, Hansen JM, Karstrup S. High incidence of normal thyroid gland volume in patients with Graves' disease. *Clin Endocrinol*. 1983;19:603-607.

104. Hegedus L, Hansen JEM, Veiergang D, Karstrup S. Thyroid size and goitre frequency in hyperthyroidism. *Dan Med Bull*. 1987;34:121-123.

105. Nordyke RA, Gilbert FI, Harada ASM. Graves' disease: Influence of age on clinical findings. *Arch Intern Med*. 1988;148:626-631.

106. Chapdelain A, Coulombe R, LeLorier J. The effects of propranolol, practolol, and placebo on the clinical manifestations of thyrotoxicosis. *Int J Clin Pharm*. 1976;14: 308-312.

107. Davis PJ, Davis FB. Hyperthyroidism in patients over the age of 60 years: Clinical features in 85 patients. *Medicine*. 1974;53:161-181.

108. Healy JF, Brault T. Enlargement of the superior thyroid artery: An unusual cause for a cervical bruit. *Angiology*. 1984;35:579-580.

109. Cooper WW. On protrusion of the eyes, in connexion with anaemia, palpitation, and goitre. *Lancet*. 1849;1:551-554.

110. Ruedemann AD. Ocular changes associated with hyperthyroidism. In: Crile G, ed. *Diagnosis and treatment of diseases of the thyroid gland*. Philadelphia: W.B. Saunders; 1932:196-208.

111. Miller NR. *Walsh and Hoyt's clinical neuro-ophthalmology*, Vol 2, 4th ed. Baltimore: Williams and Wilkins; 1985:945-957.

112. Duke-Elder S. Lid-retraction. In: Duke-Elder S, ed. *System of ophthalmology: Neuro-ophthalmology*, Vol 12. London: Henry Kimpton; 1971:905-915.

113. Gladstone GJ. Ophthalmologic aspects of thyroid-related orbitopathy. *Endocrinol Metab Clin North Am*. 1998;27:91-100.

114. Murchison L, Bewsher PD, Chesters MI, Ferrier WR. Comparison of propanolol and practolol in the management of hyperthyroidism. *Br J Clin Pharm*. 1976;3: 273-277.

115. Hall R, Storey E, Farmer FT. Ophthalmic Graves' disease: Clinical and laboratory features. *Proc Soc Med*. 1968;61:1305-1306.

116. Bartley GB, Fatourechi V, Kadrmas EF, et al. Clinical features of Graves' ophthalmopathy in an incidence cohort. *Am J Ophthalmol*. 1996;121:284-290.

117. Feldon SE, Levin L. Graves' ophthalmopathy: V. Aetiology of upper eyelid retraction in Graves' ophthalmopathy. *Br J Ophthalmol*. 1990;74:484-485.

118. Hallin ES, Feldon SE. Graves' ophthalmopathy: II. Correlation of clinical signs with measures derived from computed tomography. *Br J Ophthalmol*. 1988;72:678-682.

119. Bartley GB. The differential diagnosis and classification of eyelid retraction. *Ophthalmology*. 1996;103:168-176.

120. Lepore FE. Unilateral ptosis and Hering's law. *Neurology*. 1988;38:319-322.

121. Schmidtke K, Buettner-Ennever JA. Nervous control of eyelid function: A review of clinical, experimental and pathological data. *Brain.* 1992;115:227-247.

122. Bahn RS, Heufelder AE. Pathogenesis of Graves' ophthalmopathy. *N Engl J Med.* 1993;329:1468-1475.

123. Grove AS. Evaluation of exophthalmos. *N Engl J Med.* 1974;292:1005-1013.

124. Feldon SE, Muramatsu S, Weiner JM. Clinical classification of Graves' ophthalmopathy: Identification of risk factors for optic neuropathy. *Arch Ophthalmol.* 1984;102:1469-1472.

125. Shanks RG, Lowe DC, Hadden DR, et al. Controlled trial of propranolol in thyrotoxicosis. *Lancet.* 1969;1:993-994.

126. Woeber KA. Thyrotoxicosis and the heart. *N Engl J Med.* 1992;327:94-98.

127. van Olshausen K, Bischoff S, Kahaly G, et al. Cardiac arrhythmias and heart rate in hyperthyroidism. *Am J Cardiol.* 1989;63:930-933.

128. Forfar JC, Muir AL, Sawers SA, Toft AD. Abnormal left ventricular function in hyperthyroidism: Evidence for a possible reversible cardiomyopathy. *N Engl J Med.* 1982;307:1165-1170.

129. Lerman J, Means JH. Cardiovascular symptomatology in exophthalmic goiter. *Am Heart J.* 1932;8:55-65.

130. Fatourechi V, Pajouhi M, Fransway AF. Dermopathy of Graves' disease (pretibial myxedema). *Medicine.* 1994;73:1-7.

131. Engel AG. Neuromuscular manifestations of Graves' disease. *Mayo Clin Proc.* 1972;47:919-925.

132. Williams RH. Thiouracil treatment of thyrotoxicosis: I. The results of prolonged treatment. *J Clin Endocrinol.* 1946;6:1-22.

133. Martin WH, Spina RJ, Korte E, et al. Mechanism of impaired exercise capacity in short duration experimental hyperthyroidism. *J Clin Invest.* 1991;88:2047-2053.

134. Crooks J, Murray IPC, Wayne EJ. Statistical methods applied to the clinical diagnosis of thyrotoxicosis. *Q J Med.* 1959;28:211-234.

135. Gurney C, Owen SG, Hall R, et al. Newcastle thyrotoxicosis index. *Lancet.* 1970;2:1275-1278.

136. Harvey RF. Indices of thyroid function in thyrotoxicosis. *Lancet.* 1971;2:230-233.

137. Klein I, Trzepacz PT, Roberts M, Levey GS. Symptom rating scale for assessing hyperthyroidism. *Arch Intern Med.* 1988;148:387-390.

138. Trzepacz PT, Klein I, Roberts M, et al. Graves' disease: An analysis of thyroid hormone levels and hyperthyroid signs and symptoms. *Am J Med.* 1989;87:558-561.

139. Trivalle C, Doucet J. Differences in the signs and symptoms of hyperthyroidism in older and younger patients. *J Am Geriatr Soc.* 1996;44:50-53.

140. Martin FIR, Deam DR. Hyperthyroidism in elderly hospitalised patients: Clinical features and treatment outcomes. *Med J Austral.* 1996;164:200-203.

141. Tibaldi JM, Barzel US, Albin J, Surks M. Thyrotoxicosis in the very old. *Am J Med.* 1986;81:619-622.

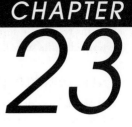

Meninges

I. THE FINDINGS

The terms "meningeal signs" and "meningismus" refer to the physical findings that develop after meningeal irritation from inflammation, tumor, or hemorrhage. Those most widely known are neck stiffness (or "nuchal rigidity"), Kernig's sign, and Brudzinski's sign.

A. NECK STIFFNESS

Neck stiffness denotes involuntary resistance to neck flexion, which the clinician perceives when trying to bend the patient's neck, bringing the chin down to the chest. Occasionally, the aggravated extensor tone of the neck and spine is so severe that the patient's entire spine is hyperextended, leaving the torso of the supine patient supported only by occiput and heels. This extreme posture is called "opisthotonus."

B. KERNIG'S SIGN (DESCRIBED BY VLADIMIR KERNIG IN 1882)

With the patient's hip and knee flexed, Kernig's sign is positive when the patient resists extension of the knee. Kernig called this a "contracture" of the hamstrings that prevented extension of the knee beyond an angle of 135 degrees, even though he found the knee extended perfectly fully if the hip was first positioned in the fully extended position (Fig. 23-1).[1] Most clinicians perform this test in the supine patient, although Kernig described the test being performed in the seated patient.

C. BRUDZINSKI'S SIGN

Jozef Brudzinski described several meningeal signs between 1909 and 1916. In his most popular sign, flexion of the supine patient's neck causes the patient to flex both hips and knees, thus retracting the legs toward the chest (see Fig. 23-1).[1]

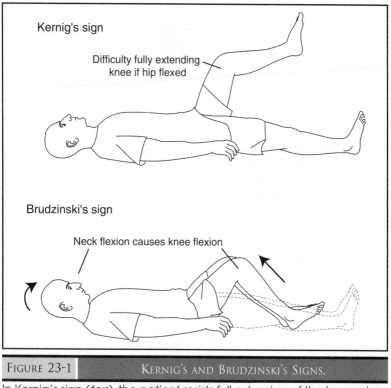

FIGURE 23-1	KERNIG'S AND BRUDZINSKI'S SIGNS.

In Kernig's sign (*top*), the patient resists full extension of the knee when the knee and hip are first flexed (patient's left leg), although the knee extends normally if the hip is extended (patient's right leg). In Brudzinski's sign (*bottom*), flexion of the patient's neck causes the hips and knees to flex, pulling both legs up toward the chest. See text.

II. PATHOGENESIS OF MENINGEAL SIGNS

The basis for all meningeal signs is the patient's natural rejection of any move-ment that stretches spinal nerves, all of which pass through the irritated sub-arachnoid space. Experiments with cadavers show that flexion of the neck pulls the spinal cord toward the head, thus stretching spinal nerves, whereas flexion of the hips with knees extended pulls on the sciatic nerve, thus displacing the conus of the spinal cord downward toward the sacrum.[2] Flexion of the hips with knees flexed, in contrast, does not stretch the sciatic nerve.

These experiments explain why patients with meningeal irritation have neck stiffness and a positive Kernig's sign, and also show that Kernig's sign does not differ from the straight-leg raising test for sciatica (see Chapter 60). Brudzinski's sign, however, is more difficult to understand. At first, it seems logical that patients with meningeal irritation would want to extend their hips and flex their knees when their neck is flexed (i.e., the position opposite Kernig's sign). Although this position removes tension from the sciatic nerve, it stretches the femoral nerve,[2] explaining why Brudzinski's test causes the patient to flex both hips and knees, thus relieving tension on both nerves.

III. CLINICAL SIGNIFICANCE

A. ACUTE BACTERIAL MENINGITIS

Table 23-1 summarizes the frequency of individual findings of 1100 adults with acute bacterial meningitis (the major organisms in these studies were *Streptococcus pneumoniae*, *Neisseria meningitidis*, and *Listeria monocytogenes*; cases of tuberculosis were excluded). This table reveals that the most frequent findings in bacterial meningitis are neck stiffness, fever, and altered mental sta-tus. Neck stiffness is a more frequent sign than Kernig's or Brudzinski's sign (sensitivity is 84% for neck stiffness vs. 61% for Kernig/Brudzinski's signs), although this difference is not significant and may reflect in part the clinician's diligence in looking for these findings. Seventy-three percent to 92% percent of patients with petechial rash have infection with *N. meningiditis*.[7,11]

Some of the heterogeneity in these studies (see Table 23-1) is due to the ages of the patients. Compared with younger patients, elderly patients (defined as >65 years old for three of four studies, >50 years for one study) have a higher frequency of mental status change (90% vs. 72%), focal neurologic signs (30% vs. 17%), and fever (94% vs. 84%) but no difference in the frequency of neck stiffness.[4,8–10]

Few studies have addressed the overall accuracy of meningeal signs. In one study of 297 patients undergoing lumbar puncture because of suspected meningitis,[15]

| Table 23-1 | Acute Bacterial Meningitis and Subarachnoid Hemorrhage* |

Finding	Frequency (%)†
Acute Bacterial Meningitis	
Neck stiffness	57–92
Fever	66–100
Altered mental status	53–96
Kernig's or Brudzinski's sign	61
Focal neurologic signs	9–37
Seizures	5–23
Petechial rash	3–52
Subarachnoid Hemorrhage	
Neck stiffness	21–86
Seizures	32
Altered mental status	29
Focal neurologic findings	13–36
Fever	8
Preretinal hemorrhages	2

*Data obtained from 1100 patients with meningitis from references 3–11 and 583 patients with subarachnoid hemorrhage from references 12–14.
Diagnostic standard: For meningitis, cerebrospinal fluid pleocytosis and appropriate microbiologic data or postmortem examination; for subarachnoid hemorrhage, computed tomography or lumbar puncture.
†Results are overall mean frequency or, if statistically heterogeneous, the range of values.

the finding of nuchal rigidity detected meningitis [i.e., cerebrospinal fluid (CSF) pleocytosis ≥1000 white blood cells (WBCs)/mL] with a sensitivity of 90%, specificity of 70%, and positive likelihood ratio (LR) of 3.0.[15] Kernig's and Brudzinski's signs were rarely observed in this study. Other studies have addressed just the specificity of meningeal signs: In one such study, nuchal rigidity was found in 35% of hospitalized elderly patients (mean age 79 years), none of whom had meningitis, (i.e., specificity 65%).[16] Also, Kernig's sign may appear in patients with sciatica and those with subarachnoid or epidural hemorrhage or tumor of the cauda equina.[17]

B. SUBARACHNOID HEMORRHAGE

Table 23-1 summarizes the findings of more than 500 patients with subarachnoid hemorrhage, 80% of whom presented with a severe precipitous headache. The most common physical finding in these patients was neck stiffness (sensitivity 21%–86%). Only 29% had altered mental status.

Box 23-1　Subarachnoid Hemorrhage*

Finding	Sensitivity (%)	Specificity (%)	Likelihood Ratio if Finding	
			Present	Absent
Neck stiffness	59	94	**10.3**	0.4
Neurologic findings not focal	64	89	**5.9**	0.4
Age ≤60 years	86	52	1.8	**0.3**
Seizures	32	86	2.2	NS

NS, not significant; likelihood ratio (LR) if finding present = positive LR; LR if finding absent = negative LR.
*Diagnostic standard: For subarachnoid hemorrhage, computed tomography or lumbar puncture.[14]

SUBARACHNOID HEMORRHAGE (IF SUDDEN NEUROLOGIC IMPAIRMENT)

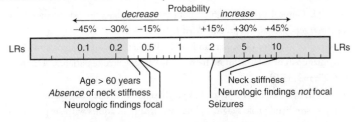

In another study of 197 patients admitted to the hospital within 24 hours of a sudden global or focal neurologic impairment (EBM Box 23-1), two findings argued strongly *for* subarachnoid hemorrhage and *against* cerebral infarction or intracranial hemorrhage: neck stiffness (LR = 10.3) and the absence of focal neurologic findings (LR = 5.9).[14]

REFERENCES

1. Verghese A, Gallemore G. Kernig's and Brudzinski's signs revisited. *Rev Inf Dis.* 1987;9:1187-1192.
2. O'Connell JEA. The clinical signs of meningeal irritation. *Brain.* 1946;69:9-21.
3. Sigurdardottir B, Bjornsson OM, Jonsdottir KE, et al. Acute bacterial meningitis in adults: A 20-year overview. *Arch Intern Med.* 1997;157:425-430.

4. Gorse GJ, Thrupp LD, Nudleman KL, et al. Bacterial meningitis in the elderly. *Arch Intern Med.* 1984;144:1603-1607.

5. Aronin SI, Peduzzi P, Quagliarello VJ. Community-acquired bacterial meningitis: Risk stratification for adverse clinical outcome and effect of antibiotic timing. *Ann Intern Med.* 1998;129:862-869.

6. Hosoglu S, Ayaz C, Geyik MF, et al. Acute bacterial meningitis in adults: Analysis of 218 episodes. *Ir J Med Sci.* 1997;166:231-234.

7. Durand ML, Calderwood SB, Weber DJ, et al. Acute bacterial meningitis in adults: A review of 493 episodes. *N Engl J Med.* 1993;328:21-28.

8. Behrman RE, Meyers BR, Mendelson MH, et al. Central nervous system infections in the elderly. *Arch Intern Med.* 1989;149:1596-1599.

9. Domingo P, Mancebo J, Blanch L, et al. Acute bacterial meningitis in the elderly. *Arch Intern Med.* 1990;150:1546-1548.

10. Massanari RM. Purulent meningitis in the elderly: When to suspect an unusual pathogen. *Geriatrics.* 1977;32(3):55-59.

11. van den Beek D, Gans JD, Spanjaard L, et al. Clinical features and prognostic factors in adults with bacterial meningitis. *N Engl J Med.* 2004;351:1849-1859.

12. Sengupta RP, McAllister VL. *Subarachnoid haemorrhage.* Berlin: Springer-Verlag; 1986.

13. Seet CM. Clinical presentation of patients with subarachnoid haemorrhage at a local emergency department. *Sing Med J.* 1999;40:383-385.

14. Talavera JO, Wacher NH, Laredo F, et al. Predictive value of signs and symptoms in the diagnosis of subarachnoid hemorrhage among stroke patients. *Arch Med Res.* 1996;27:353-357.

15. Thomas KE, Hasbun R, Jekel J, Quagliarello VJ. The diagnostic accuracy of Kernig's sign, Brudzinski's sign, and nuchal rigidity in adults with suspected meningitis. *Clin Infect Dis.* 2002;35:46-52.

16. Puxty JAH, Fox RA, Horan MA. The frequency of physical signs usually attributed to meningeal irritation in elderly patients. *J Am Geriatr Soc.* 1983;31:590-592.

17. Wartenberg R. The signs of Brudzinski and of Kernig. *J Pediatr.* 1950;37:679-684.

24

Peripheral Lymphadenopathy

I. INTRODUCTION

Lymphatic vessels are located in all tissues and organs of the body except the central nervous system. These vessels collect extracellular tissue fluid (or lymph) and carry it to the systemic venous system, traversing along the way regional collections of bean-shaped structures called lymph nodes. As these lymph nodes slowly filter the lymph fluid, they may encounter microbes, malignant cells, particulate debris, or other substances to which they react, enlarge, and harden. Should such nodes enlarge or harden enough, they may become palpable, a problem called peripheral lymphadenopathy.

Ancient Greek and Roman physicians recognized peripheral lymphadenopathy as an important sign of tuberculosis (scrofula),[1,2] and for more than a century clinicians have known that lymphadenopathy may signify serious disorders such as carcinoma, lymphoma, leukemia, and certain infectious diseases (tuberculosis, syphilis, and plague, among others).[3] How often adenopathy reflects one of these serious disorders in current practice depends on the clinical setting. In family practice clinics, peripheral lymphadenopathy is benign 99% of the time, sometimes reflecting known disorders (e.g., pharyngitis, dermatitis, or insect bites) but more often appearing and resolving without explanation.[4,5] In specialized lymph node clinics, however, 18% to 24% of referred patients are eventually diagnosed with malignancy (i.e., lymphoma or metastatic cancer) and up to 5% have a treatable infectious or granulomatous disorder [e.g., tuberculosis, human immunodeficiency virus (HIV) infection, sarcoidosis].[6-8] This chapter focuses on those physical findings that help discriminate serious causes of lymphadenopathy from more benign causes.

II. ANATOMY AND PATHOGENESIS

A. INTRODUCTION

The lymphatic drainage of the body is subdivided into seven distinct regions, all of which converge and drain into the great veins near the base of the neck (Fig. 24-1). A normal adult has approximately 400 to 450 lymph nodes, although only about a quarter are in locations that could ever become palpable: 30 in the arm and axilla, 20 in the leg, and 60 to 70 in the head and neck (the remaining lymph nodes reside deep in the thorax and abdomen and are detectable only by clinical imaging).[9] Anatomists divide lymph nodes into "superficial" and "deep" nodes, based on whether they accompany superficial or deep blood vessels. Superficial nodes lie just under the surface of the skin, accompany superficial veins, and often are visible when enlarged. Most palpable nodes are superficial nodes. The only deep nodes detectable by bedside examination are the deep cervical nodes (which accompany the carotid artery and internal jugular vein under the sternocleidomastoid muscle) and the axillary nodes (which surround the axillary vessels).

The fact that lymph nodes accompany blood vessels is helpful when searching for two nodal groups: (1) the epitrochlear nodes, which lie near the basilic vein, and (2) the vertical group of inguinal nodes, which surround the proximal saphenous vein (Fig. 24-2).

B. REGIONAL LYMPH NODE GROUPS

Maps of regional lymphatic drainage are based on older experiments in living humans and cadavers, in which injections of mercury, Prussian blue, radiocontrast materials, or other dyes were used to highlight normal lymph channels and regional nodes (lymph vessels are otherwise difficult to distinguish from small veins during dissection).[9-12] These maps of lymph drainage are helpful because they allow clinicians to predict the spread of local infections or neoplasms and, when faced with isolated adenopathy, to focus the diagnostic search to a particular region. Nonetheless, clinical experience demonstrates that disease does not always spread in an orderly way through these channels and nodes. For example, infections and malignancy may occasionally skip one

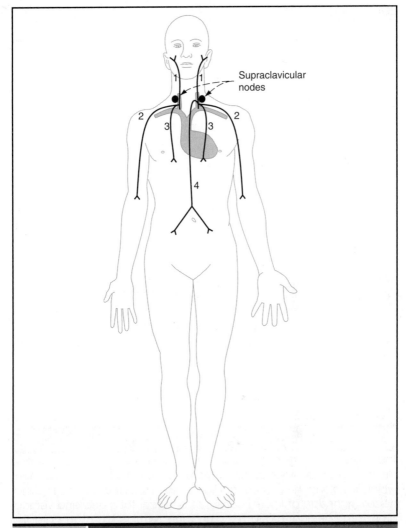

| FIGURE 24-1 | THE SEVEN REGIONS OF LYMPHATIC DRAINAGE. |

All lymphatic drainage of the body converges on the right and left junctions of the internal jugular and subclavian veins (shaded gray, along with the superior vena cava and heart). The great veins on the right side of the neck receive drainage from: the right head and neck (region 1, traversing cervical nodes); the right arm, chest wall, and breast (region 2, traversing axillary nodes); and the right lung and mediastinal structures (region 3, via mediastinal and tracheobronchial nodes but no peripheral nodes). The left great veins receive drainage from similar regions of the left upper body (regions 1–3) and, via the thoracic duct, drainage from all tissues below the diaphragm (region 4). Only the supraclavicular nodes are depicted, illustrating their strategic proximity to the confluence of these seven major lymph channels.

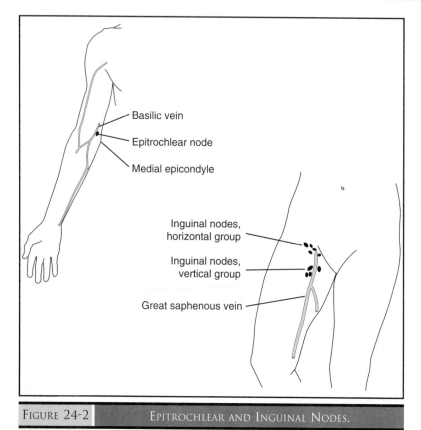

| FIGURE 24-2 | EPITROCHLEAR AND INGUINAL NODES. |

The epitrochlear nodes (left side of figure) are located 2–3 cm above the medial epicondyle of the humerus, just medial to the basilic vein, which lies along the groove medial to the biceps muscle. The inguinal nodes (right side of figure) consist of a horizontal group and vertical group: The vertical group lies along the termination of the greater saphenous vein.

regional node group to travel to another (e.g., an infection of the ring finger may involve the axillary nodes and skip the epitrochlear nodes), and malignancy may sometimes travel in a retrograde direction between nodal groups (e.g., supraclavicular adenopathy, see "Supraclavicular Nodes").[11] Also, despite the implication of these maps, isolated adenopathy does not necessarily reflect focal disease but instead may represent the sole sign of a generalized disorder (e.g., tuberculosis or lymphoma).[13,14]

1. Cervical Nodes

All structures of the head and neck drain into the deep cervical nodes, either directly or via intermediary superficial nodes (Fig. 24-3). The skin of the face and neck drains into the superficial nodes in a predictable fashion (see Fig. 24-3). The pharynx, nasal cavity, and sinuses usually drain to the upper deep cervical nodes; the mouth and teeth to the submandibular nodes and eventually the upper cervical nodes; and the larynx to both upper and lower cervical nodes.

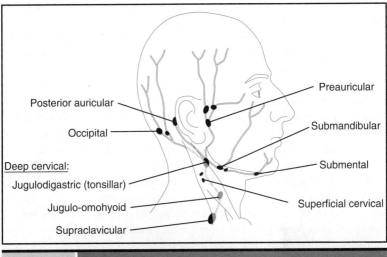

FIGURE 24-3   CERVICAL LYMPH NODES.

Superficial cervical nodes are named according to regional anatomy: occipital nodes, posterior auricular (or "mastoid") nodes, preauricular (or "parotid" nodes), submandibular nodes, submental nodes, and superficial cervical nodes. Deep cervical nodes lie along the carotid sheath and are mostly buried under the sternocleido-mastoid muscle, although the uppermost nodes appear in front of this muscle and the lowermost posterior to it. Three deep cervical nodes have specific names because of their size and clinical importance: (1) The jugulodigastric node, an upper deep cervical node at the level of the hyoid bone that becomes tender and prominent in patients with pharyngitis (i.e., the "tonsillar" node). (2) The jugulo-omohyoid node, a lower deep cervical node located where the omohyoid muscle crosses the jugular vein. This node drains the tongue and may become enlarged in patients with tongue carcinoma. (3) The supraclavicular nodes, which are the lowermost deep cervical nodes and are considered separately in the section titled "Supraclavicular Nodes."

The tongue has the most diverse drainage: efferents travel to the submental, submandibular, and upper deep cervical and lower deep cervical nodes, and disease near the midline may travel to either side.[9,11,15,16]

2. Supraclavicular Nodes

Although supraclavicular nodes actually belong to the deep cervical nodes, they are considered separately because of their strategic location in the base of the neck, close to where all lymph drainage returns to the systemic venous system (see Fig. 24-1). Because of this location, supraclavicular adenopathy may signify serious disease located in the thoracic or abdominal cavities, regions where nodes are otherwise hidden from the examiner. The anatomy depicted in Fig. 24-1 predicts that right supraclavicular adenopathy would be associated with disorders of the right thorax, arm, and neck and that the left supraclavicular adenopathy would be associated with disorders of the left thorax, arm, neck, and also the abdomen and pelvis.

Normally, lymph flows from supraclavicular nodes downward toward the confluence of lymph channels and great veins (see Fig. 24-1). Therefore, in order for intra-abdominal or intrathoracic disorders to involve the supraclavicular nodes, disease must spread in a *retrograde* direction from the thoracic duct or bronchomediastinal lymphatic vessels through the cervical efferents leaving the supraclavicular nodes. Such retrograde spread easily occurs and does not imply obstruction of lymphatic channels. In one investigation of 92 patients undergoing lymphangiography of the lower limbs, radiopaque material appeared in the supraclavicular nodes within 48 hours in 55% of the patients.[17] As expected, the dye opacified exclusively the left supraclavicular nodes in 48 of 51 patients, but it opacified both right and left supraclavicular nodes in 2 patients and exclusively the right supraclavicular nodes in 1 patient, indicating normal anatomic variation in the connections between the thoracic duct and supraclavicular nodes.[17]

Supraclavicular adenopathy appears just behind the clavicle, underneath or posterior to the sternocleidomastoid muscle. A Valsalva maneuver may make these nodes more prominent, by pushing the apical pleural surface upward against the nodes and bringing them into view.[18] In 1848, Virchow first observed the association between abdominal malignancies and metastases to supraclavicular nodes.[17,19,20] Unaware of Virchow's description, the French clinician and pathologist Trosier described the same association in 1886, emphasizing the predisposition to the left side.[17,19,20] Left supraclavicular adenopathy has been therefore called "Virchow's nodes," "Trosier's nodes," "Virchow-Trosier nodes," "sentinel nodes," or "signal nodes."

3. Epitrochlear Nodes ("Supratrochlear" or "Cubital" Nodes, see Fig. 24-2)

These superficial nodes, located on the anteromedial arm 2 to 3 cm above the medial epicondyle of the humerus, drain the ulnar side of the forearm and hand (i.e., little and ring fingers) and send efferents to the axillary nodes. A common method for palpating these nodes is for the clinician to face the patient and reach across to shake the patient's hand on the side to be examined. The examiner then places his or her free hand behind the patient's arm, just proximal to the elbow, and uses the fingertips to palpate these nodes above and anterior to the medial epicondyle.

Although epitrochlear adenopathy may indicate infection or malignancy on the ulnar side of the forearm or hand, these nodes have historically been associated with conditions causing generalized lymphadenopathy, especially when they are enlarged bilaterally (see "Epitrochlear Adenopathy"). One hundred years ago, epitrochlear adenopathy was felt to be a compelling sign of secondary syphilis, occurring in 25% to 93% of cases.[21-23] Modern examples of this specific association, however, are scarce.

4. Axillary Nodes

Axillary nodes drain the ipsilateral arm, breast, and chest wall (Fig. 24-4). To examine these nodes, the clinician should ensure that the patient's axillary skin is relaxed, by first supporting and adducting the patient's arm. Nodes are

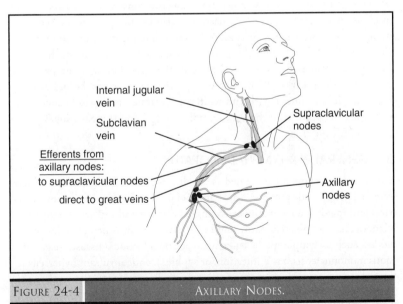

FIGURE 24-4	AXILLARY NODES.

The axillary nodes receive lymphatic drainage from the ipsilateral arm, breast, and chest wall. Efferent vessels travel to the great veins at the root of the neck, although a few vessels travel first through the supraclavicular nodal group.

located in the posterior, anterior, or medial walls of the axillary fossa or in its apex. Efferent lymph vessels travel directly to the systemic veins at the root of the neck, although a few efferents pass first through the ipsilateral supraclavicular nodes (see Fig. 24-4).[9,11]

5. Inguinal Nodes

Inguinal nodes are superficial nodes that are organized into two groups: a proximal or "horizontal" group located just below the inguinal ligament, which drains the external genitalia, perineum, and lower anterior abdominal, and a distal or "vertical" group located at the termination of the great saphenous vein, which drains the leg (see Fig. 24-2).[9]

III. THE FINDING

A. DESCRIBING ADENOPATHY

The important features to observe when describing adenopathy are the lymph node's location, size, number, hardness, and tenderness. "Fixed" nodes are immobile from attachments to adjacent structures, implying malignant invasion of these tissues. A "hard" node has the consistency of a rock, again implying malignant disease (the hardness presumably reflects the accompanying fibrosis induced by the tumor). "Shotty" adenopathy indicates multiple tiny superficial nodes, mimicking the sensation of buckshot under the skin, a finding sometimes observed in the inguinal region but without particular diagnostic significance.[24] The size of a particular node can be indicated by recording its maximal length and width or, as some investigators suggest, by recording the product of these two numbers (e.g., a node measuring 2.5 cm × 3 cm is "7.5 cm²").

B. GENERALIZED LYMPHADENOPATHY

Generalized adenopathy is defined as simultaneous enlargement of two or more regional lymph node groups.[25] Most affected patients have either combined cervical and inguinal adenopathy or combined cervical and axillary adenopathy.[26] Generalized lymphadenopathy implies a systemic disorder affecting lymph nodes, such as lymphoma or leukemia, specific infectious diseases (e.g., infectious mononucleosis, HIV infection, or syphilis), anticonvulsant hypersensitivity syndrome, sarcoidosis, or connective tissue disorders.[25,27–30]

C. "GLANDULAR" SYNDROMES

The term "glandular" refers to lymph nodes (e.g., "glandular fever" was the original name for infectious mononucleosis). Therefore, the "ulceroglandular" syndrome is the triad of fever, ulceration on the distal arm or leg (indicating the portal of entry of infectious agent), and regional adenopathy. The "oculoglandular" syndrome ("Parinaud's syndrome"*) describes the association of conjunctivitis with ipsilateral preauricular and submandibular adenopathy. Both ulceroglandular and oculoglandular syndromes have been associated with specific microbial agents (see "Ulceroglandular and Oculoglandular Syndromes").

Chapter 22 reviews the "Delphian node" and Chapter 46 discusses the "Sister Mary Joseph nodule."

IV. CLINICAL SIGNIFICANCE

A. DEFINITION OF DISEASE

EBM Box 24-1 reviews the diagnostic accuracy of physical examination in distinguishing serious causes of adenopathy from more benign disorders. All of the patients in these studies were referred to specialists because of persistent unexplained peripheral lymphadenopathy. Most patients (35%–83%) presented with cervical adenopathy, 1% to 29% with supraclavicular adenopathy, 4% to 24% with axillary adenopathy, 3% to 16% with inguinal adenopathy, and 16% to 32% with generalized adenopathy.[4,6,8,26,32,36,37]

The etiology of lymphadenopathy in these studies was determined either by fine needle or excisional biopsy or, in a few low-risk patients who did not undergo biopsy, prolonged periods of observation.[7,8] Some of these studies defined a "serious disorder" (or "disease") as any disorder in which the biopsy results would imply specific treatment or prognosis. These studies therefore included both malignancy and granulomatous disease (e.g., tuberculosis or sarcoidosis) as disease.[6,7,34–36,39,40] Other studies confined disease to the diagnosis of malignancy alone.[8,32,33,37,38] Both definitions of disease are combined in EBM Box 24-1, because analyzing the definitions separately revealed the same diagnostic accuracy, and because the overwhelming majority of patients in all studies had a malignant cause for their disease.

B. EXTRANODAL MIMICS OF LYMPH NODES

Up to 15% of patients referred for unexplained lymphadenopathy instead have extranodal explanations for their subcutaneous lumps.[8] Common mimics of lymphadenopathy at all locations are skin nodules such as lipomas[41] or epidermoid cysts. In the cervical region, thyroglossal cysts, branchial cleft cysts, and

---

*Henri Parinaud, one of the world's first neuro-ophthalmologists, was recruited to Paris by Charcot in the late 1800s. He also described the pupillary and eye movement abnormalities of the pretectal syndrome (see Chapter 19).[31]

Box 24-1 Lymphadenopathy*

Finding (Ref)[†]	Sensitivity (%)	Specificity (%)	Likelihood Ratio if Finding Present	Absent
General				
Male sex[6,7,32–34]	44–59	49–72	1.3	0.8
Age ≥40 years[6,7,32,33,35,36]	48–91	53–87	2.4	0.4
Weight loss[6,7,33,37]	19–28	90–95	**3.4**	0.8
Fever[6,7,34,37]	1–31	60–80	NS	NS
Distribution of Adenopathy				
Head and neck nodes (excluding supraclavicular nodes)[6–8,32–34,36–38]	21–79	15–69	NS	NS
Supraclavicular nodes[6–8,33,36,38]	8–61	84–98	**3.2**	0.8
Axillary nodes[6–8,32–34,36–38]	8–52	30–91	0.8	NS
Inguinal nodes[6–8,32–34,36–38]	3–22	61–96	0.6	NS
Epitrochlear nodes[34]	2	97	NS	NS
Generalized lymphadenopathy[8,32,39]	32–48	31–87	NS	NS
Characteristics of Adenopathy				
Lymph node size[6,7]				
<4 cm²	33–36	9–37	0.4	...
4–8.99 cm²	26–30	...	NS	...
≥9 cm²	37–38	91–98	**8.4**	...
Hard texture[6,7]	48–62	83–84	**3.2**	0.6
Lymph node tenderness[6,7,34,37]	3–18	50–86	0.4	1.3
Fixed lymph nodes[6,37]	12–52	97	**10.9**	NS
Other Findings				
Rash[7,34]	4–8	85–95	NS	NS
Palpable spleen[6,7,34]	5–10	92–96	NS	NS
Palpable liver[7,34]	14–16	86–89	NS	NS
Lymph Node Score[6,7]				
−3 or less	1–3	42–72	**0.04**	...
−2 or −1	1–3	...	**0.1**	...
0 to 4	23	...	NS	...
5 or 6	17–26	...	**5.1**	...
7 or more	49–56	94–99	**21.9**	...

NS, not significant; likelihood ratio (LR) if finding present = positive LR; LR if finding absent = negative LR.

*Diagnostic standard: see text.

[†]Definition of findings: see text.

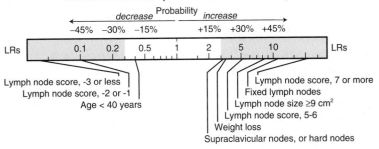

SERIOUS DISEASE (IF LYMPHADENOPATHY)

prominent carotid sinuses may be mistaken for nodes[42] (see Chapter 22). In the supraclavicular region, synovial cysts from rheumatoid arthritis of the shoulder,[43] cervical ribs, and abnormal articulations of the first rib[44,45] have all been mistaken for nodes.

C. INDIVIDUAL FINDINGS

In these studies, the symptom of generalized pruritus argued for a serious cause, probably because of its association with lymphoma [sensitivity 6%–10%, specificity 98%–100%, likelihood ratios (LR) = 4.9].[6,7] According to the LRs in EBM Box 24-1, several physical findings also argue for serious disease: fixed lymph nodes (LR = 10.9), size ≥9 cm^2 (i.e., the equivalent of 3 × 3 cm or larger, LR = 8.4), weight loss (LR = 3.4), hard texture (LR = 3.2), supraclavicular adenopathy (LR = 3.2), and age ≥40 years (LR = 2.4).

Only three findings argue against serious disease, all of them reducing probability only modestly: age younger than 40 years (LR = 0.4), lymph node size less than 4 cm^2 (i.e., 2 × 2 cm or smaller, LR = 0.4), and lymph node tenderness (LR = 0.4). Tenderness may be less specific for benign disorders than expected because hemorrhage or necrosis into neoplastic nodes also causes discomfort mimicking acute inflammatory changes. The symptom of throat soreness also argues against serious disease (sensitivity 3%–14%, specificity 23%–89%, LR = 0.2).[6,7,40]

Findings that are unhelpful in distinguishing serious from benign disease include rash, regional distribution of nodes (other than supraclavicular location), fever, a palpable spleen, and a palpable liver (all LRs either not significant or very close to the value of 1.0).

The finding of generalized adenopathy, defined as involvement of two or more regional node groups, also lacks diagnostic value (LR not significant). Even when generalized lymphadenopathy is defined as involvement of four or more regional lymph node groups, it fails to discriminate serious from benign causes (LR not significant),[39] probably because this finding appears just as often in benign disorders (e.g., infectious mononucleosis) as in serious disorders (e.g., lymphoma).

D. COMBINED FINDINGS

Based on evaluation of more than 300 patients, Vassilakopoulos and Pangalis[7] have identified six independent predictors of serious disease, creating a "lymph node score" that can easily be calculated at the bedside (Table 24-1). According to this scoring scheme, a score of −3 or less virtually excludes serious disease (LR = 0.04, EBM Box 24-1), one of −2 or −1 argues *against* a serious cause (LR = 0.1), one of 5 or 6 argues *for* a serious disorder (LR = 5.1), and one of 7 or more is practically diagnostic *for* serious disease (LR = 21.9). Scores of 0 to 4 lack diagnostic significance.

E. LYMPH NODE SYNDROMES
1. Supraclavicular Adenopathy

In studies confined to patients undergoing biopsy of supraclavicular adenopathy, 54% to 87% of patients are discovered to have malignancy, mostly metastatic carcinoma (46%–69% of all patients).[41,45–50] As expected, supradiaphragmatic carcinomas (e.g., lung or breast carcinoma) are equally distributed between the right and left sides. Most lung and breast cancers spread to the ipsilateral supraclavicular nodes, although examples of contralateral spread occur.[11,20,41,46–50]

Table 24-1	Lymph Node Score*

Finding	Points
Age >40 years	+5
Lymph node tenderness	−5
Lymph node size	
<1 cm^2	0
1–3.99 cm^2	+4
4–8.99 cm^2	+8
≥9 cm^2	+12
Generalized pruritus	+4
Supraclavicular nodes present	+3
Lymph node is hard	+2
Correction factor	−6[†]

*Based on reference 7.
[†]Included in every patient's score. For example a 55-year-old asymptomatic patient with nontender but hard supraclavicular adenopathy measuring 6 cm^2 has a score of 12 (i.e., 5 + 8 + 3 + 2 − 6).

Surprisingly, infradiaphragmatic carcinomas do not always spread to the left supraclavicular nodes as would be predicted by normal anatomy (see Fig. 24-1) and implied by Virchow's and Trosier's eponym. On average, only three quarters of infradiaphragmatic carcinomas metastatic to supraclavicular nodes go to the left side; one quarter appear on the *right* side (range = 0%–38%). Two proposed mechanisms for involvement of the right side by these tumors include (1) some patients normally have anatomic connections between the thoracic duct and the right supraclavicular nodes (see "Supraclavicular Nodes") and (2) the metastatic tumor first involves the mediastinal nodes, which via the right bronchomediastinal lymphatic vessels provide passage to the right neck. In support of the second explanation, one autopsy study of patients with infradiaphragmatic malignancies metastatic to the supraclavicular nodes documented that most patients also had mediastinal metastases.[20]

About 50% of patients whose supraclavicular node biopsies revealed malignancy were unaware of the diagnosis before biopsy,[20,47] illustrating the diagnostic importance of this node. In patients with metastases to the *right* supraclavicular node, the most common primary tumors by far are lung and breast cancer, followed by esophageal cancer and a medley of other tumors located above and below the diaphragm.[20,41,46–50] In those with metastases to the *left* side, lung, breast, gastric, and gynecologic primary tumors figure prominently in reported series of cases, although carcinoma of virtually any organ located in the thorax, abdomen, and pelvis has been associated with metastases to these nodes.[20,41,46–53]

2.   Epitrochlear Adenopathy

Epitrochlear nodes are a rare finding in normal individuals but are commonly observed in patients with disorders causing generalized lymphadenopathy.[21] They are palpable in 25% to 30% of patients with sarcoidosis, lymphoma, and chronic lymphocytic leukemia, and up to 55% of patients with infectious mononucleosis.[21] Also, in a study of hospitalized patients in Zimbabwe, where HIV infection is prevalent, the finding of epitrochlear adenopathy (i.e., epitrochlear nodes >0.5 cm diameter) distinguished patients with HIV seropositivity from those without it (sensitivity 84%, specificity 81%, positive LR = 4.5, negative LR = 0.2).[54]

3.   Staging Patients with Known Cancer

The absence of regional adenopathy is often unhelpful when staging patients with known malignancies. For example, up to 50% of patients with head and neck tumors and negative nodes by examination have nodal metastases discovered during radial neck exploration.[55–57] Similarly, up to one third of women with breast carcinoma and a negative axillary examination have axillary nodal metastases discovered at surgery,[58] and up to one quarter of patients with lung carcinoma and negative supraclavicular nodes have involvement of these nodes histologically.[59,60] Bedside examination is inaccurate because malignancy may involve regional nodes without changing their appearance. Even surgeons directly inspecting the physical characteristics of dissected nodes during staging operations often cannot distinguish metastatic nodes from normal ones.[55,57].

4.   Ulceroglandular and Oculoglandular Syndromes

Common reported causes of the ulceroglandular syndrome are tularemia, rickettsial infections, and herpes simplex infections. Important etiologies of the oculoglandular syndrome are cat scratch disease, tularemia, and viral infections (especially enterovirus and adenovirus).[61–64]

REFERENCES

1. Celsus. *De Medicina.* New York: Gryphon Editions; 1989.
2. *Hippocratic writings.* Harmondsworth, Middlesex, England: Penguin Books Ltd; 1978.
3. Brown JG. *Medical diagnosis: A manual of clinical methods.* New York: Bermingham and Company; 1884.
4. Williamson HA. Lymphadenopathy in a family practice: A descriptive study of 249 cases. *J Fam Pract.* 1985;20:449-452.
5. Linet OI, Metzler C. Incidence of palpable cervical nodes in adults. *Postgrad Med.* 1977;62(4):210-212.
6. Tokuda Y, Kishaba Y, Kato J, Nakazato N. Assessing the validity of a model to identify patients for lymph node biopsy. *Medicine.* 2003;82:414-418.
7. Vassilakopoulos TP, Pangalis GA. Application of a prediction rule to select which patients presenting with lymphadenopathy should undergo a lymph node biopsy. *Medicine.* 2000;79:338-347.
8. Chau I, Kelleher MT, Cunningham D, et al. Rapid access multidisciplinary lymph node diagnostic clinic: Analysis of 550 patients. *Br J Cancer.* 2003;88:354-361.
9. Williams PL, Warwick R, Dyson M, Bannister LH. The lymphatic system. *Gray's anatomy,* 37th ed. Edinburgh: Churchill Livingstone; 1989:821-858.
10. Jamieson JK, Dobson JF. On the injection of lymphatics by Prussian blue. *J Anat Physiol.* 1910;45:7-10.
11. Haagensen CD, Feind CR, Herter FP, et al. *The lymphatics in cancer.* Philadelphia: W.B. Saunders; 1972.
12. Rouviere H. *Anatomy of the human lymphatic system,* 1st ed. Ann Arbor, MI: Edwards Brothers, Inc; 1938.

13. Crum NF. Tuberculosis presenting as epitrochlear lymphadenitis. *Scand J Infect Dis.* 2003;35:888-890.

14. Patel DA. The supraclavicular lymph nodes: Their diagnostic significance in a swollen elbow joint. *Ann R Coll Surg Engl.* 2001;83:425-426.

15. Jamieson JK, Dobson JF. The lymphatics of the tongue: With particular reference to the removal of lymphatic glands in cancer of the tongue. *Br J Surg.* 1920;8:80-90.

16. Looney WW. Lymphatic drainage of head and neck—Emphasizing special structures. *Ann Otol Rhinol Laryngol.* 1935;44:33-41.

17. Negus D, Edwards JM, Kinmonth JB. Filling of the cervical and mediastinal nodes from the thoracic duct and the physiology of Virchow's node—Studies by lymphography. *Br J Surg.* 1970;57(6):267-271.

18. Kuiper DH, Papp JP. Supraclavicular adenopathy demonstrated by the Valsalva maneuver. *N Engl J Med.* 1969;280:1007-1008.

19. Morgenstern L. The Virchow-Trosier node: A historical note. *Am J Surg.* 1979; 138:703.

20. Viacava EP, Pack GT. Significance of supraclavicular signal node in patients with abdominal and thoracic cancer: A study of one hundred and twenty-two cases. *Arch Surg.* 1944;48:109-119.

21. Selby CD, Marcus HS, Toghill PJ. Enlarged epitrochlear lymph nodes: An old physical sign revisited. *J Roy Coll Physic London.* 1992;26:159-161.

22. Beeson BB. Epitrochelar adenopathy in secondary syphilis. *Arch Dermatol Syph.* 1935;32:746-749.

23. Evans G. Palpable epitrochlear glands: Their value as a physical sign. *Lancet.* 1937; 2:256-257.

24. Stitelman M. Shotty, not shoddy. *J Am Board Fam Pract.* 2002;15:434.

25. Libman H. Generalized lymphadenopathy. *J Gen Intern Med.* 1987;2:48-58.

26. Allhiser JN, McKnight TA, Shank JC. Lymphadenopathy in a family practice. *J Fam Pract.* 1981;12(1):27-32.

27. Jeghers H, Clark SL, Templeton AC. Lymphadenopathy and disorders of the lymphatics. In: Blacklow RS, ed. *MacBryde's signs and symptoms: Applied pathologic physiology and clinical interpretation,* 6th ed. Philadelphia Lippincott, Williams and Wilkins; 1983:467-533.

28. Harris DWS, Ostlere L, Buckley C, et al. Phenytoin-induced pseudolymphoma. A report of a case and review of the literature. *Br J Dermatol.* 1992;127:403-406.

29. Brynes RK, Chan WC, Spira TJ, et al. Value of lymph node biopsy in unexplained lymphadenopathy in homosexual men. *JAMA.* 1983;250:1313-1317.

30. Calguneri M, Ozturk MA, Ozbalkan Z, et al. Frequency of lymphadenopathy in rheumatoid arthritis and systemic lupus erythematosus. *J Int Med Res.* 2003;31: 345-349.

31. Ouvrier R. Henri Parinaud and his syndrome. *Med J Aust.* 1993;158:711-712.

32. Anthony PP, Knowles SAS. Lymphadenopathy as a primary presenting sign: A clinico-pathological study of 228 cases. *Br J Surg.* 1983;70:412-414.

33. Fijten GH, Blijham GH. Unexplained lymphadenopathy in family practice: An evaluation of the probability of malignant causes and the effectiveness of physicians' workup. *J Fam Pract.* 1988;27:373-376.

34. Slap GB, Brooks JSJ, Schwartz JS. When to perform biopsies of enlarged peripheral lymph nodes in young patients. *JAMA.* 1984;252:1321-1326.

35. Amr SS, Kamal M, Tarawneh MS. Diagnostic value of cervical lymph node biopsy: A pathological study of 596 cases. *J Surg Oncol.* 1989;42:239-243.

36. Lee YN, Terry R, Lukes RJ. Lymph node biopsy for diagnosis: A statistical study. *J Surg Oncol.* 1980;14:53-60.

37. Sriwatanawongasa V, Cardoso R, Chang P. Incidence of malignancy in peripheral lymph node biopsy. *Am Surg.* 1985;51:587-590.

38. Doberneck RC. The diagnostic yield of lymph node biopsy. *Arch Surg.* 1983;118:1203-1205.

39. Pangalis GA, Vassilakopoulos TP, Boussiotis VA, Fessas P. Clinical approach to lymphadenopathy. *Sem Oncol.* 1993;20:570-582.

40. Slap GB, Connor JL, Wigton RS, Schwartz JS. Validation of a model to identify young patients for lymph node biopsy. *JAMA.* 1986;255:2768-2773.

41. Cervin JR, Silverman JF, Loggie BW, Geisinger KR. Virchow's node revisited: Analysis with clinicopathologic correlation of 152 fine-needle aspiration biopsies of supraclavicular lymph nodes. *Arch Pathol Lab Med.* 1995;119:727-730.

42. Martin H, Morfit HM. Cervical lymph node metastasis as the first symptom of cancer. *Surg Gynecol Obstet.* 1944;78:133-159.

43. Cuende E, Vesga JC, Barrenengoa E, et al. Synovial cyst as differential diagnosis of supraclavicular mass in rheumatoid arthritis. *J Rheumatol.* 1996;23:1432-1434.

44. Zrada SE, Finkelstein JM. Anomalous articulation of the first rib mimicking supraclavicular neoplasia. *Otolaryngol Head neck Surg.* 1997;116:389-391.

45. Fakhry SM, Thomas CG. Pseudotumor of the supraclavicular fossa. *South Med J.* 1986;79:822-824.

46. Carson HJ, Candel AG, Gattuso P, Castelli MJ. Fine-needle aspiration of supraclavicular lymph nodes. *Diag Cytopathol.* 1996;14:216-220.

47. Ellison E, LaPuerta P, Martin SE. Supraclavicular masses: Results of a series of 309 cases biopsied by fine needle aspiration. *Head Neck.* 1999;21:239-246.

48. Gupta RK, Naran S, Lallu S, Fauck R. The diagnostic value of fine needle aspiration cytology (FNAC) in the assessment of palpable supraclavicular lymph nodes: A study of 218 cases. *Cytopathology.* 2003;14:201-207.

49. McHenry CR, Cooney MM, Slusapczyk SJ, Khiyami A. Supraclavicular lymphadenopathy: The spectrum of pathology and evaluation by fine-needle aspiration biopsy. *Am Surg.* 1999;65:742-747.

50. Nasuti JF, Mehrotra R, Gupta PK. Diagnostic value of fine-needle aspiration in supraclavicular lymphadenopathy: A study of 106 patients and review of literature. *Diagn Cytopathol.* 2001;25:351-355.

51. Kew MC. Virchow-Troisier's lymph node in hepatocellular carcinoma. *J Clin Gastroenterol.* 1991;13:217-219.

52. McKusick VA. Virchow-Troisier node: An occasional conspicuous manifestation of gallbladder cancer. *South Med J.* 1953;46:965-967.

53. Schwarz KO, Schwartz IS, Marchevsky A. Virchow-Troisier's lymph node as the presenting sign of hepatocellular carcinoma. *Mt Sinai J Med.* 1982;49(1):59-62.

54. Malin A, Ternouth I, Sarbah S. Epitrochlear lymph nodes as marker of HIV disease in sub-Saharan Africa. *BMJ.* 1994;309:1550-1551.

55. Finn S, Toner M, Timon C. The node-negative neck: Accuracy of clinical intraoperative lymph node assessment for metastatic disease in head and neck cancer. *Laryngoscope.* 2002;112:630-633.

56. Merritt RM, Williams MF, James TH, Porubsky ES. Detection of cervical metastasis: A meta-analysis comparing computed tomography with physical examination. *Arch Otolaryngol Head Neck Surg.* 1997;123:149-152.

57. Wein RO, Winkle MR, Norante JD, Coniglio JU. Evaluation of selective lymph node sampling in the node-negative neck. *Laryngoscope.* 2002;112:1006-1009.

58. Leidenius M, Krogerus L, Toivonen T, et al. The sensitivity of axillary staging when using sentinel node biopsy in breast cancer. *Eur J Surg Oncol.* 2003;29:849-853.

59. Brantigan JW, Brantigan CO, Brantigan OC. Biopsy of nonpalpable scalene lymph nodes in carcinoma of the lung. *Am Rev Respir Dis.* 1973;107:962-974.

60. Skinner DB. Scalene-lymph-node biopsy: Reappraisal of risks and indications. *N Engl J Med.* 1963;268:1324-1329.

61. Steinemann TL, Sheikholeslami MR, Brown HH, Bradsher RW. Oculoglandular tularemia. *Arch Ophthalmol.* 1999;117:132.

62. Thompson S, Omphroy L, Oetting T. Parinaud's oculoglandular syndrome attributable to an encounter with a wild rabbit. *Am J Ophthalmol.* 2001;131:283-284.

63. Grando D, Sullivan LJ, Flexman JP, et al. Bartonella henselae associated with Parinaud's oculoglandular syndrome. *Clin Infect Dis.* 1999;28:1156-1158.

64. Cunningham ET, Koehler JE. Ocular bartonellosis. *Am J Ophthalmol.* 2000;130:390-399.

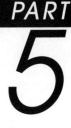

THE LUNGS

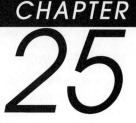

Inspection of the Chest

This chapter discusses the findings of clubbing, barrel chest, pursed-lips breathing, accessory muscle use, and inspiratory "white noise." Other relevant findings that may be detected during inspection of the respiratory system include cyanosis (Chapter 7) and abnormal respiratory rate or breathing pattern (Chapter 17).

I. CLUBBING ("ACROPACHY," "HIPPOCRATIC FINGERS")

A. INTRODUCTION

Clubbing is a painless focal enlargement of the connective tissue in the terminal phalanges of the digits.[1] Clubbing is usually symmetric, affecting the fingers more prominently than the toes. Although some persons have hereditary clubbing, the finding usually indicates serious underlying disease (see "Clinical Significance" later).

Hippocrates first described clubbing in the third century BC. He noted it in patients with empyema, commenting that "the fingernails become curved and the fingers become warm, especially at their tips."[2]

B. THE FINDING

Precise definitions of clubbing were developed in the 1960s and 1970s, prompted by reports that clinicians of that time were using at least a dozen different definitions[3] and by the observation that clubbing regresses after effective treatment of the underlying disorder, thus making accurate measures of this physical finding an important endpoint to follow. There are two substantiated definitions of clubbing: (1) an interphalangeal depth ratio greater than 1 and (2) a hyponychial angle greater than 190 degrees (Fig. 25-1). Both definitions are valid in patients of all ages, heights, and weights.

1. Interphalangeal Depth Ratio

Measurement of the interphalangeal depth ratio is described in Fig. 25-1. If this ratio exceeds 1, clubbing is present, a conclusion supported by two observations: (1) the interphalangeal depth ratio of normal persons is 0.895 ± 0.041, making the threshold of 1.0 more than 2.5 standard deviations above the normal,[4,5] and (2) a ratio of 1.0 distinguishes digits of healthy

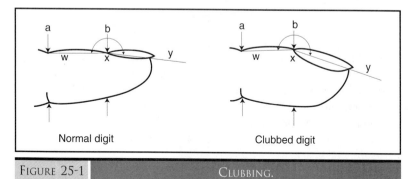

FIGURE 25-1	CLUBBING.

A, Normal digit. **B,** Clubbed digit. The distal interphalangeal joint is denoted by *a;* the junction of the nail and skin at the midline is denoted by *b.* The interphalangeal depth ratio is the ratio of the digit's depth measured at *b* divided by that at *a.* The hyponychial angle is the angle *wxy.* In the figure, the depth ratio is 0.9 for the normal digit and 1.2 for the clubbed digit (a ratio >1 indicates clubbing), and the hyponychial angle is 185 degrees for the normal digit and 200 degrees for the clubbed digit (a hyponychial angle >190 degrees indicates clubbing).

persons from those of patients with disorders traditionally associated with clubbing (such as cyanotic heart disease and cystic fibrosis). For example, studies demonstrate that 75% to 91% of patients with cystic fibrosis have an interphalangeal depth ratio exceeding 1, but only 0% to 1.5% of normal persons do.[4,5]

2. Hyponychial Angle

Measurement of the hyponychial angle is described in Fig. 25-1. If this angle exceeds 190 degrees, clubbing is present, a conclusion supported by three observations: (1) the normal hyponychial angle is 180 ± 4.2 degrees, and thus the 190 degree threshold is almost 2.5 standard deviations above normal[4,6,7]; (2) the hyponychial angle is the best parameter distinguishing plaster casts of digits labeled "definitely clubbed" by experienced clinicians from those labeled "definitely normal"[8]; and (3) studies show that 69% to 80% of patients with cystic fibrosis have hyponychial angles exceeding 190 degrees, whereas only 0% to 1.6% of normal persons have angles this large.[6,7]

A disadvantage to using the hyponychial angle is that special equipment is required for precise measurements. Historically, clinicians used an apparatus called the shadowgraph, which projects the silhouette of the finger against a screen fitted with a movable protractor.[9] Modern investigators use computerized analysis of digital photographs.[7] Neither of these instruments is widely available.

3. Shamroth's Sign

After watching his own clubbing come and go during an episode of endocarditis, the renowned electrocardiographer Leo Shamroth suggested another definition of clubbing in 1976.[10] He noted that when clubbing was absent, placing the terminal phalanges of similar fingers back to back (especially the ring fingers) formed a small diamond-shaped window, its contour outlined by the bases of the nail beds. When clubbing developed, this window disappeared. Shamroth recommended that others subject his sign to more rigorous study, but thus far this has not occurred.

4. Other Definitions

Parameters found to be not as accurate definitions of clubbing (compared with the hyponychial angle and interphalangeal depth ratio) are the distal interphalangeal *width* ratio, the longitudinal curvature of nail, the transverse curvature of the nail, and the profile angle (i.e., the angle between line *wx* in Fig. 25-1 and a second line extending from *x* to a point on the top of nail about a third of the distance from nail fold to nail tip).[8,11]

C. CLINICAL SIGNIFICANCE

1. Etiology

In one study of 350 patients with clubbed fingers, 80% had underlying respiratory disorders (e.g., lung tumor, bronchiectasis, lung abscess, empyema, interstitial fibrosis), 10% to 15% had miscellaneous disorders (congenital cyanotic heart disease, liver cirrhosis, chronic diarrhea, subacute endocarditis), and 5% to 10% were hereditary or idiopathic.[12]

2. Relationship to Hypertrophic Osteoarthropathy

Clubbing is sometimes associated with hypertrophic osteoarthropathy, which consists of painful edema and arthritis of the distal arms and legs, and periosteal elevation of the diaphysis of the distal long bones.[13] The usual cause is intrathoracic neoplasm (e.g., lung cancer or mesothelioma).

3. Clubbing and Cystic Fibrosis

In patients with cystic fibrosis, clubbing (i.e., interphalangeal depth ratio >1) predicts significant hypoxemia (i.e., $PaO_2 \leq 88$ mm Hg on room air) with a sensitivity of 91%, specificity of 72%, positive likelihood ratio (LR) of 3.2, and negative LR of 0.1^5. After lung transplantation, the clubbing of patients with cystic fibrosis regresses slowly over months.[14]

D. PATHOGENESIS

The increased volume of the clubbed digit is primarily because of increased amounts of vascular connective tissue,[15] although the cause of this fibrovascular proliferation is still debated. According to one hypothesis, clubbing results from large megakaryocytes and clumps of platelets that become trapped in the distal digits and then release growth factors causing soft tissue growth.[16,17] Normally, megakaryocytes do not appear in arterial blood: They leave the bone marrow and travel in the systemic veins to the pulmonary capillaries, where they become trapped because of their large size (20–50 microns in diameter) and fragment into smaller platelets. In most patients with clubbing, the pulmonary capillaries are either damaged (e.g., as in many inflammatory and neoplastic pulmonary disorders) or a right-to-left shunt exists (e.g., as in congenital heart disease, or the hepatopulmonary syndrome of cirrhosis), which allows the large megakaryocytes to travel freely through the lung into arterial blood and the distal digits, where they become wedged in the digital capillaries and release growth factors, causing fibrovascular proliferation and clubbing.

This hypothesis explains why clubbing accompanies endocarditis and why it is sometimes found unilaterally in the digits distal to an infected dialysis shunt. In both examples, platelet clumps are presumably released from the infected surface to travel to the digits, where they become embedded within capillaries and release growth factors.[16]

II. BARREL CHEST

A. THE FINDING

The normal chest is shaped like an oval cylinder, its anteroposterior diameter being less that it lateral diameter. The ratio of the anteroposterior to lateral diameter (called the "thoracic ratio," "thoracic index," or "chest index") is normally about 0.70 to 0.75 in adults and increases as persons grow older. The upper normal limit is about 0.9.[18-20]

The "barrel chest deformity" refers to a chest whose transverse section is more round than oval. It is traditionally a finding of chronic obstructive lung disease (i.e., chronic bronchitis, emphysema). Most patients also have dorsal kyphosis, a prominent sternum, widened intercostal spaces, elevated clavicles, and a shortened neck.[18] According to traditional teachings, the thoracic ratio of these patients exceeds 0.90, presumably because overactivity of the scalene and sternocleidomastoid muscles lift the upper ribs and sternum (see "Accessory Muscle Use" later).

B. CLINICAL SIGNIFICANCE

Evidence linking the barrel chest deformity with chronic obstructive lung disease is conflicting. Two studies did find a significant correlation between the barrel chest deformity and more severe airflow obstruction,[21,22] although another two studies found no relationship between the finding and measures of obstruction.[18,23] Additional problems with this physical sign are that the barrel chest is not specific for obstruction and also occurs in elderly persons without lung disease[18] and that, in some patients, the large anteroposterior dimension of the barrel chest is an illusion: The actual anteroposterior dimension is normal but it appears to be abnormally large because it contrasts with an abnormally thin abdominal dimension, caused by weight loss (Fig. 25-2).[24]

III. PURSED-LIPS BREATHING

Many patients with chronic obstructive lung disease instinctively learn that pursing the lips during expiration reduces dyspnea. The exact cause of the relief of dyspnea is still debated. Pursed-lips breathing significantly reduces the respiratory rate (from about 20 breaths/min to 12–15 breaths/min), increases tidal volume (by about 250–800 mL), decreases $PaCO_2$ (by 5%), and increases oxygen saturation (by 3%).[25-28] Dyspnea may be diminished because there is less work of breathing (from slower rate), less expiratory airway collapse (the pressure drop across the lips, 2–4 cm of H_2O, provides continuous expiratory positive pressure), or recruitment of respiratory muscles in a way that is less fatiguing to the diaphragm.[25,26,29]

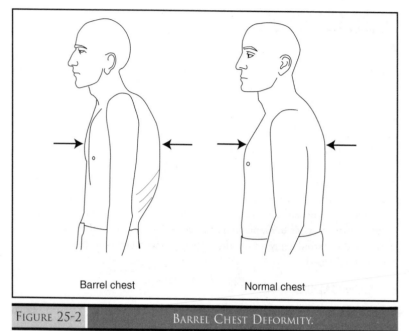

Barrel chest   Normal chest

FIGURE 25-2	BARREL CHEST DEFORMITY.

In some patients, the "large" anteroposterior dimension of the barrel chest (*left*) is an illusion, because it is no bigger that the anteroposterior dimension of the normal chest (*right*). Instead, what strikes the clinician's eyes is the barrel chest's prominent dorsal kyphosis and marked contrast between the preserved anteroposterior chest dimension and the thin abdomen.

IV. ACCESSORY MUSCLE USE

A. THE FINDING

The only muscle used in normal breathing is the diaphragm, which contracts during inspiration. Normal expiration is a passive process that relies on the elastic recoil of the lungs.[30] The term "accessory muscle use," therefore, refers to the contraction of muscles other than the diaphragm during inspiration (usually the sternocleidomastoid and scalene muscles) or to the contraction of any muscle during expiration (primarily the abdominal oblique muscles). Accessory muscle use is a common finding in patients with chronic obstructive lung disease or respiratory muscle fatigue.

B. PATHOGENESIS

Contraction of the sternocleidomastoid and scalene muscles lifts the clavicle and first rib, which helps expand the thorax of distressed patients, especially those with chronic obstructive lung disease in whom the flattened diaphragm generates only meager inspiratory movements. Contraction of the abdominal oblique muscles assists ventilation in two ways. In patients with obstructed airways, the abdominal muscles help expel air across the obstructed airways; in patients with respiratory muscle fatigue (e.g., amyotrophic lateral sclerosis), the abdominal muscles characteristically contract right at the moment expiration ends, to compress the respiratory system so that the early part of the subsequent inspiration can occur passively.[31]

C. CLINICAL SIGNIFICANCE

Accessory muscle use—defined as inspiratory contraction of the sternocleidomastoid and scalene muscles—is associated with severe obstructive disease.[21,23,32–34] More than 90% of patients hospitalized with acute exacerbations of chronic obstructive lung disease use accessory muscles, but by hospital day 5, less than half do.[35] In one study, patients whose clavicle lifted more than 5 mm during inspiration identified patients with more severe obstructive disease (mean FEV_1 0.6 L) than those whose clavicle moved smaller amounts (mean FEV_1 1.5 L, $p < .001$).*[32]

Inspection of accessory muscles also provides useful information in patients with amyotrophic lateral sclerosis. When these patients are supine, the *absence* of sternocleidomastoid and scalene contractions argues that diaphragmatic strength is *normal* (i.e., transdiaphragmatic sniff pressure ≥ 70 cm H_2O, sensitivity 83%, specificity 81%, and positive LR of 4.4).[37]

V. INTENSITY OF BREATHING SOUNDS (INSPIRATORY "WHITE NOISE"; "NOISY BREATHING")

A. THE FINDING

The breathing of normal persons is inaudible more than a few centimeters from the mouth, unless the person is sighing, panting, or gasping.[38] In three clinical settings, breathing sometimes becomes very noisy and is easily heard a distance

---

*FEV_1 is forced expiratory volume in 1 second, which is a measure of ventilatory capacity. It is normally 3.0 to 3.8 L.[36] The FEV_1 is abnormally low in obstructive lung disease and restrictive lung disease, dyspnea first appearing in these conditions when the FEV_1 falls below 2.5 L. An FEV_1 less than 1.0 L in chronic obstructive lung disease indicates severe disease.

from the bedside: in patients with lower airways obstruction, who may have audible *expiratory* wheezing (see Chapter 27); in patients with upper airway obstruction, who may have *inspiratory* stridor (see Chapter 27); and in patients with chronic bronchitis or asthma, who may have *inspiratory* white noise.[38]

White noise is an acoustical term meaning that, unlike wheezing and stridor, the sound lacks a musical pitch and therefore resembles more the static of a radio tuned between stations. In patients with chronic bronchitis and asthma, the loud inspiratory white noise heard at the patient's bedside without the stethoscope often contrasts sharply with the quiet inspiratory sounds heard through the stethoscope during auscultation (see Chapter 27).

B. PATHOGENESIS

Inspiratory white noise results from air turbulence caused by narrowed central airways,[39] a conclusion based on the observation that the sounds diminish after the patient receives effective bronchodilator treatment (which increases the patient's FEV_1) or breathes a mixture oxygen and helium (a gas mixture that reduces turbulence).[39] Inspiratory white noise is not a feature of emphysema, presumably because the inspiratory caliber of the central airways in these patients is normal.[39]

C. CLINICAL SIGNIFICANCE

Inspiratory white noise is a feature of chronic bronchitis and asthma but not emphysema. The intensity of white noise in patients with asthma and chronic bronchitis correlates inversely with the patient's FEV_1 (r = −0.60 to −0.64).[39]

REFERENCES

1. Fischer DS, Singer DH, Feldman SM. Clubbing, a review, with emphasis on hereditary acropachy. *Medicine*. 1964;43:459-479.
2. *Hippocratic writings*. Harmondsworth, Middlesex, England: Penguin Books; 1978.
3. Pyke DA. Finger clubbing: Validity as a physical sign. *Lancet*. 1954;2:352-354.
4. Waring WW, Wilkinson RW, Wiebe RA, et al. Quantitation of digital clubbing in children. *Am Rev Respir Dis*. 1971;104:166-174.
5. Nakamura CT, Ng GY, Paton JY, et al. Correlation between digital clubbing and pulmonary function in cystic fibrosis. *Pediatr Pulmonol*. 2002;33:332-338.
6. Bentley D, Moore A, Shwachman H. Finger clubbing: A quantitative survey by analysis of the shadowgraph. *Lancet*. 1976;2:164-167.
7. Husarik D, Vavricka SR, Mark M, et al. Assessment of digital clubbing in medical inpatients by digital photography and computerized analysis. *Swiss Med Wkly*. 2002; 132(11-12):132-138.
8. Regan GM, Tagg B, Thomson ML. Subjective assessment and objective measurement of finger clubbing. *Lancet*. 1967;1:530-532.

9. Bentley D, Cline J. Estimation of clubbing by analysis of shadowgraph. *Br Med J.* 1970;3:43.

10. Shamroth L. Personal experience. *South Afr Med J.* 1976;50:297-300.

11. Carroll DG. Curvature of the nails, clubbing of the fingers and hypertrophic pulmonary osteoarthropathy. *Trans Am Clin Climat Assoc.* 1971;83:198-208.

12. Coury C. Hippocratic fingers and hypertrophic osteoarthropathy: A study of 350 cases. *Br J Dis Chest.* 1960;54:202-209.

13. Hansen-Flaschen J, Nordberg J. Clubbing and hypertrophic osteoarthropathy. *Clin Chest Med.* 1987;8:287-298.

14. Augarten A, Goldman R, Laufer J, et al. Reversal of digital clubbing after lung transplantation in cystic fibrosis patients: A clue to the pathogenesis of clubbing. *Pediatr Pulmonol.* 2002;34:378-380.

15. Shneerson JM. Digital clubbing and hypertrophic osteoarthropathy: The underlying mechanisms. *Br J Dis Chest.* 1981;75:113-131.

16. Dickinson CJ. The aetiology of clubbing and hypertrophic osteoarthropathy. *Eur J Clin Invest.* 1993;23:330-338.

17. Spicknall KE, Zirwas MJ, English JC. Clubbing: An update on diagnosis, differential diagnosis, pathophysiology, and clinical experience. *J Am Acad Dermatol.* 2005; 52:1020-1028.

18. Pierce JA, Ebert RV. The barrel deformity of the chest, the senile lung and obstructive pulmonary emphysema. *Am J Med.* 1958;25:13-22.

19. Takahashi E, Atsumi H. Age differences in thoracic form as indicated by thoracic index. *Human Biol.* 1955;27:65-74.

20. Hurato A, Kaltreider NL, Fray WW, et al. Studies of total pulmonary capacity and its subdivisions. VI. Observations on cases of obstructive pulmonary emphysema. *J Clin Invest.* 1934;13:1027-1051.

21. Schneider IC, Anderson AE. Correlation of clinical signs with ventilatory function in obstructive lung disease. *Ann Intern Med.* 1965;62:477-485.

22. Ravid M, Schindler D, Shapira J, Chen B. The "ruler sign": A semiquantitative physical sign of chronic obstructive pulmonary disease. *Israel J Med Sci.* 1988;24:10-12.

23. Fletcher CM. The clinical diagnosis of pulmonary emphysema: An experimental study. *Proc Roy Soc Med.* 1952;45:577-584.

24. Kilburn KH, Asmundsson T. Anteroposterior chest diameter in emphysema. *Arch Intern Med.* 1969;123:379-382.

25. Breslin EH. The pattern of respiratory muscle recruitment during pursed-lip breathing. *Chest.* 1992;101:75-78.

26. Thoman RL, Stoker GL, Ross JC. The efficacy of pursed-lips breathing in patients with chronic obstructive pulmonary disease. *Am Rev Respir Dis.* 1966;93:100-106.

27. Mueller RE, Petty TL, Filley GF. Ventilation and arterial blood gas changes induced by pursed lips breathing. *J Appl Physiol.* 1970;28:784-789.

28. Jones AYM, Dean E, Chow CCS. Comparison of the oxygen cost of breathing exercises and spontaneous breathing in patients with stable chronic obstructive pulmonary disease. *Phys Ther.* 2003;83:424-431.

29. Barach AL. Physiologic advantages of grunting, groaning, and pursed-lip breathing: Adaptive symptoms related to the development of continuous positive pressure breathing. *Bull NY Acad Med.* 1973;49:666-673.

30. Goldman MD, Williams AJ, Soo Hoo G, Trang TTH. Asynchronous thoracoabdominal movements in chronic airflow obstruction (CAO). *Adv Exp Med Biol.* 1995;393:95-100.

31. Grinman S, Whitelaw WA. Pattern of breathing in a case of generalized respiratory muscle weakness. *Chest.* 1983;84:770-772.

32. Anderson CL, Shankar PS, Scott JH. Physiological significance of sternomastoid muscle contraction in chronic obstructive pulmonary disease. *Resp Care.* 1980;25:937-939.

33. Godfrey S, Edwards RHT, Campbell EJM, Newton-Howes J. Clinical and physiological associations of some physical signs observed in patients with chronic airways obstruction. *Thorax.* 1970;25:285-287.

34. Stubbing DG, Mathur PN, Roberts RS, Campbell EJM. Some physical signs in patients with chronic airflow obstruction. *Am Rev Respir Dis.* 1982;125:549-552.

35. O'Neill S, McCarthy DS. Postural relief of dyspnoea in severe chronic airflow limitation: relationship to respiratory muscle strength. *Thorax.* 1983;38:595-600.

36. Medical Section of the American Lung Association. Lung function testing: Selection of reference values and interpretative strategies. *Am Rev Respir Dis.* 1991;144:1202-1218.

37. Lechtzin N, Wiener CM, Shade DM, et al. Spirometry in the supine position improves the detection of diaphragmatic weakness in patients with amyotrophic lateral sclerosis. *Chest.* 2002;121:436-442.

38. Forgacs P. The functional basis of pulmonary sounds. *Chest.* 1978;73:399-412.

39. Forgacs P, Nathoo AR, Richardson HD. Breath sounds. *Thorax.* 1971;26:288-295.

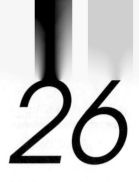

Palpation and Percussion of the Chest

PALPATION

I. INTRODUCTION

Palpation of the chest is limited because the bony rib cage hides many abnormalities of the underlying lungs. The traditional reasons to palpate the chest are to detect the following signs: (1) chest wall tenderness or masses, (2) pleural friction rubs, (3) bronchial fremitus, (4) abnormal respiratory excursion, and (5) asymmetric tactile fremitus. Bronchial fremitus is an inspiratory vibratory sensation felt in some patients with airway secretions. Respiratory excursion is assessed while the patient breathes in and out, either by simultaneously palpating symmetric areas of the chest or by measuring the changing circumference with a tape measure. According to traditional teachings, chest excursion is reduced bilaterally in chronic airflow obstruction and neuromuscular disease (see Chapter 30) and unilaterally in pleural effusion and consolidation.

II. TACTILE FREMITUS

A. THE FINDING
Tactile fremitus ("vocal fremitus") is the vibration felt by the clinician's hand resting on the chest wall of a patient who is speaking or singing.

B. TECHNIQUE
To elicit the sign, the patient usually says "one-two-three" or "ninety-nine" repeatedly and evenly while the clinician compares symmetric areas of the chest. Some early German physical diagnosticians used the word *neun-und-neuzig* (German for "ninety-nine") to elicit vocal fremitus, prompting modern English-speaking authors to suggest that the "oy" sound is necessary to elicit the finding (e.g., "toy boat" or "Toyota," to mimic the vowel sound in the German word *neun-und-neun-zig*). This is incorrect, however, and the early German diagnosticians just as often used other words, such as "one, one, one" (*eins, eins, eins*") and "one, two, three" (*eins, zwei, drei*),[1-3] or had their patients sing or scream to elicit the finding.[3]

C. FINDING
Vocal fremitus is more prominent in men than women because men have lower-pitched voices, which conduct more easily though lung tissue than do higher-pitched voices (see Pathogenesis of Vocal Resonance in Chapter 27). Tactile fremitus, therefore, may be absent in some healthy persons, especially those with high-pitched or soft voices or those with thick chest walls (which insulate the hand from the vibrating lung). Consequently, only *asymmetric* tactile fremitus is an abnormal finding: According to traditional teachings, fremitus is asymmetrically diminished whenever air, fluid, or tumor pushes the lung away from the chest wall (*unilateral* pneumothorax, pleural effusion, neoplasm) and is asymmetrically increased when there is consolidation of the underlying lung (i.e., *unilateral* pneumonia).

The pathogenesis of tactile fremitus is discussed in Chapter 27 (see "Vocal Resonance").

PERCUSSION

I. INTRODUCTION

In 1761, after studying patients and cadavers at the Spanish Hospital in Vienna for 7 years, Leopold Auenbrugger[4] published a 95-page booklet containing the first detailed description of chest percussion. His work was largely ignored for half a century, until Corvisart (physician to Napoleon) translated it into French and taught the technique to his students, including Laennec, the subsequent inventor of the stethoscope.[5] The discovery of percussion was a major diagnostic advance because, for the first time, clinicians could reliably distinguish empyema from tuberculosis and other pneumonias.[5] Until the discovery of roentgen rays in 1895, percussion and auscultation were the only methods to investigate and define diseases of the lungs during the patient's life.

II. TECHNIQUE

A. DIRECT VERSUS INDIRECT METHOD

In the direct method, the percussion blow lands directly on the body wall (the method of Auenbrugger and Laennec). In the indirect method, the blow falls instead on an intervening substance, called a "pleximeter," placed against the body wall. Historically, pleximeters were made of ivory or wood, or a coin was used, although today most clinicians use the middle finger of their left hand.

B. TYPES OF PERCUSSION

There are three ways to percuss the patient: (1) comparative percussion (the original method of Auenbrugger and Laennec), (2) topographic percussion (invented by Piorry of France in 1828),[6,7] and (3) auscultatory percussion (introduced by the Americans Camman and Clark in 1840).[5,8] Today, most clinicians use the indirect method with comparative and topographic percussion and the direct method with auscultatory percussion.

1. Comparative Percussion

Comparative percussion identifies disease by comparing the right and left sides of the chest. Prominent dullness or unusual hyperresonance over one side indicates disease in that part. Bilateral disease, by definition, is difficult to identify using comparative percussion.

2. Topographic Percussion

Topographic percussion attributes any dullness in the chest or abdomen to airless intrathoracic tissue lying directly beneath the percussion blow. Topographic percussion differs from comparative percussion in implying the clinician can precisely outline the borders of underlying organs and then measure their span. The technique is still used today to measure excursion of the diaphragm (and to identify an enlarged heart or liver; see Chapters 33 and 47).

When using topographic percussion to determine diaphragm excursion, the clinician locates the point of transition between dullness and resonance on the lower posterior chest, first during full inspiration and then during full expiration. The diaphragm excursion is the vertical distance between these two points. The reported normal excursion of healthy persons ranges from 3 to 6 cm (for comparison, the corresponding excursion on the chest radiograph is about 5 to 7 cm in normal persons and 2 to 3 cm in patients with lung disease).[5,9,10]

3.   Auscultatory Percussion

Auscultatory percussion was introduced to further refine the goals of topographic percussion.[8] Instead of listening to sounds as they resonate off the chest into the surrounding room, the clinician using auscultatory percussion places the stethoscope on the body wall and listens through it to the sounds transmitted by nearby percussive blows.

Over the last 150 years, auscultatory percussion of the chest has repeatedly fallen out of favor and then resurfaced as a "new sign."[5] In the most recent version of auscultatory percussion of the chest, introduced in 1974, the clinician taps lightly over the manubrium and listens over the posterior part of the chest with the stethoscope.[11,12] Using this technique, the clinician should find identical sounds at corresponding locations of the two sides of the chest; a note of decreased intensity on one side supposedly indicates ipsilateral disease between the tapping finger and stethoscope.

The technique of using auscultatory percussion to detect pleural fluid, first developed in 1927,[13] is slightly different. The clinician places the stethoscope on the posterior chest of the seated patient, 3 cm below the 12th rib and percusses the posterior chest from apex to base. At some point the normal dull note changes to an unusually loud note: If this occurs with strokes above the 12th rib, the test is abnormal, indicating pleural fluid.[14]

C.   THE PERCUSSION BLOW

1.   Force

Each percussion blow should strike the same part of the pleximeter with identical force, and the pleximeter finger should be applied with the same force and orientation when comparing right and left sides. Consistent technique is important because both the percussion force and the pleximeter govern the percussion sound produced. Lighter strokes produce sounds that are duller than those produced by stronger strokes. Lifting the pleximeter finger, even slightly, can transform a resonant note into a dull one.

Even though a consistent technique is important, the force and speed of percussion blows vary threefold among different clinicians,[15] which probably explains why interobserver agreement for topographic percussion is poor compared with that for other physical findings (see Chapter 3).

2. Rapid Withdrawal of Plexor

The traditional teaching is that the plexor finger should be promptly withdrawn after a blow, mimicking the action of a piano key striking a string. The only study of this found that clinicians could not distinguish the note created by a rapid withdrawal from one in which the plexor finger lightly rested on the pleximeter after the blow.[16]

III.   THE FINDING

A. PERCUSSION SOUNDS

There are three percussion sounds—**tympany** (normally heard over the abdomen), **resonance** (heard over normal lung), and **dullness** (heard over the liver or thigh) (Table 26-1). Tympany differs from resonance and dullness because it contains vibrations of a dominant frequency, which allows the clinician to actually identify its musical pitch. Resonance and dullness, in contrast, are "noise" in an acoustical sense, consisting of a jumble of frequencies that prevent identification of a specific musical pitch. The three sound characteristics distinguishing resonance and dullness are intensity, duration, and frequency content: Resonance is louder and longer and contains more low-frequency energy.[5,17] Of these three sound characteristics, clinicians appreciate most easily that resonance is louder than dullness.

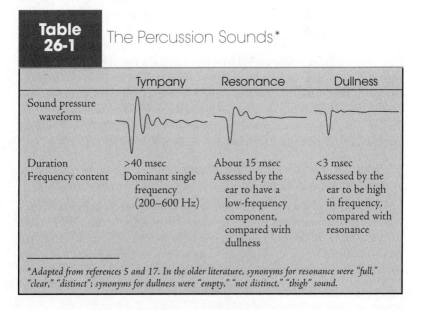

Table 26-1	The Percussion Sounds*		
	Tympany	Resonance	Dullness
Sound pressure waveform			
Duration	>40 msec	About 15 msec	<3 msec
Frequency content	Dominant single frequency (200–600 Hz)	Assessed by the ear to have a low-frequency component, compared with dullness	Assessed by the ear to be high in frequency, compared with resonance

*Adapted from references 5 and 17. In the older literature, synonyms for resonance were "full," "clear," "distinct"; synonyms for dullness were "empty," "not distinct," "thigh" sound.

Some clinicians take advantage of resonance being louder than dullness, using a technique called threshold percussion, in which percussion blows are so light that dull areas produce no sound. As the blows move along the body wall with precisely the same amount of force, a note abruptly appears the moment the blow encounters a resonant area. An old adage in percussion, attributed to Weil, is that it is much easier to distinguish "something from nothing" than to distinguish "more from less."[5]

B. SENSE OF RESISTANCE

All great teachers of percussion have emphasized that the tactile sense in the pleximeter finger provides as much information as the audible notes. Dull areas, according to these teachers, move less or offer more resistance than resonant areas (thus earning pleural effusion the descriptor "stony dullness"). Experiments using light-weight accelerometers taped to the pleximeter finger confirm that dull areas do move less than resonant areas.[18]

C. GLOSSARY OF ADDITIONAL PERCUSSION TERMS

Historically, the vocabulary of clinical percussion was diverse. Some of the more commonly used terms appear.

1. Skodaic Resonance

Skodaic resonance is a hyperresonant note produced by percussion of the chest above a pleural effusion. The cause of this finding is unknown. Skodaic resonance was originally described by Josef Skoda,[19] a champion of topographic percussion and the first to apply the principles of physics to percussion.

2. Grocco's Triangle

Grocco's triangle is a right-angled triangle of dullness found over the posterior region of the chest *opposite* a large pleural effusion. The horizontal side of the triangle follows the diaphragm for several centimeters; the vertical side lies over the spinous processes but usually ends below the top level of the effusion.[5] This finding was originally described by Koranyi (Hungary, 1897) and later by Grocco (Italy, 1902) and Rauchfuss (Germany, 1903).

3. Metallic Resonance ("Amphoric Resonance"; "Coin Test")

Metallic resonance is a pure tympanitic sound containing very high frequencies, found over large superficial pulmonary cavities or pneumothoraces.[19,20] Flicking the tense cheek while holding the mouth open mimics the sound. The sound was best elicited with a hard plexor and pleximeter (e.g., two coins) and is best perceived through the stethoscope or with the examiner's ear near the patient's chest.[5]

4. Krönig's Isthmus

Krönig's isthmus is a narrow band of resonance over each lung apex that lies between the dullness from the neck and the dullness from the shoulder muscles. Diseases of the lung apex, such as tuberculosis, supposedly reduced the width of the band.[5] Georg Krönig (Germany) described the finding in 1889.[21]

5. Cracked-Pot Resonance

Cracked-pot resonance is a percussion sound over superficial tubercular cavities, mimicked by pressing the palms together and hitting the back of one hand against the knee.[19,22] To detect the sound in patients, the clinician delivers a strong percussion blow and listens near the patient's open mouth.[2,23] Although the sound was traditionally attributed to the sudden efflux of air through bronchi communicating with a tubercular cavity, the only published pathologic study found no bronchial communication in 11 patients with this sound.[24]

IV. PATHOGENESIS

A. TOPOGRAPHIC PERCUSSION VERSUS CAGE RESONANCE THEORY

From the earliest days of percussion, two opposing theories have explained the genesis of percussion sounds: the "topographic percussion theory" and the "cage resonance theory." The topographic percussion theory argued that only the physical characteristics of the soft tissues directly beneath the percussion blow controlled whether resonance or dullness was produced. This theory emphasized that the body wall itself contributed little to the resulting sound but acted merely to convey the vibrations from the underlying tissues (much like a diaphragm in a microphone transmits the sound vibrations imparted to it). A fundamental tenet of the topographic percussion theory was the "several centimeter rule," advanced by Weil[25] in 1880, which stated that the percussion stroke penetrated only the most superficial 4 to 6 cm of tissue, and only anatomic abnormalities in this layer influenced the sound produced.

In contrast, the cage resonance theory argued that the percussion sound reflected the ease with which the body wall vibrates, which in turn was influenced by many variables, including the strength of the stroke, the condition and state of the body wall, and the underlying organs. Advocates of the cage resonance theory argued that precise topographic percussion was impossible because underlying organs or disease could cause dullness to occur at distant sites.

The topographic percussion theory became very popular—largely through the persuasive efforts of renowned clinical teachers, including Piorry; Skoda; Mueller; and Mueller's pupil, Ralph Major, who wrote one of the most popular

American physical diagnosis textbooks.[1] Nonetheless, the evidence cited to support this theory and the several centimeter rule was meager and of uncertain relevance[5]: It included only a few experiments with cadavers [25] and some sound recordings of exenterated lung slices as they were being percussed.[26]

In contrast, considerable evidence supports the cage resonance theory.

1. Analysis of Sound Recordings

The percussion sound contains more frequencies than can be explained by vibrations of just the area of the body wall percussed.[18,27–29] Areas of the body wall distant to the blow must also vibrate and contribute to the sound.

2. Condition and State of the Body Wall

External pressure on the chest—from a pillow, a stretcher, or an extra hand placed near the point of percussion—impedes chest wall motion and dampens the percussion note.[20,30]

Pressure against the inner wall of the chest of cadavers also causes dullness, even in areas of the body wall distant from where the pressure is applied.[20] The best clinical example of the distant effects of internal pressure is Grocco's triangle, a right-angled triangle of dullness found over the posterior region of the chest *opposite* a large pleural effusion (see previous). Grocco's triangle proves that pressure on the chest wall at one point (e.g., from pleural fluid) may cause dullness at sites distant to that pressure (i.e., over the opposite chest). Even in patients without pleural fluid, external pressure on one side of the posterior chest from a hand or water bottle will produce Grocco's triangle on the opposite chest.[31,32]

Heavier patients have larger liver spans than patients who weigh less,[33] not because the livers of heavier patients are larger but instead because the excess subcutaneous fat influences the cage resonance and dampens the vibrations, resulting in more dullness and larger spans.

3. The Strength of the Percussion Blow

The strength of the blow influences whether resonance or dullness is produced, especially near areas of the body wall marking the transition between resonance and dullness. For example, in percussion of the liver, the span of the liver is about 3 cm smaller when using strong strokes than it is when using light strokes (see Chapter 47).[33–35] This occurs because the heavy stroke, when located near where the liver touches the body wall, more easily generates the vibrations necessary for the resonant note, whereas the light stroke is insufficient until further removed. These findings contradict the assertion of topographic percussionists, who taught that stronger blows penetrated tissues more deeply than softer ones; if this were true, percussion of the liver with heavy strokes should produce a larger span than with light strokes (because heavier strokes would detect the dome of the liver, which is removed from the body wall).

B. AUSCULTATORY PERCUSSION

The advocates of auscultatory percussion believe that sound waves travel directly from the tapping finger through the lung to the stethoscope and are altered along the way by diseased tissue. It is much more likely, however, that these sounds are conducted circumferentially in the chest wall, for several reasons: (1) The technique fails to detect the heart, which should render some notes of the left chest more dull if sound waves traveled directly to the stethoscope; (2) sound recordings during auscultatory percussion are the same whether the patient breathes room air or a mixture of helium and oxygen.[36] Because sound characteristics depend on the gas density of the conducting medium, which is different for the two gas mixtures, it is unlikely sound travels through the lung; (3) the characteristics of the sound change during the Valsalva and Mueller maneuvers, which increase tension in the chest wall but do not alter the underlying lung[36]; and (4) contour maps reveal that the loudest sounds during auscultatory percussion appear over bony prominences, such as the scapula, indicating that the sound produced depends on the contour of the chest wall. The intervening lung contributes less to the sound heard because these sound maps do not change even when there is a large underlying tumor.[37]

V. CLINICAL SIGNIFICANCE

A. COMPARATIVE PERCUSSION

EBM Box 26-1 shows that asymmetric dullness is a helpful though infrequent finding, arguing for pneumonia in patients with fever and cough [likelihood ratio (LR) = 3.0] and for underlying abnormalities on the chest radiograph of unselected patients (LR = 3.0). In these studies, percussion detected all large pleural effusions (sensitivity 100%), but very few consolidations (sensitivity 0–15%) and no intraparenchymal nodules or granulomata. The finding of normal percussion sounds is common in patients with significant lung disease and can never be used as an argument against the presence of disease (all negative LRs are not significant, see EBM Box 26-1).

In chronic smokers, hyperresonance of the upper right anterior chest is a valuable finding arguing for chronic airflow obstruction (positive LR = 5.1, see EBM Box 26-1).[46]

B. TOPOGRAPHIC PERCUSSION OF THE DIAPHRAGM

In patients with lung disease, clinicians usually overestimate the actual movements of the diaphragm and differ from the chest film by 1 to 3 cm.[9,47] The correlation between actual and percussed movements is poor in the only study of this finding (r = 0.14–0.42, not significant half the time).[9] Another study showed that a percussed diaphragm excursion of less than 2 cm is an infrequent and unreliable diagnostic sign of chronic obstructive lung disease (both LRs not significant).[46]

Box 26-1 — Diagnostic Accuracy of Percussion of the Chest*

Finding (Ref)[†]	Sensitivity (%)	Specificity (%)	Likelihood Ratio if Finding Present	Absent
COMPARATIVE PERCUSSION				
Percussion dullness				
Detecting pneumonia in patients with fever and cough[38–42]	4–26	82–99	**3.0**	NS
Detecting any abnormality on chest radiograph[43–45]	8–15	94–98	**3.0**	NS
Hyperresonance				
Detecting chronic airflow obstruction[46]	33	94	**5.1**	NS
TOPOGRAPHIC PERCUSSION				
Diaphragm excursion <2 cm				
Detecting chronic airflow obstruction[46]	13	98	NS	NS
AUSCULTATORY PERCUSSION				
Abnormal dullness				
Detecting any abnormality on chest radiograph[43–45]	16–69	74-88	NS	NS
Detecting pleural fluid[14]	96	95	**18.6**	**0.04**

NS, not significant; likelihood ratio (LR) if finding present = positive LR; LR if finding absent = negative LR.
*Diagnostic standard: For pneumonia or pleural effusion-infiltrate or effusion on chest radiograph; for chronic airflow obstruction, FEV_1 <60% predicted or the FEV_1/FVC ratio <0.6.
†Definition of findings: For hyperresonance, hyperresonance of the upper right anterior chest[46]; for abnormal dullness during auscultatory percussion for chest radiograph abnormalities, asymmetric dullness, with stethoscope on posterior chest and while directly percussing sternum anteriorly; for abnormal dullness during auscultatory percussion for pleural fluid, transition to unusually loud note above 12th rib posteriorly in midclavicular line, with stethoscope 3 cm below 12th rib and while directly percussing posterior chest from apex to base.[14]

PERCUSSION OF THE CHEST

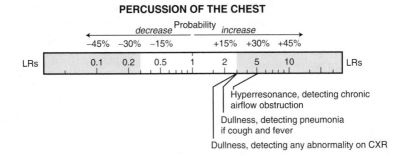

Hyperresonance, detecting chronic airflow obstruction

Dullness, detecting pneumonia if cough and fever

Dullness, detecting any abnormality on CXR

C. AUSCULTATORY PERCUSSION

Studies of auscultatory percussion have widely varying results, usually showing the technique has greater sensitivity than comparative percussion but also lower specificity. Overall, the pooled results show that this technique is an unreliable diagnostic sign (both positive and negative LRs not significant; see EBM Box 26-1).

Like conventional percussion, auscultatory percussion identifies almost all pleural effusions (sensitivity 96%, see EBM Box 26-1).[14] The technique used in the study cited in EBM Box 26-1 (see "Auscultatory Percussion" for definition) was specific for pleural fluid and resulted in few positive findings among patients with underlying lung masses, pneumonia, or other underlying diseases.

REFERENCES

1. Major R. *Physical diagnosis*, 3rd ed. Philadelphia: W.B. Saunders; 1945.
2. Sahli H. *A treatise on diagnostic methods of examination*. Philadelphia: W.B. Saunders; 1911.
3. Guttman P. *A handbook of physical diagnosis: Comprising the throat, thorax, and abdomen*. New York: William Wood and Co; 1880.
4. Auenbrugger L. *On percussion of the chest (1761), being a translation of Auenbrugger's original treatise entitled "Inventum novum ex percussione thoracis humani, ut signo abstrusos interni pectoris morbos detegendi"* (facsimile edition by Johns Hopkins Press). Baltimore: Johns Hopkins Press; 1936.
5. McGee S. Percussion and physical diagnosis: Separating myth from science. *Disease-a-Month*. 1995;41:643-692.
6. Risse GB. Pierre A. Piorry (1794-1879): The French "master of percussion". *Chest*. 1971;60:484-488.
7. Sakula A. Pierre Adolphe Piorry (1794-1879): Pioneer of percussion and pleximetry. *Thorax*. 1979;34:575-581.
8. Camman GP, Clark A. A new mode of ascertaining the dimensions, form, and condition of internal organs by percussion. *N Y J Med Surg*. 1840;3:62-96.

9. Williams TJ, Ahmad D, Morgan WKC. A clinical and roentgenographic correlation of diaphragmatic movement. *Arch Intern Med.* 1981;141:878-880.

10. Young DA, Simon G. Certain movements measured on inspiration-expiration chest radiographs correlated with pulmonary function studies. *Clin Radiol.* 1972;23:37-41.

11. Guarino JR. Auscultatory percussion: A new aid in the examination of the chest. *J Kans Med Soc.* 1974;75:193-194.

12. Guarino JR. Auscultatory percussion of the chest. *Lancet.* 1980;1:1332-1334.

13. Webb GB. Auscultatory percussion in the diagnosis of pleural fluid. *JAMA.* 1927; 88:99.

14. Guarino JR, Guarino JC. Auscultatory percussion: A simple method to detect pleural effusion. *J Gen Intern Med.* 1994;9:71-74.

15. Burger HC, Casteleyn G, Jordan FLJ. How is percussion done? *Acta Med Scand.* 1952;142:106-112.

16. Coleman W. The alleged dullness over the apex of the normal right lung. *Am J Med Sci.* 1939;197:141-145.

17. Murray A, Neilson JMM. Diagnostic percussion sounds. I. A qualitative analysis; II. Computer-automated parameter measurement for quantitative analysis. *Med Biol Eng.* 1975;13:19-38.

18. Murray A, Neilson JMM. Diagnostic percussion: A study of chest-wall motion and the associated tactile sensation. *Med Biol Eng Comput.* 1978;16:269-278.

19. Skoda J. *Auscultation and percussion.* Philadelphia: Lindsay and Blakiston; 1854.

20. Mazoon JF. Die Theorie der Perkussion der Brust auf Grundlage directer Versuche und zahlreicher Beobachtungen. *Vierteljahrschrift Prakt Heilkd.* 1852;36:1-59.

21. Krönig G. Zur Topographie der Lungenspitzen und ihrer Perkussion. *Berl Klin Wochenschr.* 1889;26:809-812.

22. Barth M, Roger MH. *A manual of auscultation and percussion.* Philadelphia: Lindsay and Blakiston; 1866.

23. Cabot R. *Physical diagnosis of diseases of the chest.* New York: William Wood; 1900.

24. Walsh J. Necropsy findings under cracked-pot tympany. *Am Rev Tuberc.* 1928;18:202-204.

25. Weil A. *Handbuch und Atlas der topographischen Perkussion.* Leipzig: F. C. W. Vogel; 1880.

26. Martini P. Studien über Perkussion und Auskultation. *Dtsch Arch Klin Med.* 1922;139:65-98, 167-190, 257-184.

27. Bishop FW, Lee YW, Scott WJM, Lyman RS. Studies on pulmonary acoustics. IV. Notes on percussion and on forced vibrations. *Am Rev Tuberc Pulm Dis.* 1930;22: 347-378.

28. Fahr G, Brandi B. Weitere Studien über Perkussion und Auskultation. *Dtsch Arch Klin Med.* 1929;164:1-33.

29. Metildi PF, Bishop FW, Morton JJ, Lyman RS. Studies on pulmonary acoustics. III. The transmission of vibrations from percussion along ribs. *Am Rev Tuberc Pulm Dis.* 1930;21:711-744.

30. Gilbert VE. Detection of pneumonia by auscultation of the lungs in the lateral decubitus positions. *Am Rev Respir Dis.* 1989;140:1012-1016.

31. Turban K. Paralipomena der Tuberkuloseforschung. *Munch Med Wochschr.* 1927;74:1399-1404.

32. Hamburger F. Ueber die Oberflächenwirkung des Perkussionstosses. *Munch Med Wochenschr.* 1906;53:2283-2286.

33. Castell DO, O'Brien KD, Muench H, Chalmers TC. Estimation of liver size by percussion in normal individuals. *Ann Intern Med.* 1969;70:1183-1189.

34. Sullivan S, Krasner N, Williams R. The clinical estimation of liver size: A comparison of techniques and an analysis of the source of error. *Br Med J.* 1976;2:1042-1043.

35. Sapira JD, Williamson DL. How big is the normal liver? *Arch Intern Med.* 1979;139:971-973.

36. Bohadana AB, Kraman SS. Transmission of sound generated by sternal percussion. *J Appl Physiol.* 1989;66:273-277.

37. Bohadana AB, Patel R, Kraman SS. Contour maps of auscultatory percussion in healthy subjects and patients with large intrapulmonary lesions. *Lung.* 1989;167:359-372.

38. Heckerling PS, Tape TG, Wigton RS, et al. Clinical prediction rule for pulmonary infiltrates. *Ann Intern Med.* 1990;113:664-670.

39. Melbye H, Straume B, Aasebo U, Brox J. The diagnosis of adult pneumonia in general practice. *Scand J Prim Health Care.* 1988;6:111-117.

40. Gennis P, Gallagher J, Falvo C, et al. Clinical criteria for the detection of pneumonia in adults: Guidelines for ordering chest roentgenograms in the emergency department. *J Emerg Med.* 1989;7:263-268.

41. Melbye H, Straume B, Aasebo U, Dale K. Diagnosis of pneumonia in adults in general practice. *Scand J Prim Health Care.* 1992;10:226-233.

42. Diehr P, Wood RW, Bushyhead J, et al. Prediction of pneumonia in outpatients with acute cough: A statistical approach. *J Chron Dis.* 1984;37(3):215-225.

43. Nelson RS, Rickman LS, Mathews WC, et al. Rapid clinical diagnosis of pulmonary abnormalities in HIV-seropositive patients by auscultatory percussion. *Chest.* 1994;105:402-407.

44. Bourke S, Nunes D, Stafford F, et al. Percussion of the chest re-visited: A comparison of the diagnostic value of ausculatory and conventional chest percussion. *Ir J Med Sci.* 1989;158(4):82-84.

45. Bohadana AB, Coimbra FTV, Santiago JRF. Detection of lung abnormalities by auscultatory percussion: A comparative study with conventional percussion. *Respiration.* 1986;50:218-225.

46. Badgett RG, Tanaka DJ, Hunt DK, et al. Can moderate chronic obstructive pulmonary disease be diagnosed by historical and physical findings alone? *Am J Med.* 1993;94:188-196.

47. Cole MB, Hammel JV, Manginelli VW, Lawton AH. Bedside versus laboratory estimations of timed and total vital capacity and diaphragmatic height and movement. *Dis Chest.* 1970;38:519-521.

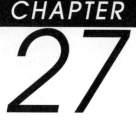

Auscultation of the Lungs

The three categories of auscultatory findings of the lungs are breath sounds, vocal resonance (i.e., the sound of the patient's voice through the stethoscope), and adventitious sounds (i.e., sounds other than breath sounds or vocal resonance). Almost all of the findings discussed in this chapter were originally described in 1819 by Laennec, in his masterpiece *A Treatise on the Disease of the Chest*.[1]

I. BREATH SOUNDS

A. FINDING

1. Vesicular Versus Bronchial Breath Sounds

There are two types of breath sounds: (1) vesicular breath sounds, which are normally heard over the posterior chest, and (2) bronchial breath sounds, which are normally heard over the trachea and right apex. These sounds are distinguished by their timing, intensity, and pitch (Table 27-1). Vesicular sounds are mostly inspiratory sounds that have a soft, breathy quality, which Laennec

	Table 27-1 Comparison of Vesicular and Bronchial Breath Sounds	
	Vesicular	**Bronchial**
Timing*	Inspiration longer than expiration:	Expiration longer than inspiration:
Intensity	Soft, breathy	Loud, harsh, tubular
Pitch	Low (100 Hz)	High (300–400 Hz)
Location they normally are heard	Posterior bases	Trachea, right apex

Based on information from references 2–6.
*Bronchial breath sounds have a short gap between the inspiratory and expiratory sound; vesicular sounds do not.

likened to the sound of leaves rustling in a gentle breeze. Bronchial sounds have a prominent expiratory component and much harsher quality, which sounds like air blowing forcibly through a tube (hence, they are sometimes called tubular breath sounds).

Bronchial breath sounds are abnormal when they occur over the posterior or lateral chest (especially the lower parts). According to traditional teachings, which in turn are based on postmortem examination, bronchial breath sounds occur in these locations only if solid, collapsed, or consolidated lung is contiguous with the chest wall and extends some distance toward the hilum.[7-9] The usual causes are pneumonia and pleural effusion (large pleural effusions presumably compress the underlying lung just enough to alter its acoustic properties).[10]

2.   Breath Sound Score

One important feature of vesicular breath sounds is the sound's intensity, which can be graded using a scoring system developed by Pardee.[11] According to this system, the clinician listens sequentially to six locations on the patient's chest: bilaterally over the upper anterior portion of the chest, in the midaxillae, and at the posterior bases. At each site the clinician grades the *inspiratory* sound as absent (0 points), barely audible (1 point), faint but definitely heard (2 points), normal (3 points), or louder than normal (4 points). The patient's total score may range from 0 (absent breath sounds) to 24 (very loud breath sounds).

B. PATHOGENESIS

1. Vesicular Sounds

a. *Origin*

The *inspiratory* component of vesicular breath sounds originates in the peripheral portions of the lung near where the stethoscope is placed. It does not represent simple filtration of tracheal sounds by the intervening inflated lung. The *expiratory* component of vesicular sounds probably originates in more proximal, larger airways. Several lines of evidence support these statements:

1. In experiments performed with sheep's and calf's lungs more than a century ago, Bullar kept the airways of both lungs patent but rhythmically inflated only one of the two lungs using negative pressure.[12] He showed that vesicular sounds occurred only if the lung contiguous to the stethoscope filled with air; if it remained airless, it simply transmitted the upper airway bronchial sounds.
2. The intensity of the inspiratory component of breath sounds, corrected for flow rate at the mouth, is roughly proportional to regional ventilation.[13]
3. The inspiratory component of vesicular sounds remains the same as the stethoscope is moved progressively from the upper to lower posterior chest, although the expiratory component becomes softer.[14]
4. Vesicular sounds contain low-frequency components lacking in tracheal sounds, which cannot be reproduced in experiments interposing inflated lung between the trachea and stethoscope.[2–4]

b. *Intensity*

The intensity of vesicular sounds is proportional to the flow rate of air at the mouth, which in turn depends on the patient's effort and ventilatory capacity.[11,15,16] Breath sounds are thus louder if a normal person breathes hard after exercise and they are faint if obstructive lung disease diminishes flow rates.[17] Breath sounds are also reduced when air or fluid is interposed between the chest wall and lung, as in patients with pneumothorax and pleural effusion.

2. Bronchial Sounds

Bronchial breath sounds originate in larger, proximal airways. They are normally heard over the right upper chest posteriorly but not over the left upper chest, because the trachea is contiguous with the right lung near the first thoracic vertebra but separated from the left lung by most of the mediastinum.[18] The glottis is not necessary to the sound, because bronchial sounds may occur in patients after laryngectomy or after intubation.[19] The pathogenesis of bronchial breath sounds in pneumonia and pleural effusion is discussed in Section II.B later.

C. CLINICAL SIGNIFICANCE

1. Breath Sound Intensity

A breath sound score ≤9 is a compelling argument *for* chronic airflow obstruction (likelihood ratio [LR] = 10.2, EBM Box 27-1) and a score ≥16 is a compelling argument *against* the diagnosis (LR = 0.1). The importance of developing some objective scoring system of breath sound intensity is demonstrated by two other studies relying just on general impressions of breath sound intensity: One study showed that reduced breath sounds strongly argued for obstructive lung disease (LR = 16.5),[27] whereas another showed the finding to have no significance.[28]

In patients with acute respiratory distress syndrome receiving mechanical ventilation, the absence of breath sounds over a specific region of the chest argues for underlying pleural fluid (LR = 4.3, see EBM Box 27-1). Also, the appearance of reduced breath sounds during methacholine challenge argues for asthma (LR = 4.2), and the general impression of diminished breath sounds in patients with fever and cough modestly suggests pneumonia (LR = 2.3).

2. Bronchial Breath Sounds

In patients with cough and fever, bronchial breath sounds argues for pneumonia (LR = 3.3), although the sign is infrequent (sensitivity = 14%).

II. VOCAL RESONANCE

A. THE FINDING

Vocal resonance refers to the sound of the patient's voice heard through a stethoscope placed on the patient's chest. Normally, the voice sounds muffled, weak, and indistinct over most of the inferior and posterior chest, and words are unintelligible. Abnormal vocal resonance is usually classified as either bronchophony, pectoriloquy, or egophony, all terms originally introduced by Laennec.[1] Although these abnormalities have distinct definitions, the pathogenesis for all three is the same and all may appear simultaneously in the same patient. Bronchial breath sounds often accompany abnormal vocal resonance.

1. Bronchophony

Bronchophony describes a voice that is much louder than normal, as if the sounds were emitted directly into the stethoscope. The patient's words are not necessarily intelligible.

2. Pectoriloquy

Pectoriloquy implies that the patient's words are intelligible. Most clinicians test this by having the patient whisper words like "one-two-three"; intelligible whispered speech is called "whispered pectoriloquy."

Box 27-1 Breath Sounds and Vocal Resonance*

Finding (Ref)[†]	Sensitivity (%)	Specificity (%)	Likelihood Ratio if Finding	
			Present	Absent
Breath sound score				
Detecting chronic airflow obstruction[11,15]				
≤ 9	23–46	96–97	**10.2**	...
10–12	34–63	...	**3.6**	...
13–15	11–16	...	NS	...
≥ 16	3–10	33–34	**0.1**	...
Diminished breath sounds				
Detecting underlying pleural effusion in mechanically ventilated patient[20]	42	90	**4.3**	0.6
Detecting asthma during methacholine challenge [21]	78	81	**4.2**	**0.3**
Detecting pneumonia in patients with cough and fever[22–25]	15–49	73–95	2.3	0.8
Bronchial breath sounds				
Detecting pneumonia in patients with cough and fever[22]	14	96	**3.3**	NS
Egophony				
Detecting pneumonia in patients with cough and fever[22,24,26]	4–16	96–99	**4.1**	NS

NS, not significant; likelihood ratio (LR) if finding present = positive LR; LR if finding absent = negative LR.
*Diagnostic standard: For chronic airflow obstruction, FEV_1 < 40% predicted (studies on breath sound intensity[11,15]) or FEV_1/FVC (%) ratio <0.6[27]; for underlying pleural effusion (in mechanically ventilated patients), computed tomography[20]; for asthma, FEV_1 decreases ≥ 20% during methacholine challenge; and for pneumonia, infiltrate on chest radiograph.
†Definition of findings: For breath sound score, see text.

BREATH SOUNDS AND VOCAL RESONANCE

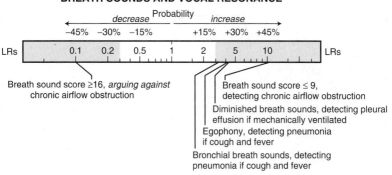

3. Egophony

Egophony is a peculiar nasal quality to the sound of the patient's voice, which Laennec likened to the "bleating of a goat."[1] Clinicians usually elicit the finding by having the patient vocalize the vowel "EE" and then listening for the abnormal transformation of the sound into a loud nasal "AH" (the "AH" sound ranges from the "a" of the word hat to the "a" of the word cart; this finding is sometimes called "E-to-A" change).* Although all vowel sounds are altered by the lung (even healthy lungs), what makes egophony distinctive is the intensity of the change and the suddenness with which it appears over a small area on *one* side of the chest.[31] Before concluding a patient has egophony, therefore, the clinician should confirm that a similar change of sound is absent over the identical location of the opposite chest.

B. PATHOGENESIS

Figure 27-1 depicts the transmission of sound from the larynx to the chest wall in normal persons and in those with pneumonia or pleural effusion. A normal lung behaves like a low-pass filter, which means it transmits low-frequency sounds (100–200 Hz) easily but filters out high-frequency sounds (>300 Hz), which include most upper airway sounds (e.g., bronchial breath sounds).[6,32–34] Consolidated lungs transmit all sound very well, both low and high frequencies. Large pleural effusions, but not small ones, reduce the transmission of frequencies less than 200 to 300 Hz but augment those more than 400 Hz.[6,10,32–34]

---

*The E-to-A change was simultaneously discovered in 1922 by Shibley[29] and Fröschels.[30] Shipley discovered it while testing for pectoriloquy in Chinese patients. He asked the patients to say "one-two-three" in the local dialect ("ee-er-san"), and he noted that the long "EE" of "one" acquired a loud nasal "AH" quality over areas of pneumonia or effusion.[29]

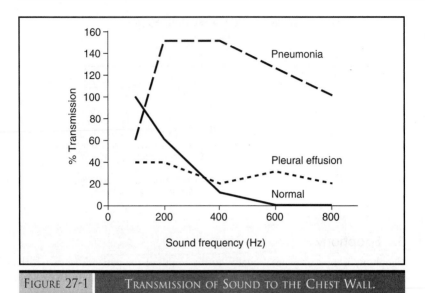

| FIGURE 27-1 | TRANSMISSION OF SOUND TO THE CHEST WALL. |

In this experiment, a speaker emitting pure musical tones of different frequencies was placed in the mouth of patients with normal lungs (*solid line*), pneumonia (*long dashes*), or massive pleural effusion (*short dashes*). Microphones on the chest wall recorded the transmission of each frequency (for purposes of comparison, "100% transmission" is the transmission of 100 Hz in normal persons). Adapted from Buller AJ, Dornshorst AC. The physics of some pulmonary signs. *Lancet.* 1956;2:649-651.

These observations explain why both pneumonia and large effusions cause abnormal vocal resonance and bronchial breath sounds, yet pneumonia increases tactile fremitus, whereas effusion decreases it. Tactile fremitus consists of low-frequency vibrations (100–200 Hz), explaining why it is more prominent over the chests of healthy men than healthy women (i.e., men's voices are lower pitched and therefore more likely to generate low-frequency vibrations than women's voices) and why tactile fremitus progressively diminishes as a healthy person sings an ascending scale. According to Fig. 27-1, pneumonia amplifies these low frequencies and thus increases tactile fremitus on the overlying chest wall. Large effusions, in contrast, reduce the transmission of low frequencies and thus diminish tactile fremitus.

Both pneumonia and large effusions transmit high frequencies much better than do healthy lungs (see Fig. 27-1), explaining why the high-frequency bronchial breath sounds, which are poorly transmitted to the peripheral chest wall of healthy lungs, occur in both disorders. Most acoustic speech consists of frequencies less than 300 Hz, although understanding whispered speech requires the transmission of frequencies higher than 400 Hz, thus explaining why whispering pectoriloquy occurs in both pneumonia and large effusions. The sound "AH" contains more high-frequency energy than the sound "EE," explaining how consolidated lungs alter the "EE" by amplifying its small amount of high-frequency energy and rendering it into a nasal "AH."[6,33]

C. CLINICAL SIGNIFICANCE

Abnormal vocal resonance has the same significance (and pathogenesis) as bronchial breath sounds. In patients with cough and fever, the finding of egophony argues *for* the diagnosis of pneumonia (LR = 4.1, see EBM Box 27-2). According to traditional teachings, an obstructed bronchus should diminish vocal resonance, although this teaching is probably incorrect, based on the more modern observations that some patients with egophony and pneumonia have obstructed bronchi from tumors and on experiments showing that sound conducts down the substance of the porous lung itself to the chest wall, not down the airway ducts.*[34,35]

III. ADVENTITIOUS SOUNDS

A. INTRODUCTION

Adventitious sounds are all sounds heard during auscultation other than breath sounds or vocal resonance. The common adventitious sounds are crackles, rubs, wheezes, rhonchi, and stridor.

Adventitious sounds have the most ambiguous and confusing nomenclature in all of physical diagnosis, and studies show clinicians use up to 16 different terms in scientific publications to describe similar sounds.[36] This confusion stems from the earliest days of auscultation and the writings of Laennec, who, in the first edition of his treatise, identified five adventitious sounds but called them all "rales," distinguishing them further only by adding adjectives (e.g., "moist crepitus rale" for a crackling sound or "dry sibilus rale" for a whistling sound).[1,37] In later editions, Laennec substituted "rhonchus" for "rale" because he became worried that patients hearing "rale" would mistake it for the death rattle ("rale" means "rattle"). In 1831, a British editor introduced the Anglo-Saxon term "wheeze," again to refer to all lung sounds.[37] Finally, Robertson in 1957 proposed using "crackling sounds" for discontinuous sounds and "wheezes" for

---

*The acoustic characteristics of the transmitted sound are the same whether the patient breathes air or a mixture of oxygen and helium. If sound were conducted down the airways, its characteristics would change with different gas mixtures.[35]

continuous, musical sounds, and suggested eliminating "rale" and "rhonchus" altogether.[38]

According to the American Thoracic Society, the recommended terms for lung sounds, based on their acoustic characteristics,[39] are "crackle" for discontinuous sounds and "wheeze" or "rhonchus" for continuous sounds (Table 27-2).

B. THE FINDING

1. Crackles

Crackles are discontinuous sounds, resembling the sound produced by rubbing strands of hair together in front of the ear or by pulling apart strips of Velcro. There are **coarse crackles,** which are loud, low-pitched, and fewer in number per breath, and **fine crackles,** which are soft, high-pitched, and greater in number per breath. Crackles that appear early during inspiration and do not continue beyond mid-inspiration are called **early inspiratory** crackles; those that continue into the second half of inspiration are called **late inspiratory** crackles.[42] Many American clinicians still use the word "rale" as a synonym for "crackle," although British clinicians more often use "crackle."[43,44]

Table 27-2	Terminology for Lung Sounds		
Recommended ATS term	**Acoustic Characteristics**	**Terms in Some Textbooks**	**British Usage**
Coarse crackle	Discontinuous sound: loud, low in pitch	Coarse rale	Crackle
Fine crackle	Discontinuous sound: soft, higher pitch, shorter duration	Fine rale	Crackle
Wheeze	Continuous sound: high-pitched, dominant frequency ≥ 400 Hz	Sibilant rhonchus	High-pitched wheeze
Rhonchus	Continuous sound: low-pitched, dominant frequency ≤ 200 Hz	Sonorous rhonchus	Low-pitched wheeze

Adapted from references 39–41.
ATS, American Thoracic Society.

The finding **posturally induced crackles**, which may have significance after myocardial infarction (see "Clinical Significance" later) indicates crackles that are present in the supine position but absent in the sitting position. To elicit the finding, the clinician listens to the lower chest wall near the posterior axillary line with the patient in three sequential positions: sitting, supine, and supine with legs elevated 30 degrees.[45] The clinician listens only after the patient has been in each position for 3 minutes. If crackles are absent when upright but appear either when supine or with legs elevated, the test is positive (i.e., the patient has posturally induced crackles).

2. Wheezes and Rhonchi

According to the American Thoracic Society, a wheeze is a high-pitched, continuous musical sound and a rhonchus is a low-pitched one (see Table 27-2). This distinction may be superfluous because both sounds have the same pathophysiology and there is no proven clinical importance to separating them. The term rhonchus is probably best avoided, not only for these reasons but because many use the term to refer to the coarse discontinuous sounds often heard in patients with airway secretions.[43]

3. Stridor

Stridor is a loud, musical sound of definite and constant pitch (usually about 400 Hz) that indicates upper airway obstruction.[34,41] It is identical acoustically to wheezing in every way except for two characteristics: (1) stridor is confined to inspiration whereas wheezing is either confined entirely to expiration (30%–60% of patients) or occurs during both expiration and inspiration (40%–70% of patients)[46,47]; (2) stridor is always louder over the neck, whereas wheezing is always louder over the chest.[47]

In some patients with upper airway obstruction, stridor does not appear until the patient breathes rapidly through an open mouth.[48]

4. Pleural Rub

Pleural rubs are loud grating or rubbing sounds associated with breathing that occur in patients with pleural disease. Sometimes, a pleural rub has a crackling character ("pleural crackling rub") and acoustically resembles the crackles heard in patients with parenchymal disease.[49,50] The timing of the crackling sound best distinguishes the pleural crackling rub from parenchymal crackles: the pleural crackling rub is predominately *expiratory* (i.e., 65% of crackling sound occurs during expiration), but parenchymal crackles are predominately *inspiratory* (i.e., only 10% of crackling sound occurs during expiration).[51]

5. Inspiratory Squawk

The "squawk" is a short, late-inspiratory musical sound that is associated with parenchymal crackles in patients with interstitial lung disease.[52] It is best heard over the upper anterior chest when the patient is semirecumbent and breathing deeply. Because the sound is sometimes found in patients with bird-fancier's lung (a cause of hypersensitivity pneumonitis), the synonym "chirping rale" has been proposed.[53]

In patients with hypersensitivity pneumonitis, the squawk tends to be shorter, high-pitched, and later in inspiration than the squawk of patients with diffuse pulmonary fibrosis.[52]

C. PATHOGENESIS

1. Crackles[34,42,49,54,55]

Crackles were initially attributed by Laennec and early auscultators to air bubbling through airway secretions. Although some crackles result from secretions, these promptly clear after the patient coughs. All remaining crackling sounds are believed to represent the sounds of distal airways, collapsed from the previous exhalation, as they abruptly open during inspiration. Several lines of evidence support this conclusion: (1) crackles are predominantly heard during inspiration, whereas air bubbling though secretions would cause both inspiratory and expiratory sounds; (2) the number of crackles has no relationship to the amount of sputum the patient produces (the disease with the most crackles, interstitial fibrosis, produces scant sputum or no sputum at all)[56]; (3) crackles have a stereotypic pattern with each respiratory cycle (i.e., in a single patient at a single location on the chest, they are always early-, late-, or paninspiratory, and individual crackles occur at the same esophageal (transpulmonary) pressure in consecutive respiratory cycles[57]; and (4) crackles are loudest in the lower portions of the chest, even when the lung disease is distributed diffusely.

Coarse crackles are believed to originate in larger, more proximal airways than fine crackles, based on the observations that distinct patterns of coarse crackles (identified by their fingerprint of identical timing and number) radiate to a larger area of the chest wall than do distinct patterns of fine crackles.[58,59]

2. Wheezes

Wheezes are caused by vibrations of the opposing walls of narrowed airways.[49,54,60] They are not due to resonance of air in the airways (i.e., like the sound of a flute or pipe organ) because (1) if they were due to resonance of air in a hollow pipe, the length of pipe for some low-pitched wheezes would be several feet, far exceeding the length of human airways; (2) the pitch of a wheeze may change between inspiration and expiration; and (3) the pitch of the wheeze remains the same when inspired air is replaced with a gas mixture of oxygen and helium (if because of resonance of air, the pitch should change).

D. CLINICAL SIGNIFICANCE

1. Crackles

The crackles discussed later refer only to crackling sounds that persist after the patient coughs.

a. Normal Persons

Crackles are rare in healthy persons during normal tidal breathing.[61,62] Fine crackling sounds, however, may appear in up to 60% of healthy persons, especially over the anterior chest, if the person first exhales as much as possible and breathes in from residual volume instead of functional residual capacity.[61,62]

b. Crackles and Disease

(1) Presence of Crackles   EBM Box 27-2 indicates that the finding of crackles suggests pulmonary fibrosis in asbestos workers (LR = 5.9), elevated left atrial pressure in patients with known heart disease (LR = 3.4), myocardial infarction in patients with chest pain (LR = 2.1), and pneumonia in patients with cough and fever (LR = 1.8).

Some interstitial lung diseases produce more crackles than others. For example, crackles are found in 100% of patients in idiopathic pulmonary fibrosis but only 5% to 20% of patients with fibrosis from sarcoidosis.[56,76] This suggests that the *absence* of crackles argues *against* idiopathic fibrosis. The only finding from computed tomography that seems to predict crackles in interstitial fibrosis is the degree of subpleural fibrosis.[76]

Although the finding of posturally induced crackles after myocardial infarction has been associated with higher pulmonary capillary wedge pressures and worse survival,[45] it is clear that any crackles in patients with acute coronary syndromes portends a worse prognosis. In one study of patients with acute sustained ischemic chest pain, crackles predicted 30-day mortality with a sensitivity of 36%, specificity of 92%, and a positive LR of 4.5.[77] The extent of crackles in patients with newly diagnosed congestive heart failure also predicts future cardiovascular mortality.[78]

(2) Characteristics of Crackles[51,71,79–81]   Table 27-3 describes the characteristic number, timing, and type of crackles in common crackling disorders, such as pulmonary fibrosis, congestive heart failure, pneumonia, and chronic obstructive lung disease. The crackles of interstitial fibrosis are characteristically fine, have a large number of individual crackling sounds each inspiration (6–14), and persist to the end of inspiration (i.e., they are "late inspiratory"). Crackles of chronic airflow obstruction are coarse or fine, have the smallest number of crackling sounds (1–4), and are confined to the first half of inspiration ("early inspiratory"). The crackles of heart failure and pneumonia lie between these

Box 27-2   Crackles and Wheezes*

Finding (Ref)	Sensitivity (%)	Specificity (%)	Likelihood Ratio if Finding	
			Present	Absent
Crackles				
Detecting pulmonary fibrosis in asbestos workers[63]	81	86	**5.9**	**0.2**
Detecting elevated left atrial pressure in patients with cardiomyopathy[64–66]	19–64	82–94	**3.4**	NS
Detecting myocardial infarction in patients with chest pain[67,68]	20–38	82–91	2.1	NS
Detecting pneumonia in patients with cough and fever[22–26,69,70]	19–67	36–94	1.8	0.8
Early inspiratory crackles				
Detecting chronic airflow obstruction in patients with crackles[42,71]	25–77	97–98	**14.6**	NS
Detecting severe disease in patients with chronic airflow obstruction[42]	90	96	**20.8**	**0.1**
Unforced wheezing				
Detecting chronic airflow obstruction[27,28,72–75]	13–56	86–99	2.8	0.8
Wheezing during methacholine challenge testing				
Detecting asthma[21]	44	93	**6.0**	0.6

NS, not significant; likelihood ratio (LR) if finding present = positive LR; LR if finding absent = negative LR.

*Diagnostic standard: For pulmonary fibrosis, fibrosis on high-resolution computed tomography; for elevated left atrial pressure, pulmonary capillary wedge pressure > 20 mm Hg[65] or > 22 mm Hg[64]; for myocardial infarction, development of new electrocardiographic Q waves, elevations of cardiac biomarkers (CK-MB or troponin), or both[67,68]; for pneumonia, infiltrate on chest radiograph; for chronic airflow obstruction, $FEV_1/FVC < 0.6$,[27] < 0.7,[72,75] < 0.75,[42] or less than lower 95% confidence interval for age, gender, and height[28,71,73,74]; for severe obstruction, $FEV_1/FVC < 0.44$[42]; and for asthma, FEV_1 decrease $\geq 20\%$ during methacholine challenge.[21]

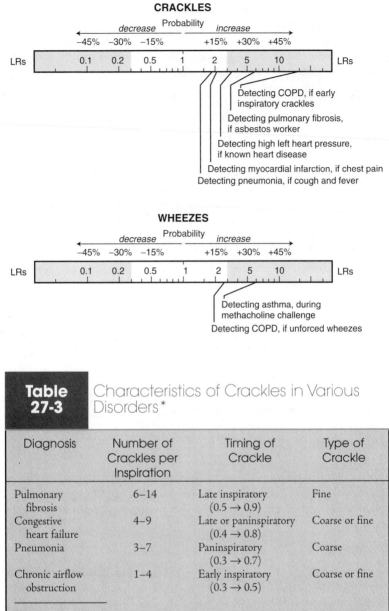

CRACKLES

decrease ← Probability → increase

−45% −30% −15%   +15% +30% +45%

LRs 0.1 0.2 0.5 1 2 5 10 LRs

Detecting COPD, if early
inspiratory crackles

Detecting pulmonary fibrosis,
if asbestos worker

Detecting high left heart pressure,
if known heart disease

Detecting myocardial infarction, if chest pain

Detecting pneumonia, if cough and fever

WHEEZES

decrease ← Probability → increase

−45% −30% −15%   +15% +30% +45%

LRs 0.1 0.2 0.5 1 2 5 10 LRs

Detecting asthma, during
methacholine challenge

Detecting COPD, if unforced wheezes

Table 27-3 Characteristics of Crackles in Various Disorders*

Diagnosis	Number of Crackles per Inspiration	Timing of Crackle	Type of Crackle
Pulmonary fibrosis	6–14	Late inspiratory (0.5 → 0.9)	Fine
Congestive heart failure	4–9	Late or paninspiratory (0.4 → 0.8)	Coarse or fine
Pneumonia	3–7	Paninspiratory (0.3 → 0.7)	Coarse
Chronic airflow obstruction	1–4	Early inspiratory (0.3 → 0.5)	Coarse or fine

*Number of crackles is mean number of crackles ± one standard deviation, after the patient first coughs to clear airway secretions. The descriptors early-, late-, paninspiratory, coarse, and fine are observations made by clinicians listening with the stethoscope; the numbers under timing refer to when crackles begin and end during a full inspiration (e.g., 0.5 → 0.9 means that crackles first appear at midinspiration (i.e., 0.5) and end when the patient has reached 90% of full inspiration (i.e., 0.9). Based on references 51, 71, and 79.

extremes; with treatment, the crackles of pneumonia become more fine and move more toward the end of inspiration.[80,81]

EBM Box 27-2 indicates the finding of early inspiratory crackles strongly suggests chronic obstructive lung disease (LR = 14.6). Most patients with these crackles have severe obstruction (LR = 20.8).

2. Wheezes

a. Presence of Wheezes

EBM Box 27-2 indicates that the finding of unforced wheezing increases the probability of chronic obstructive lung disease a small amount (LR = 2.8). If wheezing appears during methacholine challenge testing, asthma is likely (LR = 6.0). The absence of wheezing in either setting is unhelpful.

In contrast, the finding of *forced* wheezing lacks diagnostic value, because it can be produced by most healthy persons if they exhale forcibly enough.[72,82]

b. Characteristics of Wheezing

The characteristics of wheezes are their length, pitch, and amplitude. Of these, only length and pitch vary with severity of obstruction. The longer the wheeze, the more severe the obstruction (r = −0.89 between the proportion of the respiratory cycle occupied by wheezing and the patient's FEV_1*, $p <$ .001).[46,83,84] High-pitched wheezes indicate worse obstruction than low-pitched ones, and effective bronchodilator therapy reduces the pitch of the patient's wheeze.[46,83]

The amplitude of the wheeze, however, does not reflect the severity of obstruction, primarily because many patients with severe obstruction have faint or no wheezes.[46,72,83,84] This finding supports the old adage that, in a patient with asthma, the quiet chest is not necessarily a favorable sign and may instead indicate the patient is tiring and unable to push air across the obstructed airways.

The "slide whistle" sound, a unique wheezing sound whose pitch rises during inspiration and falls during expiration, has been described in a patient with a spherical tumor arising from the carina that nearly completely obstructed the trachea.[85]

3. Stridor

In patients with tracheal stenosis after tracheostomy, stridor is a late finding, usually appearing after symptoms like dyspnea, irritative cough, or difficulty clearing the throat.[48] Stridor indicates that the airway diameter is less than 5 mm.[48]

---

*See Chapter 25 for definition of FEV_1.

REFERENCES

1. Laennec RTH. *A treatise on the diseases of the chest* (facsimile edition by Classics of Medicine library). London: T. and G. Underwood; 1821.
2. Hannon RR, Lyman RS. Studies on pulmonary acoustics. II. The transmission of tracheal sounds through freshly exenterated sheep's lung. *Am Rev Tuberc.* 1929;19: 360-375.
3. Gavriely N, Palti Y, Alroy G. Spectral characteristics of normal breath sounds. *J Appl Physiol.* 1981;50:307-314.
4. Gavriely N, Nissan M, Rubin AHE, Cugell DW. Spectral characteristics of chest wall breath sounds in normal subjects. *Thorax.* 1995;50:1292-1300.
5. Cabot RC, Dodge HF. Frequency characteristics of heart and lung sounds. *JAMA.* 1925;84:1793-1795.
6. McKusick VA, Jenkins JT, Webb GN. The acoustic basis of the chest examination: Studies by means of sound spectrography. *Am Rev Tuberc.* 1955;72:12-34.
7. Martini P, Mueller H. Studien über das Bronchialatmen. *Deut Archiv Klin Med.* 1923;143:159-172.
8. Skoda J. *Auscultation and percussion.* Philadelphia: Lindsay and Blakiston; 1854.
9. Flint A. *A manual of percussion and auscultation.* Philadelphia: Henry C. Lea; 1876.
10. Bernstein A, White FZ. Unusual physical findings in pleural effusion: Intrathoracic manometric studies. *Ann Intern Med.* 1952;37:733-738.
11. Pardee NE, Martin CJ, Morgan EH. A test of the practical value of estimating breath sound intensity: Breath sounds related to measured ventilatory function. *Chest.* 1976;70:341-344.
12. Bullar JF, Cantab MB. Experiments to determine the origin of the respiratory sounds. *Proc R Soc London Series B: Biol Sci.* 1884;37:411-422.
13. Leblanc P, Macklem PT, Ross WRD. Breath sounds and distribution of pulmonary ventilation. *Am Rev Respir Dis.* 1970;102:10-16.
14. Kraman SS. Determination of the site of production of respiratory sounds by subtraction phonopneumography. *Am Rev Respir Dis.* 1980;122:303-309.
15. Bohadana AB, Peslin R, Uffholtz H. Breath sounds in the clinical assessment of airflow obstruction. *Thorax.* 1978;33:345-351.
16. Kraman SS. The relationship between airflow and lung sound amplitude in normal subjects. *Chest.* 1984;86:225-229.
17. Schreur HJW, Sterk PJ, Vanderschoot J, et al. Lung sound intensity in patients with emphysema and in normal subjects at standardised airflows. *Thorax.* 1992;47:674-679.
18. Kraman SS, Austrheim O. Comparison of lung sound and transmitted sound amplitude in normal men. *Am Rev Respir Dis.* 1983;128:451-454.
19. Fahr G. The acoustics of the bronchial breath sounds: Application to phenomena of auscultation as heard in lobar pneumonia. *Arch Intern Med.* 1926;39:286-302.
20. Lichtenstein D, Goldstein I, Mourgeon E, et al. Comparative diagnostic performance of auscultation, chest radiography, and lung ultrasonography in acute respiratory distress syndrome. *Anesthesiology.* 2004;10:9-15.

21. Purohit A, Bohadana A, Kopferschmitt-Kubler MC, et al. Lung auscultation in airway challenge testing. *Resp Med.* 1997;91:151-157.

22. Heckerling PS, Tape TG, Wigton RS, et al. Clinical prediction rule for pulmonary infiltrates. *Ann Intern Med.* 1990;113:664-670.

23. Melbye H, Straume B, Aasebo U, Brox J. The diagnosis of adult pneumonia in general practice. *Scand J Prim Health Care.* 1988;6:111-117.

24. Gennis P, Gallagher J, Falvo C, et al. Clinical criteria for the detection of pneumonia in adults: Guidelines for ordering chest roentgenograms in the emergency department. *J Emerg Med.* 1989;7:263-268.

25. Melbye H, Straume B, Aasebo U, Dale K. Diagnosis of pneumonia in adults in general practice. *Scand J Prim Health Care.* 1992;10:226-233.

26. Diehr P, Wood RW, Bushyhead J, et al. Prediction of pneumonia in outpatients with acute cough: A statistical approach. *J Chron Dis.* 1984;37:215-225.

27. Badgett RG, Tanaka DJ, Hunt DK, et al. Can moderate chronic obstructive pulmonary disease be diagnosed by historical and physical findings alone? *Am J Med.* 1993;94:188-196.

28. Holleman DR, Simel DL, Goldberg JS. Diagnosis of obstructive airways disease from the clinical examination. *J Gen Intern Med.* 1993;8:63-68.

29. Shibley GS. A new auscultatory sign found in consolidation, or the collection of fluid, in pulmonary disease. *China Med J.* 1922;36:1-9.

30. Fröschels E, Stockert FG. Ueber ein neues Symptom bei Lungen-und Pleuraerkrankungen. *Wien Klin Wochenschr.* 1922;22:500-501.

31. Stokes W. *An introduction to the use of the stethoscope* (facsimile edition by the Classics of Cardiology Library). Edinburgh: Maclachlin and Stewart; 1825.

32. Buller AJ, Dornshorst AC. The physics of some pulmonary signs. *Lancet.* 1956;2:649-651.

33. Baughman RP, Loudon RG. Sound spectral analysis of voice-transmitted sound. *Am Rev Respir Dis.* 1986;134:167-169.

34. Forgacs P. The functional basis of pulmonary sounds. *Chest.* 1978;73:399-412.

35. Mahagnah M, Gavriely N. Gas density does not affect pulmonary acoustic transmission in normal men. *J Appl Physiol.* 1995;78:928-937.

36. Bunin NJ, Loudon RG. Lung sound terminology in case reports. *Chest.* 1979;76:690-692.

37. Andrews JL, Badger TL. Lung sounds through the ages: from Hippocrates to Laënnec to Osler. *JAMA.* 1979;241:2625-2630.

38. Robertson AJ. Râles, rhonchi, and Laënnec. *Lancet.* 1957;2:417-423.

39. Murphy RLH, Holford SK, Knowler WC. Visual lung-sound characterization by time-expanded wave-form analysis. *N Engl J Med.* 1977;296:968-971.

40. Cugell D, George R, Murphy R, Teirstein A. Updated nomenclature for membership reaction: Reports from the ATS Ad Hoc Committee on Pulmonary Nomenclature. *ATS News.* 1977;3:5-6.

41. Loudon RG. The lung exam. *Clin Chest Med.* 1987;8:265-272.

42. Nath AR, Capel LH. Inspiratory crackles: Early and late. *Thorax.* 1974;29: 223-227.
43. Wilkins RL, Dexter JR, Murphy RLH, DelBono EA. Lung sound nomenclature survey. *Chest.* 1990;98:886-889.
44. Wilkins RL, Dexter JR, Smith JR. Survey of adventitious lung sound terminology in case reports. *Chest.* 1984;85:523-525.
45. Deguchi F, Hirakawa S, Gotoh K, et al. Prognostic significance of posturally induced crackles: Long-term follow-up of patients after recovery from acute myocardial infarction. *Chest.* 1993;103:1457-1462.
46. Shim CS, Williams MH. Relationship of wheezing to the severity of obstruction in asthma. *Arch Intern Med.* 1983;143:890-892.
47. Baughman RP, Loudon RG. Stridor: Differentiation from asthma or upper airway noise. *Am Rev Respir Dis.* 1989;139:1407-1409.
48. Geffin B, Grillo HC, Cooper JD, Pontoppidan H. Stenosis following tracheostomy for respiratory care. *JAMA.* 1971;216:1984-1988.
49. Forgacs P. Crackles and wheezes. *Lancet.* 1967;2:203-205.
50. Forgacs P. Lung sounds. *Br J Dis Chest.* 1969;63:1-12.
51. Al Jarad N, Davies SW, Logan-Sinclair R, Rudd RM. Lung crackle characteristics in patients with asbestosis, asbestos-related pleural disease and left ventricular failure using a time-expanded waveform analysis: A comparative study. *Resp Med.* 1994; 88:37-46.
52. Earis JE, Marsh K, Pearson MG, Ogilvie CM. The inspiratory "squawk" in extrinsic allergic alveolitis and other pulmonary fibroses. *Thorax.* 1982;37:923-926.
53. Reich JM. Chirping rales in bird-fancier's lung. *Chest.* 1993;104:326-327.
54. Forgacs P. The functional significance of clinical signs in diffuse airway obstruction. *Br J Dis Chest.* 1971;65:170-177.
55. Forgacs P. *Lung sounds.* London: Bailliere Tindall; 1978.
56. Epler GR, Carrington CB, Gaensler EA. Crackles (rales) in the interstitial pulmonary diseases. *Chest.* 1978;73:333-339.
57. Nath AR, Capel LH. Inspiratory crackles and mechanical events of breathing. *Thorax.* 1974;29:695-698.
58. Murphy RLH. Discontinuous adventitious lung sounds. *Semin Respir Med.* 1985;6:210-219.
59. Loudon R, Murphy RLH. Lung sounds. *Am Rev Resp Dis.* 1984;130:663-673.
60. Gavriely N, Shee TR, Cugell DW, Grotberg JB. Flutter in flow-limited collapsible tubes: A mechanism for generation of wheezes. *J Appl Physiol.* 1989;66: 2251-2261.
61. Thacker RE, Kraman SS. The prevalence of auscultatory crackles in subjects without lung disease. *Chest.* 1982;81:672-674.
62. Workum P, Holford SK, Delbono EZ, Murphy RLH. The prevalence and character of crackles (rales) in young women without significant lung disease. *Am Rev Respir Dis.* 1982;126:921-923.

63. Al Jarad N, Strickland B, Bothamley G, et al. Diagnosis of asbestosis by a time expanded wave form analysis, auscultation and high resolution computed tomography: A comparative study. *Thorax.* 1993;48:347-353.

64. Stevenson LW, Perloff JK. The limited reliability of physical signs for estimating hemodynamics in chronic heart failure. *JAMA.* 1989;261:884-888.

65. Chakko S, Woska D, Martinez H, et al. Clinical, radiographic, and hemodynamic correlations in chronic congestive heart failure: Conflicting results may lead to inappropriate care. *Am J Med.* 1991;90:353-359.

66. Butman SM, Ewy GA, Standen JR, et al. Bedside cardiovascular examination in patients with severe chronic heart failure: Importance of rest or inducible jugular venous distension. *J Am Coll Cardiol.* 1993;22:968-974.

67. Baxt WG. Use of an artificial neural network for the diagnosis of myocardial infarction. *Ann Intern Med.* 1991;115:843-848.

68. Tierney WM, Fitzgerald J, McHenry R, et al. Physicians' estimates of the probability of myocardial infarction in emergency room patients with chest pain. *Med Decis Making.* 1986;6:12-17.

69. Singal BM, Hedges JR, Radack KL. Decision rules and clinical prediction of pneumonia: Evaluation of low-yield criteria. *Ann Emerg Med.* 1989;18:13-20.

70. Mehr DR, Binder EF, Kruse RL, et al. Clinical findings associated with radiographic pneumonia in nursing home residents. *J Fam Pract.* 2001;50:931-937.

71. Bettencourt PE, Del Bono EA, Spiegelman D, et al. Clinical utility of chest auscultation in common pulmonary diseases. *Am J Respir Crit Care Med.* 1994;150: 1291-1297.

72. Marini JJ, Pierson DJ, Hudson LD, Lakshminarayan S. The significance of wheezing in chronic airflow obstruction. *Am Rev Respir Dis.* 1979;120:1069-1072.

73. Straus SE, McAlister FA, Sackett DL, Deeks JJ. The accuracy of patient history, wheezing, and laryngeal measurements in diagnosing obstructive airway disease. *JAMA.* 2000;283:1853-1857.

74. Straus S, McAlister FA, Sackett DL, Deeks JJ. Accuracy of history, wheezing, and forced expiratory time in the diagnosis of chronic obstructive pulmonary disease. *J Gen Intern Med.* 2002;17:684-688.

75. Garcia-Pachon E. Paradoxical movement of the lateral rib margin (Hoover sign) for detecting obstructive airway disease. *Chest.* 2002;122:651-655.

76. Baughman RP, Shipley RT, Loudon RG, Lower EE. Crackles in interstitial lung disease: Comparison of sarcoidosis and fibrosing alveolitis. *Chest.* 1991;100:96-101.

77. Boersma E, Pieper KS, Steyerberg EW, et al. Predictors of outcome in patients with acute coronary syndromes without persistent ST-segment elevation: Results from an international trial of 9461 patients. *Circulation.* 2000;101:2557-2567.

78. Cowie MR, Wood DA, Coats AJS, et al. Survival of patients with a new diagnosis of heart failure: A population based study. *Heart.* 2000;83:505-510.

79. Piirila P, Sovijarvi ARA, Kaisla T, et al. Crackles in patients with fibrosing alveolitis, bronchiectasis, COPD, and heart failure. *Chest.* 1991;99:1076-1083.

80. Piirila P. Changes in crackle characteristics during the clinical course of pneumonia. *Chest.* 1992;102:176-183.

81. Sovijarvi ARA, Piirila P, Luukkonen R. Separation of pulmonary disorders with two-dimensional discriminant analysis of crackles. *Clin Physiol.* 1996;16:171-181.

82. King DK, Thompson BT, Johnson DC. Wheezing on maximal forced exhalation in the diagnosis of atypical asthma: Lack of sensitivity and specificity. *Ann Intern Med.* 1989;110:451-455.

83. Baughman RP, Loudon RG. Quantitation of wheezing in acute asthma. *Chest.* 1984;86:718-722.

84. Baughman RP, Loudon RG. Lung sound analysis for continuous evaluation of air-flow obstruction in asthma. *Chest.* 1985;88:364-368.

85. Kraman SS, Harper P, Pasterkamp H, Wodicka GR. `Slide whistle' breath sounds: acoustical correlates of variable tracheal obstruction. *Physiol Meas.* 2002;23:449-455.

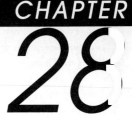

Ancillary Tests

I. FORCED EXPIRATORY TIME

A. TECHNIQUE

To measure the forced expiratory time, the clinician places the stethoscope bell over the trachea of the patient in the suprasternal notch and asks the patient to take a deep breath and blow it all out as fast as possible.[1] Using a stopwatch, the duration of the audible expiratory sound is determined to the nearest half second.

Rosenblatt introduced this test in 1962 as a test of obstructive lung disease.[2]

B. PATHOGENESIS

The forced expiratory time should be prolonged in obstructive disease simply because, by definition, the forced expiratory volume in 1 second divided by forced vital capacity (i.e., the ratio of FEV_1 to FVC) is reduced in this disorder. Slower flow rates prolong expiratory times.

C. CLINICAL SIGNIFICANCE

EBM Box 28-1 summarizes the accuracy of this finding, showing that a forced expiratory time less than 3 seconds is a compelling argument *against* obstructive disease (likelihood ratio [LR] = 0.2, see EBM Box 28-1) and a time ≥9 seconds argues *for* disease (LR = 4.1).

Box 28-1   Ancillary Tests

Finding (Ref)	Sensitivity (%)	Specificity (%)	Likelihood Ratio if Finding	
			Present	Absent
Forced expiratory time				
Detecting chronic airflow obstruction[1,3,4]				
<3 seconds	8–10	26–62	**0.2**	...
3–9 seconds	42–54	...	NS	...
≥9 seconds	29–50	86–98	**4.1**	...
Unable to blow out the match (Snider test)				
Detecting FEV_1 of ≤1.6L[5,6]	62–90	91–93	**9.6**	**0.2**

NS, not significant; FEV_1, forced expiratory volume in 1 second; likelihood ratio (LR) if finding present = positive LR; LR if finding absent = negative LR.
*Diagnostic standard: For chronic airflow obstruction, $FEV_1/FVC < 0.7$.

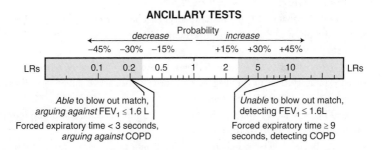

ANCILLARY TESTS

Able to blow out match, arguing against $FEV_1 ≤ 1.6$ L
Forced expiratory time < 3 seconds, arguing against COPD

Unable to blow out match, detecting $FEV_1 ≤ 1.6$L
Forced expiratory time ≥ 9 seconds, detecting COPD

The forced expiratory time is a specific test for obstruction. Patients with restrictive lung disease, despite having reductions in the FEV_1 similar to those seen in obstructive lung disease, usually have forced expiratory times ≤4 seconds.[1,2]

II.   BLOW-OUT-THE-MATCH TEST

A.   TECHNIQUE

The clinician lights a match and holds it 10 to 15 cm in front of the sitting patient, who then attempts to extinguish it by blowing as forcibly as possible.

It is important that the patient hold the mouth open and not purse the lips. Inability to extinguish the burning match is the positive finding.

The "match test" was introduced by Snider in 1959, who reasoned that the ability to extinguish a match was related to the velocity of exhaled air.[5] The test is now often called the "Snider test."

B. CLINICAL SIGNIFICANCE

EBM Box 28-1 indicates that a positive Snider test (i.e., unable to extinguish the match) argues that the patient's FEV_1 is at least moderately reduced to 1.6 L or less (LR = 9.6, see EBM Box 28-1). Being able to extinguish the match argues against an FEV_1 this low (LR = 0.2). Unlike the forced expiratory time, the Snider test is abnormal in both obstructive and restrictive lung disease, which probably explains why the Snider test performs less well in studies using it as a specific sign of obstructive disease.[7]

REFERENCES

1. Lal S, Ferguson AD, Campbell EJM. Forced expiratory time: A simple test for airways obstruction. *Br Med J.* 1964;1:814-817.
2. Rosenblatt G, Stein M. Clinical value of the forced expiratory time measured during auscultation. *N Engl J Med.* 1962;267:432-435.
3. Schapira RM, Schapira MM, Funahashi A, et al. The value of the forced expiratory time in the physical diagnosis of obstructive airways disease. *JAMA.* 1993;270: 731-736.
4. Straus S, McAlister FA, Sackett DL, Deeks JJ. Accuracy of history, wheezing, and forced expiratory time in the diagnosis of chronic obstructive pulmonary disease. *J Gen Intern Med.* 2002;17:684-688.
5. Snider TH, Stevens JP, Wilner FM, Lewis BM. Simple bedside test of respiratory function. *JAMA.* 1959;170:1691-1692.
6. Marks A, Bocles J. The match test and its significance. *South Med J.* 1960;53: 1211-1216.
7. Badgett RG, Tanaka DJ, Hunt DK, et al. Can moderate chronic obstructive pulmonary disease be diagnosed by historical and physical findings alone? *Am J Med.* 1993;94:188-196.

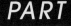

SELECTED PULMONARY DISORDERS

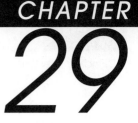
Pneumonia

I. INTRODUCTION

Like most of the pulmonary examination, the traditional findings of lobar pneumonia were described in 1819 by Laennec, who wrote that clinicians using his newly invented stethoscope could detect acute pneumonia "in every possible case."[1] According to traditional teachings, the earliest findings of pneumonia are crackles and diminished breath sounds, followed by dullness to percussion, increased tactile fremitus and vocal resonance, and bronchial breath sounds.[2]

II. CLINICAL SIGNIFICANCE

A. INDIVIDUAL FINDINGS

EBM Box 29-1 reviews the findings from more than 6000 patients presenting with acute fever, cough, sputum production, or dyspnea, all of whom underwent chest radiography (the diagnostic standard for pneumonia). In these patients, the findings arguing *for* the pneumonia were, in descending order of their positive likelihood ratios (LRs), egophony (LR = 4.1), cachexia (LR = 4.0), bronchial breath sounds (LR = 3.3), percussion dullness (LR = 3.0), diminished breath sounds (LR = 2.3), temperature greater than 37.8°C (LR = 2.0),

Box 29-1 Pneumonia*

Finding (Ref)[†]	Sensitivity (%)	Specificity (%)	Likelihood Ratio if Finding	
			Present	Absent
General appearance				
Cachexia[3]	10	97	**4.0**	NS
Abnormal mental status[4–6]	12–14	92–95	1.9	NS
Vital signs				
Temperature >37.8°C[3–8]	27–69	49–94	2.0	0.7
Respiratory rate >28/min[7]	36	82	2.0	0.8
Heart rate >100/min[3–7]	17–65	60–92	1.6	0.8
Lung findings				
Percussion dullness[3–5,9,10]	4–26	82–99	**3.0**	NS
Diminished breath sounds[4,5,9,10]	15–49	73–95	2.3	0.8
Bronchial breath sounds[4]	14	96	**3.3**	NS
Egophony[3–5]	4–16	96–99	**4.1**	NS
Crackles[3–6,8–10]	19–67	36–94	1.8	0.8
Wheezing[4–6,8–10]	15–36	50–85	0.8	NS
Diagnostic score (Heckerling et al.)[4,11]				
0 or 1 findings	7–29	33–65	**0.3**	...
2 or 3 findings	48–55	...	NS	...
4 or 5 findings	38–41	92–97	**8.2**	...

NS, not significant; likelihood ratio (LR) if finding present = positive LR; LR if finding absent = negative LR.

*Diagnostic standard: For pneumonia, infiltrate on chest radiograph.

[†]Definition of findings: For Heckerling's diagnostic score, the clinician scores 1 point for each of the following five findings that are present: temperature >37.8°C, heart rate >100/min, crackles, diminished breath sounds, and absence of asthma.

PNEUMONIA

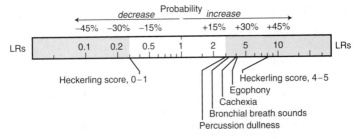

respiratory rate greater than 28/minute (LR = 2.0), abnormal mental status (LR = 1.9), and crackles (LR = 1.8). The *absence* of sore throat (LR = 1.8) and *absence* of rhinorrhea (LR = 2.2) also argue *for* pneumonia among patients with acute cough.[3,9]

No individual finding argues convincingly *against* the diagnosis of pneumonia (i.e., no LR < 0.5). In many studies, wheezing was found more often in patients *without* pneumonia, primarily because in these patients, the cause of the acute respiratory complaints was asthma not pneumonia.[4,5,9,10]

B. LAENNEC VERSUS MODERN STUDIES

There are three reasons why the studies in EBM Box 29-1 contradict Laennec's assertion that physical diagnosis is the perfect diagnostic tool: (1) The diagnosis of pneumonia today includes patients with more mild disease than in Laennec's time, when the only available diagnostic standard was postmortem examination (i.e., his conclusions were drawn from patients with only the most severe disease). (2) Many traditional findings appear only after several days of illness, times when the modern clinician, already familiar with the chest radiograph, often examines patients in a more cursory fashion. In contrast, Laennec examined each of his patients diligently day after day, concluding that bronchial breath sounds and bronchophony usually appeared only after 1 to 3 days of hospitalization, and dullness to percussion appeared only after day 4.[1,12] (3) Antimicrobial medications probably alter the course of the physical findings. For example, in the preantibiotic era, fever usually lasted 7 days in patients with lobar pneumonia[13]; now, it usually lasts only 3 or 4 days.[14,15]

Even so, many great clinicians of the past tempered Laennec's enthusiasm and taught that auscultation was an imperfect diagnostic tool. Writing just 20 years after Laennec's treatise, Thomas Addison* stated it was high time "to strip the stethoscope of the extravagant and meretricious pretensions thrust upon it . . . and to state fairly what it will not, as well as what it will do . . ."[16]

---

*Thomas Addison, the discoverer of adrenal insufficiency, was also a recognized master of percussion and auscultation.

C.   COMBINED FINDINGS

Combining findings improves the accuracy of bedside examination. One of the best models, validated in four different populations,[4,11] scores 1 point for each of the following five findings: (1) temperature greater than 37.8°C, (2) heart rate greater than 100/minute, (3) crackles, (4) diminished breath sounds, and (5) *absence* of asthma. EBM Box 29-1 shows that a score of 4 or 5 argues compellingly *for* pneumonia (LR = 8.2), whereas a score of 0 or 1 argues *against* pneumonia (LR = 0.3), which, in some groups of patients, may lower the probability of pneumonia enough that a chest radiograph becomes unnecessary (e.g., in patients presenting to a community office with cough, in whom the probability of pneumonia is 10% or less, a score of 0 or 1 reduces the probability of pneumonia to 3% or less).

D.   PNEUMONIA AND PROGNOSIS

In studies of immunocompetent adults hospitalized with community-acquired pneumonia, the 30-day mortality rate is about 10%. Of the individual findings that predict an increased risk of death (EBM Box 29-2), the most compelling ones are hypotension (LR = 10.0) and hypothermia (LR = 3.5).

Several different scoring schemes combine bedside findings to predict mortality in patients with pneumonia. One of the best validated is the "Pneumonia Severity Index,"[19,26,29] which unfortunately has the disadvantage of requiring knowledge of 20 different clinical variables, making it difficult to recall and apply at the bedside. A much simpler rule is the *CURB* score, based on four prognostic variables* identified decades ago by the British Thoracic Society[21]: (1) confusion, (2) blood urea nitrogen (BUN) greater than 19 mg/dL (>7 mmol/L), (3) respiratory rate ≥30/minute, and (4) hypotension (i.e., diastolic blood pressure ≤60 mm Hg or systolic blood pressure ≤90 mm Hg). The presence of 3 or more of these *CURB* variables is associated with increased hospital mortality (LR= 4.7 for 3 findings and LR = 10.2 for 4 findings, EBM Box 29-2), whereas the absence of all CURB variables is associated with decreased hospital mortality (LR = 0.3 for 0 findings).

E.   HOSPITAL COURSE

Among survivors of pneumonia, abnormalities of the vital signs—fever, tachycardia, tachypnea, and hypotension—usually become normal within 2 to 4 days.[14,15] Once this occurs, subsequent clinical deterioration is rare, and fewer than 1% of patients will require subsequent intensive care, coronary care, or telemetry monitoring.[14] If patients are discharged from the hospital before normalization of vital signs, there is an increased risk of readmission and death.[30]

---

*CURB is an acronym for Confusion, Urea, Respiratory rate, and Blood pressure.[28]

Box 29-2 Pneumonia: Predictors of Hospital Mortality

Finding (Ref)*	Sensitivity (%)	Specificity (%)	Likelihood Ratio if Finding Present	Absent
General appearance				
Abnormal mental status[17-20]	48–65	70–87	2.8	0.6
Vital signs				
Respiratory rate >30/min[18,19,21-23]	41–85	63–87	2.1	0.6
Systolic blood pressure <90 mm Hg[18,24,25]	11–35	97–99	**10.0**	NS
Heart rate >100/min[17]	45	78	2.1	NS
Hypothermia[18,25]	14–43	93	**3.5**	NS
"CURB" prognostic score[26-28]				
0 findings	5–19	49–68	**0.3**	...
1 finding	18–41	...	NS	...
2 findings	17–37	...	1.9	...
3 findings	8–32	...	**4.7**	...
4 findings	2–13	99–100	**10.2**	...

NS, not significant; BUN, blood urea nitrogen; likelihood ratio (LR) if finding present = positive LR; LR if finding absent = negative LR.
*Definition of findings: For hypothermia, body temperature < 36.1 °C[18] or < 37.0 °C[25]; for CURB prognostic score, the clinician scores 1 point for each of the following findings that are present: confusion, BUN >19 mg/dL, respiratory rate ≥30/min, and low blood pressure (either systolic blood pressure ≤90 mm Hg or diastolic blood pressure ≤60 mm Hg.

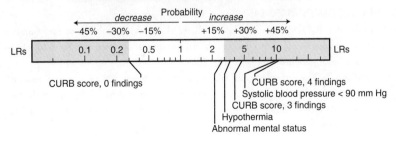

PNEUMONIA : PREDICTORS OF MORTALITY

REFERENCES

1. Laennec RTH. *A treatise on the diseases of the chest* (facsimile edition by Classics of Medicine library). London: T. and G. Underwood; 1821.
2. Cabot RC. *Physical diagnosis*. New York: William Wood and Co.; 1926.
3. Diehr P, Wood RW, Bushyhead J, et al. Prediction of pneumonia in outpatients with acute cough: A statistical approach. *J Chron Dis*. 1984;37:215-225.
4. Heckerling PS, Tape TG, Wigton RS, et al. Clinical prediction rule for pulmonary infiltrates. *Ann Intern Med*. 1990;113:664-670.
5. Gennis P, Gallagher J, Falvo C, et al. Clinical criteria for the detection of pneumonia in adults: Guidelines for ordering chest roentgenograms in the emergency department. *J Emerg Med*. 1989;7:263-268.
6. Mehr DR, Binder EF, Kruse RL, et al. Clinical findings associated with radiographic pneumonia in nursing home residents. *J Fam Pract*. 2001;50:931-937.
7. Heckerling PS. The need for chest roentgenograms in adults with acute respiratory illness: Clinical predictors. *Arch Intern Med*. 1986;146:1321-1324.
8. Singal BM, Hedges JR, Radack KL. Decision rules and clinical prediction of pneumonia: Evaluation of low-yield criteria. *Ann Emerg Med*. 1989;18:13-20.
9. Melbye H, Straume B, Aasebo U, Dale K. Diagnosis of pneumonia in adults in general practice. *Scand J Prim Health Care*. 1992;10:226-233.
10. Melbye H, Straume B, Aasebo U, Brox J. The diagnosis of adult pneumonia in general practice. *Scand J Prim Health Care*. 1988;6:111-117.
11. Emerman CL, Dawson N, Speroff T, et al. Comparison of physician judgment and decision aids for ordering chest radiographs for pneumonia in outpatients. *Ann Emerg Med*. 1991;20:1215-1219.
12. Auenbrugger L. *On percussion of the chest (1761), being a translation of Auenbrugger's original treatise entitled "Inventum novum ex percussione thoracis humani, ut signo abstrusos interni pectoris morbos detegendi"* (facsimile edition by Johns Hopkins Press). Baltimore: The Johns Hopkins Press; 1936.
13. Sahli H. *A treatise on diagnostic methods of examination*. Philadelphia: W. B. Saunders; 1911.
14. Halm EA, Fine MJ, Marrie TJ, et al. Time to clinical stability in patients hospitalized with community-acquired pneumonia: Implications for practice guidelines. *JAMA*. 1998;279:1452-1457.
15. Menendez R, Torres A, de Castro FR, et al. Reaching stability in community-acquired pneumonia: The effects of the severity of disease, treatment, and the characteristics of patients. *Clin Infect Dis*. 2004;39:1783-1790.
16. Addison T. The difficulties and fallacies attending physical diagnosis of diseases of the chest. In: Wilks, Daldy, eds. *A collection of the published writings of the late Thomas Addison* (facsimile edition by Classics of Medicine library). London: The New Sydenham society; 1846:242.

17. Starczewski AR, Allen SC, Vargas E, Lye M. Clinical prognostic indices of fatality in elderly patients admitted to hospital with acute pneumonia. *Age Ageing.* 1988;17:181-186.

18. Conte HA, Chen YT, Mehal W, et al. A prognostic rule for elderly patients admitted with community-acquired pneumonia. *Am J Med.* 1999;106:20-28.

19. Ewig S, Kleinfeld T, Seifert K, et al. Comparative validation of prognostic rules for community-acquired pneumonia in an elderly population. *Eur Respir J.* 1999;14: 370-375.

20. Neill AM, Martin IR, Weir R, et al. Community acquired pneumonia: Aetiology and usefulness of severity criteria on admission. *Thorax.* 1996;51:1010-1016.

21. Research Committee of the British Thoracic Society. Community-acquired pneumonia in adults in British hospitals in 1982-1983: A survey of aetiology, mortality, prognostic factors and outcome. *Q J Med.* 1987;62:195-220.

22. Farr BM, Sloman AJ, Fisch MJ. Predicting death in patients hospitalized for community-acquired pneumonia. *Ann Intern Med.* 1991;115:428-436.

23. Brancati FL, Chow JW, Wagener MM, et al. Is pneumonia really the old man's friend? Two-year prognosis after community-acquired pneumonia. *Lancet.* 1993;342:30-33.

24. Fedullo AJ, Swinburne AJ. Relationship of patient age to clinical features and outcome for in-hospital treatment of pneumonia. *J Gerontol.* 1985;40:29-33.

25. Allen SC. Lobar pneumonia in Northern Zambia: Clinical study of 502 adult patients. *Thorax.* 1984;39:612-616.

26. Aujesky D, Auble TE, Yealy DM, et al. Prospective comparison of three validated prediction rules for prognosis in community-acquired pneumonia. *Am J Med.* 2005;118:384-392.

27. Ewig S, de Roux A, Bauer T, et al. Validation of predictive rules and indices of severity for community acquire pneumonia. *Thorax.* 2004;59:421-427.

28. Lim WS, Macfarlane JT, Boswell TCJ, et al. Study of community acquired pneumonia aetiology (SCAPA) in adults admitted to hospital: implications for management guidelines. *Thorax.* 2001;56:296-301.

29. Fine MJ, Auble TE, Yealy DM, et al. A prediction rule to identify low-risk patients with community-acquired pneumonia. *N Engl J Med.* 1997;336:243-250.

30. Halm EA, Fine MJ, Kapoor WN, et al. Instability on hospital discharge and the risk of adverse outcomes in patients with pneumonia. *Arch Intern Med.* 2002;162: 1278-1284.

30

Chronic Obstructive Lung Disease

I. INTRODUCTION

Although descriptions of emphysema date to autopsy reports from the 1600s, it was Laennec who, in 1819, recorded the clinical features associated with the disease, including dyspnea, hyperresonance, faint breath sounds, and wheezes.[1] Over the last 200 years, others have embellished Laennec's description, but the principal bedside findings are the same. Writing in 1892, Osler stated that emphysema could be recognized "at a glance" from its characteristic features, including rounded shoulders; barrel chest; prominent epigastric cardiac impulse; hyperresonant chest; loss of cardiac, liver, and splenic dullness; enfeebled breath sounds; and prolonged expiration.[2]

In the 1920s, clinicians began to recognize that these traditional physical signs had shortcomings.[3] In 1927, Cabot wrote that only about 5% of patients with emphysema at autopsy were recognized during life and that, of patients diagnosed with emphysema during life, only 25% actually had it at autopsy.[4] Spirometry, invented in 1846 and used in many forms ("stethometers," "pneumatometers," "doppelstethograms") to supplement bedside diagnosis, gained favor because of these deficiencies and eventually became the favored diagnostic tool.[1]

This chapter compares the traditional physical signs with spirometry. As a general rule, the most accurate physical signs are also infrequent, occurring in fewer than 50% of affected patients, usually only those with the most severe disease.[5,6] For decades or longer, patients may harbor mild and moderate disease that is hidden from the eyes of the bedside examiner but is detectable by spirometry.

II. THE FINDINGS

Most of the traditional findings of chronic obstructive lung disease result from a hyperinflated chest and the great effort necessary to move air across obstructed airways. Some of these physical signs are discussed in other chapters: asynchronous breathing (Chapter 17); barrel chest, pursed lips breathing, and accessory muscle use (Chapter 25); hyperresonance to percussion (Chapter 26); pulsus paradoxus (Chapter 13); diminished breath sounds and wheezing (Chapter 27); and prolonged forced expiratory times (Chapter 28).

Additional findings are discussed in the following.

A. INSPECTION

1. Inspiratory Recession of Supraclavicular Fossa and Intercostal Spaces

Some patients with respiratory distress from obstructive lung disease have recession or indrawing of the soft tissues of the intercostal spaces and supraclavicular fossa. This finding is attributed to excess inspiratory resistance, which introduces a delay between the generation of large negative pleural pressures and subsequent increase in lung volume.[7]

2. Costal Paradox ("Hoover's Sign" or "Costal Margin Paradox")

The costal paradox is an abnormal movement of the costal angle, which is the angle formed by both costal margins as they approach the xiphoid process on the anterior body wall. The clinician assesses costal movements by placing his hands on each costal margin and observing how the hands move with respect to each other as the patient breathes. In a normal person, inspiration causes the lateral aspects of the lower ribs to move outward, like the handle of a bucket, and the clinician's hands separate as the costal angle widens. In patients with the costal paradox, in contrast, the hyperinflated chest can expand no further and the flattened diaphragm instead pulls the costal margins and the clinician's hands together.

3. Leaning Forward on Arms Propped Up on Knees[8,9]

Many patients with obstructive disease experience prompt relief of their dyspnea if they lean forward, which allows them to generate greater inspiratory force with fewer accessory muscles. This position probably diminishes dyspnea because it compresses the abdominal contents and pushes the diaphragm upward, helping restore the normal domed appearance necessary for efficient and strong inspiratory movements.

B. PALPATION: LARYNGEAL HEIGHT AND DESCENT

According to traditional teachings, the distance between the thyroid cartilage and suprasternal notch ("laryngeal height" or "tracheal length") is shorter than normal in obstructive lung disease, because the clavicles and sternum are positioned abnormally high (see "Barrel Chest" in Chapter 25). Patients with severe obstruction also have more forceful diaphragmatic contractions that, although ineffective in moving large amounts of air, may pull the trachea abnormally downward during inspiration ("laryngeal descent," "tracheal descent," or "tracheal tug").

III. CLINICAL SIGNIFICANCE

A. INDIVIDUAL FINDINGS

EBM Box 30-1 shows that several findings argue for the presence of obstructive lung disease: early inspiratory crackles (likelihood ratio [LR] = 14.6), absence of cardiac dullness (LR = 11.8), a breath sound score ≤9 (LR = 10.2), a subxiphoid cardiac impulse (LR = 7.4), hyperresonance of the chest (LR = 5.1), and forced expiratory time ≥9 seconds (LR = 4.1). Among patients with known obstructive lung disease, early inspiratory crackles also imply that the disease is severe (i.e., forced expiratory volume in 1 second divided by forced vital capacity [FEV_1/FVC] < 0.44; LR = 20.8).[15]

Only two findings argue convincingly *against* the diagnosis of obstructive disease: a breath sound score ≥ 16 (LR = 0.1) and a forced expiratory time < 3 seconds (LR = 0.2).

The evidence supporting the chest wall signs of obstructive lung disease is meager and conflicting (see also the "Barrel Chest" in Chapter 25). One study showed that indrawing of the soft tissues correlated with severity of obstruction,[20] whereas another did not.[21] In two studies, Hoover's sign (LR = 4.2, see EBM Box 30-1) and maximum laryngeal height ≤4 cm (LR = 3.6) argued for obstructive lung disease, but in two other studies these signs correlated poorly with measures of obstruction.[20,22] The degree of laryngeal descent is an unhelpful finding (LR not significant).

Box 30-1

Chronic Obstructive Pulmonary Disease*

Finding (Ref)†	Sensitivity (%)	Specificity (%)	Likelihood Ratio if Finding	
			Present	Absent
INSPECTION				
Maximum laryngeal height ≤4 cm[10]	36	90	**3.6**	0.7
Laryngeal descent >3 cm[10]	17	80	NS	NS
Hoover's sign[11]	58	86	**4.2**	0.5
PALPATION				
Subxiphoid cardiac impulse[5,6]	4–27	97–99	**7.4**	NS
PERCUSSION				
Absent cardiac dullness left lower sternal border[5]	15	99	**11.8**	NS
Hyperresonance upper right anterior chest[5]	33	94	**5.1**	NS
Diaphragm excursion percussed <2 cm[5]	13	98	NS	NS
AUSCULTATION				
Breath sound score[12,13]				
≤9	23–46	96–97	**10.2**	...
10–12	34–63	...	**3.6**	...
13–15	11–16	...	NS	...
≥16	3–10	33–34	**0.1**	...
Early inspiratory crackles[14,15]	25–77	97–98	**14.6**	NS
Any unforced wheeze[5,6,10,11,16,17]	13–56	86–99	2.8	0.8
ANCILLARY TESTS				
Forced expiratory time[17–19]				
<3 seconds	8–10	26–62	**0.2**	...
3–9 seconds	42–54	...	NS	...
≥9 seconds	29–50	86–98	**4.1**	...

(Continued)

Box 30-1   Chronic Obstructive Pulmonary Disease*—Cont'd

Finding (Ref)[†]	Sensitivity (%)	Specificity (%)	Likelihood Ratio if Finding	
			Present	Absent
COMBINED FINDINGS				
2 out of the following 3 present: (1) smoked 70 pack years or more, (2) self-reported history of chronic bronchitis or emphysema, (3) diminished breath sounds[5]	67	97	**25.7**	**0.3**

NS, not significant; likelihood ratio (LR) if finding present = positive LR; LR if finding absent = negative LR.

*Diagnostic standards: For chronic obstructive lung disease, FEV_1/FVC ratio < 0.6–0.7 (palpation, percussion, and combined findings), $FEV_1/FVC < 0.7$–0.75 (inspection, crackles, wheezes, and forced expiratory time), or $FEV_1 < 40\%$ predicted (breath sound score).

[†]Definition of finding: For maximal laryngeal height, distance between the top of the thyroid cartilage and suprasternal notch at the end of expiration; for laryngeal descent, difference in laryngeal height between end inspiration and end expiration; for Hoover's sign, paradoxical indrawing of the lateral rib margin during inspiration, noted when the patient is standing; for breath sound score, see Chapter 27; for forced expiratory time, see Chapter 28.

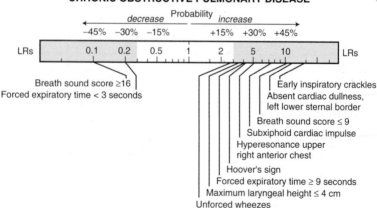

CHRONIC OBSTRUCTIVE PULMONARY DISEASE

The chest excursion of patients with obstructive disease (mean, 3–4 cm, measured as change in circumference between maximum inspiration and maximum expiration, using a tape measure at the level of the fourth intercostal space) is less than that of normal persons (mean, 6–7 cm), but the lower limit observed in normal persons (2–3 cm) makes it impossible to draw significant conclusions in a single person.[22,23]

B. COMBINED FINDINGS

Of the many successful diagnostic schemes that combine findings,[17,24] one of the simplest asks just three questions: (1) Has the patient smoked more than 70 pack-years? (2) Has the patient been previously diagnosed with chronic bronchitis or emphysema? and (3) Are breath sounds diminished in intensity? Answering "yes" to two or three of these questions is a compelling argument for obstructive disease (LR = 25.7, see EBM Box 30-1).

Although using the self-reported history of emphysema as a diagnostic indicator seems to be a circular argument, the specificity of this question is only 74%, which means that 26% of patients *without* obstructive lung disease actually remembered such a history. This question is more discriminatory than other symptoms (i.e., dyspnea, sputum production, age, or use of theophylline, steroids, inhalers, or home oxygen) and many other findings (i.e., hyperresonant chest, absence of cardiac dullness, and wheezes).[5]

REFERENCES

1. Rosenblatt MB. Emphysema in the nineteenth century. *Bull Hist Med.* 1969;43:533-552.
2. Osler W. *The principles and practice of medicine* (facsimile by Classics of Medicine library). New York: D. Appleton and Co; 1892.
3. Snider GL. Emphysema: The first two centuries—And beyond. *Am Rev Respir Dis.* 1992;146:1334-1344.
4. Cabot R. *Physical diagnosis of diseases of the chest.* New York: William Wood; 1900.
5. Badgett RG, Tanaka DJ, Hunt DK, et al. Can moderate chronic obstructive pulmonary disease be diagnosed by historical and physical findings alone? *Am J Med.* 1993;94:188-196.
6. Holleman DR, Simel DL, Goldberg JS. Diagnosis of obstructive airways disease from the clinical examination. *J Gen Intern Med.* 1993;8:63-68.
7. Stubbing DG. Physical signs in the evaluation of patients with chronic obstructive pulmonary disease. *Pract Cardiol.* 1984;10:114-120.
8. Sharp JT, Drutz WS, Moisan T, et al. Postural relief of dyspnea in severe chronic obstructive pulmonary disease. *Am Rev Respir Dis.* 1980;122:201-211.

9. O'Neill S, McCarthy DS. Postural relief of dyspnoea in severe chronic airflow limitation: Relationship to respiratory muscle strength. *Thorax*. 1983;38:595-600.

10. Straus SE, McAlister FA, Sackett DL, Deeks JJ. The accuracy of patient history, wheezing, and laryngeal measurements in diagnosing obstructive airway disease. *JAMA*. 2000;283:1853-1857.

11. Garcia-Pachon E. Paradoxical movement of the lateral rib margin (Hoover sign) for detecting obstructive airway disease. *Chest*. 2002;122:651-655.

12. Pardee NE, Martin CJ, Morgan EH. A test of the practical value of estimating breath sound intensity: Breath sounds related to measured ventilatory function. *Chest*. 1976;70:341-344.

13. Bohadana AB, Peslin R, Uffholtz H. Breath sounds in the clinical assessment of airflow obstruction. *Thorax*. 1978;33:345-351.

14. Bettencourt PE, Del Bono EA, Spiegelman D, et al. Clinical utility of chest auscultation in common pulmonary diseases. *Am J Respir Crit Care Med*. 1994;150:1291-1297.

15. Nath AR, Capel LH. Inspiratory crackles: Early and late. *Thorax*. 1974;29:223-227.

16. Marini JJ, Pierson DJ, Hudson LD, Lakshminarayan S. The significance of wheezing in chronic airflow obstruction. *Am Rev Respir Dis*. 1979;120:1069-1072.

17. Straus S, McAlister FA, Sackett DL, Deeks JJ. Accuracy of history, wheezing, and forced expiratory time in the diagnosis of chronic obstructive pulmonary disease. *J Gen Intern Med*. 2002;17:684-688.

18. Lal S, Ferguson AD, Campbell EJM. Forced expiratory time: A simple test for airways obstruction. *Br Med J*. 1964;1:814-817.

19. Schapira RM, Schapira MM, Funahashi A, et al. The value of the forced expiratory time in the physical diagnosis of obstructive airways disease. *JAMA*. 1993;270:731-736.

20. Godfrey S, Edwards RHT, Campbell EJM, Newton-Howes J. Clinical and physiological associations of some physical signs observed in patients with chronic airways obstruction. *Thorax*. 1970;25:285-287.

21. Stubbing DG, Mathur PN, Roberts RS, Campbell EJM. Some physical signs in patients with chronic airflow obstruction. *Am Rev Respir Dis*. 1982;125:549-552.

22. Schneider IC, Anderson AE. Correlation of clinical signs with ventilatory function in obstructive lung disease. *Ann Intern Med*. 1965;62:477-485.

23. Pierce JA, Ebert RV. The barrel deformity of the chest, the senile lung and obstructive pulmonary emphysema. *Am J Med*. 1958;25:13-22.

24. Holleman DR, Simel DL. Does the clinical examination predict airflow limitation? *JAMA*. 1995;273:313-319.

Pulmonary Embolism

31

I. INTRODUCTION

The diagnosis of pulmonary embolism is a difficult one that has frustrated clinicians for more than a century. In up to half of hospitalized patients who die of pulmonary embolism, the diagnosis is not even considered.[1,2] Even when pulmonary embolism is suspected, however, clinicians have great difficulty making the diagnosis based just on bedside findings and instead rely on technologic tests such as computed tomography, ventilation-perfusion lung scanning, pulmonary angiography, or venous ultrasonography. The principal role of bedside examination is to determine the patient's overall probability of pulmonary embolism, which, often combined with D-dimer levels, is then used to select which, if any, confirmatory tests are necessary.

II. THE FINDINGS

Most patients with pulmonary embolism present with dyspnea (61%–83% of patients), pleuritic chest pain (40%–48% of patients), hemoptysis (5%–22% of patients), or syncope (4%–25% of patients).[3–9] Syncope is more common (affecting 20%–80% of patients) when pulmonary embolism is "massive," meaning that it obstructs more than half of the pulmonary circulation.[10–12]

In recent years, several different investigators have applied multivariate analysis to identify which combination of bedside findings best identify a patient's overall probability of pulmonary embolism.[7,8,13] One of the simplest and best validated of these rules is the Wells Pulmonary Embolism Score (Table 31-1),* which has an advantage over other rules by not requiring laboratory tests (which are sometimes unavailable during the initial evaluation). To use this rule, the clinician simply adds the points corresponding to each of the seven independent predictors that are present (see Table 31-1) and uses the total score to determine overall probability: 0 or 1 point indicates *low* probability of pulmonary embolism; 2 to 6 points, *moderate* probability; and 7 or more points, *high* probability.

III.   CLINICAL SIGNIFICANCE

A.   INDIVIDUAL FINDINGS

The studies included in EBM Box 31-1 enrolled more than 2000 patients with suspected pulmonary embolism referred to centers having considerable experi-

---

*This score evolved from the earlier but more complicated Wells "extended rule"[14] that was presented in the first edition of *Evidence-Based Physical Diagnosis.*

Table 31-1	Wells Score for Pulmonary Embolism	

Characteristic	Points
Risk factors	
Previous pulmonary embolism or deep venous thrombosis	1.5
Immobilization or surgery in the previous 4 weeks	1.5
Cancer	1
Clinical findings	
Hemoptysis	1
Heart rate >100/min	1.5
Clinical signs of deep venous thrombosis	3
Other	
Alternative diagnosis is less likely than pulmonary embolism	3

From reference 13. Interpretation of total score: 0 or 1 point, low probability; 2–6 points, moderate probability; 7 or more points, high probability.

Box
31-1

Pulmonary Embolism *

Finding (Ref)	Sensitivity (%)	Specificity (%)	Likelihood Ratio if Finding Present	Absent
INDIVIDUAL FINDINGS				
Vital signs				
Temperature >38°C[4,6–8]	1–9	78–97	0.4	NS
Pulse >100/min[6–8]	25–43	69–75	NS	NS
Respiratory rate >30/min[8]	21	90	2.0	0.9
Systolic blood pressure ≤100 mm Hg[8]	8	95	1.9	NS
Lung				
Cyanosis[4]	3	97	NS	NS
Accessory muscle use[4]	17	89	NS	NS
Crackles[3]	59	49	NS	NS
Wheezes[7]	3	89	**0.2**	1.1
Pleural friction rub[4]	14	91	NS	NS
Heart				
Elevated neck veins[4]	3	96	NS	NS
Left parasternal heave[4]	1	99	NS	NS
Loud P_2[3]	19	84	NS	NS
New gallop (S_3 or S_4)[3]	30	89	NS	NS
Other				
Chest wall tenderness[4,15]	11–17	79–80	NS	NS
Unilateral calf pain or swelling[5–7,16]	9–29	89–95	2.3	NS
COMBINED FINDINGS				
Wells score[6,17–19]				
Low probability, 0–1 points	6–27	31–54	**0.2**	...
Moderate probability, 2–6 points	56–69	...	1.7	...
High probability, 7 or more points	14–38	90–100	**5.0**	...

NS, not significant; likelihood ratio (LR) if finding present = positive LR; LR if finding absent = negative LR.
*Diagnostic standard: For pulmonary embolism, pulmonary angiography[3,4,6,7,16] or various diagnostic strategies combining tests that either confirm thromboembolism (i.e., positive ventilation-perfusion scanning, computed tomography, pulmonary angiography, or venous ultrasound) or exclude the diagnosis (i.e., negative imaging or nondiagnostic imaging and >3 months of follow-up without thromboembolism while receiving no anticoagulation).[5,8,15,17–19]

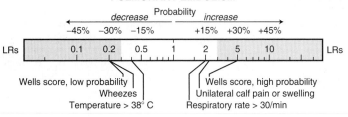

ence with venous thromboembolism. In these studies, only one of five patients suspected of pulmonary embolism actually had the diagnosis.[4,6,8,14,17,19]

Very few individual findings help the clinician distinguish patients with pulmonary embolism from those without it. The only individual symptoms arguing for pulmonary embolism are *sudden* dyspnea [likelihood ratio (LR) = 2.4],[6,7] hemoptysis (LR = 2.0),[3–8] and syncope (LR = 2.0).[4,5,7] The presence of orthopnea (LR = 0.1)[7] decreases the probability of embolism.*

The only individual physical findings arguing for pulmonary embolism are unilateral calf pain or swelling (LR = 2.3, see EBM Box 31-1) and a respiratory rate greater than 30/minute (LR = 2.0). The presence of wheezes (LR = 0.2) and fever greater than 38°C (LR = 0.4) decrease the probability of pulmonary embolism (the LR for wheezing is based on a single study). The presence or absence of a pulse rate greater than 100/minute as an isolated finding is overall unhelpful (LR not significant), although in one study the finding of a pulse less than 90/minute argued against pulmonary embolism (LR = 0.3).[3]

Other individual findings in isolation are unhelpful. Chest wall tenderness is found in 11% to 17% of patients in pulmonary embolism and has a LR that is not significant, emphasizing that this sign is not diagnostic of costochondritis. The presence of hypoxemia, defined either as room air pO_2 less than 80 mm Hg (LR = 1.2)[3,8,20] or as increased alveolar-arterial gradient (LR not significant),[20,21] also contributes little overall to diagnosis.

B. COMBINING FINDINGS TO DETERMINE CLINICAL PROBABILITY OF EMBOLISM

In contrast to the modest accuracy of individual findings, EBM Box 31-1 indicates that a Wells score of 7 or more points (*high* probability) significantly

---

*In these studies, the following risk factors and symptoms were found just as often in patients with embolism as in those without it: female sex, older age, cancer, previous heart disease, previous lung disease, estrogen use, dyspnea, chest pain (pleuritic or nonpleuritic), and cough. A few individual risk factors have LRs between 1.3 and 1.7 and thus increase probability a small amount: recent immobilization, recent surgery, recent trauma, and prior venous thromboembolism.

increases the probability of embolism (LR = 5.0), whereas a Well's score of 0 to 1 point (*low* probability) significantly decreases it (LR = 0.2).

The Wells score emphasizes that accurate assessment of a patient's probability combines both risk factors and clinical findings. The probability of embolism is high if the patient has typical signs (tachycardia, leg swelling) and risk factors (e.g., cancer, immobilization) and lacks an alternative diagnosis. The probability is low if the presentation is atypical, there are no risk factors, and there *is* a likely alternative diagnosis (e.g., angina, congestive heart failure). Many studies have shown that the probability of pulmonary embolism in patients presenting with both low clinical probability (using the Wells score) and normal D-dimer levels is so low that further imaging is unnecessary and anticoagulation can safely be withheld.[18,22,23]

REFERENCES

1. Ryu JH, Olson EJ, Pellikka PA. Clinical recognition of pulmonary embolism: Problem of unrecognized and asymptomatic cases. *Mayo Clin Proc.* 1998;73:873-879.
2. Morgenthaler TI, Ryu JH. Clinical characteristics of fatal pulmonary embolism in a referral hospital. *Mayo Clin Proc.* 1995;70:417-424.
3. Hoellerich VL, Wigton RS. Diagnosing pulmonary embolism using clinical findings. *Arch Intern Med.* 1986;146:1699-1704.
4. Hull RD, Raskob GE, Carter CJ, et al. Pulmonary embolism in outpatients with pleuritic chest pain. *Arch Intern Med.* 1988;148:838-844.
5. Kline JA, Nelson RD, Jackson RE, Courtney DM. Criteria for the safe use of D-dimer testing in emergency department patients with suspected pulmonary embolism: A multicenter US study. *Ann Emerg Med.* 2002;39:144-152.
6. Miniati M, Bottai M, Monti S. Comparison of 3 clinical models for predicting the probability of pulmonary embolism. *Medicine.* 2005;84:107-114.
7. Miniati M, Monti S, Bottai M. A structured clinical model for predicting the probability of pulmonary embolism. *Am J Med.* 2003;114:173-179.
8. Wicki J, Perneger TV, Junod AF, et al. Assessing clinical probability of pulmonary embolism in the emergency ward: A simple score. *Arch Intern Med.* 2001;161: 92-97.
9. Stein PD, Henry JW. Clinical characteristics of patients with acute pulmonary embolism stratified according to their presenting syndromes. *Chest.* 1997;112:974-979.
10. Stein PD, Willis PW, DeMets DL. History and physical examination in acute pulmonary embolism in patients without preexisting cardiac or pulmonary disease. *Am J Cardiol.* 1981;47:218-223.
11. Bell WR, Simon TL, DeMets DL. The clinical features of submassive and massive pulmonary emboli. *Am J Med.* 1977;62:355-360.
12. Sutton GC, Honey M, Gibson RV. Clinical diagnosis of acute massive pulmonary embolism. *Lancet.* 1969;1:271-273.

13. Wells PS, Anderson DR, Rodger M, et al. Derivation of a simple clinical model to categorize patients probability of pulmonary embolism: Increasing the models utility with the SimpliRED D-dimer. *Thromb Haemost.* 2000;83:416-420.

14. Wells PS, Ginsberg JS, Anderson DR, et al. Use of a clinical model for safe management of patients with suspected pulmonary embolism. *Ann Intern Med.* 1998;129:997-1005.

15. Le Gal G, Testuz A, Righini M, et al. Reproduction of chest pain by palpation: Diagnostic accuracy in suspected pulmonary embolism. *BMJ.* 2005;330:452-453.

16. Stein PD, Henry JW, Gopalakrishnan D, Relyea B. Asymmetry of calves in the assessment of patients with suspected acute pulmonary embolism. *Chest.* 1995;107: 936-939.

17. Chagnon I, Bounameaux H, Aujesky D, et al. Comparison of two clinical prediction rules and implicit assessment among patients with suspected pulmonary embolism. *Am J Med.* 2002;113:269-275.

18. Wells PS, Anderson DR, Rodger M, et al. Excluding pulmonary embolism at the bedside without diagnostic imaging: Management of patients with suspected pulmonary embolism presenting to the emergency department by using a simple clinical model and D-dimer. *Ann Intern Med.* 2001;135:98-107.

19. Wolf SJ, McCubbin TR, Feldhaus KM, et al. Prospective validation of Wells criteria in the evaluation of patients with suspected pulmonary embolism. *Ann Emerg Med.* 2004;44:503-510.

20. Stein PD, Goldhaber SZ, Henry JW, Miller AC. Arterial blood gas analysis in the assessment of suspected acute pulmonary embolism. *Chest.* 1996;109:78-81.

21. McFarlane MJ, Imperiale TF. Use of the alveolar-arterial oxygen gradient in the diagnosis of pulmonary embolism. *Am J Med.* 1994;96:57-62.

22. Leclercq MGL, Lutisan JG, Kooy MVM, et al. Ruling out clinical suspected pulmonary embolism by assessment of clinical probability and D-dimer levels: a management study. *Thromb Haemost.* 2003;89:97-103.

23. Kruip MJHA, Leclercq MGL, van der Heul C, et al. Diagnostic strategies for excluding pulmonary embolism in clinical outcome studies: A systematic review. *Ann Intern Med.* 2003;138:941-951.

7

THE HEART

CHAPTER 32

Inspection of the Neck Veins

I. INTRODUCTION

Clinicians should inspect the neck veins (1) to detect elevated central venous pressure (CVP) and (2) to detect specific abnormalities of the venous waveforms, which are characteristic of certain arrhythmias and some valvular, pericardial, and myocardial disorders.

Clinicians first associated conspicuous neck veins with heart disease about 3 centuries ago.[1,2] In the late 1800s, Sir James Mackenzie described venous waveforms of arrhythmias and various heart disorders, using a mechanical polygraph applied over the patient's neck or liver. His labels for the venous waveforms—A, C, and V waves—are still used today.[3,4] Clinician began to estimate venous pressure at the bedside routinely in the 1920s, after the introduction of the glass manometer and after Starling's experiments linking venous pressure to cardiac output.[5]

II.   VENOUS PRESSURE

A.   DEFINITIONS

1.   Central Venous Pressure

CVP is mean vena caval or right atrial pressure, which, in the absence of tricuspid stenosis, equals right ventricular end-diastolic pressure. Disorders that increase diastolic pressures of the right side of the heart—left heart disease, lung disease, primary pulmonary hypertension, and pulmonic stenosis—all increase the CVP and make the neck veins abnormally conspicuous. CVP is expressed in millimeters of mercury (mm Hg) or centimeters of water (cm H_2O) above atmospheric pressure (1.36 cm H_2O = 1.0 mm Hg).

Estimations of CVP are most helpful in patients with ascites or edema, in whom an elevated CVP indicates heart or lung disease and a normal CVP suggests alternative diagnoses, such as chronic liver disease (Despite prevailing opinion, the CVP is normal in patients with liver disease; the edema in these patients results from hypoalbuminemia and the weight of ascites compressing veins to the legs.)[6–9]

2.   Physiologic Zero Point

Physiologists have long assumed that a location in the cardiovascular system (presumed to be the right atrium in humans) tightly regulates venous pressure so that it remains the same even when the person changes position.[5,10–12] All measurements of CVP—whether by the clinician inspecting neck veins or by the catheter in intensive care units—attempt to identify the pressure at this zero point (e.g., if a manometer connected to a systemic vein supports a column of saline 8 cm above the zero point, with the top of the manometer open to atmosphere, the recorded pressure in that vein is 8 cm H_2O). Estimates of CVP are related to the zero point because interpretation of this value does not need to consider the hydrostatic effects of different patient positions, and any abnormal value thus indicates disease.

3.   External Reference Point

Clinicians require some external reference point to reliably locate the level of the zero point. Of the many such reference points that have been proposed over the last century,[5] only two are commonly used today: the sternal angle and the phlebostatic axis.

a.   *Sternal Angle*

In 1930, Sir Thomas Lewis, a pupil of Mackenzie, proposed a simple bedside method for measuring venous pressure designed to replace the manometer, which he found too burdensome for general use.[13] He observed that the top of the jugular veins of normal persons (and the top of the fluid in the manometer) always came to lie within 1 to 2 cm of vertical distance from the sternal angle, whether the person was supine, semiupright, or upright (an observation since confirmed by others).[14] Neck veins whose top level is more than 3 cm above the sternal angle, according to Lewis, indicates that venous pressure is elevated.

Others have modified this method, stating that the CVP equals the vertical distance between the top of the neck veins and a point 5 cm below the sternal angle (Fig. 32-1).[15] This variation is commonly called the "method of Lewis," even though Lewis never made such a claim.

b. Phlebostatic Axis

The phlebostatic axis is the midpoint between the anterior and posterior surfaces of the chest at the level of the fourth intercostal space. This reference point, the most common landmark used in intensive care units and cardiac catheterization laboratories, was originally proposed in the 1940s, when studies showed

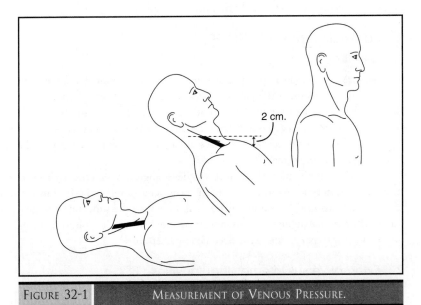

2 cm.

FIGURE 32-1	MEASUREMENT OF VENOUS PRESSURE.

The clinician should vary the patient's position until the top of the neck veins become visible. In this patient, who has normal central venous pressure (CVP), the neck veins are fully distended when supine and completely collapsed when upright. A semiupright position, therefore, is used to estimate pressure. In this position, the top of the neck veins is 2 cm above the sternal angle, and according to the method of Lewis, the patient's CVP is 2 + 5 = 7 cm H_2O.

that using it as the zero point minimized variation in venous pressure of normal persons as they changed position between 0 and 90 degrees.[11]

c. Relative Merits of Sternal Angle and Phlebostatic Axis

Obviously, the measurement of venous pressure is only as good as the reference point used. The phlebostatic axis locates a point in the right atrium several centimeters posterior to the point identified by the method of Lewis (i.e., the zero point using the phlebostatic axis is 9–10 cm posterior to the sternal angle; that using the method of Lewis is 5 cm below the sternal angle).[16,17] This means that clinicians using the phlebostatic axis will estimate the CVP to be several cm H_2O higher than those using the method of Lewis, even if these clinicians completely agree on the location of the neck veins.

The sternal angle is a better reference point for bedside examination, simply because clinicians can reproducibly locate it more easily than the phlebostatic axis. Even using flexible right-angle triangles and a standard patient position, intensive care nurses trying to locate a point similar to the phlebostatic axis disagreed by several centimeters in both horizontal and vertical directions.[18]

B. ELEVATED VENOUS PRESSURE

1. Technique

To measure the patient's venous pressure, the clinician should examine the veins on the right side of the patient's neck, because these veins have a direct route to the heart. Veins in the left side of the neck reach the heart by crossing the mediastinum, where the normal aorta may compress them, causing left jugular venous pressure to be sometimes elevated even when CVP and right venous pressure are normal.[19,20]

The patient should be positioned at whichever angle between the supine and upright position best reveals the top of the neck veins (see Fig. 32-1). The top of the neck veins is indicated by the point above which the subcutaneous conduit of the external jugular vein disappears or above which the pulsating waveforms of the internal jugular wave become imperceptible.

2. External Versus Internal Jugular Veins

Either the external or internal jugular veins may be used to estimate pressure, because measurements in both are similar.[21] Traditionally, clinicians have been taught to use only the internal jugular vein because the external jugular vein contains valves, which purportedly interfere with the development of a hydrostatic column necessary to measure pressure. This teaching is erroneous for two reasons: (1) The internal jugular vein also contains valves, a fact known to anatomists for centuries.[22–24] These valves are essential during cardiopulmonary resuscitation, preventing blood from flowing backward during chest compression,[25] (2) Valves in the jugular veins do not interfere with pressure measurements because flow is normally toward the heart. In fact, they probably act like a transducer membranes (e.g., the diaphragm of a speaker), which amplify right atrial pressure pulsations and make the venous waveforms easier to see.[22]

3. Definition of Elevated CVP

After locating the top of the external or internal jugular veins, the clinician should measure vertical distance between the top of the veins and one of the external reference points discussed previously (see Fig. 32-1). The venous pressure is abnormally elevated if (1) the top of the neck veins are more than 3 cm above the sternal angle, (2) the CVP exceeds 8 cm H_2O using the "method of Lewis" (i.e. >3 cm above the sternal angle + 5 cm), or (3) more than 12 cm H_2O using the phlebostatic axis.

C. BEDSIDE ESTIMATES OF VENOUS PRESSURE VERSUS CATHETER MEASUREMENTS

1. Diagnostic Accuracy*

In studies employing a standardized reference point, bedside estimates of CVP were within 4 cm H_2O of catheter measurements 85% of the time.[21,29] According to these studies, the finding of an elevated CVP (i.e., top of neck veins >3 cm H_2O above sternal angle or >8 cm H_2O using method of Lewis) is a strong argument *for* an elevated catheter measurement [likelihood ratio (LR) = 9.0, EBM Box 32-1]. If the clinician believes the CVP is normal, it almost certainly is less than 12 cm H_2O by catheter measurement (LR = 0.1, see EBM Box 32-1), although some of these patients have catheter measurements that are mildly elevated, between 8 and 12 cm H_2O.[†]

This tendency to slightly underestimate measured values, which is explained further later, explains why estimates made during expiration are slightly more accurate than those made during inspiration: During expiration, the neck veins move upward in the neck, increasing the bedside estimate and minimizing the error.[21]

2. Why Clinicians Underestimate Measured Values

Of the many reasons why clinicians tend to underestimate measured values of CVP, the most important one is that the vertical distance between the sternal

*Studies that test the diagnostic accuracy of bedside estimates of CVP are difficult to summarize because they often fail to standardize which external reference point was used.[26-28]

†For purposes of comparison, "measured pressure" here is in cm H_2O using the method of Lewis. Most catheterization laboratories measure pressure in mm Hg using the phlebostatic axis as the reference point.

Box 32-1 — Inspection of the Neck Veins*

Finding (Ref)[†]	Sensitivity (%)	Specificity (%)	Likelihood Ratio if Finding	
			Present	Absent
Elevated venous pressure at the bedside				
Detecting measured CVP >8 cm H_2O[21,29]	47–92	93–96	**9.0**	NS
Detecting measured CVP >12 cm H_2O[21,29]	78–95	89–93	**10.4**	**0.1**
Detecting elevated left heart diastolic pressures[30–32]	10–58	96–97	**3.9**	NS
Detecting low left ventricular ejection fraction[33,34]	7–18	98	**7.9**	NS
Predicting postoperative pulmonary edema[35,36]	19	98	**11.3**	NS
Predicting postoperative myocardial infarction or cardiac death[35,36]	17	98	**9.4**	NS
Positive abdominojugular test				
Detecting elevated left heart diastolic pressures[30,37,38]	55–84	83–98	**8.0**	**0.3**

NS, not significant; likelihood ratio (LR) if finding present = positive LR; LR if finding absent = negative LR.

*Diagnostic standards: for measured CVP, measurement by catheter in supine patient using method of Lewis[21,29]; for elevated left heart diastolic pressures, pulmonary capillary wedge pressure (PCWP) >15 mm Hg[30,37,38] or left ventricular end diastolic pressure >15 mm Hg[31,32]; for low left ventricular ejection fraction, radionuclide left ventricular ejection fraction <0.53[33] or left ventricular fractional shortening <25% by echocardiography.[34]

†Definition of findings: for elevated venous pressure, bedside estimate >8 cm H_2O using method of Lewis,[21,29] >12 cm H_2O using phlebostatic axis,[35,36] or unknown method[30–33]; for positive abdominojugular test, see text.

angle and physiologic zero point varies as the patient shifts position (Fig. 32-2).[5,39] Catheter measurements of venous pressure are always made while the patient is lying supine, whether the venous pressure is high or low. Bedside estimates of venous pressure, however, must be made in the semiupright or upright positions if the venous pressure is high, because only these positions reveal the top

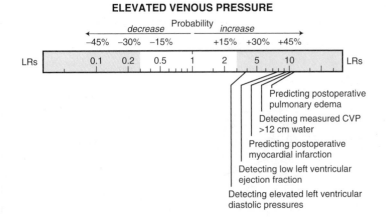

of distended neck veins. Figure 32-2 shows that the semiupright position increases the vertical distance between the right atrium and sternal angle about 3 cm, compared with the supine position, which effectively lowers the bedside estimate by the same amount. The significance of this is that patients with mildly elevated CVP by catheter measurements (i.e., 8–12 cm H_2O), whose neck veins are interpretable only in more upright positions, may have bedside estimates that are normal (i.e., < 8 cm H_2O).

In support of this, even catheter measurements using the sternal angle as reference point are about 3 cm lower when the patient is in the semiupright position than when the patient is supine.[40–42]

D. CLINICAL SIGNIFICANCE OF ELEVATED VENOUS PRESSURE

1. Differential Diagnosis of Ascites and Edema

In patients with ascites and edema, an elevated venous pressure implies that the heart or pulmonary circulation is the problem; a normal venous pressure indicates another diagnosis is the cause.

2. Elevated Venous Pressure and Left Heart Disease

EBM Box 32-1 shows that, in patients with symptoms of angina or dyspnea, the finding of elevated venous pressure argues for elevated left atrial pressure (LR = 3.9, see EBM Box 32-1)* and depressed ejection fraction (LR = 7.9). The opposite finding (normal neck veins) provides no diagnostic information about left heart pressure or function (negative LRs not significant, see EBM Box 32-1).

---

*During cardiac catheterization, a measured right atrial pressure ≥10 mm Hg detects a measured pulmonary capillary wedge pressures of ≥22 mm Hg with an LR of 4.5, which is similar to that derived from bedside examination (LR = 3.9).[43]

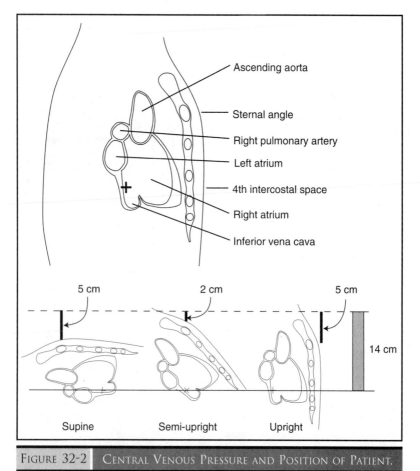

FIGURE 32-2   CENTRAL VENOUS PRESSURE AND POSITION OF PATIENT.

The top half of the figure shows the sagittal section of a 43-year-old man, just to the right of the midsternal line, demonstrating the relationship between the sternal angle, right atrium, and phlebostatic axis (indicated by the black cross in the posterior right atrium). The bottom half of the figure illustrates the changing vertical distance between the phlebostatic axis (solid horizontal line) and sternal angle in the supine (0 degrees), semiupright (45 degrees), and upright (90 degrees) positions. The venous pressure is the same in each position (14 cm above the phlebostatic axis, gray bar on right), but the vertical distance between the sternal angle and the top of the neck veins changes in the different positions: The vertical distance is 5 cm in the supine and upright positions but only 2 cm in the semiupright position. Using the method of Lewis (see text), therefore, the estimate of venous pressure from the semiupright position (7 cm = 2 + 5) is 3 cm *lower* than estimates from the supine or upright positions (10 cm = 5 + 5 cm). (Adapted from McGee SR. Physical examination of venous pressure: A critical review. *Am Heart J.* 1998;136:10-18.)

3. Elevated Venous Pressure During Preoperative Consultation

The finding of elevated venous pressure during preoperative consultation is a compelling finding predicting that the patient, without any intervening diuresis or other treatment, will develop postoperative pulmonary edema (LR = 11.3; see EBM Box 32-1) or myocardial infarction (LR = 9.4).

4. Elevated Venous Pressure and Pericardial Disease

Elevated venous pressure is a cardinal finding of cardiac tamponade (100% of cases) and constrictive pericarditis (98% of cases). Therefore, the absence of elevated neck veins is a conclusive argument against these diagnoses. In every patient with elevated neck veins, the clinician should search for other findings of tamponade (i.e., pulsus paradoxus; prominent x' descent but no y descent in venous waveforms) and constrictive pericarditis (pericardial knock, prominent x' and y descents in venous waveforms) (see Chapter 43).

5. Unilateral Elevation of Venous Pressure

Distention of the left jugular veins with normal right jugular veins sometimes occurs because of kinking of the left innominate vein by a tortuous aorta.[19,20] In these patients, the elevation often disappears after a deep inspiration.

Persistent unilateral elevation of the neck veins usually indicates local obstruction by a mediastinal lesion, such as aortic aneurysm or intrathoracic goiter.[44]

III. ABDOMINOJUGULAR TEST

A. THE FINDING

During the abdominojugular test, the clinician observes the neck veins while pressing firmly over the patient's mid abdomen for 10 seconds, a maneuver that probably increases venous return by displacing splanchnic venous blood toward the heart.[38] The CVP of normal persons usually remains unchanged during this maneuver or rises for a beat or two before returning to normal or below normal.[29,37,38,45,46] If the CVP rises more than 4 cm H_2O and remains elevated for the entire 10 seconds, the abdominojugular test is positive.[30,38] Most clinicians recognize the positive response by observing the neck veins at the moment the abdominal pressure is released, regarding a *fall* more than 4 cm as positive.

The earliest version of the abdominojugular test was the "hepatojugular reflux," introduced by Pasteur in 1885 as a pathognomonic sign of tricuspid regurgitation.[47] In 1898, Rondot discovered that patients with normal tricuspid valves could develop the sign, and by 1925, clinicians realized that pressure anywhere over the abdomen, not just over the liver, would elicit the sign.[45] Several investigators have contributed to the current definition of the abdominojugular test.[29,38,48]

B. CLINICAL SIGNIFICANCE

In patients presenting for cardiac catheterization (presumably because of chest pain or dyspnea), a positive abdominojugular test is an accurate sign of elevated left atrial pressure (i.e., ≥15 mm Hg, LR = 8.0, see EBM Box 32-1). Therefore, a positive abdominojugular test is an important finding in patients with dyspnea, indicating that at least some of the dyspnea is due to disease in the left side of the heart. A negative abdominojugular test argues against the presence of left atrial hypertension (LR = 0.3, see EBM Box 32-1).

IV. KUSSMAUL'S SIGN

Kussmaul's sign is the paradoxical elevation of CVP during inspiration. In healthy persons venous pressure falls during inspiration, because pressures in the right heart decrease as intrathoracic pressures fall. Kussmaul's sign is classically associated with constrictive pericarditis, but it occurs in only the minority of patients with constriction[49,50] and is found in other disorders such as severe heart failure,[50,51] pulmonary embolus,[52] and right ventricular infarction.[53–56]

V. PATHOGENESIS OF ELEVATED VENOUS PRESSURE, ABDOMINOJUGULAR TEST, AND KUSSMAUL'S SIGN

The peripheral veins of normal persons are distensible vessels that contain about two thirds of the total blood volume and can accept or donate blood with relatively little change in pressure. In contrast, the peripheral veins of patients with heart failure are abnormally constricted from tissue edema and intense sympathetic stimulation, a change that reduces extremity blood volume and increases central blood volume. Because constricted veins are less compliant, the added central blood volume causes CVP to be abnormally increased.[5]

In addition to causing an elevated CVP, venoconstriction probably also contributes to the positive abdominojugular test and Kussmaul's sign, two signs that often occur together. Most patients with constrictive pericarditis and Kussmaul's sign also have a notably positive abdominojugular test; many patients with severe heart failure and a markedly positive abdominojugular test also have Kussmaul's sign.[50] The venous pressure of these patients, unlike that of healthy persons, is very susceptible to changes in venous return. Maneuvers that increase venous return—exercise, leg elevation, or abdominal pressure—increase the venous pressure of patients with the abdominojugular test and Kussmaul's sign but not that of healthy persons.[5] Kussmaul's sign may be nothing more than an inspiratory abdominojugular test, the downward movement of the diaphragm compressing the abdomen and increasing venous return.[57]

Even so, an abnormal right ventricle probably also contributes to Kussmaul's sign, because all of the disorders associated with Kussmaul's sign are characterized by a right ventricle that is unable to accommodate more blood during inspiration (i.e., in constrictive pericarditis the normal ventricle is constrained by the diseased pericardium, and in severe heart failure, acute cor pulmonale, or right ventricular infarction, the dilated right ventricle is constrained by the normal pericardium). A right side of the heart thus constrained only exaggerates inspiratory increments of CVP, making Kussmaul's sign more prominent.[5]

VI.   VENOUS WAVEFORMS

A.   IDENTIFYING THE INTERNAL JUGULAR VEIN

Venous waveforms are usually only conspicuous in the internal jugular vein, which lies under the sternocleidomastoid muscle and therefore becomes evident by causing pulsating movements of the soft tissues of the neck (i.e., it does not resemble a subcutaneous vein). Because the carotid artery also pulsates in the neck, the clinician must learn to distinguish the carotid artery from internal jugular vein, using the principles outlined in Table 32-1.

Of the distinguishing features listed in Table 32-1, the most conspicuous one is the character of the movement. Venous pulsations have a prominent *inward* or *descending* movement, the outward one being slower and more diffuse. Arterial pulsations, in contrast, have a prominent *ascending* or *outward* movement, the inward one being slow and diffuse.

B.   COMPONENTS OF VENOUS WAVEFORMS

Although venous pressure tracings reveal three positive and negative waves (Fig. 32-3), the clinician at the bedside usually sees only two descents, a more prominent x′ descent and a less prominent y descent (Fig. 32-4). Figure 32-3 discusses the physiology of these waveforms.

C.   TIMING THE X′ AND Y DESCENTS

The best way to identify the individual venous waveforms is to time their *descents*, by simultaneously listening to the heart tones or palpating the carotid pulsation (see Fig. 32-4).

Table 32-1	Distinguishing Internal Jugular Waveforms from Carotid Pulses*	
Characteristic	Internal Jugular Vein	Carotid Artery
Character of movement	Descending movement most prominent	Ascending movement most prominent
Number of pulsations per ventricular systole	Two, usually	One
Palpability of pulsations	Not palpable or only slight undulation	Easily palpable
Change with respiration	During inspiration, pulsations become more prominent but drop lower in neck	No change
Change with position	Pulsations lower in neck as patient sits up	No change
Change with abdominal pressure	Pulsations may temporarily become more prominent and move higher in neck	No change
Change with pressure applied to the neck just below pulsations	Pulsations become less prominent	No change

*Based on references 58–61.

1. Using Heart Tones

The x' descent ends just *before* S_2, as if it were a collapsing hill that slides into S_2 lying at the bottom. In contrast, the y descent begins just *after* S_2.

2. Using the Carotid Artery

The x' descent is a systolic movement that coincides with the tap from the carotid pulsation. The y descent is a diastolic movement beginning after the carotid tap, with a delay roughly equivalent to the interval between the patient's S_1 and S_2.[60,65]

D. CLINICAL SIGNIFICANCE

The normal venous waveform has a prominent x' descent and a small or absent y descent; there are no abrupt outward movements.[65]

Abnormalities of the venous waveforms become conspicuous at the bedside for one of two reasons: (1) the descents are abnormal or (2) there is a sudden outward movement in the neck veins.

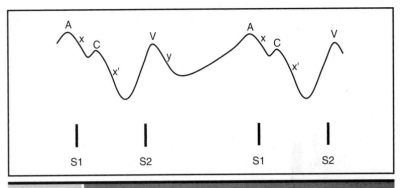

FIGURE 32-3	VENOUS WAVEFORMS ON PRESSURE TRACINGS.

There are three positive waves (A, C, and V) and three negative waves (x, x', and y descents). The A wave represents right atrial contraction; the x descent, right atrial relaxation. The C wave—named "C" because Mackenzie originally thought it was a carotid artifact—probably instead represents right ventricular contraction and closure of the tricuspid valve, which then bulges upward toward the neck veins.[62,63] The x' descent occurs because the floor of the right atrium (i.e., the A-V valve ring) moves downward, pulling away from the jugular veins, as the right ventricle contracts (physiologists call this movement the "descent of the base").[64] The V wave represents right atrial filling, which eventually overcomes the descent of the base and causes venous pressure to rise (most atrial filling normally occurs during ventricular systole, not diastole). The y descent begins the moment the tricuspid valve opens at the beginning of diastole, causing the atrium to empty into the ventricle and venous pressure to abruptly fall.

1. Abnormal Descents

There are three abnormal patterns: (**1**) **The "W" or "M" pattern** (x' = y pattern). The y descent becomes unusually prominent, which, along with the normal x' descent, creates two prominent descents per systole and traces a "W" or "M" pattern in the soft tissues of the neck; (**2**) **The diminished X' descent pattern** (x' < y pattern). The x' descent diminishes or disappears, making the y descent most prominent. This is the most common abnormal pattern, occurring both in atrial fibrillation (loss of A wave) and many different cardiomyopathies (more sluggish "descent of the base"); and (**3**) **The absent y descent pattern.** This pattern is only relevant in patients with elevated venous pressure, because healthy persons with normal CVP also have a diminutive y descent.

The etiologies of each of these patterns are presented in Table 32-2.

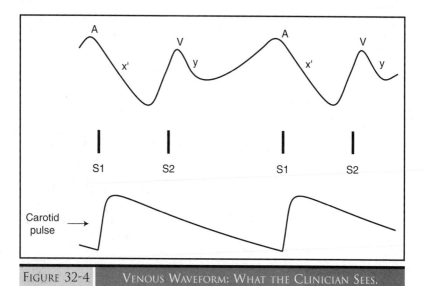

FIGURE 32-4 VENOUS WAVEFORM: WHAT THE CLINICIAN SEES.

Although tracings of venous waveforms display three positive and three negative waves (see Fig. 32-3), the C wave is too small to see. Instead, the clinician sees two descents per cardiac cycle: The first represents merging of the x and x′ descents and is usually referred to as the x′ descent (i.e., "x-prime" descent). The second is the y descent, which is smaller than the x′ descent in normal persons. The clinician identifies the descents by timing them with the heart tones or carotid pulsation (see text).

2. Abnormally Prominent Outward Waves

If the clinician detects an abnormally abrupt and conspicuous outward movement in the neck veins, he should determine if the outward movement begins just before S_1 (presystolic giant A waves) or after S_1 (tricuspid regurgitation and cannon A waves).

a. Giant A Waves (Abrupt Presystolic Outward Waves)

Giant A waves have two requirements: (1) sinus rhythm and (2) some obstruction to right atrial or ventricular emptying, usually from pulmonary hypertension, pulmonic stenosis, or tricuspid stenosis.[58,59,71] Nonetheless, many patients with severe pulmonary hypertension lack this finding, because their atria contract too feebly or at a time in the cardiac cycle when venous pressures are falling.[69,75]

Some patients with giant A waves have an accompanying abrupt presystolic sound that is heard with the stethoscope over the jugular veins.[76]

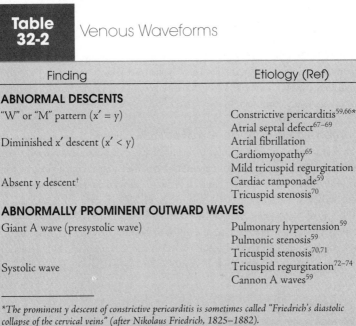

Table 32-2	Venous Waveforms

Finding	Etiology (Ref)
ABNORMAL DESCENTS	
"W" or "M" pattern (x' = y)	Constrictive pericarditis[59,66]*
	Atrial septal defect[67–69]
Diminished x' descent (x' < y)	Atrial fibrillation
	Cardiomyopathy[65]
	Mild tricuspid regurgitation
Absent y descent[†]	Cardiac tamponade[59]
	Tricuspid stenosis[70]
ABNORMALLY PROMINENT OUTWARD WAVES	
Giant A wave (presystolic wave)	Pulmonary hypertension[59]
	Pulmonic stenosis[59]
	Tricuspid stenosis[70,71]
Systolic wave	Tricuspid regurgitation[72–74]
	Cannon A waves[59]

*The prominent y descent of constrictive pericarditis is sometimes called "Friedrich's diastolic collapse of the cervical veins" (after Nikolaus Friedrich, 1825–1882).
[†]If venous pressure is normal, the absence of a y descent is a normal finding; if venous pressure is elevated, however, the absence of the y descent is abnormal and suggests impaired early diastolic filling.

b. Systolic Waves

(1) Tricuspid Regurgitation   In patients with tricuspid regurgitation and pulmonary hypertension, the neck veins are elevated (more than 90% of patients) and consist of a single outward systolic movement that coincides with the carotid pulsation and collapses after S_2 (i.e., prominent y descent).[72–74] Some patients have an accompanying midsystolic clicking sound over the jugular veins.[77] Because the jugular valves often become incompetent in chronic tricuspid regurgitation, the arm and leg veins also may pulsate with each systolic regurgitant wave (see Chapter 42)

(2) Cannon A Waves   Cannon A waves represent an atrial contraction that occurs just after ventricular contraction, when the tricuspid valve is closed.* Instead of ejecting blood into the right ventricle, the contraction forces blood

---

*The electrocardiographic correlate of the cannon A wave is a P wave (atrial contraction) falling between the QRS and T waves (ventricular systole).

upward into the jugular veins. Cannon A waves may be regular (i.e., with every arterial pulse) or intermittent.

(A)   Regular cannon A waves

This finding occurs in many paroxysmal supraventricular tachycardias (fast heart rates) and junctional rhythms (normal heart rates), both of which have retrograde P waves buried within or just after the QRS complex.[59]

(B)   Intermittent cannon A waves

If the arterial pulse is regular but cannon A waves are intermittent, only one mechanism is possible: atrioventricular dissociation (see Chapter 14). In patients with ventricular tachycardia, the finding of intermittently appearing cannon A waves detects atrioventricular dissociation with a sensitivity of 96%, specificity of 75%, positive LR of 3.8, and negative LR of 0.1[78] (see Chapter 14).

If the arterial pulse is irregular, intermittent cannon A waves have less importance because they commonly accompany ventricular premature contractions and, less commonly, atrial premature contractions (see Chapter 14).

REFERENCES

1. Lancisi GM. *De Aneurysmatibus (1745)*. New York: Macmillan Co; 1952.
2. Morgagni JB. *The seats and causes of diseases* (facsimile edition by Classics of Medicine library). Vol 1. London: Millar, Cadell, Johnson, and Payne; 1769.
3. Mackenzie J. *The study of the pulse: Arterial, venous, and hepatic and of the movements of the heart* (facsimile by the Classics of Cardiology Library). Edinburgh: Young J. Pentland; 1902.
4. Mackenzie J. The venous and liver pulses, and the arrhythmic contraction of the cardiac cavities. *J Path Bacteriol.* 1894;2:84-154, 273-345.
5. McGee SR. Physical examination of venous pressure: A critical review. *Am Heart J.* 1998;136:10-18.
6. Hussey HH, Jeghers H. Practical considerations of venous pressure. *N Engl J Med.* 1947;237:776-782; 812-778.
7. Reynolds TB, Redeker AG, Geller HM. Wedged hepatic venous pressure: A clinical evaluation. *Am J Med.* 1957;22:341-350.
8. Rössle M, Haag K, Ochs A, et al. The transjugular intrahepatic portosystemic stent-shunt procedure for variceal bleeding. *N Engl J Med.* 1994;330:165-171.
9. Reynolds TB, Balfour DC, Levinson DC, et al. Comparison of wedged hepatic vein pressure with portal vein pressure in human subjects with cirrhosis. *J Clin Invest.* 1955;34:213-218.
10. Guyton AC, Greganti FP. A physiologic reference point for measuring circulatory pressures in the dog: Particularly venous pressure. *Am J Physiol.* 1956;185:137-141.

11. Winsor T, Burch GE. Phlebostatic axis and phlebostatic level, reference levels for venous pressure measurements in man. *Proc Soc Exp Biol Med.* 1945;58:165-169.

12. Holt JP. The measurement of venous pressure in man eliminating the hydrostatic factor. *Am J Physiol.* 1940;130:635-641.

13. Lewis T. Early signs of cardiac failure of the congestive type. *Br Med J.* 1930;1:849-852.

14. Jaikaran SMN, Sagay E. Normal central venous pressure. *Br J Surg.* 1968;55:609-612.

15. Borst JGG, Molhuysen JA. Exact determination of the central venous pressure by a simple clinical method. *Lancet.* 1952;2:304-309.

16. Pedersen A, Husby J. Venous pressure measurement. I. Choice of zero level. *Acta Med Scand.* 1951;141:185-194.

17. Debrunner F, Buehler F. "Normal central venous pressure," significance of reference point and normal range. *Br Med J.* 1969;3:148-150.

18. Drake JJ. Locating the external reference point for central venous pressure determination. *Nurs Res.* 1974;23:475-482.

19. Sleight P. Unilateral elevation of the internal jugular pulse. *Br Heart J.* 1962;24:726-730.

20. Fred HL, Wukasch DC, Petrany Z. Transient compression of the left innominate vein. *Circ.* 1964;29:758-761.

21. Davison R, Cannon R. Estimation of central venous pressure by examination of jugular veins. *Am Heart J.* 1974;87:279-282.

22. Fisher J. Jugular venous valves and physical signs. *Chest.* 1984;85:685-686.

23. Fisher J, Vaghaiwalla F, Tsitlik J, et al. Determinants and clinical significance of jugular venous valve competence. *Circulation.* 1982;65:188-196.

24. Silva MA, Deen KI, Fernando DJS, Sheriffdeen AH. The internal jugular vein valve may have a significant role in the prevention of venous reflux: evidence from live and cadaveric human subjects. *Clin Physiol Func Im.* 2002;22:202-205.

25. Goetting MG, Paradis NA. Right atrial-jugular venous pressure gradients during CPR in children. *Ann Emerg Med.* 1991;20:27-30.

26. Eisenberg PR, Jaffe AS, Schuster DP. Clinical evaluation compared to pulmonary artery catheterization in the hemodynamic assessment of critically ill patients. *Crit Care Med.* 1984;12:549-553.

27. Connors AF, McCaffree DR, Gray BA. Evaluation of right-heart catheterization in the critically ill patient without acute myocardial infarction. *N Engl J Med.* 1983;308:263-267.

28. Cook DJ. Clinical assessment of central venous pressure in the critically ill. *Am J Med Sci.* 1990;299(3):175-178.

29. Ducas J, Magder S, McGregor M. Validity of the hepatojugular reflux as a clinical test for congestive heart failure. *Am J Cardiol.* 1983;52:1299-1303.

30. Butman SM, Ewy GA, Standen JR, et al. Bedside cardiovascular examination in patients with severe chronic heart failure: Importance of rest or inducible jugular venous distension. *J Am Coll Cardiol.* 1993;22:968-974.

31. Zema MJ, Restivo B, Sos T, et al. Left ventricular dysfunction: Bedside Valsalva manoeuvre. *Br Heart J.* 1980;44:560-569.

32. Harlan WR, Oberman A, Grim R, Rosati RA. Chronic congestive heart failure in coronary artery disease: Clinical criteria. *Ann Intern Med.* 1977;86:133-138.

33. Gadsboll N, Hoilund-Carlsen PF, Nielsen GG, et al. Interobserver agreement and accuracy of bedside estimation of right and left ventricular ejection fraction in acute myocardial infarction. *Am J Cardiol.* 1989;63:1301-1307.

34. Davie AP, Caruana FL, Sutherland GR, McMurray JJV. Assessing diagnosis in heart failure: Which features are any use? *Q J Med.* 1997;90:335-339.

35. Goldman L, Caldera DL, Nussbaum SR, et al. Multifactorial index of cardiac risk in noncardiac surgical procedures. *N Engl J Med.* 1977;297:845-850.

36. Goldman L, Caldera DL, Southwick FS, et al. Cardiac risk factors and complications in non-cardiac surgery. *Medicine.* 1978;57(4):357-370.

37. Sochowski RA, Dubbin JD, Naqvi SZ. Clinical and hemodynamic assessment of the hepatojugular reflux. *Am J Cardiol.* 1990;66:1002-1006.

38. Ewy GA. The abdominojugular test: Technique and hemodynamic correlates. *Ann Intern Med.* 1988;109:456-460.

39. Seth R, Magner P, Matzinger F, van Walraven C. How far is the sternal angle from the mid-right atrium? *J Gen Intern Med.* 2002;17:861-865.

40. Haywood GA, Joy MD, Camm AJ. Influence of posture and reference point on central venous pressure measurement. *Br Med J.* 1991;303:626-627.

41. Amoroso P, Greenwood RN. Posture and central venous pressure measurement in circulatory volume depletion. *Lancet.* 1989;2:258-260.

42. Haywood GA, Camm AJ. Posture and central venous pressure measurement in circulatory volume depletion (letter). *Lancet.* 1989;2:555-556.

43. Drazner MH, Hamilton MA, Fonarow G, et al. Relationship between right and left-sided filling pressures in 1000 patients with advanced heart failure. *J Heart Lung Transplant.* 1999;18:1126-1132.

44. Klassen-Udding LM, van Lijf JH, Napel HHT. Substernal goitre, deep venous thrombosis of the arm, and Pemberton's sign. *Neth J Med.* 1983;26:228-231.

45. Matthews MB. Hepatojugular reflux. *Lancet.* 1958;1:873-876.

46. Hitzig WM. Venous pressure curves in normal and abnormal circulatory states. I. Normal venous pressure curves and the negative "hepato-jugular reflux phenomenon". *J Mt Sinai Hosp.* 1945;12:309-334.

47. Pasteur W. Note on a new physical sign of tricuspid regurgitation. *Lancet.* 1885; 2:524.

48. Constant J, Lippschutz EJ. The one-minute abdominal compression test or "the hepatojugular reflux," a useful bedside test. *Am Heart J.* 1964;67:701-708.

49. Lange RL, Botticelli JT, Tsagaris TJ, et al. Diagnostic signs in compressive cardiac disorders: Constrictive pericarditis, pericardial effusion, and tamponade. *Circulation.* 1966;33:763-777.

50. Hitzig WM. On mechanisms of inspiratory filling of the cervical veins and pulsus paradoxus in venous hypertension. *J Mt Sinai Hosp.* 1941;8:625-644.

51. Wood P. Chronic constrictive pericarditis. *Am J Cardiol.* 1961;7:48-61.

52. Burdine JA, Wallace JM. Pulsus paradoxus and Kussmaul's sign in massive pulmonary embolism. *Am J Cardiol.* 1965;15:413-415.

53. Cintron GB, Hernandez E, Linares E, Aranda JM. Bedside recognition, incidence and clinical course of right ventricular infarction. *Am J Cardiol.* 1981;47:224-227.

54. Dell'Italia IJ, Starling MR, O'Rourke RA. Physical examination for exclusion of hemodynamically important right ventricular infarction. *Ann Intern Med.* 1983;99: 608-611.

55. Lorell B, Leinbach RC, Pohost GM, et al. Right ventricular infarction: Clinical diagnosis and differentiation from cardiac tamponade and pericardial constriction. *Am J Cardiol.* 1979;43:465-471.

56. Mittal SR, Garg S, Lalgarhia M. Jugular venous pressure and pulse wave form in the diagnosis of right ventricular infarction. *Int J Cardiol.* 1996;53:253-256.

57. Meyer TE, Sareli P, Marcus RH, et al. Mechanism underlying Kussmaul's sign in chronic constrictive pericarditis. *Am J Cardiol.* 1989;64:1069-1072.

58. Wood P. *Diseases of the heart and circulation,* 2nd ed. London: Eyre and Spottiswoode; 1956.

59. Benchimol A, Tippit HC. The clinical value of the jugular and hepatic pulses. *Prog Cardiovasc Dis.* 1967;10:159-186.

60. Constant J. *Bedside cardiology.* Boston: Little, Brown and Company; 1985.

61. Colman AL. *Clinical examination of the jugular venous pulse.* Springfield: Charles C. Thomas; 1966.

62. Rich LL, Tavel ME. The origin of the jugular C wave. *N Engl J Med.* 1971;284: 1309-1311.

63. Bonner AJ, Tavel ME. The relationship of the jugular "C" wave to changing diastolic intervals. *Am Heart J.* 1972;84:441-445.

64. Constant J. The X prime descent in jugular contour nomenclature and recognition. *Am Heart J.* 1974;88:372-379.

65. Sivaciyan V, Ranganathan N. Transcutaneous Doppler jugular venous flow velocity recording: Clinical and hemodynamic correlates. *Circulation.* 1978;57: 930-939.

66. El-Sherif A, El-Said G. Jugular, hepatic, and praecordial pulsations in constrictive pericarditis. *Br Heart J.* 1971;33:305-312.

67. Tavel ME. The use of the jugular pulse in the diagnosis of atrial septal defect. *Dis Chest.* 1968;54(6):58-59.

68. Tavel ME, Bard RA, Franks LC, et al. The jugular venous pulse in atrial septal defect. *Arch Intern Med.* 1968;121:524-529.

69. Hartman H. The jugular venous tracing. *Am Heart J.* 1960;59:698-717.

70. Wood P. An appreciation of mitral stenosis: Part 1. Clinical features. Part 2. Investigations and results. *Br Med J.* 1954;1:1051-1063, 1113-1024.

71. Puddu V. Rheumatic heart disease with normal rhythm and very large "a" waves in the jugular pulse. *Am Heart J.* 1951;41:708-717.

72. Salazar E, Levine HD. Rheumatic tricuspid regurgitation: The clinical spectrum. *Am J Med.* 1962;33:111-129.

73. Cha SD, Gooch AS. Diagnosis of tricuspid regurgitation. *Arch Intern Med.* 1983;143:1763-1768.

74. Lingamneni R, Cha SD, Maranhao V, et al. Tricuspid regurgitation: Clinical and angiographic assessment. *Cath Cardiovasc Diag.* 1979;5:7-17.

75. Whitaker W. Clinical diagnosis of pulmonary hypertension in patients with mitral stenosis. *Q J Med.* 1954;23:105-112.

76. Dock W. Loud presystolic sounds over the jugular veins associated with high venous pressure. *Am J Med.* 1956;20:853-859.

77. Abinader EG. Systolic venous reflux sounds. *Am Heart J.* 1973;85:452-457.

78. Garratt CJ, Griffith MJ, Young G, et al. Value of physical signs in the diagnosis of ventricular tachycardia. *Circulation.* 1994;90:3103-3107.

33

Percussion of the Heart

I. INTRODUCTION

Percussion of the heart has its roots in the 1820s, when a student of Laennec, Pierre Piorry, enthusiastically introduced topographic percussion, a technique purportedly allowing clinicians to precisely outline the borders of the underlying organs, including those of the heart.[1-3] Although many of Piorry's claims seem extraordinary today—he declared, for example, that he could outline pulmonary cavities, the spleen, hydatid cysts, and even individual heart chambers—many of his innovations persist, including indirect percussion, the pleximeter (Piorry used an ivory plate, but most clinicians now use the left middle finger), and the current practice of using percussion to locate the border of the diaphragm on the posterior chest or the span of the liver on the anterior body wall.[4]

In 1899, only 4 years after the discovery of roentgen rays, Williams challenged the accuracy of cardiac percussion, showing that many patients with moderately large hearts (autopsy weight of 350–500 g) had normal findings during cardiac percussion.[5] Cardiac percussion suffered another setback in 1907 when Moritz published the composite outlines of cardiac dullness according to various authorities, showing that these authorities not only disagreed with each other but also with the true roentgenographic outline.[4,6] By the 1930s, many leading clinicians began to regard percussion of the heart as unreliable and often inaccurate.[4,7]

II. CLINICAL SIGNIFICANCE

Studies of cardiac percussion have several limitations, the most important of which is selectively enrolling only healthy patients lacking chest deformities or

 Box 33-1 Percussion of the Heart*

Finding (Ref)	Sensitivity (%)	Specificity (%)	Likelihood Ratio if Finding	
			Present	Absent
Dullness extends more than 10.5 cm from midsternal line, patient supine				
Detecting cardiothoracic ratio >0.5[13]	97	61	2.5	**0.05**
Detecting increased left ventricular end-diastolic volume[14]	94	32	1.4	NS
Dullness extends beyond midclavicular line, patient upright				
Detecting cardiothoracic ratio >0.5[8]	97	60	2.4	**0.1**

NS, not significant; likelihood ratio (LR) if finding present = positive LR; LR if finding absent = negative LR.
*Diagnostic standards: Cardiothoracic ratio is maximal transverse diameter of heart on chest radiography divided by maximal transverse diameter of thoracic cage. Increased left ventricular end-diastolic volume is volume >186 mL by ultrafast computed tomography.[14]

PERCUSSION OF THE HEART

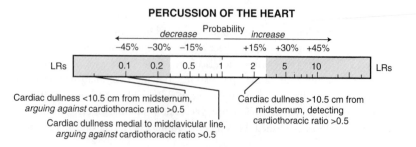

emphysema. Nonetheless, even these studies show that the percussed outline of the heart correlates only moderately with the true cardiac border. Whether the patient is supine or upright, the average error in locating the cardiac border is 1 to 2 cm (the standard deviation of this error is ~ 1 cm). The clinician usually overestimates the left border by placing it too far lateral and underestimates the right border by placing it too near the sternum (these errors tend to cancel each other if the study's endpoint is total transverse diameter of the heart).[8–11] In patients with emphysema, the errors are even greater.[12]

The traditional sign of an enlarged heart by percussion is cardiac dullness that extends too far laterally. The finding of cardiac dullness extending beyond the midclavicular line or more that 10.5 cm from the midsternal line argues modestly for an enlarged cardiothoracic ratio (likelihood ratio [LR] = 2.4–2.5, EBM Box 33-1). If cardiac dullness does *not* extend beyond these points, the patient probably does *not* have an enlarged cardiothoracic ratio (LRs = 0.05–0.1, see EBM Box 33-1). It is unlikely, however, that this information is clinically useful because the cardiothoracic ratio has uncertain clinical significance.

REFERENCES

1. Buzzi A. Piorry on percussion of the heart. *Am J Cardiol.* 1960;5:703-705.
2. Risse GB. Pierre A. Piorry (1794-1879): The French "master of percussion". *Chest.* 1971;60:484-488.
3. Sakula A. Pierre Adolphe Piorry (1794-1879): Pioneer of percussion and pleximetry. *Thorax.* 1979;34:575-581.
4. McGee S. Percussion and physical diagnosis: Separating myth from science. *Disease-a-Month.* 1995;41:643-692.
5. Jarcho S. Percussion of the heart contrasted with Roentgen examination (Williams, 1899). *Am J Cardiol.* 1969;23:845-849.
6. Moritz F. Einige Bemerkungen zur Frage der perkutorischen Darstellung der gesamten Vorderfläche des Herzens. *Dtsch Arch Klin Med.* 1907;88:276-285.
7. Parkinson J. Enlargement of the heart. *Lancet.* 1936;1:1337-1391.
8. Kurtz CM, White PD. The percussion of the heart borders and the Roentgen ray shadow of the heart. *Am J Med Sci.* 1928;176:181-195.
9. Mainland D, Stewart CB. A comparison of percussion and radiography in locating the heart and superior mediastinal vessels. *Am Heart J.* 1938;15:515-527.
10. Karnegis JN, Kadri N. Accuracy of percussion of the left cardiac border. *Int J Cardiol.* 1992;37:361-364.
11. Stroud WD, Stroud MW, Marshall DS. Measurement of the total transverse diameter of the heart by direct percussion. *Am Heart J.* 1948;35:780-786.
12. Dietlen H. Die Perkussion der wahren Herzgrenzen. *Dtsch Arch Klin Med.* 1906-1907;88:286-301.

13. Heckerling PS, Wiener SL, Moses VK, et al. Accuracy of precordial percussion in detecting cardiomegaly. *Am J Med.* 1991;91:328-334.

14. Heckerling PS, Wiener SL, Wolfkiel CJ, et al. Accuracy and reproducibility of precordial percussion and palpation for detecting increased left ventricular end-diastolic volume and mass: A comparison of physical findings and ultrafast computed tomography of the heart. *JAMA.* 1993;270:1943-1948.

34

Palpation of
the Heart

I. INTRODUCTION

Much of the science of heart palpation is based on impulse cardiography and kinetocardiography, research tools from the 1960s that precisely timed normal and abnormal precordial movements and compared them with hemodynamic data and angiograms of the right and left ventricles. These precise and sensitive instruments could detect very small movements of the body wall, many of which are inconspicuous to the clinician's hand. Although this chapter refers to these studies to make certain points, only those movements easily palpable at the bedside are discussed.

Palpation of the heart is among the oldest physical examination technique, having been recorded as early as 1550 BC by ancient Egyptian physicians (along with palpation of the peripheral pulses).[1] In the early 19th century, Jean-Nicolas Corvisart, personal physician to Napoleon and teacher of Laennec, was the first to correlate cardiac palpation with postmortem findings and point out the distinguishing features of right and left ventricular enlargement.[2-4] During animal experiments performed in 1830, James Hope proved that the cause of the apical impulse was ventricular contraction, which threw the heart up against the chest wall.[5]

II. TECHNIQUE

When palpating the chest, the clinician should describe the location, size, timing, and type of precordial movements.[6]

A. PATIENT POSITION

The clinician should first palpate the heart when the patient is lying supine and again with the patient lying on his or her left side. The supine position is used to locate all precordial movements and to identify whether these movements are abnormally hyperkinetic, sustained, or retracting (see later). The left lateral decubitus position is used to measure the diameter of the apical impulse and to detect additional abnormal diastolic filling movements (i.e., palpable third or fourth heart sounds).[7]

Because the left lateral decubitus position distorts the systolic apical movement, including those of healthy subjects (i.e., up to half of healthy patients have "abnormal" sustained movements in the lateral decubitus position), only the supine position should be used to characterize the patient's outward systolic movement.[8]

B. LOCATION OF ABNORMAL MOVEMENTS

Complete palpation of the heart includes four areas on the chest wall (Figure 34-1).[1,6,9–12]

1. Apex Beat

The "apex beat" or "apical impulse" is the palpable cardiac impulse farthest away from the sternum and farthest down on the chest wall, usually caused by the left ventricle and located near the midclavicular line in the fifth intercostal space.

The clinician should also palpate the areas above and medial to the apex beat, where ventricular aneurysms sometimes become palpable.

2. Left Lower Sternal Area (Fourth Intercostal Space near Left Edge of Sternum)

Abnormal right ventricular and left atrial movements appear at this location.

3. Left Base (Second Intercostal Space near the Left Sternum)

Abnormal pulmonary artery movements or a palpable P_2 appear at this location.

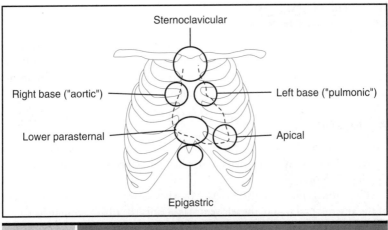

| FIGURE 34-1 | LOCATIONS OF PRECORDIAL MOVEMENTS. |

The principal areas of precordial pulsations are the apical area, lower parasternal area, left base (i.e., second left intercostal parasternal space, "pulmonic area"), right base (i.e., second right intercostal parasternal space, "aortic area"), and sternoclavicular areas. In some patients, especially those with chronic lung disease, right ventricular movements may appear in the epigastric area. The best external landmark is the sternal angle, which is where the second rib joins the sternum.

4. Right Base (Second Intercostal Space near Right Edge of Sternum) and Sternoclavicular Joint

Movements from an ascending aortic aneurysm may become palpable here.

C. MAKING PRECORDIAL MOVEMENTS MORE CONSPICUOUS

Two teaching techniques are often used to bring out precordial movements and make them easier to time and characterize. In the first technique, the clinician puts a dot of ink on the area of interest, whose direction and timing then become easy to see. In the second technique, the clinician holds a cotton-tipped applicator stick against the chest wall, with the wooden end of the stick just off the center of the area of interest (the stick should be several inches long). The stick becomes a lever and the pulsating chest wall a fulcrum, causing the free end of the stick to trace in the air a magnified replica of the precordial movement. A folded paper Post-it® may substitute for the applicator stick.[13]

III. THE FINDINGS

Precordial movements are timed by simultaneously listening to the heart tones and noting the relationship between outward movements on the chest wall and the first and second heart sounds. There are four types of systolic movement: normal, hyperkinetic, sustained, and retracting.[1,6,9–11]

A. NORMAL

The normal systolic movement is a small outward movement that begins with S_1, ends by midsystole, and then retracts inward, returning to its original position long before S_2.

The normal apical impulse is caused by a brisk early systolic anterior motion of the anteroseptal wall of the left ventricle against the ribs.[14] Despite its name, the apex beat bears no consistent relationship to the anatomic apex of the left ventricle.[14] In the supine position, the apex beat is palpable in only 25% to 40% of adults.[15–18] In the lateral decubitus position, it is palpable in only about 50% of adults.[15,19] The apex beat is more likely to be palpable in patients who have less body fat and who weigh less.[20] Some studies show that the apical impulse is more likely to be present in women than men, but this difference disappears after controlling for the participant's weights.[17]

B. HYPERKINETIC

The hyperkinetic (or "overacting" movement) is a movement identical in timing to the normal movement, although its amplitude is exaggerated. Distinguishing normal from hyperkinetic amplitude is a subjective process, even on precise tracings from impulse cardiography. This probably explains why the finding has minimal diagnostic value, appearing both in patients with volume overload of the left ventricle (e.g., aortic regurgitation, ventricular septal defect) and in some normal persons who have thin chests or increased cardiac output.

C. SUSTAINED

The sustained movement is an abnormal outward movement that begins at S_1 but, unlike normal and hyperkinetic movements, extends to S_2 or even past it before beginning to descend to its original position. The amplitude of the sustained movement may be normal or increased. Sustained apical movements are always abnormal, indicating either pressure overload of the left ventricle (e.g., aortic stenosis), volume overload (e.g., aortic regurgitation, ventricular septal defect), a combination of pressure and volume overload (combined aortic stenosis and regurgitation), severe cardiomyopathy, or ventricular aneurysm.

D. RETRACTING

In the retracting movement, inward motion begins at S_1 and outward motion does not start until early diastole. Because retracting movements are sometimes identical to normal movements in every characteristic except for timing, they are easily overlooked unless the clinician listens to the heart tones when palpating the chest. Only two diagnoses cause the retracting impulse, constrictive pericarditis and severe tricuspid regurgitation.[1,8,11]

E. HEAVES, LIFTS, AND THRUSTS

The words "heave" and "lift" sometimes refer to sustained movements and "thrust" to hyperkinetic ones, but these terms, often used imprecisely, are best avoided.[1,9–11]

IV. CLINICAL SIGNIFICANCE

A. APEX BEAT

1. Location

A traditional sign of an enlarged heart is an abnormally displaced apical impulse, which means it is located lateral to some external reference point. The three traditional reference points are (1) midclavicular line, (2) a set distance from the midsternal line (the traditional upper limit of normal is 10 cm), and (3) nipple line.

Of these three landmarks, the midclavicular line is the best, as long as the clinician locates it carefully by palpating the acromioclavicular and sternoclavicular joints and marking the midpoint between them with a ruler.[21,22] In the supine patient, an apical impulse located outside the midclavicular line argues that the heart is enlarged on the chest radiograph [likelihood ratio (LR) = 3.4; EBM Box 34-1], the ejection fraction is depressed (LR = 10.1), the left ventricular end-diastolic volume is increased (LR = 8.0), and the pulmonary capillary wedge pressure is increased (LR = 5.8). Other studies confirm the relationship between displaced apical impulse and depressed ejection fraction.[29]

Using a point 10 cm from the midsternal line to define the displaced impulse is not a useful predictor of the enlarged heart (positive LR not significant, negative LR = 0.5; see EBM Box 34-1), probably because the 10 cm threshold is set too low (the midclavicular line usually lies 10.5 to 11.5 cm from the midsternal line).[21] Finally, the nipple line is the least reliable of the three landmarks, bearing no consistent relationship to the apical impulse or to the size of the chest, even in men. The distance of the nipple line from the midsternum or midclavicular line varies greatly.[30]

2. Diameter of the Apical Impulse

As measured in the left lateral decubitus position at 45 degrees, an apical impulse with a diameter ≥ 4 cm argues that the patient has a dilated heart (LR = 4.7 for

Box 34-1   Size and Position of Palpable Apical Impulse*

Finding (Ref)[†]	Sensitivity (%)	Specificity (%)	Likelihood Ratio if Finding Present	Absent
POSITION OF APICAL BEAT				
Supine apical impulse lateral to MCL				
Detecting cardiothoracic ratio >0.5[18,20,23]	39–60	76–93	**3.4**	0.6
Detecting low ejection fraction[24–26]	24–66	93–98	**10.1**	0.6
Detecting increased left ventricular end-diastolic volume[27]	33	96	**8.0**	0.7
Detecting pulmonary capillary wedge pressure >12 mm Hg[27]	42	93	**5.8**	NS
Supine apical impulse >10 cm from midsternal line				
Detecting cardiothoracic ratio >0.5[16,20,23]	61–80	28–97	NS	0.5
SIZE OF APICAL BEAT				
Apical beat diameter ≥4 cm in left lateral decubitus position at 45 degrees				
Detecting increased left ventricular end-diastolic volume[19,28]	48–85	79–96	**4.7**	NS

MCL, midclavicular line; NS, not significant; likelihood ratio (LR) if finding present = positive LR; LR if finding absent = negative LR.

*Diagnostic standards: Cardiothoracic ratio is maximal transverse diameter of heart on chest radiography divided by maximal transverse diameter of thoracic cage; low ejection fraction, radionuclide left ventricular ejection fraction < 0.50[25] or < 0.53,[24] or left ventricular fractional shortening < 25% by echocardiography[26]; increased left ventricular end-diastolic volume by echocardiography: >90 mL/M[2],[27] >138 mL,[28] or upper fifth percentile of normal measurements by age and body surface area[19].

[†]Definition of findings: These data apply to all patients, whether or not an apical beat is palpable (i.e., if the apex beat is not palpable, the test is regarded as "negative"). The only exception is the data for "apical beat diameter," which applies only to patients who have a measurable apical beat in the left lateral decubitus position (i.e., apical beat diameter ≥4 cm = test positive; < 4 cm = test negative; unable to measure diameter = unable to evaluate using these data).

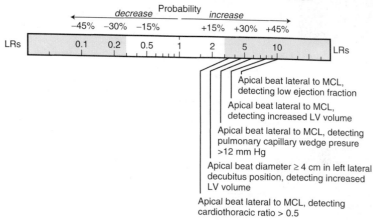

SIZE AND POSITION OF PALPABLE APICAL IMPULSE

increased left ventricular end-diastolic volume; see EBM Box 34-1). Smaller thresholds (e.g., 3 cm) discriminate between dilated and normal hearts in some studies but not others.[19,28]

3.   Abnormal Movements

a.   Hyperkinetic Apical Movements

The hyperkinetic apical movement is an important finding in one setting. In patients with mitral stenosis, left ventricular filling is impaired, causing the apical impulse to be normal or even reduced.[31] Therefore, if patients with the murmur of mitral stenosis also have a hyperkinetic apical impulse, an abnormality other than mitral stenosis also must be present, such as mitral regurgitation or aortic regurgitation (LR = 11.2; EBM Box 34-2).

b.   Sustained Apical Movements

In patients with aortic flow murmurs, the finding of a sustained apical impulse argues that the murmur represents severe aortic stenosis (LR = 4.1; see EBM Box 34-2). In patients with the early diastolic murmur of aortic regurgitation, the sustained impulse is less helpful (LR = 2.4 for significant regurgitation), although the finding of a normal or absent apical impulse (i.e., not sustained or hyperkinetic) in these patients argues strongly *against* moderate-to-severe aortic regurgitation (LR = 0.1; see EBM Box 34-2).

In patients without murmurs, the sustained apical impulse is a sign of cardiomyopathy. In one study of consecutive patients on general medicine service, patients with a sustained apical impulse had a significantly lower ejection fraction (37%) than those with a normal or absent apical beat (49%).[29]

Box 34-2 — Abnormal Palpable Movements*

Finding (Ref)[†]	Sensitivity (%)	Specificity (%)	Likelihood Ratio if Finding	
			Present	Absent
Hyperkinetic apical movement				
Detecting associated mitral regurgitation or aortic valve disease in patients with mitral stenosis[31]	74	93	**11.2**	**0.3**
Sustained apical movement				
Detecting severe aortic stenosis in patients with aortic flow murmurs[32]	78	81	**4.1**	**0.3**
Detecting moderate-to-severe aortic regurgitation in patients with basal early diastolic murmurs[33]	97	60	2.4	**0.1**
Sustained left lower parasternal movement				
Detecting right ventricular peak pressure ≥50 mm Hg[34]	71	80	**3.6**	0.4
Palpable P$_2$				
Detecting pulmonary hypertension in patients with mitral stenosis[35]	96	73	**3.6**	**0.05**

Likelihood ratio (LR) if finding present = positive LR; LR if finding absent = negative LR.
Diagnostic standards: for severe aortic stenosis and moderate-to-severe aortic regurgitation, see tables in Chapters 40 and 41; for pulmonary hypertension, mean pulmonary artery pressure ≥50 mm Hg.[35]
[†]*Definition of findings: For abnormal apical movement "apical impulse heave or enlarged,"[33] "sustained,"[32] or "thrust"[31]; for abnormal parasternal movement, "movement extending to or past S$_2$,"[34]; for palpable P$_2$ "palpable late systolic tap in second left intercostal space next to sternum, which frequently followed parasternal lift."[35]*

ABNORMAL PALPABLE MOVEMENTS

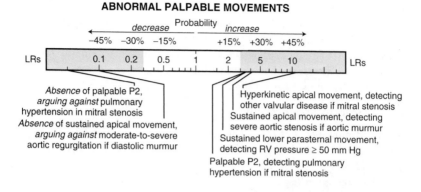

c. Retracting Apical Impulse

(1) Constrictive Pericarditis In up to 90% of patients with constrictive pericarditis, the apical impulse retracts during systole (sometimes accompanied by systolic retraction of the left parasternal area).[8,36] In these patients, the diseased pericardium prevents the normal outward systolic movement of the ventricles but allows rapid and prominent early diastolic filling of the ventricle. The prominent diastolic filling causes a palpable diastolic outward movement, which contributes to the overall impression that the apical impulse retracts during systole (see Chapter 43).

The first clinician to recognize the retracting apical impulse as a sign of "adhesive" pericarditis was Skoda in 1852.[37]

(2) Tricuspid Regurgitation In severe tricuspid regurgitation, a dilated right ventricle, occupying the apex, ejects blood into a dilated right atrium and liver, located nearer the sternum.[8] This causes a characteristic rocking motion, the apical area retracting inward during systole and the lower left or right parasternal area moving outward during systole.[38]

B. LEFT LOWER PARASTERNAL MOVEMENTS

In normal persons, the clinician either palpates no movement or only a tiny inward one during systole at this location. Abnormal movements at this location are classified as "hyperkinetic" or "sustained," depending on their relationship to S_2.

1. Hyperkinetic Movements

Hyperkinetic movements of the left lower parasternal area occur in up to 50% of patients with atrial septal defect, which causes volume overload of the right ventricle.[39] Nonetheless, this finding has limited diagnosis value without other findings of atrial septal defect—exaggerated y descent in the neck veins, wide and fixed S_2 splitting, and midsystolic murmur at the left second intercostal space (usually of grade 2/6)—because it is also sometimes found in patients without heart disease, such as those with thin chests, pectus excavatum, fever, or other high output states.[34,39]

2. Sustained Movements

Sustained movements of the left lower sternal area may represent either an abnormal right ventricle (e.g., pressure overload from pulmonary hypertension or pulmonic stenosis or volume overload from atrial septal defect) or an enlarged left atrium (e.g., severe mitral regurgitation). Both right ventricular and left atrial parasternal movements are outward movements that begin to move inward only at S_2 or just after it and therefore are classified as "sustained"; they are distinguished by when the outward movement *begins*.

a. Right Ventricle

Outward right ventricular movements begin at the first heart sound. If the clinician can exclude volume overload of the right ventricle and mitral regurgitation (both of which also cause parasternal movements), the finding of a sustained left parasternal movement is a modest sign of pulmonary hypertension. In patients with mitral stenosis, the duration of the sustained lower parasternal movement correlates well with pulmonary pressures.[31] In patients with a wide variety of valvular and congenital heart lesions (excluding mitral regurgitation), the sustained lower left parasternal movement is a modest discriminator between those with peak right ventricular pressures greater than 50 mm Hg and those with lower pressures (positive LR = 3.6, negative LR 0.4; see EBM Box 34-2). Up to 30% of patients with atrial septal defect, whether or not there is associated pulmonary hypertension, also have sustained lower left parasternal movements.[39]

b. Left Atrium and Mitral Regurgitation

In patients with severe mitral regurgitation, ventricular contraction forces blood backward into a dilated left atrium, which lies on the posterior surface of the heart and acts like an expanding cushion to lift up the heart, including the left parasternal area. This sustained movement, most easily palpated in the fourth or fifth intercostal space near the sternum,[40,41] differs from those caused by the right ventricle, because outward movement begins in the second half of systole (it parallels the V wave on the left atrial pressure tracing).

In patients with isolated mitral regurgitation, the degree of the late systolic outward movement at the lower sternal edge correlates well with the severity of mitral regurgitation ($r = 0.93$, $p < .01$; the correlation is much worse if there is associated mitral stenosis, which may cause parasternal movements from pulmonary hypertension).[40,41] In pure mitral regurgitation, as in atrial septal defect, the parasternal movement has no relationship to right ventricular pressures.[42]

C.   ANEURYSMS

In one study of consecutive patients with ventricular aneurysms identified by angiography, 33% had abnormal precordial movements.[43] Typical findings were (1) a double cardiac impulse, the first component representing the normal apical outward movement and second the bulging of the aneurysm during peak ventricular pressures later in systole,[44,45] and (2) a sustained impulse that extended superiorly or medially from the usual location of the apical impulse.[43] If detectable by palpation, the aneurysm originates in the anterior wall or apex of the left ventricle; aneurysms originating from the inferior or lateral wall are too distant from the anterior chest wall to be detectable by palpation.[43]

D.   DIFFUSE PRECORDIAL MOVEMENTS

Diffuse outward movements of the entire precordium, from the apex to lower parasternal area, may result from (1) right ventricular enlargement (which dilates to occupy the apical area), (2) left ventricular enlargement (which rotates to occupy the lower parasternal area), or (3) biventricular enlargement.[11] Palpation alone cannot distinguish these different etiologies—even sensitive recordings from impulse cardiography or kinetocardiography could not do this—and the clinician must look to other findings to determine which chamber is most likely causing the diffuse movement.

E.   RIGHT LOWER PARASTERNAL MOVEMENTS

Abnormal systolic outward movements appear in the right lower parasternal area from tricuspid regurgitation (ejection of blood into the right atrium and liver, which lies under the right side of the sternum) or from mitral regurgitation (ejection of blood in a dilated left atrium).[11,38,46]

F.   PALPABLE P$_2$

A palpable P$_2$ (i.e., the pulmonic component of second heart sound) is a sharp, brief snapping sensation felt over the left base, coincident with S$_2$. It is much briefer than other precordial movements. In patients with mitral stenosis, a palpable P$_2$ argues somewhat *for* the diagnosis of pulmonary hypertension (LR = 3.6 for mean pulmonary pressure >50 mm Hg). More importantly, the absence of a palpable P$_2$ in these patients argues strongly *against* a pulmonary pressure this high (LR = 0.05; see EBM Box 34-2).

G.   PALPABLE THIRD AND FOURTH HEART SOUNDS

Some patients with rapid early ventricular filling (e.g., mitral regurgitation) have a palpable early diastolic movement at the apex. Other patients with strong atrial contractions into stiff ventricles (e.g., hypertensive or ischemic heart disease) have palpable presystolic apical movements. These movements have the same significance as their audible counterparts, the third and fourth heart sound (i.e., S_3 and S_4, see Chapter 37). They are usually called "palpable S_3" and "palpable S_4."

The S_4 is much more likely to be palpable than the S_3, and both are more likely to be felt when the patient is in the lateral decubitus position.[7,9,10] The palpable S_4 causes either a double outward impulse near S_1 (a common analogy is the "grace note" in music) or single outward movement, consisting of the palpable S_4 and apical beat together, which is distinguished from the apical beat alone because the outward movement begins slightly before S_1.[10,11]

REFERENCES

1. Basta LL, Bettinger JJ. The cardiac impulse: A new look at an old art. *Am Heart J.* 1979;97:96-111.
2. Stokes W. *An introduction to the use of the stethoscope* (facsimile edition by the Classics of Cardiology Library). Edinburgh: Maclachlin and Stewart; 1825.
3. Corvisart JN. *An essay on the organic diseases and lesions of the heart and great vessels* (facsimile edition by New York Academy of Medicine). Boston: Bradford and Read; 1812.
4. Willius FA, Dry TJ. *A history of the heart and the circulation.* Philadelphia: W.B. Saunders Co; 1948.
5. McCrady JD, Hoff HE, Geddes LA. The contributions of the horse to knowledge of the heart and circulation. IV. James Hope and the heart sounds. *Conn Med.* 1966;30:126-131.
6. Feinstein AR, Hochstein E, Luisada AA, et al. Glossary of cardiologic terms related to physical diagnosis and history. Part III. Anterior chest movements. *Dis Chest.* 1969;56:231-232.
7. Bethell HJN, Nixon PGF. Examination of the heart in supine and left lateral positions. *Br Heart J.* 1973;35:902-907.
8. Boicourt OW, Nagle RE, Mounsey JPD. The clinical significance of systolic retraction of the apical impulse. *Br Heart J.* 1965;27:379-391.
9. Mounsey JPD. Inspection and palpation of the cardiac impulse. *Prog Cardiovasc Dis.* 1967;10:187-206.
10. Mounsey P. Praecordial pulsations in health and disease. *Postgrad Med J.* 1968; 44:134-139.
11. Stapleton JF, Groves BM. Precordial palpation. *Am Heart J.* 1971;81:409-427.
12. Willis PW. Analysis of precordial movements. *Heart Dis Stroke.* 1993;2:284-289.
13. Shindler D. Post-it apexcardiography. *N Engl J Med.* 2004;351:1364.
14. Deliyannis AA, Gillam PMS, Mounsey JPD, Steiner RE. The cardiac impulse and the motion of the heart. *Br Heart J.* 1964;26:396-411.

15. Heckerling PS, Wiener SL, Wolfkiel CJ, et al. Accuracy and reproducibility of precordial percussion and palpation for detecting increased left ventricular end-diastolic volume and mass: A comparison of physical findings and ultrafast computed tomography of the heart. *JAMA*. 1993;270:1943-1948.

16. Heckerling PS, Wiener SL, Moses VK, et al. Accuracy of precordial percussion in detecting cardiomegaly. *Am J Med*. 1991;91:328-334.

17. Niehaus FW, Wright WD. Facts and fallacies about the normal apex beat. *Am Heart J*. 1945;30:604-609.

18. Mulkerrin E, Saran R, Dewar R, et al. The apex cardiac beat: Not a reliable clinical sign in elderly patients. *Age Ageing*. 1991;20:304-306.

19. Dans AL, Bossone EF, Guyatt GH, Fallen EL. Evaluation of the reproducibility and accuracy of apex beat measurement in the detection of echocardiographic left ventricular dilation. *Can J Cardiol*. 1995;11:493-497.

20. O'Neill TW, Smith M, Barry M, Graham IM. Diagnostic value of the apex beat. *Lancet*. 1989;1:410-411.

21. Naylor CD, McCormack DG, Sullivan SN. The midclavicular line: A wandering landmark. *Can Med Assoc J*. 1987;136:48-50.

22. Ryand DA. The midclavicular line: Where is it? *Ann Intern Med*. 1968;69:329-330.

23. O'Neill TW, Barry MA, Smith M, Graham IM. Diagnostic value of the apex beat. *Lancet*. 1989;2:499.

24. Gadsboll N, Hoilund-Carlsen PF, Nielsen GG, et al. Interobserver agreement and accuracy of bedside estimation of right and left ventricular ejection fraction in acute myocardial infarction. *Am J Cardiol*. 1989;63:1301-1307.

25. Mattleman SJ, Hakki AH, Iskandrian AS, et al. Reliability of bedside evaluation in determining left ventricular function: Correlation with left ventricular ejection fraction determined by radionuclide ventriculography. *J Am Coll Cardiol*. 1983;1:417-420.

26. Davie AP, Caruana FL, Sutherland GR, McMurray JJV. Assessing diagnosis in heart failure: Which features are any use? *Q J Med*. 1997;90:335-339.

27. Gadsboll N, Hoilund-Carlsen PF, Nielsen GG, et al. Symptoms and signs of heart failure in patients with myocardial infarction: Reproducibility and relationship to chest X-ray, radionuclide ventriculography and right heart catheterization. *Eur Heart J*. 1989;10:1017-1028.

28. Eilen SD, Crawford MH, O'Rourke RA. Accuracy of precordial palpation for detecting increased left ventricular volume. *Ann Intern Med*. 1983;99:628-630.

29. Eagle KA, Quertermous T, Singer DE, et al. Left ventricular ejection fraction: Physician estimates compared with gated blood pool scan measurements. *Arch Intern Med*. 1988;148:882-885.

30. Kurtz CM, White PD. The percussion of the heart borders and the Roentgen ray shadow of the heart. *Am J Med Sci*. 1928;176:181-195.

31. Wood P. An appreciation of mitral stenosis. Part 1. Clinical features. Part 2. Investigations and results. *Br Med J*. 1954;1:1051-1063, 1113-1024.

32. Forssell G, Jonasson R, Orinius E. Identifying severe aortic valvular stenosis by bed-side examination. *Acta Med Scand.* 1985;218:397-400.

33. Frank MJ, Casanegra P, Migliori AJ, Levinson GE. The clinical evaluation of aortic regurgitation. *Arch Intern Med.* 1965;116:357-365.

34. Gillam PMS, Deliyannis AA, Mounsey JPD. The left parasternal impulse. *Br Heart J.* 1964;26:726-736.

35. Whitaker W. Clinical diagnosis of pulmonary hypertension in patients with mitral stenosis. *Q J Med.* 1954;23:105-112.

36. El-Sherif A, El-Said G. Jugular, hepatic, and praecordial pulsations in constrictive pericarditis. *Br Heart J.* 1971;33:305-312.

37. Skoda J. *Auscultation and percussion.* Philadelphia: Lindsay and Blakiston; 1854.

38. Salazar E, Levine HD. Rheumatic tricuspid regurgitation: The clinical spectrum. *Am J Med.* 1962;33:111-129.

39. Fukumoto T, Ito M, Arita M, et al. Right parasternal lift in atrial septal defect. *Am Heart J.* 1977;94:699-704.

40. James TM, Swatzell RH, Eddleman EE. Hemodynamic significance of the precordial late systolic outward movement in mitral regurgitation. *Ala J Med Sci.* 1978;15:55-64.

41. Basta LL, Wolfson P, Eckberg DL, Abboud FM. The value of left parasternal impulse recordings in the assessment of mitral regurgitation. *Circulation.* 1973;48:1055-1065.

42. Manchester GH, Block P, Gorlin R. Misleading signs in mitral insufficiency. *JAMA.* 1965;191:99-100.

43. Gorlin R, Klein MD, Sullivan JM. Prospective correlative study of ventricular aneurysm: Mechanistic concept and clinical recognition. *Am J Med.* 1967;42:512-531.

44. El-Sherif A, Saad Y, El-Said G. Praecordial tracings of myocardial aneurysms. *Br Heart J.* 1969;31:357-364.

45. Eddleman EE, Langley JO. Paradoxical pulsation of the precordium in myocardial infarction and angina pectoris. *Am Heart J.* 1962;63:579-581.

46. El-Sherif N, El-Ramly Z. External left atrial pulse tracings in extreme left atrial dilation. *Am Heart J.* 1972;84:387-394.

35

Auscultation of the Heart: General Principles

I. CHARACTERISTICS OF HEART SOUNDS AND MURMURS

Different heart sounds and murmurs are distinguished by four characteristics: (1) their timing (i.e.., systolic or diastolic), (2) intensity (i.e., loud or soft), (3) duration (i.e., long or short), and (4) pitch (i.e., low or high frequency). A fifth characteristic, the sound's quality, is also sometimes included in descriptions of sounds (e.g., "musical," "whoop," "honk"). Almost all heart sounds contain a mixture of frequencies (i.e., they are not "musical" in the acoustical sense, but instead are "noise," like the static of a radio). Therefore, the descriptors "low frequency" and "high frequency" do not indicate that a sound has a pure musical tone of a certain low or high pitch but instead that the bulk of the sound's energy is within the low or high range.

411

Although the human ear can hear sounds with frequencies from 20 to 20,000 cycles per second (Hz), the principal frequencies of heart sounds and murmurs are at the lower end of this range, from 20 to 500 Hz.[1,2] Low-frequency sounds, therefore, are those whose dominant frequencies are less than 100 Hz, such as third and fourth heart sounds and the diastolic murmur of mitral stenosis. These sounds are usually difficult to hear because the human ear perceives lower frequencies relatively less well than higher frequencies. The murmur containing the highest frequency sound is aortic regurgitation, whose dominant frequencies are about 400 Hz. The principal frequencies of other sounds and murmurs are between 100 and 400 Hz.

II. THE STETHOSCOPE

A. BELL AND DIAPHRAGM

The stethoscope has two different heads to receive sound, the bell and the diaphragm. The bell is used to detect low-frequency sounds; the diaphragm, high-frequency sounds.

The traditional explanation that the bell selectively transmits low-frequency sounds and the diaphragm selectively filters out low-frequency sounds is probably incorrect. Actually, the bell transmits all frequencies well, but in some patients with high-frequency murmurs (e.g., aortic regurgitation), any additional low-frequency sound masks the high-frequency sound and makes the murmur difficult to detect.[3] The diaphragm does not selectively filter out low-frequency sounds, but instead attenuates all frequencies equally, thus dropping the barely audible low-frequency ones below the threshold of human hearing.[3]

B. PERFORMANCE OF DIFFERENT STETHOSCOPE MODELS

Many studies have examined the acoustics of stethoscopes, but the clinical relevance of this research has never been formally tested. In general, these studies show that shallow bells transmit sound as well as deeper bells and that double tube stethoscopes are equivalent to single tube models.[3] The optimal internal bore of a stethoscope is somewhere between 1/8 and 3/16 inch, because smaller bores diminish transmission of the higher frequency sounds.[1,4,5] Compared with shorter lengths of stethoscope tubing, longer tubes also impair the conduction of high-frequency sounds.[1]

Most modern stethoscopes, however, transmit sound equally well, the differences among various models for single frequencies being very small.[3] The most important source of poor acoustic performance is an air leak, which typically results from poorly fitting ear pieces. Even a tiny air leak with a diameter of only 0.015 inch will diminish transmission of sound by as much as 20 dB,* particularly for those sounds less than 100 Hz.[6]

III. USE OF THE STETHOSCOPE

Between the 1950s and late 1970s, cardiac auscultation was at its peak.† During this time cardiologists perfected their skills by routinely comparing the bedside findings to the patient's phonocardiogram, angiogram, and surgical findings, which allowed clinicians to make precise and accurate diagnoses from bedside findings alone. The principles of bedside diagnosis used by these clinicians are included elsewhere in this book. How these clinicians specifically used the stethoscope to examine the patient is presented in the following.

A. THE ROOM SHOULD BE QUIET

Many faint heart sounds and murmurs are inaudible unless there is complete silence in the room. The clinician should close the door to the examination room, turn off the television and radio, and ask that all conversation stop.

B. VARYING PRESSURE ON THE BELL

To detect low-frequency sounds, the bell should be applied to the body wall with only enough pressure to create an air seal and exclude ambient noise. Excessive pressure with the bell stretches the skin, which then acts like a diaphragm and makes low-frequency sounds more difficult to hear. By selectively varying the pressure on the stethoscope bell, the clinician can easily distinguish low- from high-frequency sounds: if a sound is audible with the bell using light pressure but disappears with firm pressure, it is a low-frequency sound. This technique is often used to confirm that an early diastolic sound is indeed a third heart sound (i.e., third heart sounds are low-frequency sounds, whereas other early diastolic sounds like the pericardial knock are high-frequency sounds) and to distinguish the combined fourth and first heart sounds (S_4-S_1) from the split S_1 (the S_4 is a low-frequency sound but the S_1 is not; firm pressure renders the S_4-S_1 into a single sound but does not affect the double sound of the split S_1).

---

*Decibels describe relative intensity (or loudness) on a logarithmic scale.
†In the late 1970s, two events initiated the decline of cardiac auscultation: the widespread introduction of echocardiography and the decision by insurance companies to no longer reimburse phonocardiography.

C.   PATIENT POSITION

The clinician should listen to the patient's heart with the patient in three positions: supine, left lateral decubitus, and seated upright. The lateral decubitus position is best for detection of the third and fourth heart sounds and the diastolic murmur of mitral stenosis (to detect these sounds, the clinician places the bell lightly over the apical impulse or just medial to the apical impulse).[7] The seated upright position is necessary to further evaluate audible expiratory splitting of S_2 (see Chapter 36) and to detect some pericardial rubs and murmurs of aortic regurgitation (see Chapters 41 and 43).

D.   ORDER OF EXAMINATION

Routine auscultation of the heart should include the right upper sternal area, the entire left sternal border, and the apex. Some cardiologists recommend proceeding from base to apex[2]; others from apex to base.[8] The diaphragm of the stethoscope should be applied to all areas, especially at the upper left sternal area to detect S_2 splitting and at all areas to detect other murmurs and sounds. After using the diaphragm to listen to the lower left sternal area and apex, the bell should also be applied to these areas to detect diastolic filling sounds (S_3 and S_4) and diastolic rumbling murmurs (e.g., mitral stenosis).

In selected patients, the clinician also should listen over the carotid arteries and axilla (in patients with systolic murmurs, to clarify radiation of murmur), the lower right sternal area (in patients with diastolic murmur of aortic regurgitation, to detect aortic root disease), the back (in young patients with hypertension, to detect the continuous murmur of coarctation), or other thoracic sites (in patients with central cyanosis, to detect the continuous murmur of pulmonary arteriovenous fistula).

E.   DESCRIBING THE LOCATION OF SOUNDS

When describing heart sounds and murmurs, the clinician should identify where on the chest wall the sound is loudest. Traditionally, the second right intercostal space next to the sternum is called the "aortic area" or "right base"; the second left intercostal space next to the sternum, the "pulmonary area" or "left base"; the fourth or fifth left parasternal space, the "tricuspid area" or "left lower sternal border", and; the most lateral point of the palpable cardiac impulse, the "mitral area" or "apex" (see Fig. 34-1 in Chapter 34).

The terms "aortic area," "pulmonary area," "tricuspid area," and "mitral area" are ambiguous, however, and are best avoided. Many patients with aortic stenosis have murmurs loudest in the "mitral area," and many with mitral regurgitation have murmurs loudest in the "pulmonary" or "aortic area." A more precise way to describe the location of sounds is to use the apex and the parasternal areas as reference points, the parasternal location being further specified by the intercostal space (first, second, third, or lower sternal border), and whether it is the right or left edge of the sternum. For example, a sound might be loudest at the "apex," the "second left intercostal space" (i.e., next to the left sternal edge in the second intercostal space), or "between the apex and left lower sternal border."

F. TECHNIQUE OF FOCUSING

The human brain has an uncanny ability to isolate and focus on one type of sensory information, by repressing awareness of all other sensations. A common example of this phenomenon is the person reading a book in a room in which a clock is ticking. The person can read long passages of the book without even hearing the clock but hears the ticking clock immediately after putting the book down. When listening to the heart, the clinician's attention is quickly drawn to the most prominent sounds, but this occurs at the expense of detecting the fainter sounds. Therefore, to avoid missing these fainter sounds or subtle splitting, the clinician should concentrate sequentially on each part of the cardiac cycle, asking the following questions at each location: (1) Is S_1 soft or loud? (2) Is S_2 split and, if so, how is it split? (3) Are there are any extra sounds or murmurs during systole? and (4) Are there any extra sounds or murmurs during diastole?

G.   IDENTIFYING SYSTOLE AND DIASTOLE

Because all auscultatory findings are characterized by their timing, distinguishing systole from diastole accurately is essential. Three principles help the clinician distinguish these events.

1.   Systole is Shorter than Diastole

If the heart rate is normal or slow, systole can be easily distinguished from diastole because systole is much shorter. The normal cadence of the heart tones, therefore, is

> *lub dup   lub dup   lub dup   lub dup*

(*lub* is S_1 and *dup* is S_2). When the heart rate accelerates, however, diastole shortens and, at a rate of 100 or more, the cadence of S_1 and S_2 resembles a "tic toc" rhythm:

> *lub dup lub dup lub dup lub dup lub dup lub dup*

In these patients, other techniques are necessary to distinguish systole from diastole.

2.   Characteristics of the First and Second Heart Sounds

At the second left intercostal space, S_2 is generally louder, shorter and sharper than S_1 (S_2 has more high-frequency energy than S_1, which is why *dup*, a snappier sound than *lub*, is used to characterize S_2). If the timing of extra heart sounds and murmurs is confusing at the lower sternal edge or apex (as it often is in patients with fast heart rhythms), the clinician can return the stethoscope to the second left intercostal space, identify S_2 by its louder and sharper sound, and then inch slowly back to the area of interest, keeping track of S_2 along the way.

3. Carotid Impulse

The palpable impulse from the carotid usually occurs just after S_1, which the clinician detects by simultaneously listening to the heart tones and palpating the carotid artery. In elderly patients with tachycardia, however, this rule is sometimes misleading because the carotid impulse seems to fall closer to S_2, although even in these patients the carotid impulse still falls between S_1 and S_2.

REFERENCES

1. Ongley PA, Sprague HB, Rappaport MB, Nadas AS. *Heart sounds and murmurs: A clinical and phonocardiographic study.* New York: Grune and Stratton; 1960.

2. Leatham A. *Auscultation of the heart and phonocardiography,* 2nd ed. Edinburgh: Churchill Livingstone; 1975.

3. Kindig JR, Beeson TP, Campbell RW, et al. Acoustical performance of the stethoscope: A comparative analysis. *Am Heart J.* 1982;104:269-275.

4. Rappaport MB, Sprague HB. The effects of tubing bore on stethoscope efficiency. *Am Heart J.* 1951;42:605-609.

5. Ravin A, Craddock LD, Wolf PS, Shander D. *Auscultation of the heart,* 3rd ed. Chicago: Year Book Medical Publishers, Inc; 1977.

6. Rappaport MB, Sprague HB. The effects of improper fitting of stethoscope to ears on auscultatory efficiency. *Am Heart J.* 1952;43:713-715.

7. Bethell HJN, Nixon PGF. Examination of the heart in supine and left lateral positions. *Br Heart J.* 1973;35:902-907.

8. Perloff JK. *Physical examination of the heart and circulation,* 1st ed. Philadelphia: W. B. Saunders; 1982.

36

The First and Second Heart Sounds

INTRODUCTION

The first and second heart sounds (S_1 and S_2) define systole and diastole and therefore form the framework for analyzing all other auscultatory physical signs, including the third and fourth heart sounds, clicks and ejection sounds, knocks and opening snaps, and systolic and diastolic murmurs. In his classic treatise describing the discovery of the circulatory system, written in 1628, Harvey described both S_1 and S_2, comparing them to the gulping sound made by a horse drinking water.[1] The first person to state that S_1 and S_2 were the sounds of closing heart valves was Rouanet of France, who wrote in his 1832 M.D. thesis that S_1 occurred when the atrioventricular (i.e., mitral and tricuspid) valves closed, and S_2 occurred when the semilunar (i.e., aortic and pulmonic) valves closed.[2]

THE FIRST HEART SOUND (S₁)

I. THE FINDING

S_1 is heard well across the entire precordium, both with the bell and diaphragm of the stethoscope. It is usually loudest at or near the apex and contains more low-frequency energy than does S_2, which explains why, when mimicking the sound, the term "lub" is used for S_1 and the sharper term "dup" for S_2.*

II. PATHOGENESIS

A. CAUSE OF S₁

The precise cause of S_1 has been debated for decades. Although its two recordable components coincide with closure of the mitral and tricuspid valves, the force of valve closure itself is insufficient to generate sound.[4] Instead, their closure probably causes moving columns of blood to abruptly decelerate, which sets up vibrations in the chordae tendineae, ventricles, and blood as a unit (i.e., "cardiohemic" system).[4,5]

B. INTENSITY OF S₁

The most important abnormalities of S_1 relate to its intensity: The sound can be abnormally loud, abnormally faint, or vary in intensity abnormally from beat to beat. The primary variables governing intensity of S_1 are strength of ventricular contraction and the position of the atrioventricular leaflets at the onset of ventricular systole.

1. Ventricular Contractility

The stronger the ventricular contraction, the louder the S_1. Strong contractions, which have a high dP/dT (i.e., large increase in pressure with respect to time), intensify S_1 because the valves close with more force and generate more vibrations in the cardiohemic system.[6]

2. Position of the Valve Leaflets at Onset of Ventricular Systole

If the mitral valve is wide open at the onset of ventricular systole, it will take longer to close completely than if it had been barely open. Even this small delay in closure intensifies S_1, because closure occurs on a later and steeper portion of the left ventricular pressure curve (i.e., dP/dT is greater).[7]

---

*It was Williams in 1840 who invented the "lub dup" onomatopoeia.[3]

The PR interval is the main variable determining the position of the valves at the beginning of ventricular systole. If the PR interval is short, ventricular systole immediately follows atrial systole (i.e., the R wave immediately follows the P wave). Because atrial systole kicks the valve open, a short PR guarantees that the valve will be wide open at the onset of ventricular systole. In contrast, a long PR interval allows time for the cusps of the atrioventricular valves to float back together before ventricular systole occurs. Studies show that, with PR intervals less than 0.20 seconds, the intensity of S_1 varies inversely with the PR interval (the shorter the PR interval the louder the sound). With intervals greater than 0.20 seconds, S_1 is faint or absent.[7,8]

III. CLINICAL SIGNIFICANCE

A. LOUD S_1

S_1 may be abnormally loud because of unusually vigorous ventricular contractions or because of delayed closure of the mitral valve.

1. Vigorous Ventricular Contractions

Vigorous contractions, such as those occurring from fever and sympathetic stimulation (e.g., beta-adrenergic inhalers, thyrotoxicosis), increase dP/dT and intensify S_1.[6]

2. Delayed Closure of the Mitral Valve
a. Prolapsed Mitral Valve

In patients with the murmur of mitral regurgitation, a loud S_1 is a clue to the diagnosis of early prolapse of the mitral valve (most patients with mitral regurgitation have a normal or soft S_1).[9,10] S_1 is loud in these patients because the prolapsing leaflets stop moving and tense later than normal, when dP/dT in the ventricle is greater.[9]

b. Mitral Stenosis

Ninety percent of patients with pure uncomplicated mitral stenosis have a loud S_1.[11] Because the murmur of mitral stenosis is often difficult to hear, a traditional teaching is that clinicians should suspect mitral stenosis in any patient with a loud, unexplained S_1 and listen carefully for the murmur with the patient lying on the left side.

Mitral stenosis delays closure of the mitral valve because the pressure gradient between the left atrium and left ventricle keeps the leaflets open until the moment of ventricular systole. After successful valvuloplasty, the loud S_1 becomes softer.[11]

c. Left Atrial Myxoma

Many patients with left atrial myxoma (seven of nine in one series) also have a loud S_1 because the tumor falling into the mitral orifice during diastole delays closure of the valve.[12]

B. FAINT OR ABSENT S_1

S_1 is unusually faint if ventricular contractions are weak or if the mitral valve is already closed when ventricular systole occurs.

1. Weak Ventricular Contractions (low dP/dT)

Common examples of weak contractions causing a faint S_1 are myocardial infarction and left bundle branch block.[13]

2. Early Closure of the Mitral Valve

Common causes of early mitral closure causing the faint S_1 include the following.

a. Long PR Interval (<0.20 Seconds)

See "Intensity of S_1" section.

b. Acute Aortic Regurgitation

In patients with the murmur of aortic regurgitation, the faint or absent S_1 is an important clue that the regurgitation is acute (e.g., endocarditis) and not chronic. Patients with acute aortic regurgitation have much higher left ventricular end diastolic pressures than those with chronic regurgitation, because the acutely failing valve has not allowed time for the ventricle to enlarge, as it does to compensate for chronic regurgitation. The high pressures in the ventricle eventually exceed diastolic left atrial pressures, closing the mitral valve before ventricular systole and thus making S_1 faint or absent.[14]

C. VARYING INTENSITY OF S_1

If the rhythm is *regular* but S_1 varies in intensity, the only possible explanation is that the PR interval is changing from beat to beat, which means the patient has atrioventricular dissociation. In contrast, in patients with *irregular* rhythms, changing intensity of S_1 has no diagnostic significance, because ventricular filling and dP/dT—and therefore S_1 intensity—depend completely on cycle length.

In patients with pacer-induced regular rhythms, an S_1 that varies in intensity is compelling evidence for atrioventricular dissociation (likelihood ratio [LR] = 24.4; EBM Box 36-1). Presumably, the finding is also as accurate in patients with native rhythms. In patients with complete heart block, S_1 intensity is predictable, varying inversely with the PR interval for intervals less than 0.2 seconds, becoming inaudible for intervals 0.2 to 0.5 seconds, and becoming louder again with intervals greater than 0.5 seconds (because the mitral valve reopens).[8]

Box 36-1 The First and Second Heart Sounds*

Finding (Ref)[†]	Sensitivity (%)	Specificity (%)	Likelihood Ratio if Finding	
			Present	Absent
FIRST HEART SOUND				
Varying intensity S_1				
Detecting atrioventricular dissociation[15]	58	98	**24.4**	0.4
SECOND HEART SOUND				
Fixed wide splitting				
Detecting atrial septal defect[16]	92	65	2.6	**0.1**
Paradoxic splitting				
Detecting significant aortic stenosis[17]	50	79	NS	NS
Loud P_2				
Detecting pulmonary hypertension[18,19]	58–96	19–46	NS	NS
Palpable P_2				
Detecting pulmonary hypertension[18]	96	73	**3.6**	**0.05**

NS, not significant; likelihood ratio (LR) if finding present = positive LR; LR if finding absent = negative LR.

*Diagnostic standard: For atrioventricular dissociation, ventricles were paced independently of atria; for atrial septal defect, right heart catheterization; for significant aortic stenosis, peak gradient >50 mm Hg; for pulmonary hypertension, mean pulmonary arterial pressure ≥50 mm Hg.

†Definition of findings: For loud P_2, splitting heard with loud second component[18] or S_2 louder at left second interspace than right second interspace[19]; the figures for fixed splitting of S_2 apply only to patients having audible expiratory splitting.

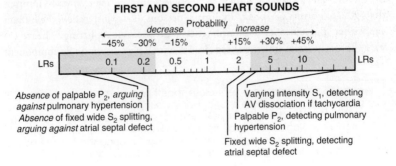

FIRST AND SECOND HEART SOUNDS

D.   PROMINENT SPLITTING OF S₁

Any delay in the closure of the tricuspid valve, the second component of S_1, accentuates splitting of S_1. This finding therefore occurs in patients with right bundle branch block or in left ventricular ectopic or paced beats, all of which delay the onset of right ventricular systole and also cause wide physiologic splitting of S_2 (see later).[5,20]

How to distinguish the split S_1 from other double sounds occurring around S_1, such as $S_4 + S_1$ and S_1 + ejection sound, is discussed in Chapter 37.

THE SECOND HEART SOUND (S₂)

I.   INTRODUCTION

The most important diagnostic feature of S_2 is its "splitting," which refers to how the aortic and pulmonic components of S_2 vary in timing during the respiratory cycle. The intensity of S_2 has less diagnostic importance (this contrasts with S_1, in which intensity is more important than splitting). Splitting of S_2 was first recognized by Potain in 1865, and its importance to cardiac auscultation was described by Leatham in the 1950s, who called S_2 the "key to auscultation of the heart."[21,22] The correct explanation for normal splitting—increased "hangout" in the pulmonary circulation—was discovered in the 1970s.[23,24]

II.   NORMAL SPLITTING OF S₂

A.   THE FINDING

In normal persons, the first component of S_2 is caused by closure of the aortic valve (A_2); the second, by closure of the pulmonic valve (P_2). During inspiration the interval separating A_2 and P_2 increases by about 20 to 30 msec (Fig. 36-1).[16,22,24]

Although the phonocardiogram almost always records both components of S_2, the human ear perceives them as a single sound *during expiration* in more than 90% of normal persons.[25] In normal persons *during inspiration*, the human ear either perceives two components ("physiologic splitting," heard in 65%–75% of normal adults; see Fig. 36-1)* or still perceives a single component

---

*These two components are very close together, bordering the threshold of being perceived as a single sound. Harvey suggests mimicking the normal expiratory sound by striking a single knuckle against a tabletop and mimicking inspiratory physiologic splitting by striking two knuckles almost simultaneously.[26] Constant suggests mimicking inspiratory splitting by rolling the tongue as in a Spanish *dr* or *tr*, or saying "pa-da" as quickly and sharply as possible.[27]

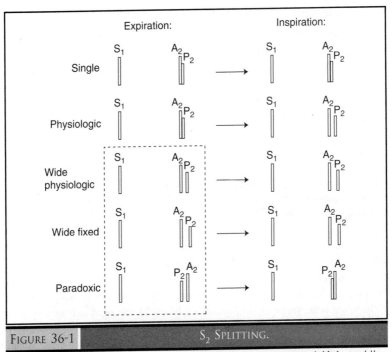

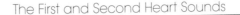

FIGURE 36-1 | S₂ SPLITTING.

Splitting refers to the separation of the aortic component (A_2) and the pulmonic component (P_2) during expiration (left column) and inspiration (right column). There are two normal patterns ("single" and "physiologic") and three abnormal patterns ("wide physiologic," "wide fixed," and "paradoxic"). The dotted lines indicate that all three abnormal forms of splitting are distinguished having by audible expiratory splitting. See text.

("single S_2," heard in 25%–35% of normal adults). The older the person, the more likely S_2 will be single instead of physiologic.[25,28]

In a minority of normal persons, expiratory splitting is heard in the supine position, although S_2 becomes single during expiration in these patients when they sit up.[29]

B. LOCATION OF SOUND

S_2 splitting is usually heard only in the second or third intercostal space, next to the left sternum.[28] It is sometimes heard at a slightly lower location, especially in patients with chronic pulmonary disease, and at a slightly higher location in those who are obese.[28] Splitting is not heard at other locations normally because P_2 is too faint.

C.   TECHNIQUE

It is important that the patient breathe regularly in and out when evaluating S_2 splitting, because held inspiration or held expiration tends to make the two components drift apart, thus making it impossible to interpret the sound.[16]

D.   PHYSIOLOGY OF SPLITTING

The normal delay in P_2 results from a long "hangout" interval in the normal pulmonary circulation (it is not because right ventricular systole ends later than left ventricular systole; they actually end at the same moment, Fig. 36-2). Hangout means that the pulmonary circulation offers so little resistance to blood flow that flow continues for a short period even after completion of right ventricular mechanical systole.[23,24] At the aortic valve, there is little hangout, causing flow to cease and the valve to close immediately after completion of left ventricular contraction.

A_2 and P_2 move apart during inspiration, primarily because inspiration delays P_2 even more. About half of the inspiratory augmentation of the A_2-P_2 interval is due to a further increase in the hangout interval in the pulmonary circulation. About 25% of inspiratory augmentation is due to lengthening of right ventricular systole (from increased filling of the right side of the heart during inspiration), and the remaining 25% is due to shortening of left ventricular systole (from a reduction of filling of the left side of the heart during inspiration).[24]

III.   ABNORMAL SPLITTING OF S_2

A.   THE FINDING

There are three abnormalities of S_2 splitting (see Fig. 36-1).

1.   Wide Physiologic Splitting

Wide physiologic splitting means that splitting occurs during inspiration and expiration, although the A_2P_2 interval widens further during inspiration.

2.   Wide Fixed Splitting

Wide fixed splitting means that splitting occurs during inspiration and expiration, but the A_2P_2 interval remains constant.

3.   Paradoxic Splitting (Also Called "Reversed Splitting")

Paradoxic splitting means that audible expiratory splitting narrows or melds into a single sound during inspiration. Paradoxic splitting occurs because the order of the S_2 components has reversed: A_2 now follows P_2, and as P_2 is delayed during inspiration, the sounds move together.

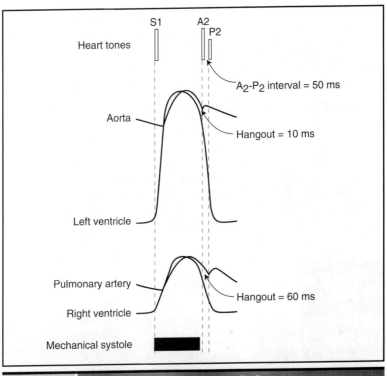

FIGURE 36-2 MECHANISM OF S_2 SPLITTING.

The timing of heart tones (*top*) is correlated with pressure tracings from the left side of the heart (i.e., "aorta" and "left ventricle," *top pressure tracings*) and right side of the heart (i.e., "pulmonary artery" and "right ventricle," *bottom pressure tracings*). The solid rectangle at the bottom of the figure depicts the duration of mechanical systole, which is the same for the right and left ventricles. A_2 coincides with the incisura (i.e., notch) on the aorta tracing, P_2 coincides with the incisura on the pulmonary artery tracing, and both sounds occur a short interval after completion of mechanical systole (the interval between the end of mechanical systole and valve closure is called "hangout"). On the left side of the heart, hangout is very short (10 msec, i.e., the aortic valve closes almost immediately after completion of mechanical systole). On the right side of the heart, however, hangout is longer (60 msec) because the compliant pulmonary circulation offers so little resistance to continued forward flow. The difference between these numbers explains why P_2 normally occurs after A_2 (i.e., A_2-P_2 interval in this patient = 60 − 10 = 50 msec). Changes in hangout also explain in part why splitting normally increases during inspiration and why most patients with pulmonary hypertension have a single S_2. See text.

B. SCREENING FOR ABNORMAL SPLITTING OF S₂

Figure 36-1 reveals that all three abnormal second heart sounds—wide physiologic, fixed, and paradoxic—have audible splitting *during expiration* (dotted lines in Fig. 36-1). Therefore, the best screening tool for the abnormal S_2 is audible expiratory splitting that persists when the patient sits up.[29–32]

C. CLINICAL SIGNIFICANCE AND PATHOGENESIS

Table 36-1 lists the common causes of abnormal S_2 splitting.

1. Wide Physiologic Splitting

Wide physiologic splitting may result from P_2 appearing too late or A_2 too early (see Table 36-1).[16,30] The most common cause is right bundle branch block.

In pulmonic stenosis, the A_2P_2 interval correlates well with severity of stenosis (gauged by the right ventricular systolic pressure, $r = 0.87$, $p < .001$),[33]

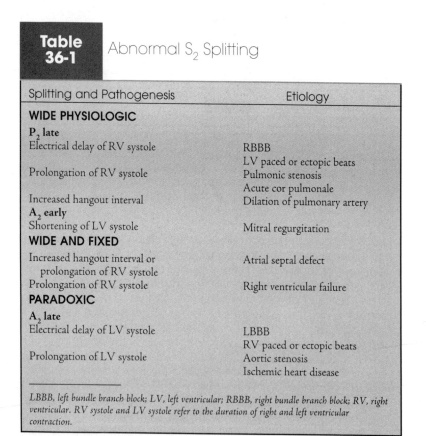

Table 36-1 Abnormal S_2 Splitting

Splitting and Pathogenesis	Etiology
WIDE PHYSIOLOGIC	
P₂ late	
Electrical delay of RV systole	RBBB
	LV paced or ectopic beats
Prolongation of RV systole	Pulmonic stenosis
	Acute cor pulmonale
Increased hangout interval	Dilation of pulmonary artery
A₂ early	
Shortening of LV systole	Mitral regurgitation
WIDE AND FIXED	
Increased hangout interval or prolongation of RV systole	Atrial septal defect
Prolongation of RV systole	Right ventricular failure
PARADOXIC	
A₂ late	
Electrical delay of LV systole	LBBB
	RV paced or ectopic beats
Prolongation of LV systole	Aortic stenosis
	Ischemic heart disease

LBBB, left bundle branch block; LV, left ventricular; RBBB, right bundle branch block; RV, right ventricular. RV systole and LV systole refer to the duration of right and left ventricular contraction.

although in many patients the clinician must listen at the third interspace to hear splitting because the murmur is too loud at the second interspace.

In most patients with pulmonary hypertension, the normal hangout interval disappears and S_2 is single. S_2 becomes wide in these patients only if there is associated severe right ventricular dysfunction and prolonged right ventricular systole.[23,24,34] Most patients with pulmonary hypertension and a wide S_2 have either long-standing severe pulmonary hypertension[23,24,34] or massive pulmonary embolism (the wide S_2 of pulmonary embolism is temporary, usually lasting hours to days).[35]

2.   Wide and Fixed Splitting

Patients with atrial septal defect have wide fixed splitting of S_2, although this is true only when their pulse is regular (if the patient has atrial fibrillation or frequent extrasystoles, the degree of splitting varies directly with the preceding cycle length).[22,36] The reason S_2 is wide is not the same in every patient: in some, hangout is increased; in others, right ventricular mechanical systole is prolonged.[36] S_2 is fixed because hangout remains constant during respiration[36] and because the presence of a common left and right atrial chamber interrupts the normal respiratory variation of right ventricular filling.[22]

In patients with audible expiratory splitting (and regular rhythm), the *absence* of fixed splitting argues strongly *against* the diagnosis of atrial septal defect (LR = 0.1; see EBM Box 36-1), whereas the presence of fixed splitting increases the probability of atrial septal defect only modestly (LR = 2.6; see EBM Box 36-1). Patients with false-positive results (i.e., fixed splitting without atrial septal defect) commonly have the combination of right ventricular failure and audible expiratory splitting from bundle branch block or some other cause.[16]

3.   Paradoxic Splitting

In elderly adults with aortic flow murmurs, the finding of paradoxic splitting does not distinguish significant aortic stenosis from less severe disease (see EBM Box 36-1).

D. S_2 SPLITTING VERSUS OTHER DOUBLE SOUNDS[32]

Other double sounds that mimic S_2 splitting include the following (see also Chapter 38).

1. S_2-Opening Snap

In contrast to the split S_2, the S_2-opening snap interval is slightly wider, the opening snap is loudest at the apex, and the opening snap ushers in the diastolic rumble of mitral stenosis at the apex. Patients with S_2-opening snap sometimes have a triple sound (split S_2 + opening snap) during inspiration at the upper sternal border.

2. S$_2$-Pericardial Knock

In contrast to the split S$_2$, the S$_2$-knock interval is slightly wider, the pericardial knock is loudest at or near apex, and the knock is always accompanied by elevated neck veins.

3. S$_2$-Third Heart Sound

In contrast to the split S$_2$, the S$_2$-S$_3$ interval is two to three times wider, and S$_3$ is a low-frequency sound heard best with the bell.

4. Late Systolic Click-S$_2$

Clicks are loudest at or near apex and are often multiple. Their timing changes with maneuvers (see Chapter 42).

IV. INTENSITY OF S$_2$

Despite traditional teachings, no evidence supports a loud P$_2$ as a sign of pulmonary hypertension. Whether defined as an S$_2$ that is louder at the left side of the upper sternum compared with the right side[19] or as a split S$_2$ with a louder second component,[18] the finding does not accurately discriminate patients with pulmonary hypertension from those without it (see EBM Box 36-1). Even when A$_2$ and P$_2$ are precisely identified by phonocardiography (e.g., A$_2$ corresponds to aortic incisura on simultaneous aortic pressure tracing), the relative intensities of the two components do not correlate well with pulmonary pressure.[37] Another suggested sign of pulmonary hypertension is audible splitting at the apex, which is based on the observation that P$_2$ normally is not heard at the apex[25] and the assumption that splitting at this location therefore indicates P$_2$ is abnormally loud. However, even this finding correlates better with the etiology of heart disease—it is common in atrial septal defect and primary pulmonary hypertension—than it does with measurements of pulmonary pressure.[34,37]

Nonetheless, the *palpable* S$_2$ does accurately detect pulmonary arterial pressures ≥50 mm Hg in patients with mitral stenosis (positive LR = 3.6, negative LR = 0.05; see EBM Box 36-1). In this study, the palpable P$_2$ was defined as an abrupt tapping sensation coincident with S$_2$ at the second left intercostal space.

REFERENCES

1. Harvey W. *De Motu Cordis* (facsimile edition by Classics of Medicine library). London: Nonesuch; 1926.
2. McKusick VA. Rouanet of Paris and New Orleans. *Bull Hist Med.* 1958;32: 137-151.

3. McCrady JD, Hoff HE, Geddes LA. The contributions of the horse to knowledge of the heart and circulation. IV. James Hope and the heart sounds. *Conn Med.* 1966;30(2):126-131.

4. Luisada AA, Portaluppi F. The main heart sounds as vibrations of the cardiohemic system: Old controversy and new facts. *Am J Cardiol.* 1983;52:1133-1136.

5. Ronan JA. Cardiac auscultation: The first and second heart sounds. *Heart Dis Stroke.* 1992;1:113-116.

6. Sakamoto T, Kusukawa R, MacCanon DM, Luisada AA. Hemodynamic determinants of the amplitude of the first heart sound. *Circ Res.* 1965;16:45-57.

7. Leech G, Brooks N, Green-Wilkinson A, Leatham A. Mechanism of influence of PR interval on loudness of first heart sound. *Br Heart J.* 1980;43:138-142.

8. Burggraf GW, Craige E. The first heart sound in complete heart block: Phono-echocardiographic correlations. *Circulation.* 1974;50:17-24.

9. Tei C, Shah PM, Cherian G, et al. The correlates of an abnormal first heart sound in mitral-valve-prolapse syndrome. *N Engl J Med.* 1982;307:334-339.

10. Perloff JK, Harvey WP. Auscultatory and phonocardiographic manifestations of pure mitral regurgitation. *Prog Cardiovasc Dis.* 1962;5:172-194.

11. Wood P. An appreciation of mitral stenosis: I. Clinical features. II. Investigations and results. *Br Med J.* 1954;1:1051-1063, 1113-1024.

12. Gershlick AH, Leech G, Mills PG, Leatham A. The loud first heart sound in left atrial myxoma. *Br Heart J.* 1984;52:403-407.

13. Stein PD, Sabbah HN, Barr I. Intensity of heart sounds in the evaluation of patients following myocardial infarction. *Chest.* 1979;75:679-684.

14. Meadows WR, van Praagh S, Indreika M, Sharp JT. Premature mitral valve closure: A hemodynamic explanation for absence of the first sound in aortic insufficiency. *Circulation.* 1963;28:251-258.

15. Garratt CJ, Griffith MJ, Young G, et al. Value of physical signs in the diagnosis of ventricular tachycardia. *Circulation.* 1994;90:3103-3107.

16. Perloff JK, Harvey WP. Mechanisms of fixed splitting of the second heart sound. *Circulation.* 1958;18:998-1009.

17. Aronow WS, Kronzon I. Correlation of prevalence and severity of valvular aortic stenosis determined by continuous-wave Doppler echocardiography with physical signs of aortic stenosis in patients aged 62 to 100 years with aortic systolic ejection murmurs. *Am J Cardiol.* 1987;60:399-401.

18. Whitaker W. Clinical diagnosis of pulmonary hypertension in patients with mitral stenosis. *Q J Med.* 1954;23:105-112.

19. Fowler NO, Noble WJ, Giarratano SJ, Mannix EP. The clinical estimation of pulmonary hypertension accompanying mitral stenosis. *Am Heart J.* 1955;49:237-249.

20. Leatham A. *Auscultation of the heart and phonocardiography,* 2nd ed. Edinburgh: Churchill Livingstone; 1975.

21. Leatham A. The second heart sound: Key to auscultation of the heart. *Acta Cardiol.* 1964;19:395-416.

22. Aygen MM, Braunwald E. The splitting of the second heart sound in normal subjects and in patients with congenital heart disease. *Circulation.* 1962;25:328-345.

23. Shaver JA, Nadolny RA, O'Toole JD, et al. Sound pressure correlates of the second heart sound: An intracardiac sound study. *Circulation.* 1974;49:316-325.

24. Curtiss EI, Matthews RG, Shaver JA. Mechanism of normal splitting of the second heart sound. *Circulation.* 1975;51:157-164.

25. Harris A, Sutton G. Second heart sound in normal subjects. *Br Heart J.* 1968;30:739-742.

26. Levine SA, Harvey WP. *Clinical auscultation of the heart.* Philadelphia: W.B. Saunders; 1959.

27. Constant J. *Bedside cardiology.* Boston: Little, Brown and Company; 1985.

28. Nelson WP, North RL. Splitting of the second heart sound in adults forty years and older. *Am J Med Sci.* 1967;234:805-807.

29. Breen WJ, Rekate AG. Effect of posture on splitting of the second heart sound. *JAMA.* 1960;173:1326-1328.

30. Shaver JA, O'Toole JD. The second heart sound: Newer concepts. I. Normal and wide physiologic splitting. *Mod Concept Cardiovasc Dis.* 1977;46(2):7-12.

31. Shaver JA, O'Toole JD. The second heart sound: Newer concepts. II. Paradoxical splitting and narrow physiological splitting. *Mod Concept Cardiovasc Dis.* 1977;46(3):13-16.

32. Adolph RJ, Fowler NO. The second heart sound: A screening test for heart disease. *Mod Concept Cardiovasc Dis.* 1970;39(4):91-96.

33. Leatham A, Weitzman D. Auscultatory and phonocardiographic signs of pulmonary stenosis. *Br Heart J.* 1957;19:303-317.

34. Perloff JK. Auscultatory and phonocardiographic manifestations of pulmonary hypertension. *Prog Cardiovasc Dis.* 1967;9:303-340.

35. Cobbs BW, Logue RB, Dorney ER. The second heart sound in pulmonary embolism and pulmonary hypertension. *Am Heart J.* 1966;71:843-844.

36. O'Toole JD, Reddy PS, Curtiss EI, Shaver JA. The mechanism of splitting of the second heart sound in atrial septal defect. *Circulation.* 1977;56:1047-1053.

37. Sutton G, Harris A, Leatham A. Second heart sound in pulmonary hypertension. *Br Heart J.* 1968;30:743-756.

37

The Third and Fourth Heart Sounds

I. INTRODUCTION

Although the third and fourth heart sounds (S_3 and S_4) are both sounds that originate in the ventricle from rapid diastolic filling, they differ in timing and clinical significance. S_3 appears in early diastole and, if the patient is older than 40 years, the sound indicates severe systolic dysfunction or valvular regurgitation. In persons younger than 40 years, S_3 may be a normal finding (i.e., the "physiologic S_3").[1] S_4 appears in late diastole, immediately before S1, indicating that the patient's ventricle is abnormally stiff from hypertrophy or fibrosis. If discovered in persons of any age, the S_4 is an abnormal finding.

In the late 19th century, the great French clinician Potain accurately described most features of S_3 and S_4, their pathogenesis, and their distinction from other double sounds such as the split S_1 or split S_2.[2] In his writings he called them "gallops," a term he attributed to his teacher Bouillard.[2,3]

II.   DEFINITIONS

Several different terms have been used to describe these diastolic sounds.

A.   GALLOP

A gallop is a triple rhythm with an extra sound in diastole (an S_3, an S_4, or their summation). The term refers only to pathologic sounds (i.e., it excludes physiologic S_3), and, despite its connotation, a patient may have a gallop whether the heart rate is fast or slow.[2,4]

B.   THIRD HEART SOUND (S_3)

The third heart sound is sometimes called the "ventricular gallop" or "protodiastolic gallop."[2] It appears in early diastole, 120 to 180 msec after S_2.[5] To mimic the sound, the clinician should first establish the cadence of the normal S_1 (*lub*) and S_2 (*dup*):

    lub   *dup*   *lub*   *dup*   *lub*   *dup*

and then add an early diastolic sound (*bub*)*:

    lub   *du bub*   *lub*   *du bub*   *lub*   *du bub*

    The overall cadence of the S_3 gallop (*lub du bub*) is similar to the cadence of the word "Kentucky."

C.   FOURTH HEART SOUND (S_4)

The fourth heart sound is sometimes called the "atrial gallop" or "presystolic gallop."[2] To mimic the sound, the clinician establishes the cadence of S_1 and S_2 (*lub dup*) and then adds a presystolic sound (*be*):

    be lub   *dup*   *be lub*   *dup*   *be lub*   *dup*

    The cadence of S_4 gallop (*be lub dup*) is similar to the cadence of "Tennessee."

D.   SUMMATION GALLOP

The summation gallop is a loud gallop that occurs in patients with tachycardia. In fast heart rhythms, diastole shortens, causing the events that produce S_3 (rapid early diastolic filling) to coincide with those producing S_4 (atrial systole). The resulting sound sometimes is louder than the patient's S_1 or S_2.

    Not all gallop rhythms in patients with tachycardia are summation gallops. The only way to confirm the finding is to observe the patient after the heart rate slows. (In the past, slowing was often induced by carotid artery massage,

---

*To pronounce the S_3 gallop with correct timing, the "p" of *dup* (S_2) must be dropped. In most patients the accent is on S_2 (*lub **du** bub*), although in others it falls on S_1 or S_3. The clinician can practice all three versions, always maintaining the same cadence, to become familiar with the varying sounds of S_3.

although in elderly patients this is not recommended. See Chapter 14). If slowing causes the gallop to disappear or evolve into two distinct but fainter sounds (i.e., S_3 and S_4), it was a genuine summation gallop. If the sound evolves instead into a single S_3 or single S_4, it was not a summation gallop.[4,6]

E. QUADRUPLE RHYTHM

The quadruple rhythm consists of S_1, S_2, and both S_3 and S_4.[4] It is an uncommon finding, usually only evident in patients with slow heart rates. It is sometimes called the "train wheel" rhythm, because the sound resembles that produced by the two pairs of wheels from adjacent train cars as they cross the coupling of a railroad track.[3,6]

be lub   du bup   be lub   du bub   be lub   du bub

III. TECHNIQUE

A. LOCATION OF SOUND AND USE OF STETHOSCOPE

S_3 and S_4 are both low-frequency sounds (20–70 Hz), bordering on the threshold of hearing.[7] They therefore are best heard with the bell of the stethoscope, applied lightly to the body wall with only enough force to create an air seal.[2,5] Gallops that originate in the left ventricle are best heard with the bell over the apical impulse or just medial to it. They are sometimes only audible with the patient lying in the left lateral decubitus position.[8] Gallops from the right ventricle are best heard with the bell over the left lower sternal border or, in patients with chronic lung disease, the subxiphoid area.[2,5]

B. RIGHT VERSUS LEFT VENTRICULAR GALLOPS

Aside from their different locations, other distinguishing features of right and left ventricular gallops are their response to respiration and association with other findings in the neck veins and precordium. Right ventricular gallops become louder during inspiration; left ventricular gallops become softer during inspiration.[9] The right ventricular S_4 may be associated with giant A waves in the neck veins and sometimes a loud presystolic jugular sound (see Chapter 32).[10] The left ventricular S_4 may be associated with a palpable presystolic movement of the apical impulse (see Chapter 34).

C. DISTINGUISHING THE S_4-S_1 SOUND FROM OTHER SOUNDS

Three combinations of heart sounds produce a double sound around S_1: (1) the S_4-S_1 sound, (2) the split S_1, and (3) the S_1-ejection sound. The following characteristics distinguish these sounds.[9]

1. Use of the Bell

The S_4 is a low-frequency sound, best heard with the bell. Firm pressure with the bell on the skin—which tends to remove low-frequency sounds—will cause the S_4-S_1 combination to evolve into a single sound, in contrast to the split S_1 and the S_1-ejection sound, which remain double.

2. Location

The S_4-S_1 sound is heard best at the apex, left lower sternal border, or subxiphoid area (see "Location of Sound and Use of Stethoscope"). The split S_1 is loudest from the apex to lower sternal border but sometimes is also heard well over the upper left sternal area. The aortic ejection sound is heard from the apex to the upper right sternal border. The pulmonary ejection sound is restricted to the upper left sternal area.[11]

3. Effect of Respiration

Although the S_4 may become louder (RV S_4) or softer (LV S_4) during inspiration, respiration does not affect the interval between S_4 and S_1. In contrast, the split S_1 interval varies with respiration in up to one third of patients.

Expiration makes the pulmonary ejection sound louder.[11] The aortic ejection sound does not vary with respiration.[12]

4. Palpation

Only the S_4-S_1 sound is accompanied by a presystolic apical impulse (see Chapter 34). The intensity of the S_4 (i.e., by auscultation) correlates moderately with the amplitude of the presystolic impulse on apexcardiography ($r = 0.46$, $p < .01$); similarly, the palpability of the presystolic impulse correlates roughly with the amplitude of S_4 on phonocardiography ($r = 0.52$, $p < .01$).[13]

IV. PATHOGENESIS

A. NORMAL VENTRICULAR FILLING CURVES

Filling of the right and left ventricles during diastole is divided into three distinct phases (Fig. 37-1). The first phase, the rapid filling phase, begins immediately after the atrioventricular valves open. During this phase, blood stored in the atria rapidly empties into the ventricles. The second phase, the plateau phase (diastasis), begins at the moment the ventricles are unable to relax passively any further. Very little filling occurs during this phase. The third phase, atrial systole, begins with the atrial contraction, which expands the ventricle further just before the next S_1.

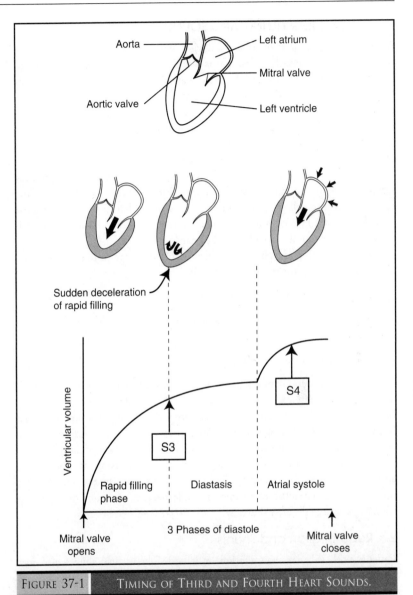

FIGURE 37-1 TIMING OF THIRD AND FOURTH HEART SOUNDS.

The figure depicts the three phases of diastolic filling of the left ventricle (y-axis on graph, ventricular volume; x-axis, time). The S_3 occurs at the end of the rapid filling phase, when passive filling suddenly decelerates. The S_4 occurs during atrial systole. Similar events on the right side of the heart may produce a right ventricular S_3 or S_4. See text.

B.   VENTRICULAR FILLING AND SOUND

Both S_3 and S_4 occur at those times during diastole when blood flow entering the ventricles temporarily stops, that is, the S_3 appears at the end of the rapid filling phase, and the S_4 toward the peak of atrial systole (see Fig. 37-1). Sounds become audible if the blood *decelerates abruptly* enough, which transmits sufficient energy to the ventricular walls and causes them to vibrate (an analogy is the tensing of a handkerchief between two hands: abrupt tensing produces sound, whereas slow tensing is silent).[14-19] Two variables govern the suddenness of this deceleration, and therefore whether a gallop becomes audible: (1) the flow rate during entry and (2) the stiffness of the ventricle. The greater the flow rate, the *louder* the sound. The stiffer the ventricle, the *higher the frequency* of the sound.[20] Because gallops consist of low frequencies that are difficult to hear (around 20–50 Hz), anything increasing its frequency content (i.e., stiff ventricles) makes the sound more likely to be heard.

Even though S_3 and S_4 both result from rapid flow rates into stiff ventricles, the diseases causing them differ completely.

C.   THE THIRD HEART SOUND (S_3)

The S_3 gallop appears when early diastolic filling is exaggerated, which occurs in two types of cardiac disorders.

1.   Congestive Heart Failure

The most common cause of the S_3 gallop is congestive heart failure from systolic dysfunction. In these patients, the S_3 indicates that atrial pressure is abnormally high, an especially important finding in patients with dyspnea, implying that heart disease is the principal cause of the shortness of breath. In addition to high atrial pressure, these patients typically have a dilated cardiomyopathy and low cardiac output.[21,22] Although both high atrial pressure (causing rapid flow rates) and cardiomyopathy (causing stiff ventricles) contribute to the sound, atrial pressure is the more important clinical variable, because the sound disappears as soon as pressure falls after diuresis.

2.   Regurgitation and Shunts

Patients with valvular regurgitation or left-to-right cardiac shunts also may develop an S_3 gallop, whether or not atrial pressure is high, because these disorders all cause excess flow over the atrioventricular valves. Patients with mitral regurgitation, ventricular septal defect, or patent ductus arteriosus may develop a left ventricular S_3 from excess diastolic flow over the mitral valve into the left ventricle (in mitral regurgitation, the excess diastolic flow simply represents the diastolic return of the regurgitant flow). Patients with atrial septal defect may develop a right ventricular S_3 from excess flow over the tricuspid valve into the right ventricle.

D. THE FOURTH HEART SOUND (S_4)

The S_4 gallop occurs in patients with hypertension, ischemic cardiomyopathy, hypertrophic cardiomyopathy, or aortic stenosis—all disorders characterized by ventricles stiffened from hypertrophy or fibrosis.[2,21-23] Patients with the sound must be in sinus rhythm and have strong atrial contractions, and most have normal atrial pressures, normal cardiac output, and normal ventricular chamber size. Unlike the S_3, the S_4 is a durable finding that does not wax and wane, although it does disappear if the patient develops atrial fibrillation (and loses the atrial kick).

E. SUMMATION GALLOP AND QUADRUPLE RHYTHM

The summation gallop occurs because fast heart rates shorten diastole, primarily by eliminating the plateau phase (see Fig. 37-1), which brings the events causing S_3 close to those causing S_4. Diastolic filling is concentrated into a single moment, thus causing a very loud sound.

The quadruple rhythm typically occurs in patients who have had a long-standing S_4 gallop from ischemic or hypertensive heart disease but who then develop cardiac decompensation, high filling pressures, and an S_3.[6]

Rarely, an intermittent summation gallop may appear in patients with slow heart rates resulting from complete heart block (or VVI pacing).[24] The gallop appears only during those moments of atrioventricular dissociation when atrial systole and early diastole coincide (i.e., the P wave on the electrocardiogram falls just after the QRS). Although the sound is technically a summation gallop, the clinician perceives what sounds like an intermittent S_3.

F. PHYSIOLOGIC S_3

Persons younger than 40 years with normal hearts may also have an S_3 sound (i.e., physiologic S_3), because normal early filling can sometimes be so rapid that it ends abruptly and causes the ventricular walls to vibrate and produce sound. Compared with healthy persons lacking the sound, those with the physiologic S_3 are leaner and have more rapid early diastolic filling.[1] The physiologic S_3 disappears by age 40, because normal aging slows ventricular relaxation and shifts filling later in diastole, thus diminishing the rate of early diastolic filling and making the sound disappear.[25]

V. CLINICAL SIGNIFICANCE

A. THE THIRD HEART SOUND

1. Congestive Heart Failure

EBM Box 37-1 shows that the presence of the S_3 gallop is a significant finding indicating depressed ejection fraction (likelihood ratio [LR] = 3.4–4.1; see

Box 37-1 The Third and Fourth Heart Sounds*

Finding (Ref)	Sensitivity (%)	Specificity (%)	Likelihood Ratio if Finding	
			Present	Absent
The third heart sound				
Detecting ejection fraction <0.5[19,26–28]	11–51	86–98	**3.4**	0.7
Detecting ejection fraction <0.3[27,28]	68–78	80–88	**4.1**	**0.3**
Detecting elevated left heart filling pressures[29–31]	12–32	95–96	**5.7**	NS
Detecting elevated BNP level[32,33]	41–65	93–97	**10.1**	0.5
Detecting myocardial infarction in patients with acute chest pain[34]	16	95	**3.2**	NS
Predicting postoperative pulmonary edema[35,36]	17	99	**14.6**	NS
Predicting postoperative myocardial infarction or cardiac death[35,36]	11	99	**8.0**	NS
The fourth heart sound				
Predicting 5-year mortality in patients after myocardial infarction[37]	29	91	**3.2**	NS
Detecting elevated left heart filling pressures[30]	71	50	NS	NS
Detecting severe aortic stenosis[38,39]	29–50	57–63	NS	NS

NS, not significant; BNP, B-type natriuretic peptide; likelihood ratio (LR) if finding present = positive LR; LR if finding absent = negative LR.
*Diagnostic standards: For ejection fraction, radionuclide left ventricular ejection fraction < 0.5 or <0.3, as indicated above; for elevated left heart filling pressures, pulmonary capillary wedge pressure >12 mm Hg[29] or left ventricular end diastolic pressure >15 mm Hg[30,31]; for elevated BNP level, ≥ 100 pg/mL[32] or > 1525 pg/mL[33]; for myocardial infarction, development of new electrocardiographic Q waves, elevations of CK-MB, or both; for severe aortic stenosis, peak gradient >50 mm Hg[38] or valve area < 0.75 cm²[39].

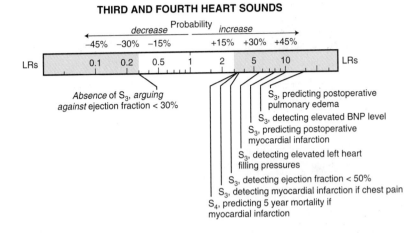

THIRD AND FOURTH HEART SOUNDS

EBM Box 37-1), elevated left atrial pressures (LR = 5.7), and elevated B-type natriuretic peptide (BNP) levels (LR = 10.1). Other studies confirm its value as a predictor of poor systolic function.[32,40] The *absence* of the S_3 gallop argues that the patient's ejection fraction is greater than 30% (i.e., negative LR for ejection fraction <30% is 0.3; see EBM Box 37-1).

In patients with a history of congestive heart failure, the S_3 predicts responsiveness to digoxin[41] and overall mortality.[42]

2. Valvular Heart Disease

In patients with mitral regurgitation, the S_3 is a poor predictor of elevated filling pressure (LR not significant) and depressed ejection fraction (LR = 1.9).[43] Some studies correlate the sound with severity of mitral regurgitation,[19] whereas others do not.[43]

In contrast, the S_3 is a helpful finding in patients with aortic valve disease. In patients with aortic stenosis, the S_3 detects both elevated filling pressures (LR = 2.3 for pulmonary capillary wedge pressures $\geq$ 12 mm Hg) and depressed ejection fraction (LR = 5.7 for EF <50%).[43] In patients with aortic regurgitation, the S_3 detects both severity of regurgitation (LR = 5.9 for regurgitant fraction $\geq$ 40%, see Chapter 41) and ejection fraction less than 50% (LR = 8.3).[19]

3. Patients with Acute Chest Pain

In patients with acute chest pain presenting to emergency departments, the finding of an S_3 increases the probability of myocardial infarction (LR = 3.2).

4. Preoperative Consultation

During preoperative consultation, the finding of S_3 is ominous, indicating that the patient, without any other intervention, has an increased risk of perioperative pulmonary edema (LR = 14.6) and myocardial infarction or cardiac death (LR = 8.0).[35]

B. THE FOURTH HEART SOUND

The finding of the S_4 gallop has less diagnostic value, simply because the disorders causing stiff ventricles are so diverse and because the S_4 does not predict the patient's hemodynamic findings. The finding does not predict ejection fraction, left heart filling pressures, or postoperative cardiac complications.[21,22,30,35,36] It also does not predict significant aortic stenosis in elderly patients with aortic flow murmurs, presumably because many patients with mild stenosis have the finding for other reasons, such as ischemic heart disease.[38,39]

Nonetheless, when detected 1 month after myocardial infarction, the S_4 is a modest predictor of 5-year cardiac mortality (LR = 3.2; see EBM Box 37-1). Experienced auscultators in the past did show that clinical deterioration in patients with ischemic disease caused the S_4-S_1 interval to widen, which could be recognized at the bedside, but proper interpretation of this finding required knowledge of the patient's PR interval, thus limiting its utility.[44] In patients with chaotic heart rhythms, the finding of a S_4 excludes atrial fibrillation and suggests other diagnoses such as multifocal atrial tachycardia.

The S_4 is rare in patients with chronic mitral regurgitation, because the dilated atrium of these patients cannot contract strongly. Therefore, finding a S_4 gallop in a patient with mitral regurgitation is an important clue to the diagnosis of *acute* mitral regurgitation (e.g., ruptured chorda tendineae; see Chapter 42).[45-47]

REFERENCES

1. Kupari M, Koskinen P, Virolainen J, et al. Prevalence and predictors of audible physiological third heart sound in a population sample aged 36 to 37 years. *Circulation*. 1994;89:1189-1195.
2. Craige E. Gallop rhythm. *Prog Cardiovasc Dis*. 1967;10:246-261.
3. Sloan AW. Cardiac gallop rhythm. *Medicine*. 1958;37:197-215.
4. Feinstein AR, Hochstein E, Luisada AA, et al. Glossary of cardiologic terms related to physical diagnosis and history. *Am J Cardiol*. 1968;21:273-274.
5. Ronan JA. Cardiac auscultation: The third and fourth heart sounds. *Heart Dis Stroke*. 1992;1:267-270.
6. Harvey WP, Stapleton J. Clinical aspects of gallop rhythm with particular reference to diastolic gallop. *Circulation*. 1958;18:1017-1024.
7. Tavel ME. *Clinical phonocardiography and external pulse recording*. 4th ed. Chicago: Year Book Publishers, Inc; 1985.

8. Bethell HJN, Nixon PGF. Examination of the heart in supine and left lateral positions. *Br Heart J.* 1973;35:902-907.

9. Fowler NO, Adolph RJ. Fourth sound gallop or split first sound? *Am J Cardiol.* 1972;30:441-444.

10. Dock W. Loud presystolic sounds over the jugular veins associated with high venous pressure. *Am J Med.* 1956;20:853-859.

11. Perloff JK. Auscultatory and phonocardiographic manifestations of pulmonary hypertension. *Prog Cardiovasc Dis.* 1967;9:303-340.

12. Leatham A. *Auscultation of the heart and phonocardiography,* 2nd ed. Edinburgh: Churchill Livingstone; 1975.

13. Jordan MD, Taylor CR, Nyhuis AW, Tavel ME. Audibility of the fourth heart sound: Relationship to presence of disease and examiner experience. *Arch Intern Med.* 1987;147:721-726.

14. Ozawa Y, Smith D, Craige E. Origin of the third heart sound. I. Studies in dogs. *Circulation.* 1983;67:393-398.

15. Ozawa Y, Smith D, Craige E. Origin of the third heart sound. II. Studies in human subjects. *Circulation.* 1983;67:399-404.

16. Kono T, Rosman H, Alam M, et al. Hemodynamic correlates of the third heart sound during the evolution of chronic heart failure. *J Am Coll Cardiol.* 1993;21: 419-423.

17. Ishimitsu T, Smith D, Berko B, Craige E. Origin of the third heart sound: Comparison of ventricular wall dynamics in hyperdynamic and hypodynamic types. *J Am Coll Cardiol.* 1985;5:268-272.

18. Van de Werf F, Boel A, Geboers J, et al. Diastolic properties of the left ventricle in normal adults and in patients with third heart sounds. *Circulation.* 1984;69: 1070-1078.

19. Tribouilloy CM, Enriquez-Sarano M, Mohty D, et al. Pathophysiologic determinants of third heart sounds: A prospective clinical and Doppler echocardiography study. *Am J Med.* 2001;111:96-102.

20. Glower DD, Murrah RL, Olsen CO, et al. Mechanical correlates of the third heart sound. *J Am Coll Cardiol.* 1992;19:450-457.

21. Shah PM, Gramiak R, Kramer DH, Yu PN. Determinants of atrial (S_4) and ventricular (S_3) gallop sounds in primary myocardial disease. *N Engl J Med.* 1968;278: 753-758.

22. Shah PM, Yu PN. Gallop rhythm: Hemodynamic and clinical correlation. *Am Heart J.* 1969;78:823-828.

23. Homma S, Bhattacharjee D, Gopal A, Correia J. Relationship of auscultatory fourth heart sound to the quantitated left atrial filling fraction. *Clin Cardiol.* 1991; 14:671-674.

24. Iga K, Konishi T. Intermittently audible the "third heart sound" as a sign of complete atrioventricular block in patients with a VVI pacemaker. *Int J Cardiol.* 1999; 71:135-139.

25. Van de Werf F, Geboers J, Kesteloot H, et al. The mechanisms of disappearance of the physiologic third heart sound with age. *Circulation*. 1986;73:877-884.

26. Gadsboll N, Hoilund-Carlsen PF, Nielsen GG, et al. Interobserver agreement and accuracy of bedside estimation of right and left ventricular ejection fraction in acute myocardial infarction. *Am J Cardiol*. 1989;63:1301-1307.

27. Mattleman SJ, Hakki AH, Iskandrian AS, et al. Reliability of bedside evaluation in determining left ventricular function: Correlation with left ventricular ejection fraction determined by radionuclide ventriculography. *J Am Coll Cardiol*. 1983;1:417-420.

28. Patel R, Bushnell DL, Sobotka PA. Implications of an audible third heart sound in evaluating cardiac function. *West J Med*. 1993;158:606-609.

29. Gadsboll N, Hoilund-Carlsen PF, Nielsen GG, et al. Symptoms and signs of heart failure in patients with myocardial infarction: Reproducibility and relationship to chest X-ray, radionuclide ventriculography and right heart catheterization. *Eur Heart J*. 1989;10:1017-1028.

30. Zema MJ, Restivo B, Sos T, et al. Left ventricular dysfunction: Bedside Valsalva manoeuvre. *Br Heart J*. 1980;44:560-569.

31. Harlan WR, Oberman A, Grim R, Rosati RA. Chronic congestive heart failure in coronary artery disease: Clinical criteria. *Ann Intern Med*. 1977;86:133-138.

32. Marcus GM, Michaels AD, de Marco T, et al. Usefulness of the third heart sound in predicting an elevated level of B-type natriuretic peptide. *Am J Cardiol*. 2004;93: 1312-1313.

33. Narain VS, Puri A, Gilhotra HS, et al. Third heart sound revisited: A correlation with N-terminal pro brain natriuretic peptide and echocardiography to detect left ventricular dysfunction. *Indian Heart J*. 2005;57:31-34.

34. Tierney WM, Fitzgerald J, McHenry R, et al. Physicians' estimates of the probability of myocardial infarction in emergency room patients with chest pain. *Med Decis Making*. 1986;6:12-17.

35. Goldman L, Caldera DL, Nussbaum SR, et al. Multifactorial index of cardiac risk in noncardiac surgical procedures. *N Engl J Med*. 1977;297:845-850.

36. Goldman L, Caldera DL, Southwick FS, et al. Cardiac risk factors and complications in non-cardiac surgery. *Medicine*. 1978;57:357-370.

37. Ishikawa M, Sakata K, Maki A, et al. Prognostic significance of a clearly audible fourth heart sound detected a month after an acute myocardial infarction. *Am J Cardiol*. 1997;80:619-621.

38. Aronow WS, Kronzon I. Correlation of prevalence and severity of valvular aortic stenosis determined by continuous-wave Doppler echocardiography with physical signs of aortic stenosis in patients aged 62 to 100 years with aortic systolic ejection murmurs. *Am J Cardiol*. 1987;60:399-401.

39. Kavalier MA, Stewart J, Tavel ME. The apical A wave versus the fourth heart sound in assessing the severity of aortic stenosis. *Circulation*. 1975;51:324-327.

40. Eagle KA, Quertermous T, Singer DE, et al. Left ventricular ejection fraction: Physician estimates compared with gated blood pool scan measurements. *Arch Intern Med.* 1988;148:882-885.

41. Lee DCS, Johnson RA, Bingham JB, et al. Heart failure in outpatients: A randomized trial of digoxin versus placebo. *N Engl J Med.* 1982;306:699-705.

42. Likoff MJ, Chandler SL, Kay HR. Clinical determinants of mortality in chronic congestive heart failure secondary to idiopathic dilated or to ischemic cardiomyopathy. *Am J Cardiol.* 1987;59:634-638.

43. Folland ED, Kriegel BJ, Henderson WG, et al. Implications of third heart sounds in patients with valvular heart disease. *N Engl J Med.* 1992;327:458-462.

44. Barlow JB. Some observations on the atrial sound. *S Afr Med J.* 1960;34:887-892.

45. Cohen LS, Mason DT, Braunwald E. Significance of an atrial gallop sound in mitral regurgitation: A clue to the diagnosis of rupture chordae tendineae. *Circulation.* 1967;35:112-118.

46. DePace NL, Nestico PF, Morganroth J. Acute severe mitral regurgitation: Pathophysiology, clinical recognition, and management. *Am J Med.* 1985;78: 293-306.

47. Hultgren HN, Hancock EW, Cohn KE. Auscultation in mitral and tricuspid valvular disease. *Prog Cardiovasc Dis.* 1968;10:298-322.

38

Miscellaneous Heart Sounds

I n addition to the first, second, third, and fourth heart sounds, several other discrete, short sounds may occur (Fig. 38-1). These sounds include early systolic sounds (e.g., the aortic or pulmonary ejection sound), midsystolic or late systolic sounds (e.g., systolic click of mitral valve prolapse), early diastolic sounds (e.g., opening snap of mitral stenosis, pericardial knock of constrictive pericarditis, and tumor plop of atrial myxoma), and prosthetic valve sounds. All are high-frequency sounds best heard with the diaphragm of the stethoscope.

EJECTION SOUNDS

I.   THE FINDING AND PATHOGENESIS

The ejection sound is the most common early systolic sound. It results from abnormal sudden halting of the semilunar cusps as they open during early systole.[2,3] Patients with aortic ejection sounds typically have aortic stenosis, bicuspid aortic valves, or a dilated aortic root.[2,3] Those with pulmonary ejection

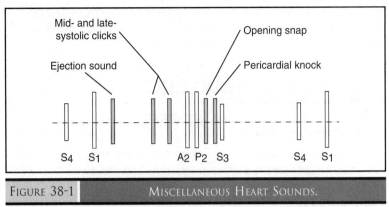

FIGURE 38-1 | MISCELLANEOUS HEART SOUNDS.

The figure shows the timing of the miscellaneous systolic sounds (ejection sounds and mid-to-late systolic clicks) and diastolic sounds (opening snap and pericardial knock), in relation to the principal heart sounds (first, second, third, and fourth heart sounds). The tumor plop of atrial myxoma, not depicted in the figure, has variable timing, ranging from 80 msec after A_2 (i.e., timing of the opening snap) to 150 msec after A_2 (i.e., timing of the third heart sound).[1]

sounds have pulmonary stenosis, pulmonary hypertension, or a dilated pulmonary trunk.[3,4]

Aortic and pulmonary ejection sounds are distinguished by their location, associated murmurs, and how they vary during respiration. An aortic ejection sound is a loud high-frequency sounds (often louder than S_1) best heard at the apex, although commonly also audible at the upper right sternal border.[5] It does not vary with respiration. Pulmonary ejection sounds are confined to the sternal edge at the second or third intercostal space; they often diminish in intensity during inspiration. Ejection sounds associated with aortic or pulmonic stenosis occur immediately before the onset of the systolic murmur.[5,6]

Chapter 37 describes how to distinguish ejection sounds from other double sounds around S_1, including the combination of S_4-S_1 and the split S_1.

II.   CLINICAL SIGNIFICANCE

The primary importance of these sounds is their etiologic associations. In patients with aortic stenosis, the ejection sound implies that the stenosis is at the valvular level and that there is some mobility to the valve. Elderly patients with calcific aortic stenosis usually do not have ejection sounds, because the calcific degeneration makes the valve leaflets inflexible. Children with noncalcific aortic stenosis, in contrast, usually have the ejection sound. In one consecutive series of 118 patients with aortic stenosis, the ejection sound was audible in 100% of patients with noncalcific valvular stenosis, in 32% with calcific valvular stenosis, and in none with subvalvular or supravalvular stenosis.[5]

MID-TO-LATE SYSTOLIC CLICKS

I. THE FINDING AND PATHOGENESIS

Mid-to-late systolic clicks occur in patients with mitral valve prolapse. These sounds, which are sometimes multiple, are caused by sudden deceleration of the billowing mitral leaflet as it prolapses backward into the left atrium during systole.[7] The click is loudest at the apex or left lower sternal border and is often associated with a late systolic murmur.[8]

The hallmark of the click of mitral valve prolapse (and also of the associated murmur) is that its timing shifts during maneuvers that change venous return. For example, the straining phase of the Valsalva maneuver or the squat-to-stand maneuver, both of which decrease venous return, cause the mitral leaflets to prolapse earlier in systole, thus shifting the click (and murmur) closer to S_1 (see Fig. 42-1 in Chapter 42).[8,9]

Clicks have been heard by clinicians for more than a century, although they were ascribed to pleuropericardial adhesions or other extracardiac causes[10] until the 1960s, when Barlow demonstrated the sound coincided with systolic prolapse of the posterior mitral leaflet.[11]

II. CLINICAL SIGNIFICANCE

The presence of the characteristic click or murmur alone is sufficient grounds for the diagnosis of mitral valve prolapse.[12,13] See Chapter 42 for further discussion of these findings.

OPENING SNAP

I. THE FINDING AND PATHOGENESIS

The opening snap is an early diastolic sound heard in patients with mitral stenosis.* The sound occurs because the stenotic mitral leaflets (although

---

*Patients with tricuspid stenosis also may have an opening snap, but all of these patients also have mitral stenosis and the mitral opening snap. Differentiating tricuspid and mitral opening snaps by auscultation alone is difficult.

fused, they are mobile) billow like a large sail into the ventricle during early diastole but then abruptly decelerate as they meet the limits of movement.[2,7] The abrupt deceleration causes a loud, medium-to-high frequency sound, which is then followed by the middiastolic rumbling murmur of mitral stenosis. The opening snap is best heard between the apex and left lower sternal border.

The clinician can mimic the sound of snap and murmur together by first setting up the cadence of S_1, S_2, and opening snap (RUP = S_1; bu = S_2; DUP = opening snap):

RU**P**   bu **DUP**   RU**P**   bu **DUP**   RU**P**   bu **DUP**

and then adding the murmur:

RU**P**   bu **DUP**rrrRRRR**UP**   bu **DUP**rrrRRRR**UP**   bu **DUP**

In some patients the opening snap is so loud it is easily heard at the second left intercostal space, where it then mimics a widely split S_2. Careful attention to inspiration in these patients, however, may reveal a *triple* sound (split S_2 and opening snap) at this location, confirming the last sound to be the opening snap.

The opening snap of mitral stenosis was first described by Bouillard in 1835.[2]

II.   CLINICAL SIGNIFICANCE

According to traditional teachings, the opening snap is inaudible in patients with mitral stenosis whose valve leaflets have become so thickened and inflexible they cannot create sound.[7,14] Although mitral stenosis is sometimes silent, no systematic studies of this teaching could be found.

The interval between the A_2 component of S_2 and the opening snap (A_2-OS interval) has been used to gauge the severity of mitral stenosis. Patients with more severe obstruction tend to have a narrower A_2-OS interval than those with milder disease. This occurs because the mitral valve opens when the pressure in the relaxing ventricle falls below the atrial pressure; the more severe the obstruction, the higher the atrial pressure and the sooner this crossover occurs. Nonetheless, determining the A_2-OS interval is primarily a phonocardiographic exercise, not an auscultatory one.[15] Furthermore, the A_2-OS interval also depends on variables other than severity of stenosis, such as ventricular relaxation time and heart rate, which further complicates interpreting it accurately at the bedside.[15]

The opening snap does indicate that the accompanying diastolic murmur represents mitral stenosis and not a flow rumble from increased flow over a nonstenotic valve (see Chapter 42 for discussion of flow rumbles).

PERICARDIAL KNOCK

The pericardial knock is a loud early diastolic sound heard in 28% to 94% of patients with constrictive pericarditis (see Chapter 43).[16-18] It is heard over a wide area between the apex and left lower sternal border. Compared with the third heart sound, the pericardial knock is a higher frequency sound (easily detected with the diaphragm of the stethoscope), appears over a wider area of the precordium, and occurs slightly earlier (although still later than the opening snap or widely split second heart sound).[17]

The pericardial knock results from the sudden deceleration of the filling ventricle as it meets the borders of the rigid pericardial sac.[17,18] In this way, it is similar to the third heart sound, although the more abrupt deceleration of constriction is what probably makes the pericardial knock higher-pitched and louder than the third heart sound (see Chapter 37).

TUMOR PLOP

The tumor plop, which may be heard in rare patients with atrial myxoma (only one of nine patients in one series), is an early diastolic sound representing prolapse of the pedunculated tumor into the ventricle after the mitral (or tricuspid) valve opens.[19,20] Characteristically, the intensity and timing of the tumor plop vary between examinations: it may be as early as the timing of an opening snap or as late as that of the third heart sound.

PROSTHETIC HEART SOUNDS

I. INTRODUCTION

Abnormal prosthetic heart sounds may be the only clue explaining the patient's dyspnea, syncope, or chest pain. To recognize these abnormal sounds simply and quickly, the clinician must first understand the normal prosthetic heart sounds. This section focuses on rigid mechanical valves, such as caged-ball valves (Starr-Edwards), single tilting disc valves (Bjork-Shiley, Medtronic-Hall), and bileaflet tilting-disc valves (St. Jude Medical).[21-23]

II. PRINCIPLES

The important observations are (1) timing and intensity of opening and closing sounds, which typically have a clicking or metallic quality and are often audible without a stethoscope, and (2) any associated murmurs. Any new or changing sound or murmur requires investigation.

A. OPENING AND CLOSING SOUNDS

In patients with caged-ball valves, the opening sound is louder than the closing sound. In patients with tilting-disc valves (both single disc and bileaflet), the closing sounds are loud and the opening sounds are only faint or inaudible (Fig. 38-2).

1. Caged Ball Valves

In the aortic position, the caged ball valve produces a loud opening sound, which is an extra systolic sound occurring just after S_1 with timing identical to the aortic ejection sound (i.e., instead of just S_1 and S_2, *lub dup . . . lub dup*, the clinician hears *ledup dup . . . ledup dup*). Caged ball valves in the mitral position produce an extra diastolic sound when they open, with timing identical to that of the opening snap (i.e., instead of S_1 and S_2, *lub bup . . . lub bup*, it is *lub budup . . .*

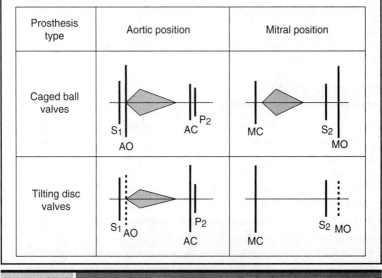

Prosthesis type	Aortic position	Mitral position
Caged ball valves	S_1 AO AC P2	MC S_2 MO
Tilting disc valves	S_1 AO AC P2	MC S_2 MO

The normal findings of prosthetic valves, based on references [21-23]. AC, closure sound of aortic prothesis; AO, opening sound of aortic prothesis; MC, closure sound of mitral prosthesis; MO, opening sound of mitral prosthesis; P_2, pulmonary component of second heart sound; S_1, first heart sound; S_2, second heart sound. See text.

lub budup). These opening sounds should always be louder than the corresponding closing sound (i.e., closing sounds are coincident with S_2 in aortic prostheses and with S_1 in mitral prostheses). The finding of an inaudible or abnormally soft opening sound indicates something is interfering with excursion of the ball, such as thrombus.

2. Tilting Disc Valves

These valves produce distinct, metallic closing sounds coincident with S_1 (mitral position) or S_2 (aortic position). Patients whose closing sounds are abnormally quiet may have significant valve dysfunction.

B. MURMURS

In the aortic position, all rigid valves (caged ball and tilting disc) typically produce short midsystolic murmurs that are best heard at the base and sometimes radiate to the neck. Diastolic murmurs in these patients suggest perivalvular regurgitation and require investigation.[21-23]

In patients with rigid valves in the mitral position, any holosystolic murmur suggests perivalvular regurgitation and requires investigation. A normal finding in patients with the caged ball valve in the mitral position (but not tilting disc valves) is an early-to-midsystolic murmur at the left sternal border. This murmur does not indicate regurgitation but instead represents turbulence caused by the cage of the valve projecting into the left ventricular outflow tract.[21,23]

REFERENCES

1. Tavel ME. *Clinical phonocardiography and external pulse recording*, 4th ed. Chicago: Year Book Publishers, Inc; 1985.
2. Leatham A. *Auscultation of the heart and phonocardiography*, 2nd ed. Edinburgh: Churchill Livingstone; 1975.
3. Perloff JK. The physiologic mechanisms of cardiac and vascular physical signs. *J Am Coll Cardiol*. 1983;1:184-198.
4. Perloff JK. Auscultatory and phonocardiographic manifestations of pulmonary hypertension. *Prog Cardiovasc Dis*. 1967;9:303-340.
5. Hancock EW. The ejection sound in aortic stenosis. *Am J Med*. 1966;40:569-577.
6. Leatham A, Weitzman D. Auscultatory and phonocardiographic signs of pulmonary stenosis. *Br Heart J*. 1957;19:303-317.
7. Ronan JA. Cardiac auscultation: Opening snaps, systolic clicks, and ejection sounds. *Heart Dis Stroke*. 1993;2:188-191.
8. Barlow JB, Bosman CK, Pocock WA, Marchand P. Late systolic murmurs and non-ejection ("mid-late") systolic clicks: An analysis of 90 patients. *Br Heart J*. 1968;30:203-218.

9. Fontana ME, Wooley CF, Leighton RF, Lewis RP. Postural changes in left ventricular and mitral valvular dynamics in systolic click: Late systolic murmur syndrome. *Circulation.* 1975;51:165-173.

10. Devereux RB, Perloff JK, Reichek N, Josephson ME. Mitral valve prolapse. *Circulation.* 1976;54:3-14.

11. Barlow JB, Pocock WA, Marchand P, Denny M. The significance of late systolic murmurs. *Am Heart J.* 1963;66:443-452.

12. Perloff JK, Child JS. Clinical and epidemiologic issues in mitral valve prolapse: Overview and perspective. *Am Heart J.* 1987;113:1324-1332.

13. Perloff JK, Child JS, Edwards JE. New guidelines for the clinical diagnosis of mitral valve prolapse. *Am J Cardiol.* 1986;57:1124-1129.

14. Wood P. An appreciation of mitral stenosis: Part 1. Clinical features. Part 2. Investigations and results. *Br Med J.* 1954;1:1051-1063, 1113-1024.

15. Hultgren HN, Hancock EW, Cohn KE. Auscultation in mitral and tricuspid valvular disease. *Prog Cardiovasc Dis.* 1968;10:298-322.

16. Harvey WP. Auscultatory findings in diseases of the pericardium. *Am J Cardiol.* 1961;7:15-20.

17. Mounsey P. The early diastolic sound of constrictive pericarditis. *Br Heart J.* 1955;17:143-152.

18. Tyberg TI, Goodyer AVN, Langou RA. Genesis of pericardial knock in constrictive pericarditis. *Am J Cardiol.* 1980;46:570-575.

19. Gershlick AH, Leech G, Mills PG, Leatham A. The loud first heart sound in left atrial myxoma. *Br Heart J.* 1984;52:403-407.

20. Pitt A, Pitt B, Schaefer J, Criley JM. Myxoma of the left atrium: Hemodynamic and phonocardiographic consequences of sudden tumor movement. *Circulation.* 1967;36:408-416.

21. Vongpatanasin W, Hillis LD, Lange RA. Prosthetic heart valves. *N Engl J Med.* 1996;335:407-416.

22. Commerford PJ, Stevens JE, Millar RS. Rumbles and prosthetic heart valves. *N Engl J Med.* 1997;336:1259-1260.

23. Smith ND, Raizada V, Abrams J. Auscultation of the normally functioning prosthetic valve. *Ann Intern Med.* 1981;95:594-598.

Heart Murmurs: General Principles

I. INTRODUCTION

During the last 170 years, the understanding of the significance of heart murmurs has evolved in three distinct stages.[1] In the first stage, brilliant clinicians, such as Hope, Steell, and Flint, attentively observed patients at the bedside, correlating the timing and quality of murmurs to the patients' clinical course and postmortem findings.[2] In the second stage, during the 1950s and 1960s, cardiac catheterization and phonocardiography helped clinicians understand the hemodynamics responsible for heart murmurs,[3,4] and the introduction of cardiac surgery increased the stakes of cardiac auscultation, stimulating clinicians to be as precise and accurate as possible. Finally, in the 1970s and 1980s, the introduction of echocardiography solved many of the remaining mysteries about murmurs, including the cause of ejection sounds in aortic stenosis and late systolic murmurs and clicks in mitral valve prolapse.

This chapter covers the principles of describing and diagnosing murmurs. Specific cardiac disorders and their associated murmurs are further discussed in Chapters 40 to 42.

II. THE FINDINGS

The important characteristics of heart murmurs are timing, intensity, frequency (or "pitch," which is high, low, or a mixture of high and low frequencies), and location (both where the murmur is loudest and in which direction its sound travels, or "radiates").[5] The terms "rough," "rumbling," "blowing," "coarse," and "musical" are also sometimes used to describe the specific tonal quality of murmurs.

A. TIMING

Murmurs are broadly classified as systolic, diastolic, and continuous (Table 39-1).[5] Systolic murmurs occur at any time from S_1 to S_2; diastolic murmurs occur at any time from S_2 to the next S_1. Continuous murmurs begin in systole but extend beyond S_2 into diastole, indicating they do not respect the confines of systole and diastole and thus do not arise within the four heart chambers. Despite their name, continuous murmurs do not necessarily occupy all of systole and diastole.

1. Systolic Murmurs

a. Etiology

There are two causes of systolic murmurs.

(1) Abnormal Flow over an Outflow Tract or Semilunar Valve (i.e., Aortic or Pulmonary Valve)
Such abnormal flow may occur for three reasons: (1) flow is obstructed (e.g., aortic stenosis, pulmonic stenosis, hypertrophic cardiomyopathy); (2) flow is normal, but the valve is abnormal without obstruction (e.g., aortic sclerosis); and (3) flow is increased over a normal valve (e.g., atrial septal defect, flow murmurs of anemia, fever, pregnancy, and thyrotoxicosis).

(2) Regurgitation from a Ventricle into a Low-Pressure Chamber
Examples are mitral regurgitation (leak between left ventricle and left atrium), tricuspid regurgitation (leak between right ventricle and right atrium), and ventricular septal defect (leak between left and right ventricles).

b. Classification

In 1958, Leatham divided all systolic murmurs into "ejection murmurs" and "regurgitant murmurs," based entirely on their relationship to S_2.[3,4] According to his classification, ejection murmurs began after S_1, had a crescendo-decrescendo

Table 39-1 Classification of Murmurs by Timing and Location

Timing	Etiology	Location Where Loudest
SYSTOLIC MURMURS		
Early systolic	Mitral regurgitation, acute	Apex or L base
	Tricuspid regurgitation, low pressure	LLSB
	Ventricular septal defect, small	LLSB
Midsystolic	Pulmonic stenosis	L base
	Atrial septal defect	L base
	Hypertrophic cardiomyopathy	LLSB
	Aortic stenosis	R base, LLSB, or apex
	Papillary muscle dysfunction*	Apex
Late systolic	Mitral valve prolapse	Apex
	Papillary muscle dysfunction*	Apex
Holosystolic	Mitral regurgitation	Apex
	Ventricular septal defect	LLSB
	Tricuspid regurgitation, high pressure	LLSB, apex
	Aortic stenosis	R base, LLSB, or apex
DIASTOLIC MURMURS		
Early diastolic	Aortic regurgitation	LLSB
	Pulmonary regurgitation, high pressure	L base
Mid diastolic	Pulmonary regurgitation, low pressure	LLSB
Mid diastolic, presystolic, or both	Mitral stenosis	Apex
	Tricuspid stenosis	LLSB
CONTINUOUS MURMURS		
	Patent ductus arteriosus	L base
	Arteriovenous fistula	Over fistula
	Venous hum	Above head of clavicle
	Mammary souffle†	Between breast and sternum
	Coarctation of the aorta	Over back

Apex, point of apical impulse; *L base,* second left intercostal space next to sternum; *LLSB,* fourth and fifth left intercostal space next to sternum; *R base,* second right intercostal space next to sternum.
*Papillary muscle dysfunction is a form of mitral regurgitation that occurs in ischemic heart disease.
†"Souffle" (French, sound or murmur) is pronounced "SOO ful."

shape, and always ended before S_2.* Ejection murmurs represented abnormal flow across the aortic or pulmonic valve. In contrast, regurgitant murmurs (e.g., mitral and tricuspid regurgitation) began with S_1, had a plateau shape, and extended up to or even slightly past S_2, thus obliterating it.

Leatham's classification is no longer widely used, for several reasons: (1) it relies entirely on phonocardiography and does not always correspond to what clinicians hear at the bedside[6]; (2) it depends entirely on the audibility of the aortic and pulmonary components of S_2, which are not always audible; (3) it assumes all "ejection" murmurs result from ejection over a semilunar valve, although experience has shown many are due to regurgitant lesions; and (4) its fundamental premise, that a murmur's intensity depends on pressure gradients, is not always true (e.g., the murmur of mitral valve prolapse is loudest during late systole, when gradients are decreasing).

Instead, systolic murmurs are now usually classified simply as "early systolic," "midsystolic," "late systolic," or "holosystolic," based only on whether the murmur obscures S_1, S_2, or both sounds.[1] Midsystolic murmurs obscure neither heart tone, holosystolic murmurs obscure both heart tones, early systolic murmurs obscure S_1 but preserve S_2, and late systolic murmurs obscure S_2 but preserve S_1.

2. Diastolic Murmurs
a. Etiology

There are two causes of diastolic murmurs: (1) abnormal backward flow across a leaking semilunar valve (e.g., aortic or pulmonic regurgitation) or (2) abnormal forward flow across an atrioventricular valve (e.g., mitral stenosis, tricuspid stenosis, and flow rumbles[†]).

b. Classification

Diastolic murmurs are further classified as "early diastolic," "mid diastolic," or "late diastolic" murmurs (the term "presystolic" murmur is synonymous with "late diastolic" murmur).

---

*More precisely, ejection murmurs end before the S_2 component belonging to the same side of the heart generating the murmur. For example, the murmur of aortic stenosis ends before A_2; the murmur of pulmonic stenosis ends before P_2.

†Flow rumbles are short low-frequency diastolic murmurs that result from increased flow over a nonobstructed atrioventricular valve. Atrial septal defects and tricuspid regurgitation may increase diastolic flow over the tricuspid valve, thus producing tricuspid flow rumbles (which resembles the murmur of tricuspid stenosis). Mitral regurgitation and ventricular septal defect may increase diastolic flow over the mitral valve, producing a mitral flow rumble (which resembles the murmur of mitral stenosis).

3. Continuous Murmurs

Continuous murmurs result from (1) abnormal connections between the aorta and pulmonary trunk (e.g., patent ductus arteriosus), (2) abnormal connections between arteries and veins (e.g., arteriovenous fistulas) (see Chapter 50), (3) abnormal flow in veins (e.g., venous hum and mammary souffle), or (4) abnormal flow in arteries (e.g., coarctation of the aorta, renal artery stenosis).

B.   GRADING THE INTENSITY OF MURMURS

The intensity of murmurs is graded on a 1 to 6 scale, based on the work of Freeman and Levine, which was later modified by Constant and Lippschutz (their work is now collectively referred to as "Levine's grading system").[7–9] Although this system was devised for systolic murmurs, it now applies to all murmurs.

The 6 categories are as follows: **(1) Grade 1** murmurs are so faint they can be heard only with special effort. **(2) Grade 2** murmurs can be recognized readily after placing the stethoscope on the chest wall. **(3) Grade 3** murmurs are very loud. Murmurs of Grades 1 through 3 all lack thrills, which are palpable vibrations on the body wall resembling the purr of a cat. Grade 4 through 6 murmurs all have associated thrills. **(4) Grade 4** murmurs are very loud, although the stethoscope must be in complete contact with the skin to hear them. **(5) Grade 5** murmurs are very loud and still audible if only the edge of the stethoscope is in contact with the skin; they are not audible after complete removal of the stethoscope from the chest wall. **(6) Grade 6** murmurs are exceptionally loud and audible even when the stethoscope is just removed from the chest wall.

C.   TIMING AND QUALITY OF MURMURS: USING ONOMATOPOEIA

Figure 39-1 presents traditional diagrams of various heart murmurs, which in turn are based on phonocardiographic tracings. Because murmurs are sounds, however, diagrams such as these often fail to convey the precise cadence and tonal qualities that distinguish murmurs. Throughout the history of cardiac auscultation, clinicians have used onomatopoeia to mimic heart sounds and murmurs, finding this to be an effective teaching tool allowing clinicians to rapidly recognize the patterns of different sounds.[2,10,11]

The system described here is based on the published work of Feinstein[12] and Adolph.[13–16] High-frequency murmurs are mimicked by sounds from the front of the mouth; low-frequency murmurs are mimicked by sounds from the back of the throat. The high-frequency murmur of mitral and tricuspid regurgitation is mimicked by saying "SHSHSHSH." The high-frequency, murmur of aortic regurgitation is mimicked by blowing air out through slightly pursed lips or

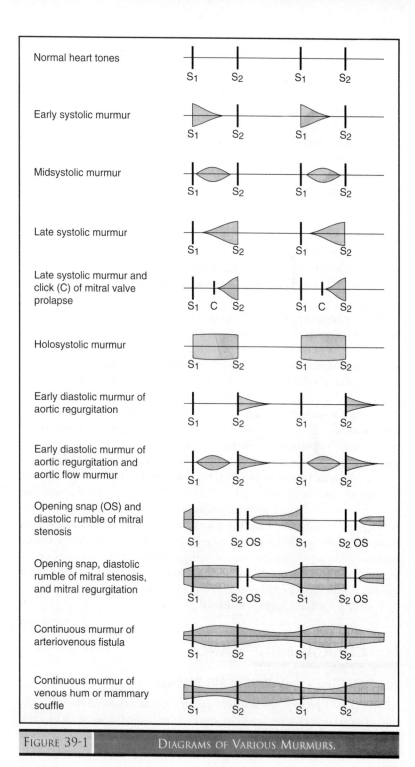

FIGURE 39-1   DIAGRAMS OF VARIOUS MURMURS.

457

whispering "PHEWEWEWEWEW" or "AHAHAHAHAH" (hence the "blowing" descriptor). The low-frequency murmurs of tricuspid or mitral stenosis are mimicked by the "RRRRR" portion of a growl (hence the "rumbling" descriptor). Murmurs containing a mixture of low and high frequencies, such as aortic stenosis, are mimicked by the sound made when clearing the throat (common descriptors are "coarse" or "harsh").

The clinician should first establish the normal cadence of S_1 and S_2 (*lub* is S_1 and *dup* is S_2):

    lub   *dup*   *lub*   *dup*   *lub*   *dup*

and then add the appropriate sound for the murmur at the appropriate time. For example, the high-frequency late systolic murmur of mitral valve prolapse preserves S_1 but obscures S_2 (i.e., dup is replaced by SHSHP):

    lub SHSHP   *lub SHSHP*   *lub SHSHP*

Figure 39-2 describes how to mimic many other common murmurs using onomatopoeia.

By using onomatopoeia, clinicians can quickly learn the cadence of murmurs, which sometimes leads to rapid recognition of complicated sounds without first having to sort out the location of S_1 and S_2. For example, if auscultation reveals a cadence consisting of a single murmur and no heart sounds:

    SHSHSHSH   *SHSHSHSH*   *SHSHSHSH*

the only possible diagnosis is a holosystolic murmur.

If instead auscultation reveals murmurs in systole and diastole, there are three possible causes: (1) a true continuous murmur, (2) a to-fro murmur, or (3) combined mitral stenosis and regurgitation. In true continuous murmurs, the cadence is uninterrupted by the cardiac cycles (*SHSHSHSHSHSHSHSHSH*). To-fro murmurs consist of two high-frequency murmurs, one in systole and another in diastole (*SHSHSHSHP PHEWEWEWEWEW*). To-fro murmurs result from isolated severe aortic regurgitation (the diastolic component representing aortic regurgitation and the systolic one representing increased systolic flow over the aortic valve) or aortic regurgitation combined with another systolic murmur, such as aortic stenosis, mitral regurgitation, or ventricular septal defect. In combined mitral stenosis and regurgitation, a high-frequency murmur is combined with a low-frequency one ("PUSHSHSHSHP DUPRRRRRRRRRUP").

III. CLINICAL SIGNIFICANCE

A. DETECTING VALVULAR HEART DISEASE

EBM Box 39-1 presents the diagnostic accuracy of murmurs. In this table, the finding refers to the characteristic murmur of that lesion (as described in Table 39-1 and Chapters 40–42). For example, the diagnostic accuracy of diastolic

Normal heart tones	**Lub**	**Dup**	**Lub**	**Dup**
	S$_1$	S$_2$	S$_1$	S$_2$
Early systolic murmur	**L**SHSHSH **Dup**		**L**SHSHSH **Dup**	
	S$_1$	S$_2$	S$_1$	S$_2$
Midsystolic murmur	**Lub** SHSH **Dup**		**Lub** SHSH **Dup**	
	S$_1$	S$_2$	S$_1$	S$_2$
Late systolic murmur	**Lub** SHSH**P**		**Lub** SHSH**P**	
	S$_1$	S$_2$	S$_1$	S$_2$
Late systolic murmur and click (C) of mitral valve prolapse	**Lub K**SHSH**P**		**Lub K**SHSH**P**	
	S$_1$ C S$_2$		S$_1$ C S$_2$	
Holosystolic murmur	SHSHSHSHSH		SHSHSHSHSH	
	S$_1$	S$_2$	S$_1$	S$_2$
Early diastolic murmur of aortic regurgitation	**Lub**	**P**EWWWww	**Lub**	**P**EWWWww
	S$_1$	S$_2$	S$_1$	S$_2$
Early diastolic murmur of aortic regurgitation and aortic flow murmur	**Lub** SHSH **P**EWWWww		**Lub** SHSH **P**EWWWww	
	S$_1$	S$_2$	S$_1$	S$_2$
Opening snap (OS) and diastolic rumble of mitral stenosis	R**UP**	bu **DUP**RRRRR**UP**		bu **DUP**RRRRR**UP**
	S$_1$	S$_2$ OS	S$_1$	S$_2$ OS
Opening snap, diastolic rumble of mitral stenosis, and mitral regurgitation	R**UP**SHSHSHS**P**	**DUP**RRRRR**UP**SHSHSHS**P**		**DUP**RRRRR**UP**
	S$_1$	S$_2$ OS	S$_1$	S$_2$ OS
Continuous murmur of arteriovenous fistula	**Pu**SHSH**SHPuSH**SHSHSHSH		**Pu**SHSH**SHPuSH**SHSHSHSH	
	S$_1$	S$_2$	S$_1$	S$_2$
Continuous murmur of venous hum or mammary souffle	**Pu**SHSHSHS**Pu**SHSH**SH**SHSH		**Pu**SHSHSHS**Pu**SHSH**SH**SHSH	
	S$_1$	S$_2$	S$_1$	S$_2$

FIGURE 39-2   MURMURS AND ONOMATOPOEIA.

Box 39-1   Murmurs and Valvular Heart Disease*

Finding (Ref)†	Sensitivity (%)	Specificity (%)	Likelihood Ratio if Finding Present	Likelihood Ratio if Finding Absent
Abnormal heart examination				
Detecting any valvular heart disease[17,18]	70–79	93–98	**18.3**	**0.3**
Characteristic systolic murmur				
Detecting aortic stenosis[19]	96	71	**3.3**	**0.1**
Detecting mild mitral regurgitation or worse[20,21]	56–75	89–93	**5.4**	0.4
Detecting moderate-to-severe mitral regurgitation[20,21]	84–93	65–76	**3.3**	**0.2**
Detecting mild tricuspid regurgitation or worse[21]	23	98	**14.6**	0.8
Detecting moderate-to-severe tricuspid regurgitation[21]	62	94	**10.1**	0.4
Detecting ventricular septal defect[18]	90	96	**24.9**	NS
Detecting mitral valve prolapse[18]	55	96	**12.1**	0.5
Characteristic diastolic murmur				
Detecting mild aortic regurgitation or worse[21–28]	54–87	75–98	**9.9**	**0.3**
Detecting moderate-to-severe aortic regurgitation[21,26–28]	88–98	52–88	**4.3**	**0.1**
Detecting pulmonary regurgitation[21]	15	99	**17.4**	NS

NS, not significant; likelihood ratio (LR) if finding present = positive LR; LR if finding absent = negative LR.

*Diagnostic standards: For all valvular lesions, Doppler echocardiography,[18,21,26,29] angiography,[20,22–24,27,28,30] or surgery.[19,25] Trivial regurgitation seen during echocardiography is classified as "absent regurgitation" (i.e., no disease).

†Definition of finding: For abnormal heart examination, see text; for all other murmurs, finding refers only to those murmurs characteristic in quality, location, and timing for that diagnosis. For example, the positive LR of 9.9 for aortic regurgitation refers to an early diastolic high-frequency blowing decrescendo murmur at the lower left sternal border, not any diastolic murmur.

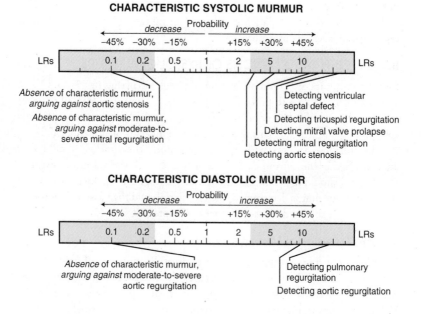

murmurs for aortic regurgitation refers not to just any diastolic murmur but instead to the finding of an early diastolic high-frequency murmur along the lower sternal border. In these studies, trivial regurgitation (a common finding at echocardiography of no clinical significance) was classified as "no regurgitation" (i.e., "no disease").

For five of the lesions in EBM Box 39-1, the finding of the characteristic murmur is a conclusive argument that that lesion is present: tricuspid regurgitation [likelihood ratio (LR) = 14.6, see EBM Box 39-1], ventricular septal defect (LR = 24.9), mitral valve prolapse (LR = 12.1), aortic regurgitation (LR = 9.9), and pulmonary regurgitation (LR = 17.4). For two murmurs, aortic stenosis and mitral regurgitation, the positive LRs are less compelling (LR = 3.3 for aortic stenosis and LR = 5.4 for mitral regurgitation), primarily because these two murmurs are often confused with each other and with other causes of systolic murmurs (see the following section).

The *absence* of the characteristic murmur is a compelling argument *against* significant left-sided valvular lesions: aortic stenosis (negative LR = 0.1), moderate-to-severe mitral regurgitation (negative LR = 0.2), and moderate-to-severe aortic regurgitation (negative LR = 0.1). On the right side of the heart, however, the *absence* of the characteristic murmur does not exclude valvular disease (negative LR for moderate-to-severe tricuspid regurgitation is 0.4; the negative LR for pulmonary regurgitation is not significant), probably because right-sided pressures, which are lower than those on the left side, generate less turbulence and softer sounds. Many patients with *mild* mitral regurgitation or *mild* aortic regurgitation also lack murmurs.

B. DIFFERENTIAL DIAGNOSIS OF SYSTOLIC MURMURS

Systolic murmurs are common bedside findings, occurring in 5% to 52% of young adults and 29% to 60% of older persons.[31] More than 90% of younger adults and more than half of older adults with systolic murmurs have a normal echocardiogram, which means the murmur is "innocent" or "functional."[31]

Therefore, in patients with systolic murmurs, the clinician should first address whether the murmur is functional or organic. If the murmur is organic, the clinician should then address which lesion is responsible. Once the cause of the organic murmur is determined, the clinician should then assess the severity of the lesion, a subject discussed further in Chapters 40 and 42.

1. The Functional Murmur

Functional murmurs are short, early or midsystolic murmurs of grade 2/6 or less. They are well-localized to the area of the left sternal border, and they diminish in intensity when the patient stands, sits up, or strains during the Valsalva maneuver. Patients with functional murmurs have normal neck veins, apical impulse, arterial pulse, and heart tones.

In EBM Box 39-1, "abnormal heart examination" refers to any murmur not meeting the definition of a functional murmur (i.e., the murmur is too long or loud, is heard away from the sternal border, intensifies during the Valsalva strain, or is associated with other abnormal cardiac findings). This definition of the abnormal murmur argues conclusively for valvular heart disease when the abnormal murmur is present (LR = 18.3). Murmurs meeting the criteria for functional murmurs argue *against* subsequently finding significant abnormalities on echocardiography (LR = 0.3).

2. Identifying the Cause of Systolic Murmurs

The following comments apply only to patients with an abnormal systolic murmur (i.e., not meeting definition of functional murmur).

a. Timing and Location

Despite classic teachings, the timing and location of a systolic murmur often do not distinguish aortic stenosis from mitral regurgitation. For example, mitral regurgitation may be early systolic (acute mitral regurgitation), midsystolic (papillary muscle dysfunction), late systolic (mitral valve prolapse or papillary muscle dysfunction), or holosystolic (chronic valvular mitral regurgitation). Aortic stenosis may be midsystolic or, when S_2 is absent, holosystolic. Mitral regurgitation is classically heard at the apex, but it also may be loudest at the right base (aortic area), especially when the posterior leaflet is abnormal.[32,33] Aortic stenosis is usually loudest over the sternum and right base, but in many older patients with calcific aortic stenosis, the murmur is loudest at the apex, the traditional area for mitral regurgitation.[34,35]

Therefore, to distinguish these two systolic murmurs from each other and other murmurs, the clinician must rely on other characteristics. Of these, the most helpful are the murmur's response to irregular rhythms and maneuvers, its tonal quality, and its relationship to S_2.

b. Changing Cycle Length

One important clue to the etiology of a systolic murmur is how it changes in intensity with changing cycle lengths, as occurs in the irregular pulse of atrial fibrillation or frequent premature beats. Mitral regurgitation remains the same loudness whether the beats are quick or delayed.[36] The intensity of aortic stenosis, in contrast, depends on cycle length: the longer the previous diastole (e.g., beat after a premature beat or after a pause in atrial fibrillation), the louder the murmur.[36,37]

Explaining why these two murmur behave differently first requires an understanding of the physiology of the pause. The pause causes diastolic filling and contractility to be greater for the next beat than it would have been if the cycle had been quicker (contractility is increased because of Starling forces and, in the case of extrasystoles, postextrasystolic accentuation of contractility). The pause also reduces afterload for the next beat, because the aortic pressures have had more time to fall before the next ventricular systole. In aortic stenosis, all three of these changes—increased filling, increased contractility, and decreased afterload—promote greater flow across the stenotic valve after pauses than after quick beats, causing the murmur to become louder.[38] In mitral regurgitation, however, the stroke volume is divided between two paths: (1) blood flowing out the aorta and (2) into the left atrium. The reduced afterload promotes the extra filling from the pause to exit into the aorta, leaving the regurgitant volume the same as with quicker beats and making the intensity of the murmur independent of cycle length.

Another systolic murmur, that of hypertrophic cardiomyopathy, responds unpredictably to changing cycle lengths: The long pause may make the murmur louder, softer, and not change it at all.[37]

c. Musical Systolic Murmurs

Almost all musical systolic murmurs are due to mitral regurgitation (mitral valve prolapse or endocarditis) or tricuspid regurgitation (congestive heart failure).[39-44] Although they are called "musical," the sound resembles more a "honk" or "whoop." The pure musical tones emanate from vibrations of the chordae tendineae, vegetations, or portions of the atrioventricular leaflets themselves, all generated during ventricular contraction.

d. Relationship to S₂

Systolic murmurs from flow over semilunar valves must end before S_2, because S_2 marks cessation of forward flow. In contrast, regurgitant murmurs can extend past S_2, because the pressure gradient between the ventricle and the low-pressure chamber may persist after S_2 (e.g., mitral regurgitation may persist until the early diastolic mitral opening sound).

This relationship to S_2, part of Leatham's original classification of systolic murmurs (see Section II.A.1.b), is still useful during auscultation, as long as the clinician is certain S_2 is audible somewhere on the chest. For example, in a patient with a long holosystolic murmur at the apex (*SHSHSH.......SHSHSH.......SHSHSH*), the clinician should return to the left second intercostal space to search for S_2. If S_2 is present (*SHSHSH dup....SHSHSH dup*), the clinician can conclude that the murmur at the apex is obliterating S_2 and thus represents regurgitation.[15,35] On the other hand, if the clinician still cannot hear S_2 at the left second intercostal space, the finding is unhelpful: S_2 could be inaudible either because the murmur is regurgitant or because S_2 has disappeared for some other reason (i.e., the aortic valve is inflexible from calcific aortic stenosis and does not make a sound).

e. Maneuvers

Several maneuvers help differentiate systolic murmurs (Table 39-2). They are classified into respiratory maneuvers, maneuvers that change venous return (e.g., Valsalva maneuver, squatting-to-standing, standing-to-squatting, passive leg elevation), and maneuvers that primarily change systemic vascular resistance (isometric hand grip, transient arterial occlusion, and inhalation of amyl nitrite).

(1) Respiration   Inspiration increases venous return to the right side of the heart and decreases it to the left side of the heart.* Therefore, murmurs that intensify during inspiration characteristically originate in the right side of the heart (e.g., tricuspid regurgitation or pulmonic stenosis; LR = 7.8; EBM Box 39-2). Murmurs that become *softer* during inspiration are most likely *not* right-sided murmurs (LR = 0.2; see EBM Box 39-2).

---

*This occurs because pressures in the right side of the heart diminish with intrathoracic pressures during inspiration, increasing the pressure gradient between the right side of the heart and systemic veins and causing filling to increase to the right side of the heart. In contrast, inspiration increases the capacitance of pulmonary veins, thus reducing flow to the left side of the heart during inspiration.

| Table 39-2 | Maneuvers and Heart Murmurs | | |

Maneuver*	Technique	When to Note Change in Murmur
Normal respiration	The patient breathes normally in and out	During inspiration and expiration
Maneuvers affecting venous return		
Valsalva maneuver (↓ venous return)	The patient exhales against closed glottis for 20 seconds	At end of the strain phase (i.e., at 20 seconds)
Squatting-to-standing (↓ venous return)	The patient squats for at least 30 seconds and then rapidly stands up	Immediately after standing
Standing-to-squatting (↑ venous return)	The patient squats rapidly from the standing position, while breathing normally to avoid a Valsalva maneuver	Immediately after squatting
Passive leg elevation (↑ venous return)	The patient's legs are passively elevated to 45 degrees while the patient is supine.	15–20 seconds after leg elevation
Maneuvers affecting systemic vascular resistance		
Isometric handgrip exercise (↑ afterload)	The patient uses one hand to squeeze the examiner's index and middle fingers together tightly[†]	After 1 minute of maximal contraction
Transient arterial occlusion (↑ afterload)	The examiner places blood pressure cuffs around both upper arms of patient and inflates them to pressures above the patient's systolic blood pressure	20 seconds after cuff inflation
Amyl nitrite (↓ afterload)	The patient takes three rapid, deep breaths from a broken amyl nitrite capsule	15–30 seconds after inhalation

From information cited in references 38, 45–48.

*Arrows indicated how maneuver affects venous return or systemic vascular resistance. The squatting-to-standing maneuver also decreases systemic vascular resistance, and amyl nitrite also diminishes pulmonary vascular resistance a small amount.

†In clinical studies, a hand dynamometer was used to confirm that at least 75% of maximal hand grip strength was sustained for 1 minute.[47]

Box 39-2   Systolic Murmurs and Maneuvers*

Finding (Ref)[†]	Sensitivity (%)	Specificity (%)	Likelihood Ratio if Finding	
			Present	Absent

RESPIRATION

Louder during inspiration

Detecting right-sided murmurs (tricuspid regurgitation or pulmonic stenosis)[46,49]	78–95	87–97	**7.8**	**0.2**

CHANGING VENOUS RETURN

Louder with Valsalva strain

Detecting hypertrophic cardiomyopathy[46]	70	95	**14.0**	**0.3**

Louder with squatting-to-standing

Detecting hypertrophic cardiomyopathy[46]	95	84	**6.0**	**0.1**

Softer with standing-to-squatting

Detecting hypertrophic cardiomyopathy[46,50]	88–95	84–97	**7.6**	**0.1**

Softer with passive leg elevation

Detecting hypertrophic cardiomyopathy[46]	90	90	**9.0**	**0.1**

CHANGING SYSTEMIC VASCULAR RESISTANCE (AFTERLOAD)

Softer with isometric hand grip

Detecting hypertrophic cardiomyopathy[46]	90	75	**3.6**	**0.1**

Louder with isometric hand grip

Detecting mitral regurgitation or ventricular septal defect[46,47]	70–76	78–93	**5.8**	**0.3**

(Continued)

Box
39-2

Systolic Murmurs and Maneuvers*—
Cont'd

Finding (Ref)[†]	Sensitivity (%)	Specificity (%)	Likelihood Ratio if Finding	
			Present	Absent
Louder with transient arterial occlusion				
Detecting mitral regurgitation or ventricular septal defect[46]	79	98	**48.7**	**0.2**
Softer with amyl nitrite inhalation				
Detecting mitral regurgitation or ventricular septal defect[46,47,51,52]	41–95	89–95	**10.5**	**0.2**

Likelihood ratio (LR) if finding present = positive LR; LR if finding absent = negative LR.
*Diagnostic standards: Doppler echocardiography or angiography.
[†]Definition of finding: See text; for amyl nitrite inhalation, the test was interpretable only if it induced tachycardia.

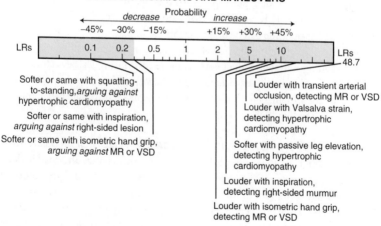

SYSTOLIC MURMURS AND MANEUVERS

Before interpreting the test, the clinician should be certain the patient is breathing evenly in and out, because breath holding during inhalation or exhalation makes interpretation impossible. To help direct the patient's breathing, the clinician can move his or her arm slowly up and down and ask the patient to breathe in when the arm is going up and out when it is going down.

Inspiratory intensification of the murmur of tricuspid regurgitation was originally described by Rivero-Carvallo in 1946 (the sign is sometimes called "Carvallo's sign").[53]

(2) *Maneuvers Changing Venous Return*   Venous return to the heart *decreases* during the straining phase of the Valsalva maneuver and the squatting-to-standing maneuver. Venous return *increases* during passive leg elevation and the standing-to-squatting maneuver (see Table 39-2 for definitions).

These maneuvers are most useful in identifying hypertrophic cardiomyopathy, which, unlike most systolic murmurs, intensifies with decreased venous return and becomes softer with increased venous return. This paradoxical response occurs because the murmur is caused by obstruction in the outflow tract, below the aortic valve and between the anterior leaflet of the mitral valve and the hypertrophied interventricular septum. Decreased venous return brings the mitral leaflet and septum closer together and aggravates the obstruction; increased return moves them apart and relieves the obstruction.

All four venous return maneuvers are useful in diagnosing hypertrophic cardiomyopathy (LRs = 6.0–14.0; see EBM Box 39-2), although the most compelling argument is a systolic murmur that intensifies during the Valsalva strain (positive LR = 14.0, see EBM Box 39-2). For three of the maneuvers (squatting-to-standing, standing-to-squatting, passive leg elevation), the *absence* of the response characteristic of hypertrophic cardiomyopathy is a compelling argument *against* the diagnosis (LR = 0.1, see EBM Box 39-2). Of these four maneuvers, only passive leg elevation can be easily performed in patients who are frail.

One other systolic murmur, mitral valve prolapse, may intensify during squatting-to-standing, although it does *not* become louder during Valsalva strain. This paradoxical finding is discussed further in Chapter 42 but is presented now to explain why the specificity for Valsalva strain (95%) is slightly higher than that for squatting-to-standing (84%).

(3) *Maneuvers Changing Systemic Vascular Resistance (or "Afterload")*   Before employing maneuvers that change afterload in diagnosing systolic murmurs, the clinician has already addressed the possibility of right-sided murmurs (respiratory maneuver) and hypertrophic cardiomyopathy (venous return maneuvers). The primary remaining diagnostic possibilities are murmurs generated by flow over the aortic valve (e.g., aortic stenosis, aortic sclerosis) and murmurs from left-sided regurgitant lesions (e.g., mitral regurgitation, ventricular septal defect).

Changing afterload is most useful in distinguishing these last two groups of lesions. The murmurs of mitral regurgitation and ventricular septal defect intensify with increased afterload, because blood leaving the ventricle, having two paths to potentially follow, encounters more resistance in the aorta and therefore flows more readily through the regurgitant lesion. Similarly, these murmurs become softer when afterload is decreased, because enhanced aortic flow reduces the regurgitant volume.

The common techniques of manipulating afterload at the bedside are isometric hand grip and transient arterial occlusion (see Table 39-2), both of which increase afterload. The finding of a systolic murmur that intensifies with either maneuver is a strong argument the murmur represents mitral regurgitation or ventricular septal defect (LR = 5.8 for isometric hand grip and 48.7 for transient arterial occlusion, see EBM Box 39-2). Another maneuver that reduces afterload, amyl nitrite inhalation, was used commonly 30 to 40 years ago but is rarely used today.

REFERENCES

1. Perloff JK. The physiologic mechanisms of cardiac and vascular physical signs. *J Am Coll Cardiol.* 1983;1:184-198.

2. Flint A. On cardiac murmurs. *Am J Med Sci.* 1862;44:29-54.

3. Leatham A. *Auscultation of the heart and phonocardiography,* 2nd ed. Edinburgh: Churchill Livingstone; 1975.

4. Leatham AM. Systolic murmurs. *Circulation.* 1958;17:601-611.

5. Soffer A, Feinstein AR, Luisada AA, et al. Glossary of cardiologic terms related to physical diagnosis and history. *Am J Cardiol.* 1967;20:285-286.

6. Tavel ME. Classification of systolic murmurs: Still in search of a consensus. *Am Heart J.* 1997;134(2 Part 1):330-336.

7. Freeman AR, Levine SA. The clinical significance of the systolic murmur: A study of 1000 consecutive "non-cardiac" cases. *Ann Intern Med.* 1933;6:1371-1385.

8. Levine SA. Notes on the gradation of the intensity of cardiac murmurs. *JAMA.* 1961;177:261.

9. Constant J, Lippschutz EJ. Diagramming and grading heart sounds and murmurs. *Am Heart J.* 1965;70:326-332.

10. Willius FA, Dry TJ. *A history of the heart and the circulation.* Philadelphia: W.B. Saunders Co; 1948.

11. Vaslef SN. Early descriptions of aortic valve stenosis. *Am Heart J.* 1993;125(5 Part 1):1465-1474.

12. Feinstein AR. Acoustic distinctions in cardiac auscultation: With emphasis on cardiophonetics, synecphonesis, the analysis of cadence, and problems of hydraulic distortion. *Arch Intern Med.* 1968;121:209-224.

13. Adolph RJ. The value of bedside examination in an era of high technology. Part 1. *Heart Dis Stroke.* 1994;3:128-131.

14. Adolph RJ. The value of bedside examination in an era of high technology. Part 2. *Heart Dis Stroke.* 1994;3:188-190.

15. Adolph RJ. The value of bedside examination in an era of high technology. Part 3. *Heart Dis Stroke.* 1994;3:236-239.

16. Adolph RJ. The value of bedside examination in an era of high technology. Part 4. *Heart Dis Stroke.* 1994;3:312-315.

17. Roldan CA, Shively BK, Crawford MH. Value of the cardiovascular physical examination for detecting valvular heart disease in asymptomatic subjects. *Am J Cardiol.* 1996;77:1327-1331.

18. Jost CHA, Turina J, Mayer K, et al. Echocardiography in the evaluation of systolic murmurs of unknown cause. *Am J Med.* 2000;108:614-620.

19. Aronow WS, Schwartz KS, Koenigsberg M. Correlation of aortic cuspal and aortic root disease with aortic systolic ejection murmurs and with mitral anular calcium in persons older than 62 years in a long-term health care facility. *Am J Cardiol.* 1986;58:651-652.

20. Meyers DG, McCall D, Sears TD, et al. Duplex pulsed Doppler echocardiography in mitral regurgitation. *J Clin Ultrasound.* 1986;14:117-121.

21. Rahko PS. Prevalence of regurgitant murmurs in patients with valvular regurgitation detected by Doppler echocardiography. *Ann Intern Med.* 1989;111:466-472.

22. Linhart JW. Aortic regurgitation: Clinical, hemodynamic, surgical, and angiographic correlations. *Ann Thorac Surg.* 1971;11:27-37.

23. Meyers DG, Sagar KB, Ingram RF, et al. Diagnosis of aortic insufficiency: Comparison of auscultation and M-mode echocardiography to angiography. *South Med J.* 1982;75:1192-1194.

24. Meyers DG, Olson TS, Hansen DA. Auscultation, M-mode, echocardiography and pulsed Doppler echocardiography compared with angiography for diagnosis of chronic aortic regurgitation. *Am J Cardiol.* 1985;56:811-812.

25. Cohn LH, Mason DT, Ross J, et al. Preoperative assessment of aortic regurgitation in patients with mitral valve disease. *Am J Cardiol.* 1967;19:177-182.

26. Aronow WS, Kronzon I. Correlation of prevalence and severity of aortic regurgitation detected by pulsed Doppler echocardiography with the murmur of aortic regurgitation in elderly patients in a long-term health care facility. *Am J Cardiol.* 1989;63:128-129.

27. Dittmann H, Karsch KR, Seipel L. Diagnosis and quantification of aortic regurgitation by pulsed Doppler echocardiography in patients with mitral valve disease. *Eur Heart J.* 1987;8 (Suppl C):53-57.

28. Grayburn PA, Smith MD, Handshoe R, et al. Detection of aortic insufficiency by standard echocardiography, pulsed Doppler echocardiography, and auscultation: A comparison of accuracies. *Ann Intern Med.* 1986;104:599-605.

29. Desjardins VA, Enriquez-Sarano M, Tajik J, et al. Intensity of murmurs correlates with severity of valvular regurgitation. *Am J Med.* 1996;100:149-156.

30. Frank MJ, Casanegra P, Migliori AJ, Levinson GE. The clinical evaluation of aortic regurgitation. *Arch Intern Med.* 1965;116:357-365.

31. Etchells E, Bell C, Robb K. Does this patients have an abnormal systolic murmur? *JAMA*. 1997;277:564-571.

32. Antman EM, Angoff GH, Sloss LJ. Demonstration of the mechanism by which mitral regurgitation mimics aortic stenosis. *Am J Cardiol*. 1978;42:1044-1048.

33. Perloff JK, Harvey WP. Auscultatory and phonocardiographic manifestations of pure mitral regurgitation. *Prog Cardiovasc Dis*. 1962;5:172-194.

34. Roberts WC, Perloff JK, Costantino T. Severe valvular aortic stenosis in patients over 65 years of age: A clinicopathologic study. *Am J Cardiol*. 1971;27:497-506.

35. Burch GE, Phillips JH. Murmurs of aortic stenosis and mitral insufficiency masquerading as one another. *Am Heart J*. 1963;66:439-442.

36. Henke RP, March HW, Hultgren HN. An aid to identification of the murmur of aortic stenosis with atypical localization. *Am Heart J*. 1960;60:354-363.

37. Kramer DS, French WJ, Criley JM. The postextrasystolic murmur response to gradient in hypertrophic cardiomyopathy. *Ann Intern Med*. 1986;104:772-776.

38. Karliner JS, O'Rourke RA, Kearnery DJ, Shabetai R. Haemodynamic explanation of why the murmur of mitral regurgitation is independent of cycle length. *Br Heart J*. 1973;35:397-401.

39. Sheikh MU, Lee WR, Mills RJ, Dais K. Musical murmurs: Clinical implications, long-term prognosis, and echo-phonocardiographic features. *Am Heart J*. 1984;108: 377-386.

40. Upshaw CB. Precordial honk due to tricuspid regurgitation. *Am J Cardiol*. 1975;35:85-88.

41. Rackley CE, Whalen RE, Floyd WL, et al. The precordial honk. *Am J Cardiol*. 1966;17:509-515.

42. Keenan TJ, Schwartz MJ. Tricuspid whoop. *Am J Cardiol*. 1973;31:642-645.

43. Kalyanasundaram V, Siegel R, Kim SJ, Allen JW. Musical murmurs: An echo-phonocardiographic study. *Am J Cardiol*. 1978;41:952-954.

44. Alam M, Garcia R, Goldstein S. Echo-phonocardiographic features of regurgitant porcine mitral and tricuspid valves presenting with musical murmurs. *Am Heart J*. 1983;105:456-460.

45. Lembo NJ, Dell'Italia LJ, Crawford MH, O'Rourke RA. Diagnosis of left-sided regurgitant murmurs by transient arterial occlusion: A new maneuver using blood pressure cuffs. *Ann Intern Med*. 1986;105:368-370.

46. Lembo NJ, Dell'Italia LJD, Crawford MH, O'Rourke RA. Bedside diagnosis of systolic murmurs. *N Engl J Med*. 1988;318:1572-1578.

47. McCraw DB, Siegel W, Stonecipher HK, et al. Response of heart murmur intensity to isometric (handgrip) exercise. *Br Heart J*. 1972;34:605-610.

48. Rothman A, Goldberger AL. Aids to cardiac auscultation. *Ann Intern Med*. 1983; 99:346-353.

49. Maisel AS, Gilpin EA, Klein L, et al. The murmur of papillary muscle dysfunction in acute myocardial infarction: Clinical features and prognostic implications. *Am Heart J*. 1986;112:705-711.

50. Nellen M, Gotsman MS, Vogelpoel L, et al. Effects of prompt squatting on the systolic murmur in idiopathic hypertrophic obstructive cardiomyopathy. *Br Med J.* 1967;3:140-143.
51. Luisada AA, Madoery RJ. Functional tests as an aid to cardiac auscultation. *Med Clin North Am.* 1966;50:73-89.
52. Barlow J, Shillingford J. The use of amyl nitrite in differentiating mitral and aortic systolic murmurs. *Br Heart J.* 1958;20:162-166.
53. Vitums VC, Gooch AS, Evans JM. Bedside maneuvers to augment the murmur of tricuspid regurgitation. *Med Ann DC.* 1969;38:533-542.

SELECTED CARDIAC DISORDERS

40

Aortic Stenosis

I. INTRODUCTION

Aortic stenosis is any disorder of the aortic valve that obstructs the ejection of blood from the left ventricle into the aorta. Its characteristic findings are a systolic murmur, abnormal carotid pulse, and sustained apical impulse.

The pathology of aortic stenosis was recognized in the 1600s, but it was James Hope who in 1832 first clearly described the characteristic murmur.[1,2]

II. THE FINDINGS

A. THE MURMUR

The murmur of aortic stenosis is midsystolic or holosystolic. It is loudest at the right second intercostal space, left sternal border, or apex, and it characteristically radiates into the neck, especially on the right side. In calcific aortic stenosis, the most common etiology of aortic stenosis today, the murmur at the upper sternal borders contains both high- and low-frequency vibrations, which gives it a harsh or rough sound, like that of clearing the throat. At the apex, in contrast, the murmur of calcific aortic stenosis often contains a narrow band of high-frequency sound, thus making it sound like mitral regurgitation. This harmonic distortion of sound—the loss of low-frequency components of the murmur when the stethoscope is moved upstream—is called the "Gallavardin phenomenon."[3]

B.   ASSOCIATED CARDIAC SIGNS

Other traditional findings of severe aortic stenosis are (1) a carotid pulse that is abnormally small in volume and delayed ("pulsus parvus et tardus"); (2) a palpable apical impulse that is abnormally sustained (see Chapter 34 for definition of sustained impulse); and (3) reduced intensity of the second heart sound, which occurs because the inflexible aortic leaflets close with less force than normal. Another traditional finding is a prominent A wave in the neck veins (i.e., the "Bernheim phenomenon"), although this wave is more often seen on pressure tracings than at the bedside. Its mechanism is still disputed.[4]

III.   CLINICAL SIGNIFICANCE

A.   DETECTING AORTIC STENOSIS

Although the *presence* of a characteristic aortic systolic murmur, anywhere from the base to apex, argues modestly *for* aortic stenosis [likelihood ratio (LR) = 3.3; see EBM Box 39-1 in Chapter 39],[5] the *absence* of a systolic murmur argues strongly *against* the diagnosis (LR = 0.1). The presence of the characteristic murmur, by itself, is less compelling, simply because this murmur is often confused with systolic murmurs from other valvular lesions. Chapter 39 discusses the differential diagnosis of systolic murmurs and how the clinician—by observing the second heart sound, quality of the murmur, and how the murmur responds to irregular heart beats and different maneuvers—can be more confident a systolic murmur indeed represents aortic stenosis or sclerosis.

B.   SEVERITY OF AORTIC STENOSIS

Once the clinician is confident the murmur is an aortic flow murmur (i.e., aortic stenosis or aortic sclerosis), he or she must decide whether the patient has significant aortic stenosis. Significant aortic stenosis refers to those lesions with such severe obstruction that, if the patient has symptoms of angina, syncope, or dyspnea, valvular replacement is indicated (see footnotes to EBM Box 40-1 for diagnostic standards used).

Many of the traditional teachings about aortic stenosis were first described at a time when congenital and rheumatic disease were more common than they are today. Because the primary cause of aortic stenosis today is calcific aortic stenosis, some of these teachings may not be as relevant as they were in the past. In comparison to congenital and rheumatic disease, calcific aortic stenosis affects older patients, who commonly have aortic flow murmurs *without* stenosis (i.e., aortic sclerosis) and who often have ischemic heart disease, a disorder complicating the bedside evaluation because patients then have two possible explanations (i.e., severe aortic stenosis or ischemic heart disease) for symptoms of angina or dyspnea.

The patients whose clinical signs are summarized in EBM Box 40-1 (more than 1000 patients in all) were all elderly (mean age 66 years) with aortic

Box 40-1   Characteristics of Severe Aortic Stenosis*

Finding (Ref)[†]	Sensitivity (%)	Specificity (%)	Likelihood Ratio if Finding Present	Absent
Arterial pulse				
Delayed carotid artery upstroke[6–9]	31–90	68–93	**3.7**	0.4
Reduced carotid artery volume[7,8]	74–80	65–67	2.3	**0.3**
Brachioradial delay[10]	97	62	2.5	**0.04**
Apical impulse				
Sustained apical impulse[7]	78	81	**4.1**	**0.3**
Apical-carotid delay[11]	97	63	2.6	**0.05**
Heart tones				
Absent A_2[6,12]	18–20	96–98	**4.5**	NS
Absent or diminished A_2[6,8,9,12]	44–90	76–98	**3.6**	0.4
S_4 gallop[9,13]	29–50	57–63	NS	NS
Murmur				
Late peaking[6,7,9]	83–90	72–88	**4.4**	**0.2**
Prolonged duration[6,9]	83–90	72–84	**3.9**	**0.2**
Loudest over aortic area[8,9]	58–75	41–73	1.8	0.6
Murmur transmits to neck[8,9]	90–98	22–36	1.4	**0.1**

NS, not significant; likelihood ratio (LR) if finding present = positive LR; LR if finding absent = negative LR.
*Diagnostic standard: For severe aortic stenosis, aortic valve area < 0.75 cm²,[10,12] < 0.8 cm²,[8,11] < 0.9 cm²[7]; peak gradient > 50 mm Hg[8,9]; or peak velocity of aortic flow > 3.6 m/sec.[6]
†Definition of findings: For late peaking murmur, murmur peaks at midsystole or beyond; for aortic area, second right intercostal space.

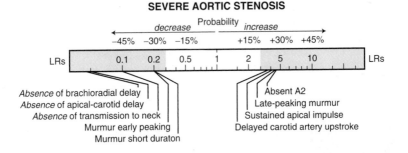

SEVERE AORTIC STENOSIS

Absence of brachioradial delay
Absence of apical-carotid delay
Absence of transmission to neck
Murmur early peaking
Murmur short duraton

Absent A2
Late-peaking murmur
Sustained apical impulse
Delayed carotid artery upstroke

ejection murmurs (largely calcific aortic stenosis and sclerosis). Although some had mild aortic regurgitation, other significant valvular disease was excluded from most of these studies.

1. Individual Findings

The following findings, in descending order of diagnostic accuracy (see EBM Box 40-1), distinguish severe aortic stenosis from other causes of aortic flow murmurs (i.e., aortic sclerosis and mild-to-moderate aortic stenosis): absent A_2 (LR = 4.5), late peaking murmur (LR = 4.4), sustained apical impulse (LR = 4.1), prolonged murmur (LR = 3.9), delayed carotid artery upstroke ("pulsus tardus," LR = 3.7), apical-carotid delay (i.e., a palpable delay between the apical impulse and carotid impulse, LR = 2.6), brachioradial delay (i.e., palpable delay between the brachial and radial artery pulses, LR = 2.5), and reduced carotid artery volume ("i.e, pulsus parvus," LR = 2.3).

The findings that best argue *against* the diagnosis of severe aortic stenosis are (see EBM Box 40-1): the absence of brachioradial delay (LR = 0.04), absence of an apical carotid delay (LR = 0.05), absence of transmission of the murmur to the neck (LR = 0.1), peaking of murmur in early systole (LR = 0.2), and short duration of the murmur (LR = 0.2). Brachioradial delay and apical-carotid delay were each investigated in only one study and therefore require confirmation by others.

Two additional bedside findings are the chest radiograph and electrocardiogram. On the chest radiograph, calcification of the aortic valve detects severe stenosis with a sensitivity of 31% to 81%, specificity of 63% to 96%, positive LR of 3.9, and negative LR of 0.5.[8,12,14,15] Left ventricular hypertrophy on the electrocardiogram detects severe stenosis with a sensitivity of 49% to 94%, specificity of 57% to 86%, positive LR of 2.1, and negative LR of 0.5.[6,8,11,12,14,15]

The following findings are not helpful in identifying patients with severe aortic stenosis: narrow pulse pressure,[16] fourth heart sound,[9,12] third heart sound,[12] reversed splitting of the second heart sound,[9] aortic ejection click,[9] and intensity of the murmur.[15]

2. Why Positive LRs Are So Low

The highest positive LR for the findings listed in EBM Box 40-1 is 4.5 (i.e., the absent A_2). In general, positive LRs are low when patients *without* disease also have the physical finding (i.e., specificity is low and there are many *false-positive* results). The cause of false-positive results in the studies of aortic stenosis is principally *moderate* aortic stenosis (defined as aortic valve area of 0.8–1.2 cm² or peak gradient of 25–50 mm Hg).

Therefore, if "disease" is instead defined as "combined moderate-to-severe aortic stenosis," the positive likelihood ratios improve dramatically, especially for delayed carotid upstroke (positive LR = 13.1, negative LR = 0.5), A_2 reduced or absent (positive LR = 10.7, negative LR = 0.4), prolonged duration of murmur (positive LR = 29.5, negative LR = 0.3), and late peaking murmur (positive LR = 29.5, negative LR = 0.3).[6,9,17]

This means that the clinician examining patients with aortic flow murmurs can easily distinguish patients with moderate-to-severe aortic stenosis from those with mild aortic stenosis and aortic sclerosis but has greater difficulty distinguishing severe stenosis from those with moderate stenosis.

3. Combined Findings

One study has validated the use of combined findings in the diagnosis of aortic stenosis.[8] According to this diagnostic scheme, the clinician evaluates five bedside findings and assigns the following points: delayed carotid upstroke (3 points), diminished carotid volume (2 points), murmur loudest at right upper sternal border (2 points), single/absent second heart sound (3 points), and calcification of the aortic valve on chest radiography (4 points).

This diagnostic scheme distinguishes moderate-to-severe aortic stenosis from other causes of aortic flow murmurs. The probability of moderate-to-severe aortic stenosis is low with 0 to 6 points (LR = 0.2) and high with 10 to 14 points (LR = 10.6). Scores from 7 to 9 points are unhelpful (LR not significant).

REFERENCES

1. Vaslef SN. Early descriptions of aortic valve stenosis. *Am Heart J*. 1993;125(5 Part 1): 1465-1474.

2. Willius FA, Dry TJ. *A history of the heart and the circulation*. Philadelphia: W.B. Saunders Co.; 1948.

3. Roberts WC, Perloff JK, Costantino T. Severe valvular aortic stenosis in patients over 65 years of age: A clinicopathologic study. *Am J Cardiol*. 1971;27:497-506.

4. Henein MY, Xiao HB, Brecker SJD, Gibson DG. Bernheim "a" wave: Obstructed right ventricular inflow or atrial cross talk? *Br Heart J.* 1993;69:409-413.

5. Aronow WS, Schwartz KS, Koenigsberg M. Correlation of aortic cuspal and aortic root disease with aortic systolic ejection murmurs and with mitral anular calcium in persons older than 62 years in a long-term health care facility. *Am J Cardiol.* 1986;58: 651-652.

6. Aronow WS, Kronzon I. Prevalence and severity of valvular aortic stenosis determined by Doppler echocardiography and its association with echocardiographic and electrocardiographic left ventricular hypertrophy and physical signs of aortic stenosis in elderly patients. *Am J Cardiol.* 1991;67:776-777.

7. Forssell G, Jonasson R, Orinius E. Identifying severe aortic valvular stenosis by bedside examination. *Acta Med Scand.* 1985;218:397-400.

8. Hoagland PM, Cook EF, Wynne J, Goldman L. Value of noninvasive testing in adults with suspected aortic stenosis. *Am J Med.* 1986;80:1041-1050.

9. Aronow WS, Kronzon I. Correlation of prevalence and severity of valvular aortic stenosis determined by continuous-wave Doppler echocardiography with physical signs of aortic stenosis in patients aged 62 to 100 years with aortic systolic ejection murmurs. *Am J Cardiol.* 1987;60:399-401.

10. Leach RM, McBrien DJ. Brachioradial delay: A new clinical indicator of the severity of aortic stenosis. *Lancet.* 1990;335:1199-1201.

11. Chun PKC, Dunn BE. Clinical clue of severe aortic stenosis: Simultaneous palpation of the carotid and apical impulses. *Arch Intern Med.* 1982;142:2284-2288.

12. Nakamura T, Hultgren HN, Shettigar UR, Fowles RE. Noninvasive evaluation of the severity of aortic stenosis in adult patients. *Am Heart J.* 1984;107:959-966.

13. Kavalier MA, Stewart J, Tavel ME. The apical A wave versus the fourth heart sound in assessing the severity of aortic stenosis. *Circulation.* 1975;51:324-327.

14. Nitta M, Nakamura T, Hulgren HN, et al. Noninvasive evaluation of the severity of aortic stenosis in adults. *Chest.* 1987;91:682-687.

15. Danielsen R, Nordrehaug JE, Vik-Mo H. Clinical and haemodynamic features in relation to severity of aortic stenosis in adults. *Eur Heart J.* 1991;12:791-795.

16. Hancock EW, Abelmann WH. A clinical study of the brachial arterial pulse form: With special reference to the diagnosis of aortic valvular disease. *Circulation.* 1957;16:572-581.

17. Etchells E, Glenns V, Shadowitz S, et al. A bedside clinical prediction rule for detecting moderate or severe aortic stenosis. *J Gen Intern Med.* 1998;13:699-704.

41

Aortic Regurgitation

I. INTRODUCTION

The principal problem in aortic regurgitation is defective closure of the aortic valve, which allows blood to return from the aorta to the left ventricle during diastole. In patients with significant chronic regurgitation, the traditional physical findings are a diastolic murmur, dilated apical impulse, and abnormally forceful and collapsing arterial pulses (pulsus celer).

In the 1700s, clinicians associated the postmortem finding of damaged aortic valves with hearts "larger than that of an ordinary ox" (the origin of the phrase "cor bovinum") and the finding during life of "violently throbbing" carotid arteries. In 1832, Sir Dominic John Corrigan, a Dublin surgeon, taught clinicians how to diagnose the disease during life, by emphasizing the importance of these dramatic arterial pulsations and the associated diastolic murmur.[1,2]

II. THE FINDINGS

A. THE MURMUR(S)

Severe aortic regurgitation may cause three distinct murmurs: (1) the early diastolic murmur of aortic regurgitation, (2) a systolic aortic flow murmur, and (3) the apical diastolic rumble of the Austin Flint murmur.

1. Early Diastolic Murmur of Regurgitation

The most important physical sign of aortic regurgitation is the early diastolic murmur, which is blowing, high-frequency, and decrescendo in shape (**Lub**   PEWWWWWWW, see Chapter 39). The murmur may occupy all of diastole or just its early part.[3] Pressing firmly against the chest wall with the diaphragm of the stethoscope brings out the murmur, which is usually loudest in the left parasternal area at the third or fourth intercostal space. In some patients, the murmur is only audible when the patient sits up, leans forward, and holds his or her breath in exhalation.

2. Systolic Aortic Flow Murmur

Severe aortic regurgitation also produces a short systolic aortic flow murmur, which results from ejection over the aortic valve of the large stroke volume characteristic of the disease. The combination of this murmur and the early diastolic one causes a characteristic "to-fro" sound near the sternum (**Lub** SHSHSH PEWWWWWWW, see Chapter 39). This murmur may superficially resemble that of aortic stenosis, although the flow murmur of pure regurgitation is shorter and associated with the peripheral pulse findings of severe regurgitation (see later).

3. Apical Diastolic Rumble: Austin Flint Murmur

a. Definition

The Austin Flint murmur is a diastolic rumbling murmur heard at the apex in patients with severe aortic regurgitation, which resembles mitral stenosis even though the mitral valve is completely normal. It was first described by the American physician Austin Flint in 1862.[4]

The Austin Flint murmur is found in up to 60% of patients with moderate or severe aortic regurgitation but is rarely heard in mild aortic regurgitation.[5,6] Austin Flint called his murmur "presystolic," but by this he meant it was loudest before S_1 and thus different from the murmur of aortic regurgitation, which began immediately after S_2 and tapered off during diastole. About half of Austin Flint murmurs have two diastolic components (middiastolic and presystolic), whereas the other half have just a presystolic component.[6,7]

b. Pathogenesis

The cause of the Austin Flint murmur is still debated. Although all hypotheses assume the murmur depends on a strong regurgitant stream of blood being directed back toward the left ventricle during diastole, these hypotheses differ in how this regurgitant stream causes an apical rumbling sound. Proposed mechanisms include fluttering of the anterior leaflet of the mitral valve, premature closure of the mitral valve from elevated left ventricular end-diastolic pressure, collision of the regurgitant stream with the anterior mitral leaflet, ventricular vibrations caused by the regurgitant stream itself, and harmonic distortion of the aortic regurgitant murmur.[6,8,9]

B.   WATER HAMMER PULSE AND INCREASED PULSE PRESSURE

Because of the large stroke volume and diastolic emptying of aortic blood into the left ventricle (i.e., "aortic runoff"), the arterial pulse wave of aortic regurgitation rises suddenly and collapses abruptly. This abnormality has many names, although the most common ones are "collapsing pulse," "Corrigan pulse," or the "water hammer pulse."* In most patients with aortic regurgitation, the collapsing pulse becomes more prominent as the examiner elevates the patient's wrist.[10,11] This occurs because elevation of the arm with respect to the heart reduces the diastolic pressure in that arm, causing the vessel to collapse more completely with each beat (The pounding sensation of the water hammer pulse is identical to the sensation felt by the examiner when palpating a person's blood pressure, with the cuff pressure just above the person's diastolic pressure. See Chapter 15.)

C.   ABNORMAL PULSATIONS OF OTHER STRUCTURES: THE AORTIC REGURGITATION EPONYMS

The large stroke volume and aortic runoff of aortic regurgitation often induce pulsations in other parts of the body, which has generated many eponyms of what is fundamentally a single physical finding (the number of eponyms for aortic regurgitation rivals those of some neurologic reflexes).[1,12-15] These various bobbings include (1) abnormally conspicuous capillary pulsation, best elicited by blanching a portion of the nail and then observing the pulsating border between the white and red color (Quincke's capillary pulsations, described in 1868, although Heinrich Quincke should be known instead for inventing the lumbar puncture); (2) anterior-posterior bobbing of the head, synchronous

---

*Corrigan actually emphasized the exaggerated *visible* pulsations of aortic regurgitation, not the palpable ones. The term "water hammer pulse" was coined in 1836 by Sir Thomas Watson, who likened the pulse to a Victorian toy called a water-hammer, which imparted to a child's hands the same sensation of a collapsing pulse of aortic regurgitation.[2]

with the arterial pulsations (de Musset's sign, named after the French poet Alfred de Musset, who was afflicted with aortic regurgitation)[16]; (3) alternate blanching and flushing of the forehead and face (Lighthouse sign); (4) pulsations of organs or their parts, including the uvula (Müller's sign, 1899), retinal arteries (Becker's sign), larynx (Oliver-Cardavelli's sign), spleen (Sailer's sign, 1928),[17] and cervix (Dennison's sign).*[18]

In many of the original descriptions of these eponymous findings, the sign was presented simply as an interesting observation, not one of particular diagnostic value.

D. HILL'S TEST

In 1909, Leonard Hill of Britain observed that patients with severe aortic regurgitation often have a systolic pressure in the foot that is much greater than a simultaneously measured systolic pressure in the arm.[19,20] "Hill's test" specifically refers to the systolic pressure of the foot minus that of the arm. The correct technique for measuring the pressure in the foot is to wrap the arm cuff around the patient's calf and to measure the systolic pressure in the dorsalis pedis and posterior tibial arteries by palpation. The higher of these two pressures is the "foot pressure."

E. AUSCULTATION OVER ARTERIES

Two auscultatory findings may appear over the peripheral arteries of patients with aortic regurgitation: pistol shot sounds and Duroziez's murmur (or Duroziez's sign).

1. Pistol Shot Sound
a. Definition

Pistol shot sounds are short, loud, snapping sounds with each pulse, heard over the femoral, brachial, or radial arteries. They are identical in quality to the Korotkoff sounds heard when measuring blood pressure. Pistol shot sounds are heard with only *light* pressure of the stethoscope and, like the water hammer pulse, may first appear only after elevation of the patient's arm.[11]

Pistol shot sounds were first described by Traube in 1872.[21,22]

b. Pathogenesis

Pistol shot sounds occur because of sudden expansion and tensing of the walls of the vessels during systole. Consequently, they are not only associated with the collapsing pulses of aortic regurgitation but also are inducible in normal

---

*The eponym does not necessarily indicate priority: Sailor gave credit for the pulsating spleen to Tulp of the 1600s,[17] and Dennison gave credit for the pulsating cervix to Shelly, one of his house officers.[18]

individuals by administering intravenous vasodilator medications.[23] The sounds are analogous to the loud, snapping notes heard when a sail or parachute suddenly fills with wind.[24] The quicker the vessel dilates, the louder the note, and in patients with aortic regurgitation, the intensity of the pistol-shot sound correlates with the height of the pulse pressure[25] and the change in pressure over time (dP/dt) of the pulse.[23]

2. Duroziez's Murmur or Sign[12,21,26–29]

a. Definition

Duroziez's sign is a *double* to-fro murmur heard over the brachial or femoral artery. It is heard only with *firm* pressure from the stethoscope. For Duroziez's sign to be positive, both a systolic and diastolic murmur must be present (many normal persons develop systolic murmurs with pressure on the stethoscope). The diastolic component often becomes louder with pressure applied distal to the stethoscope.

Although some claim Duroziez's murmur also may occur in normal individuals who have increased flow because of fever, anemia, or peripheral vasodilatation,[26] the vascular sound produced in these conditions does not have the characteristic "to-fro" sound of Duroziez's murmur, but instead resemble the continuous murmur of an arteriovenous fistula (**Pu**SHSHSHSH**Pu**SHSHSHSHSHSHSH).[28]

Duroziez described his "double intermittent murmur" in 1861.[21,30]

b. Pathogenesis

The diastolic component of Duroziez's sign results from the blood actually reversing directions in the artery during diastole.[27,28]

III. CLINICAL SIGNIFICANCE

A. DETECTING AORTIC INSUFFICIENCY

The presence of the characteristic early diastolic murmur of aortic insufficiency argues strongly that an aortic leak is actually present (likelihood ratio [LR] = 9.9, EBM Box 41-1). Although some patients with mild regurgitation have no murmur, the *absence* of the characteristic murmur does argue strongly *against* the presence of moderate-to-severe aortic regurgitation (LR = 0.1, see EBM Box 41-1).

B. DISTINGUISHING AORTIC VALVE DISEASE FROM AORTIC ROOT DISEASE

The early diastolic murmur of aortic regurgitation is usually loudest in the left parasternal area. In some patients, the murmur may be loudest to the

Box 41-1   Aortic Regurgitation*

Finding (Ref)	Sensitivity (%)	Specificity (%)	Likelihood Ratio if Finding Present	Absent
Characteristic diastolic murmur				
Detecting mild aortic regurgitation or worse[31-38]	54–87	75–98	**9.9**	**0.3**
Detecting moderate-to-severe aortic regurgitation[35-38]	88–98	52–88	**4.3**	**0.1**
Early diastolic murmur loudest on right side of sternum				
Detecting dilated aortic root or endocarditis[3]	29	96	**8.2**	0.7
Early diastolic murmur softer with amyl nitrite inhalation				
Detecting aortic regurgitation (vs. Graham Steell murmur)[39]	95	83	NS	**0.1**

NS, not significant; likelihood ratio (LR) if finding present = positive LR; LR if finding absent = negative LR.
*Diagnostic standard: For moderate-to-severe aortic regurgitation, see EBM Box 41-2.

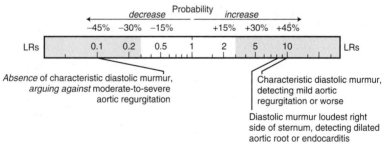

AORTIC REGURGITATION

right of the sternum, which suggest an eccentric regurgitant stream from dilation of the aortic root (e.g., Marfan syndrome, aortic dissection, syphilitic aortitis) or damage to a single aortic cusp (e.g., endocarditis). This sign, introduced by Harvey in 1963,[40] argues strongly for a dilated root or endocarditis (LR = 8.2, see EBM Box 41-1); its absence is diagnostically less helpful (LR = 0.7).*

C. DISTINGUISHING AORTIC REGURGITATION FROM PULMONARY REGURGITATION

Distinguishing aortic from pulmonary regurgitation was particularly relevant in patients with rheumatic mitral stenosis, who often had associated aortic valve disease but who also could develop pulmonary hypertension and the early diastolic murmur of pulmonary insufficiency (i.e., the Graham Steell murmur).

In patients with mitral stenosis who also have an early diastolic murmur of regurgitation heard next to the sternum, the additional lesion is aortic regurgitation at least 80% of the time. Aortic regurgitation is the most common correct diagnosis even when there are no peripheral pulse findings of aortic regurgitation and the patient shows signs of severe pulmonary hypertension.[31,41,42] In the past, reducing afterload with amyl nitrite inhalation was used to distinguish aortic from pulmonary regurgitation, because amyl nitrite should diminish the intensity of the aortic regurgitation murmur (i.e., less regurgitant flow) but not affect the pulmonary regurgitation murmur. The finding of an early diastolic murmur that instead becomes louder or does not change after amyl nitrite inhalation argues strongly *against* aortic regurgitation (LR = 0.1, see EBM Box 41-1).

D. SEVERITY OF AORTIC REGURGITATION

This section applies only to patients with the characteristic early diastolic murmur of chronic aortic regurgitation (EBM Box 41-2). It does not apply to acute aortic regurgitation (see "Acute Aortic Regurgitation" later). Many of the patients enrolled in the studies also had additional murmurs of aortic stenosis or mitral regurgitation.

1. The Diastolic Murmur

The louder the murmur, the more severe the aortic regurgitation (r = 0.67).[43] Murmurs of grade 3 or more indicate moderate-to-severe aortic regurgitation (LR = 8.2, see EBM Box 41-2).

---

*The diagnostic accuracy of Harvey's sign is based on patients from the 1960s, when most patients with aortic insufficiency had either rheumatic valvular disease or syphilitic root disease. Whether it is as accurate today is unknown.

Box 41-2

Characteristics of Moderate-to-Severe
Aortic Regurgitation*

Finding (Ref)[†]	Sensitivity (%)	Specificity (%)	Likelihood Ratio if Finding Present	Absent
DIASTOLIC MURMUR				
Murmur grade 3 or louder[34,43]	30–61	86–98	**8.2**	0.6
BLOOD PRESSURE				
Diastolic blood pressure[31,44]				
>70 mm Hg	8–21	32–55	**0.2**	...
51–70 mm Hg	42–50	...	NS	...
≤50 mm Hg	30–50	98	**19.3**	...
Pulse pressure[44]				
<60 mm Hg	21	32	**0.3**	...
60–79 mm Hg	21	...	NS	...
≥80 mm Hg	57	95	**10.9**	...
HILL'S TEST				
Hill's test[44]				
<40 mm Hg	29	13	**0.3**	...
40–59 mm Hg	29	...	NS	...
≥60 mm Hg	42	98	**17.3**	...
OTHER SIGNS				
Enlarged or sustained apical impulse[44]	97	60	2.4	**0.1**
S₃ gallop[45]	20	97	**5.9**	0.8
Duroziez's sign, femoral pistol shot, water hammer pulse[28,44]	37–55	63–98	NS	0.7

NS, not significant; likelihood ratio (LR) if finding present = positive LR; LR if finding absent = negative LR.
*Diagnostic standards: For moderate-to-severe regurgitation, regurgitation was either 3+ (moderate) or 4+ (severe) on a 0 to 4+ scale, using angiography,[31–33,37,38,44] Doppler echocardiography,[35,36,43,45] or surgery.[34] Trivial regurgitation on echocardiography was classified as "absent regurgitation."
[†]Definition of findings: See text.

MODERATE-TO-SEVERE AORTIC REGURGITATION

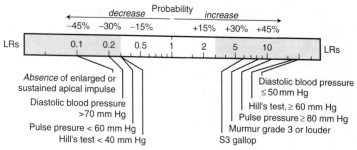

2. Blood Pressure

Two findings arguing strongly *for* moderate-to-severe regurgitation are a diastolic blood pressure ≤50 mm Hg (LR = 19.3, see EBM Box 41-2) and a pulse pressure ≥80 mm Hg (LR = 10.9, see EBM Box 41-2). Two findings arguing *against* significant regurgitation are a diastolic blood pressure greater than 70 mm Hg (LR = 0.2) and a pulse pressure less than 60 mm Hg (LR = 0.3). These signs have no diagnostic value when applied to other patients lacking the characteristic murmur of aortic regurgitation.[34]

3. Hill's Test

If the abnormal response in Hill's test is defined as a foot-arm blood pressure difference ≥60 mm Hg, the positive test argues strongly for significant regurgitation (LR = 17.3, see EBM Box 41-2).

Some doubt Hill's test is accurate, citing experiments that show the intra-arterial pressure in the *femoral arteries* of patients with aortic regurgitation to be identical to that of the brachial arteries.[46,47] Hill's test, however, measures the pressure of the pedal arteries, not the femoral arteries. It is possible that the systolic pressure is augmented in the foot, which is near the point of reflection of the abnormal pulse waveform.

4. Other Signs

The *absence* of an enlarged or sustained apical impulse argues *against* moderate-to-severe regurgitation (LR = 0.1; see EBM Box 41-2).

In one study of patients with pure aortic regurgitation, the finding of a third heart sound argued *for* severe regurgitation (LR = 5.9). The S_3 does not reliably indicate elevated left atrial pressure in these patients, however, because regurgitation alone may cause sufficiently rapid early diastolic filling to produce the sound (see Chapter 37).[48,49] Duroziez's sign, femoral pistol shots, and the water hammer pulse are all unreliable signs of the severity of regurgitation.

E. ACUTE AORTIC REGURGITATION

Compared with chronic aortic regurgitation, acute aortic regurgitation (e.g., from endocarditis or acute aortic dissection) causes a much shorter murmur, faster pulse rate (108/min vs. 71/min, mean values), smaller pulse pressure (55 vs. 105 mm Hg), and lower systolic blood pressures (110 vs. 155 mm Hg).[50] The murmur of acute aortic regurgitation is shorter because the combination of low arterial pressure and very high ventricular filling pressure eliminates the pressure gradient causing regurgitation by mid-diastole.[50] The first heart sound is faint or absent in acute aortic regurgitation, because of premature closure of the mitral valve (see Chapter 36).[51] In patients with aortic regurgitation from endocarditis, an associated pericardial rub often indicates extravalvular extension of the infection.[50]

F. DISTINGUISHING THE AUSTIN FLINT MURMUR FROM MITRAL STENOSIS

Based on an older analysis of 400 patients with severe aortic regurgitation, many of whom also had apical diastolic rumbles, the following findings argue for mitral stenosis: atrial fibrillation, a loud S_1, no S_3, and an opening snap. The findings arguing that the apical rumble is more likely the Austin Flint murmur are sinus rhythm, a faint S_1, an S_3, and no opening snap.[52] In addition, inhalation of amyl nitrite, which reduces systemic vascular resistance, makes the Austin Flint murmur (and the aortic regurgitation murmur) softer but the apical rumble of true mitral stenosis louder.[53]

REFERENCES

1. Vaslef SN, Roberts WC. Early descriptions of aortic regurgitation. *Am Heart J.* 1993;125(5 Part 1):1475-1483.
2. Dock G. I. Dominic John Corrigan: His place in the development of our knowledge of cardiac disease. II. The water-hammer pulse. *Ann Med Hist.* 1934;6:381-395.
3. Sakamoto T, Kawai N, Uozumi A, et al. The point of maximum intensity of aortic diastolic regurgitant murmur, with special emphasis to the "right-sided aortic diastolic murmur". *Jpn Heart J.* 1968;9:117-133.
4. Flint A. On cardiac murmurs. *Am J Med Sci.* 1862;44:29-54.
5. Lee D, Chen CH, Hsu TL, et al. Reappraisal of cardiac murmurs related to aortic regurgitation. *Chin Med J (Taipei).* 1995;56:152-158.
6. Rahko PS. Doppler and echocardiographic characteristics of patients having an Austin Flint murmur. *Circulation.* 1991;83:1940-1950.
7. Fortuin NJ, Craige E. On the mechanism of the Austin Flint murmur. *Circulation.* 1972;45:558-570.

8. Feinstein AR. Acoustic distinctions in cardiac auscultation: With emphasis on cardiophonetics, synecphonesis, the analysis of cadence, and problems of hydraulic distortion. *Arch Intern Med*. 1968;121:209-224.

9. Emi S, Fukuda N, Oki T, et al. Genesis of the Austin Flint murmur: Relation to mitral inflow and aortic regurgitant flow dynamics. *J Am Coll Cardiol*. 1993;21: 1399-1405.

10. Warnes CA, Harris PC, Fritts HW. Effect of elevating the wrist on the radial pulse in aortic regurgitation: Corrigan revisited. *Am J Cardiol*. 1983;51:1551-1553.

11. Palfrey FW. Auscultation of the Corrigan or water-hammer pulse. *N Engl J Med*. 1952;247:771-772.

12. Sapira JD. Quincke, de Musset, Duroziez, and Hill: Some aortic regurgitations. *South Med J*. 1981;74:459-467.

13. Kishan CV, Talley JD. Hill's sign: A non-invasive clue of the severity of chronic aortic regurgitation. *J Ark Med Soc*. 1999;95:501-502.

14. Cheng TO. Twelve eponymous signs of aortic regurgitation, one of which was named after a patient instead of a physician. *Am J Cardiol*. 2004;93:1332-1333.

15. Babu AN, Kymes SM, Fryer SMC. Eponyms and the diagnosis of aortic regurgitation: What says the evidence? *Ann Intern Med*. 2003;138:736-742.

16. Delpeuch A. Le signe de Musset: secousses rhythmées de la téte chez les aortiques. *Presse Méd*. 1900;8:237-238.

17. Sailer J. Pulsating spleen in aortic insufficiency. *Am Heart J*. 1928;3:447-453.

18. Dennison AD. Aortic regurgitation: Multiple eponyms, physical signs and etiologies. *J Ind State Med Assoc*. 1959;52:1283-1289.

19. Hill L. The measurement of systolic blood pressure in man. *Heart*. 1909;1:73-82.

20. Hill L, Rowlands RA. Systolic blood pressure: (1) In change of posture. (2) In cases of aortic regurgitation. *Heart*. 1911;3:219-232.

21. Luisada AA. On the pathogenesis of the signs of Traube and Duroziez in aortic insufficiency. *Am Heart J*. 1943;26:721-736.

22. Luft FC. Traube's double tone. Invited comment on: `Reports from the clinic of Privy Councilor Traube: two peculiar phenomena regarding aortic insufficiency". *J Mol Med*. 2002;80:687.

23. Lange RL, Hecht HH. Genesis of pistol-shot and Korotkoff sounds. *Circulation*. 1958;18:975-978.

24. McGee SR, Adcox M. Unilateral femoral pistol-shot sounds: A clue to aortic dissection. *West J Med*. 1995;162:547-548.

25. Boudoulas H, Triposkiadis F, Dervenagas S, et al. Mechanisms of pistol shot sounds in aortic regurgitation. *Acta Cardiologica*. 1991;46:139-145.

26. Blumgart HL, Erstene AC. Two mechanisms in the production of Duroziez's sign: Their diagnostic significance and a clinical test for differentiating between them. *JAMA*. 1933;100:173-177.

27. Rowe GG, Afonso S, Castillo CA, McKenna DH. The mechanism of the production of Duroziez's murmur. *N Engl J Med*. 1965;272:1207-1210.

28. Folts JD, Young WP, Rowe GG. A study of Duroziez's murmur of aortic insufficiency in man utilizing an electromagnetic flowmeter. *Circulation.* 1968;38:426-431.

29. MacAlpin RN, Kattus AA. Brachial-artery bruits in aortic-valve disease and hypertrophic subaortic stenosis. *N Engl J Med.* 1965;273:1012-1018.

30. Willius FA, Keys TE. *Classics of cardiology: A collection of classic works on the heart and circulation with comprehensive biographic accounts of the authors,* Vol 2. New York: Henry Schuman, Inc; 1941.

31. Linhart JW. Aortic regurgitation: Clinical, hemodynamic, surgical, and angiographic correlations. *Ann Thorac Surg.* 1971;11:27-37.

32. Meyers DG, Sagar KB, Ingram RF, et al. Diagnosis of aortic insufficiency: Comparison of auscultation and M-mode echocardiography to angiography. *South Med J.* 1982;75:1192-1194.

33. Meyers DG, Olson TS, Hansen DA. Auscultation, M-mode, echocardiography and pulsed Doppler echocardiography compared with angiography for diagnosis of chronic aortic regurgitation. *Am J Cardiol.* 1985;56:811-812.

34. Cohn LH, Mason DT, Ross J, et al. Preoperative assessment of aortic regurgitation in patients with mitral valve disease. *Am J Cardiol.* 1967;19:177-182.

35. Rahko PS. Prevalence of regurgitant murmurs in patients with valvular regurgitation detected by Doppler echocardiography. *Ann Intern Med.* 1989;111:466-472.

36. Aronow WS, Kronzon I. Correlation of prevalence and severity of aortic regurgitation detected by pulsed Doppler echocardiography with the murmur of aortic regurgitation in elderly patients in a long-term health care facility. *Am J Cardiol.* 1989;63:128-129.

37. Dittmann H, Karsch KR, Seipel L. Diagnosis and quantification of aortic regurgitation by pulsed Doppler echocardiography in patients with mitral valve disease. *Eur Heart J.* 1987;8 (Suppl C):53-57.

38. Grayburn PA, Smith MD, Handshoe R, et al. Detection of aortic insufficiency by standard echocardiography, pulsed Doppler echocardiography, and auscultation: A comparison of accuracies. *Ann Intern Med.* 1986;104:599-605.

39. Luisada AA, Madoery RJ. Functional tests as an aid to cardiac auscultation. *Med Clin North Am.* 1966;50:73-89.

40. Harvey WP, Corrado MA, Perloff JK. "Right-sided" murmurs of aortic insufficiency (diastolic murmurs better heard to the right of the sternum rather than to the left). *Am J Med Sci.* 1963;245:533-543.

41. Cohn KE, Hultgren HN. The Graham Steell murmur re-evaluated. *N Engl J Med.* 1966;274:486-489.

42. Runco V, Molnar W, Meckstroth CV, Ryan JM. The Graham Steell murmur versus aortic regurgitation in rheumatic heart disease: Results of aortic valvulography. *Am J Med.* 1961;31:71-80.

43. Desjardins VA, Enriquez-Sarano M, Tajik J, et al. Intensity of murmurs correlates with severity of valvular regurgitation. *Am J Med.* 1996;100:149-156.

44. Frank MJ, Casanegra P, Migliori AJ, Levinson GE. The clinical evaluation of aortic regurgitation. *Arch Intern Med.* 1965;116:357-365.
45. Tribouilloy CM, Enriquez-Sarano M, Mohty D, et al. Pathophysiologic determinants of third heart sounds: A prospective clinical and Doppler echocardiographi study. *Am J Med.* 2001;111:96-102.
46. Pascarelli EF, Bertrand CA, Lopez M. Comparison of arm and leg blood pressure in aortic insufficiency: an appraisal of Hill's sign. *Br Med J.* 1965;2:73-75.
47. Kutryk M, Fitchett D. Hills sign in aortic regurgitation: Enhanced pressure wave transmission or artefact? *Can J Cardiol.* 1997;13:237-240.
48. Abdulla AM, Frank MJ, Erdin RA, Canedo MI. Clinical significance and hemodynamic correlates of the third heart sound gallop in aortic regurgitation: A guide to optimal timing of cardiac catheterization. *Circulation.* 1981;64:464-471.
49. Folland ED, Kriegel BJ, Henderson WG, et al. Implications of third heart sounds in patients with valvular heart disease. *N Engl J Med.* 1992;327:458-462.
50. Mann T, McLaurin L, Grossman W, Craige E. Assessing the hemodynamic severity of acute aortic regurgitation due to infective endocarditis. *N Engl J Med.* 1975;293:108-113.
51. Meadows WR, van Praagh S, Indreika M, Sharp JT. Premature mitral valve closure: A hemodynamic explanation for absence of the first sound in aortic insufficiency. *Circ.* 1963;28:251-258.
52. Segal JP, Harvey WP, Corrado MA. The Austin Flint murmur: Its differentiation from the murmur of rheumatic mitral stenosis. *Circulation.* 1958;18:1025-1033.
53. Nasser W, Tavel ME, Feigenbaum H, Fisch C. Austin-Flint murmur versus the murmur of organic mitral stenosis. *N Engl J Med.* 1966;275:1007-1009.

42

Miscellaneous Heart Murmurs

HYPERTROPHIC CARDIOMYOPATHY

I. THE MURMUR

The murmur of hypertrophic cardiomyopathy is usually midsystolic, harsh in quality, and loudest at the lower left sternal border or between the lower left sternal border and apex.[1] The murmur may obliterate the second heart sound and become late systolic, especially if mitral regurgitation is associated. The intensity of the murmur behaves in distinctive ways during maneuvers altering venous return to the heart (see Chapter 39).

II. ASSOCIATED FINDINGS

The palpable apex beat may be sustained and the arterial pulse hyperkinetic (see Chapters 13 and 34). Although pulsus bisferiens has been described in hypertrophic cardiomyopathy,[2] this refers to a finding on intra-arterial pressure tracings, not a palpable finding at the bedside.[3] The second heart sound is usually single or physiologically split, although in 10% splitting it is paradoxic or reversed.[1] More than half of patients have audible fourth heart sound.[1]

MITRAL REGURGITATION

I. THE FINDING

A. THE MURMUR

The murmur of chronic mitral regurgitation is usually holosystolic, high in frequency, and loudest at the apex.[4] It radiates to the axilla and inferior angle of the left scapula, although in some patients with isolated incompetence of the medial portion of the posterior leaflet, the murmur radiates instead to the right base and even into the neck, thus mimicking aortic stenosis.[4,5]

In 1832, James Hope was the first to describe the apical systolic murmur of mitral regurgitation.[4,6]

B. ASSOCIATED FINDINGS

In chronic mitral regurgitation, the intensity of S_1 is normal 75% of the time, loud 12% of the time, and soft 12% of the time. In 50% of patients, S_2 splitting is wide and physiologic.[4] An associated S_3 is common, appearing in 89% with severe regurgitation. S_4 is rare.

Associated cardiac findings are an enlarged, laterally displaced palpable apical movement,[7] a palpable lower parasternal movement from an enlarged left atrium (see Chapter 34),[8] and a hyperkinetic arterial pulse (see Chapter 13).[9] Neck veins are normal unless the patient has decompensated heart failure.

II. CLINICAL SIGNIFICANCE

A. DETECTING MITRAL REGURGITATION

The presence of the characteristic murmur of mitral regurgitation argues that regurgitation is present, at least to a mild degree (likelihood ratio [LR] = 5.4, see Chapter 39). Although 25% to 50% of patients with *mild* regurgitation lack a murmur, the absence of the characteristic murmur does argues against the presence of *moderate-to-severe* mitral regurgitation (LR = 0.2, see Chapter 39).

B. SEVERITY OF MITRAL REGURGITATION

1. The Murmur

In a very general way, the intensity of the murmur of mitral regurgitation correlates with the severity of regurgitation, especially for rheumatic mitral regurgitation

($r = 0.67$) but less so for ischemic or functional* mitral regurgitation ($r = 0.45$).[10-12] A murmur of grade 3 intensity or louder argues moderately for severe mitral regurgitation (LR = 4.4, EBM Box 42-1).

2. Other Findings

Patients with severe mitral regurgitation may have a late systolic, sustained left lower parasternal impulse from a dilated left atrium (Chapter 34 discusses how to distinguish this impulse from a right ventricular one). The degree of this movement correlates well with severity of regurgitation ($r = 0.93$, $p < .01$), as long as the patient does not have associated mitral stenosis (the presence of mitral stenosis confounds analyzing the parasternal impulse of patients with mitral regurgitation because the impulse could be due to either a large left atrium from severe regurgitation or a hypertensive right ventricle from mitral stenosis).[8,13]

Some studies correlate the third heart sound with severity of mitral regurgitation,[14] whereas others do not,[15] Overall, the pooled LR is not significant (see EBM Box 42-1).

C. DISTINGUISHING ACUTE FROM CHRONIC MITRAL REGURGITATION

The physical signs of acute and chronic mitral regurgitation differ in several ways: In acute lesions, the patient is acutely ill with elevated neck veins and signs of pulmonary edema; in chronic lesions, these signs may be absent. In acute lesions the pulse is rapid and regular; in chronic lesions, it may be slow and commonly is irregular (from atrial fibrillation).[17] In acute lesions, the murmur may be short and confined to early systole (40% of patients in one series), because the left atrial pressures are so high they equal ventricular pressures by mid-to-late systole and thus eliminate the regurgitation gradient.[18,19] In chronic lesions, the murmur is holosystolic, late systolic, or midsystolic but not early systolic. In acute lesions, the fourth heart sound is common (80% in one series); in chronic lesions, the fourth heart sound is rare, because there is either no atrial contraction (i.e., atrial fibrillation) or the atrium is so dilated it cannot contract strongly.[10,17,20]

D. PAPILLARY MUSCLE DYSFUNCTION

Papillary muscle dysfunction refers to the murmur of mitral regurgitation that develops in the setting of myocardial ischemia. The murmur, which is usually transient, may be holosystolic, midsystolic, or late systolic. It appears in up to

---

*Functional mitral regurgitation implies that the primary problem is cardiomyopathy, which dilates the atrioventricular ring and renders the valve incompetent. Because of their low ejection fraction, these patients often tolerate valve replacement poorly.

Box 42-1   Severity of Mitral and Tricuspid Regurgitation*

Finding (Ref)	Sensitivity (%)	Specificity (%)	Likelihood Ratio if Finding	
			Present	Absent
MITRAL REGURGITATION				
Systolic murmur grade 3 or louder				
Detecting moderate-to-severe mitral regurgitation, in patients with characteristic systolic murmur[12]	85	81	**4.4**	**0.2**
Third heart sound				
Detecting moderate-to-severe mitral regurgitation, in patients with characteristic systolic murmur[14,15]	24–41	77–98	NS	0.8
TRICUSPID REGURGITATION				
Pulsatile liver				
Detecting moderate-to-severe tricuspid regurgitation, in patients with characteristic systolic murmur[16]	30	92	**3.9**	NS
Systolic regurgitant wave in neck veins				
Detecting moderate-to-severe tricuspid regurgitation, in patients with characteristic systolic murmur[16]	51	66	NS	NS

NS, not significant; likelihood ratio (LR) if finding present = positive LR; LR if finding absent = negative LR.

*Diagnostic standard: For moderate-to-severe mitral regurgitation, regurgitant fraction > 40% by Doppler echocardiography[12,14] or as assessed visually from angiogram[15]; for moderate-to-severe tricuspid regurgitation, 3+ or 4+ by angiography.[16]

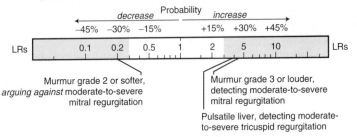

SEVERITY OF MITRAL AND TRICUSPID REGURGITATION

Murmur grade 2 or softer, *arguing against* moderate-to-severe mitral regurgitation

Murmur grade 3 or louder, detecting moderate-to-severe mitral regurgitation

Pulsatile liver, detecting moderate-to-severe tricuspid regurgitation

20% of patients with myocardial infarction,[21] in whom it is associated with a higher incidence of persistent chest pain in the intensive care unit (45% vs. 26% without murmur) and a higher 1-year mortality (18% vs. 10%).[21]

MITRAL VALVE PROLAPSE

I. INTRODUCTION

Mitral valve prolapse describes an abnormal posterosuperior movement of the mitral valve leaflets into the left atrium after they close at the beginning of systole. It is an important cause of mitral regurgitation and the physical findings of late systolic murmurs and mid-to-late systolic clicks.[22-24]

At the beginning of the 20th century, most clinicians believed that all late systolic murmurs were benign and that late systolic clicks were generated outside of the heart.[22,23] In 1963, Barlow performed angiograms in several patients with late systolic murmurs and proved the cause of the murmur was mitral prolapse and regurgitation.[25]

II. THE FINDINGS

A. THE MURMUR

The murmur of mitral valve prolapse is loudest at the apex and is sometimes musical (see Chapter 39). It is characteristically late systolic because the mitral leaflets are well supported by their chordae tendineae and competent during early systole but lose this support as the ventricle becomes smaller during late systole. The leaflets then buckle backward toward the left atrium and create a regurgitant leak.[22-24]

B. THE CLICKS

The clicks of mitral valve prolapse occur during mid-to-late systole and are loudest at the apex or left lower sternal border.[22] They are sometimes multiple. In patients with both a click and a murmur, the click introduces the murmur 65% of the time and occurs just after the beginning of the murmur 35% of the time.[22] Sudden deceleration of the billowing mitral leaflet, as it prolapses into the left atrial cavity, causes the sound, thus resembling the sound produced by a parachute or sail that suddenly tenses as it fills with wind.[26]

C. RESPONSE OF MURMURS AND CLICKS TO MANEUVERS

Bedside maneuvers that alter venous return or afterload (i.e., systemic vascular resistance) change both the timing of the clicks and murmurs and the intensity of the murmur, although they affect timing and intensity independently.

The *timing* of clicks and murmur depends on the venous return to the heart (Fig. 42-1). Reductions in venous return—by straining during the Valsalva maneuver or moving from squatting-to-standing—causes the ventricular chamber to become smaller and the mitral leaflets to prolapse earlier during systole, thus moving the click closer to S_1 and making the murmur longer.[22,24]

In contrast, the *intensity* of the murmur depends more on afterload, and in this way the response resembles that of chronic mitral regurgitation (see Chapter 39). As afterload is reduced with amyl nitrite inhalation, the murmur of mitral valve prolapse becomes fainter.[22] The Valsalva strain also usually makes the murmur *softer*. Squatting-to-standing, however, makes the murmur *louder*, perhaps because the standing position invokes sufficient sympathetic tone to preserve afterload while making ventricular contractions more vigorous, thus intensifying the sound.*[22]

III. CLINICAL SIGNIFICANCE

A. DETECTION OF MITRAL VALVE PROLAPSE

The presence of the characteristic click and murmur of mitral valve prolapse argues strongly that prolapse will be found by echocardiography (LR = 12.1, see Chapter 39). In fact, some have argued that the auscultatory criteria alone are sufficient for diagnosis.[27,28] The criteria for diagnosing mitral valve prolapse are the reproducible finding in a young patient of a mid-to-late systolic click or late systolic murmur at or near the apex. These sounds should shift their

---

*Mitral valve prolapse is therefore an important cause of the false-positive result when using the squatting-to-standing maneuver to diagnose obstructive cardiomyopathy (see Chapter 39).

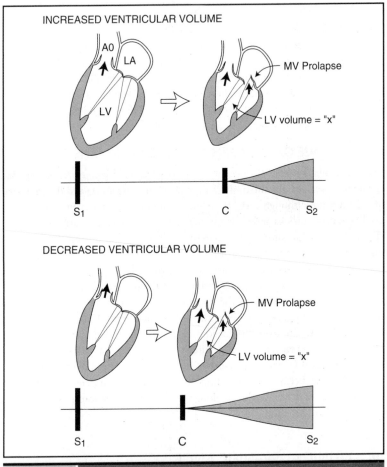

INCREASED VENTRICULAR VOLUME

MV Prolapse

LV volume = "x"

S₁   C   S₂

DECREASED VENTRICULAR VOLUME

MV Prolapse

LV volume = "x"

S₁   C   S₂

FIGURE 42-1   TIMING OF MITRAL VALVE PROLAPSE.

In each example, the left ventricle is ejecting blood during systole and prolapse of the mitral valve occurs at the moment ventricular volume = "x." If ventricular systole begins with a relatively large ventricular volume (*top row*), the ventricular volume of "x" is delayed until late systole. If ventricular systole instead begins with a smaller ventricular volume (e.g., by straining during the Valsalva maneuver or moving from squatting-to-standing, *bottom row*), the ventricular volume of "x" is reached earlier during systole, causing the click and murmur to move toward S_1. Ao, aorta; C, click; LA, left atrium; LV, left ventricle; MV, mitral valve.

timing with respect to S_1 and S_2 in response to the Valsalva and squatting-to-standing maneuvers (see "Response of Murmurs and Clicks to Maneuvers" and Fig. 42-1). These criteria require the patient to be young to avoid confusion with papillary muscle dysfunction, which is a common cause of late systolic murmurs in older patients.[27] The click should be mobile and occur in mid-to-late systole to eliminate confusion with other short systolic sounds, such as the split S_1 and the aortic ejection sound (Chapters 37 and 38 further discuss the differentiation of these sounds).[27,28]

B. RISK OF SIGNIFICANT MITRAL REGURGITATION

The risk of significant mitral regurgitation in mitral valve prolapse is low. In one study of 291 patients with a click or murmur presenting to a cardiologist (which biases selection toward more severe cases), none of the patients with an isolated click developed significant mitral regurgitation during 8 years of follow-up, and only 3% of those with murmurs ever required mitral valve replacement.[29]

TRICUSPID REGURGITATION

I. THE FINDINGS

The physical findings of tricuspid regurgitation depend on the patient's pulmonary pressure, which may be high ("high-pressure" tricuspid regurgitation) or normal ("low-pressure" tricuspid regurgitation). High-pressure tricuspid regurgitation is commonly due to left-sided heart disease; low-pressure tricuspid regurgitation commonly results from endocarditis of the tricuspid valve.

A. THE MURMUR

Whether pulmonary pressures are high or low, the murmur of tricuspid regurgitation is typically loudest at the lower left sternal border, becomes louder during inspiration, and may radiate below the xiphoid process.[30]

1. High-Pressure Tricuspid Regurgitation

The murmur of high-pressure tricuspid regurgitation is holosystolic because the elevated right ventricular pressures exceed right atrial pressures throughout systole. The murmur becomes louder during inspiration (Carvallo's sign) in 75% of patients and during manual pressure over the liver in 60% of patients.[15,31–35]

In some patients with high-pressure tricuspid regurgitation, the murmur is loudest at the apex because the enlarged right ventricle has replaced the normal position of the left ventricle. At this location, the resulting holosystolic apical murmur resembles mitral regurgitation, which, in the 1950s, led to the significant bedside error of misdiagnosing mitral regurgitation in some patients with mitral stenosis, thus inappropriately denying them valvuloplasty (a procedure contraindicated with severe mitral regurgitation).[36] Clues that help the clinician correctly recognize the apical holosystolic murmur as tricuspid regurgitation are the associated findings of an identical murmur at the lower sternal border, inspiratory augmentation of the murmur, elevated neck veins, and pulsatile liver.[36]

2. Low-Pressure Tricuspid Regurgitation

If pulmonary and right ventricular pressures are normal, the murmur of tricuspid regurgitation is confined to early systole, because by mid systole right atrial and right ventricular pressure are the same, thus eliminating the gradient causing the murmur.[37]

B. OTHER FINDINGS
1. High-Pressure Tricuspid Regurgitation

Other important cardiac findings are elevated neck veins (more than 90% of patients), a systolic regurgitant wave in the neck veins (51%–83% of patients), and systolic retraction of the apical impulse (22% of patients).[15,32,34] Thirty percent to 91% of patients have a pulsatile liver, and 90% have edema, ascites, or both.[15,30,32,34]

2. Low-Pressure Tricuspid Regurgitation

In these patients, the neck veins and apical impulse are normal, and there is no edema, pulsatile liver, or ascites.

C. ESTIMATING VENOUS PRESSURE IN TRICUSPID REGURGITATION

Estimates of venous pressure are useful because they indicate right ventricular *diastolic* pressures (or filling pressures), which provides important clues to the etiology of ascites and edema (see Chapter 32). In tricuspid regurgitation, however, the neck veins characteristically reveal a large *systolic* wave, raising the question of whether these bedside estimates of venous pressure still reliably indicate the right heart filling pressures.

In patients with tricuspid regurgitation (and no tricuspid stenosis), catheter measurements of the *mean* pressure in the right atrium correlate closely with right ventricular end-diastolic pressure ($r = 0.94$, $p < .001$, slope 1.0).[32] Mean atrial pressure is estimated at the bedside by identifying which patient position brings out the regurgitant waves. If the regurgitant waves are visible when the patient is supine, then the diastolic pressure in the veins must be very low (i.e., the waves collapse and become visible because the diastolic venous pressure is below the level of the sternum, or very low). The mean atrial pressure (i.e., central venous pressure) in these patients is probably normal. On the other hand, if the regurgitant waves are only visible in the upright position, the diastolic pressure in the veins must be high (otherwise the neck veins would collapse and be visible in lower positions). The mean atrial and central venous pressure of these patients is probably high.

II. CLINICAL SIGNIFICANCE

A. DETECTING TRICUSPID REGURGITATION

The presence of the characteristic systolic murmur of tricuspid regurgitation is a strong argument that some degree of tricuspid regurgitation is present (LR = 14.6, see Chapter 39). Many patients with tricuspid regurgitation, however, lack a murmur, which means that the *absence* of a murmur has less diagnostic significance (negative LR is 0.8 for detecting mild regurgitation or worse and 0.4 for detecting moderate-to-severe regurgitation, Chapter 39).

B. SEVERITY OF TRICUSPID REGURGITATION

In patients with the murmur of tricuspid regurgitation, the finding of a pulsatile liver argues for moderate-to-severe regurgitation (LR = 3.9, see EBM Box 42-1). Its absence is unhelpful.

The association between prominent jugular pulsations and severity of tricuspid regurgitation is more controversial. The only clinical study addressing this question found that prominent jugular systolic waves did not accurately predict severe regurgitation (LR NS, see EBM Box 42-1), but unfortunately this study failed to indicate whether the patients were supine or seated during examination. As discussed previously, many patients with mild tricuspid regurgitation have systolic waves that appear when they are supine but disappear when upright, and other patients with severe tricuspid regurgitation have prominent jugular pulsations when upright but lack them when supine. Cardiac catheterization data indicate that a CV wave greater than 15 mm Hg does detect moderate-to-severe tricuspid regurgitation (sensitivity of 48%, specificity of 93%, positive LR = 6.8),[38] and the comparable bedside observation—venous pulsations conspicuous in the *seated* patient—would presumably have similar accuracy.

PULMONIC REGURGITATION

I. THE FINDING

The murmur of pulmonic regurgitation is a diastolic murmur heard best at the second left intercostal space. Its timing and frequency depend on pulmonary pressures.

A. HIGH-PRESSURE PULMONIC REGURGITATION

Sustained pulmonary hypertension may cause the pulmonic valve to become incompetent, producing an early diastolic, high-frequency murmur at the second left intercostal space. The murmur begins immediately with a loud S_2, and most patients have elevated neck veins and other auscultatory findings of pulmonary hypertension, such as the pulmonary ejection sound, abnormal S_2 splitting, and right ventricular gallops (see Chapters 36–38).[39] Chapter 41 discusses how to distinguish this murmur from that of aortic regurgitation.

The high-pressure pulmonic regurgitation murmur was first described by the British clinician Graham Steell in 1888[40] and is often called the "Graham Steell" murmur.

B. LOW-PRESSURE PULMONIC REGURGITATION

When pulmonary pressures are normal, pulmonic regurgitation represents primary valvular disease (e.g., endocarditis). This murmur is mid diastolic and contains a mixture of low- and high-frequency sound. It begins with a short delay after S_2.[37]

II. CLINICAL SIGNIFICANCE

A. DETECTING PULMONIC REGURGITATION

Although the presence of the characteristic murmur is diagnostic (LR = 17.4, see Chapter 39), the absence of the murmur is unhelpful (LR not significant, see Chapter 39).

B. HEMODIALYSIS PATIENTS

A common cause of an early diastolic murmur at the sternal border in patients with end-stage renal disease is pulmonic regurgitation.[41] This murmur presumably occurs because of volume overload, because it is loudest immediately before dialysis and often disappears just after dialysis.

MITRAL STENOSIS

I. THE FINDINGS

A. THE MURMUR

Mitral stenosis causes a low-frequency, rumbling mid-diastolic murmur, which is usually heard with the bell lightly applied to the apex, often only after the patient has turned to the left lateral decubitus position. The murmur peaks during mid-diastole and again immediately before the first heart sound ("presystolic accentuation"). The mid-diastolic peak occurs because the mitral leaflets move backward toward the left atrium at this time, narrowing the mitral orifice and causing more turbulence (an analogy is the difficulty whistling with the mouth open).[42,43] The importance of these movements to the sound may explain why some patients with severe calcific mitral stenosis and inflexible leaflets have no murmur.[43]

The traditional explanation for presystolic accentuation is atrial systole, but this is probably incorrect because presystolic accentuation also occurs in patients with atrial fibrillation.[44] Instead, there is some evidence that presystolic accentuation is actually caused by *ventricular* contraction: The crescendo sound occurs because the closing movement of the mitral leaflets, induced by ventricular systole, occurs when a pressure gradient is still maintaining forward flow across the valve. The sound continues and crescendos up until the moment the valve completely closes, at the first heart sound (therefore, the "presystolic" accentuation is not presystolic at all, but instead is systolic).[42–44]

Because the sound vibrations of mitral stenosis border on the threshold of human hearing, this murmur is indistinct and the most difficult to detect, as reflected in metaphors used to describe the sound: "the faint sound of distant thunder," "the rumbling sound of a ball rolling down a bowling alley," and "the absence of silence."[45]

B. OTHER CARDIAC FINDINGS

Other cardiac findings in mitral stenosis include an irregular pulse (atrial fibrillation); a loud first heart sound; opening snap (early diastolic sound); and associated findings of pulmonary hypertension, including elevated neck veins with an exaggerated A wave, right ventricular parasternal impulse, and a palpable P_2 (see Chapters 32, 34, and 36).[9] The palpable apical impulse is small or absent, because of obstruction of blood flow into the left ventricle.[9]

II. CLINICAL SIGNIFICANCE

A. THE MURMUR

Not all apical diastolic rumbles are due to mitral stenosis, which has become a rare diagnosis in developed countries. Other causes of this murmur include mitral annular calcification; the Austin Flint murmur; atrial myxoma; and increased flow over a nonobstructed mitral valve from mitral regurgitation, ventricular septal defect, or high output states (see Chapter 37). In one study of 529 elderly patients living in the United States, an apical diastolic rumble detected *mitral annular calcification* on echocardiography with a sensitivity of 10%, specificity of 99%, and positive LR = 7.5 (90% of patients with this murmur had *no* mitral stenosis).[46]

B. OTHER CARDIAC FINDINGS

In patients with mitral stenosis, the apical impulse should be absent or small and the arterial pulse should be normal or reduced. Consequently, the finding of a hyperkinetic apical movement in patients with mitral stenosis suggests additional mitral or aortic regurgitation (LR = 11.2, EBM Box 42-2), and the finding of a hyperkinetic arterial pulse strongly suggests additional mitral regurgitation (LR = 14.2, see EBM Box 42-2).

ARTERIOVENOUS FISTULAE: THE HEMODIALYSIS FISTULA

The hemodialysis fistula provides a good example of the continuous murmur typical of arteriovenous fistulae: it is a high-frequency murmur, persisting throughout systole and diastole but peaking during late systole (**Pu**SHSHSH**SHPu**SHSHSHSHSHSHSH; venous hums, in contrast peak during diastole, see Chapter 39). Moving the stethoscope progressively away from the fistula and toward the heart makes the diastolic component of the murmur fainter until only a systolic murmur remains.[48]

Box 42-2   Other Cardiac Findings in Mitral Stenosis*

Finding (Ref)†	Sensitivity (%)	Specificity (%)	Likelihood Ratio if Finding	
			Present	Absent
Graham Steell murmur				
Detecting pulmonary hypertension[47]	69	83	**4.2**	0.4
Hyperkinetic apical movement				
Detecting associated mitral regurgitation or aortic valve disease[9]	74	93	**11.2**	**0.3**
Hyperkinetic arterial pulse				
Detecting associated mitral regurgitation[9]	71	95	**14.2**	**0.3**

Likelihood ratio (LR) if finding present = positive LR; LR if finding absent = negative LR.
*Diagnostic standard: For pulmonary hypertension, mean pulmonary pressure >50 mm Hg [47]
†Definition of findings: For Graham Steell murmur, early diastolic decrescendo murmur of high pressure pulmonic regurgitation at 2nd left intercostal space; for hyperkinetic apical movement, apical "thrust"[9] (see Chapter 34); for hyperkinetic pulse, arterial pulse strikes fingers abruptly and strongly (see Chapter 13).

OTHER CARDIAC FINDINGS IN MITRAL STENOSIS

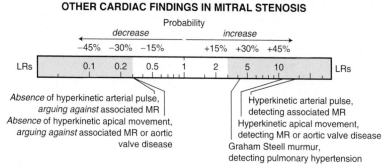

The importance of this murmur is that its systolic remnants are transmitted to the upper sternal border, where they can be mistaken for cardiac murmurs unless the clinician traces them to the fistula.[48]

REFERENCES

1. Tucker RBK, Zion MM, Pocock WA, Barlow JB. Auscultatory features of hypertrophic obstructive cardiomyopathy: A study of 90 patients. *S Afr Med J.* 1975;49: 179-186.

2. Frank S, Braunwald E. Idiopathic hypertrophic subaortic stenosis: Clinical analysis of 126 patients with emphasis on the natural history. *Circulation.* 1968;37: 759-788.

3. Perloff JK. Clinical recognition of aortic stenosis: The physical signs and differential diagnosis of the various forms of obstruction to left ventricular outflow. *Prog Cardiovasc Dis.* 1968;10:323-352.

4. Perloff JK, Harvey WP. Auscultatory and phonocardiographic manifestations of pure mitral regurgitation. *Prog Cardiovasc Dis.* 1962;5:172-194.

5. Antman EM, Angoff GH, Sloss LJ. Demonstration of the mechanism by which mitral regurgitation mimics aortic stenosis. *Am J Cardiol.* 1978;42:1044-1048.

6. Willius FA, Dry TJ. *A history of the heart and the circulation.* Philadelphia: WB Saunders; 1948.

7. Sutton GC, Craige E, Grizzle JE. Quantitation of precordial movement. II. Mitral regurgitation. *Circulation.* 1967;35:483-491.

8. Basta LL, Wolfson P, Eckberg DL, Abboud FM. The value of left parasternal impulse recordings in the assessment of mitral regurgitation. *Circulation.* 1973;48: 1055-1065.

9. Wood P. An appreciation of mitral stenosis. I. Clinical features. II. Investigations and results. *Br Med J.* 1954;1:1051-1063, 1113-1024.

10. Hultgren HN, Hancock EW, Cohn KE. Auscultation in mitral and tricuspid valvular disease. *Prog Cardiovasc Dis.* 1968;10:298-322.

11. Rahko PS. Prevalence of regurgitant murmurs in patients with valvular regurgitation detected by Doppler echocardiography. *Ann Intern Med.* 1989;111:466-472.

12. Desjardins VA, Enriquez-Sarano M, Tajik J, et al. Intensity of murmurs correlates with severity of valvular regurgitation. *Am J Med.* 1996;100:149-156.

13. James TM, Swatzell RH, Eddleman EE. Hemodynamic significance of the precordial late systolic outward movement in mitral regurgitation. *Ala J Med Sci.* 1978; 15(1):55-64.

14. Tribouilloy CM, Enriquez-Sarano M, Mohty D, et al. Pathophysiologic determinants of third heart sounds: A prospective clinical and Doppler echocardiographic study. *Am J Med.* 2001;111:96-102.

15. Folland ED, Kriegel BJ, Henderson WG, et al. Implications of third heart sounds in patients with valvular heart disease. *N Engl J Med.* 1992;327:458-462.

16. Cha SD, Gooch AS. Diagnosis of tricuspid regurgitation. *Arch Intern Med.* 1983;143:1763-1768.

17. DePace NL, Nestico PF, Morganroth J. Acute severe mitral regurgitation: Pathophysiology, clinical recognition, and management. *Am J Med.* 1985;78: 293-306.

18. Friedman AW, Stein L. Pitfalls in bedside diagnosis of severe acute mitral regurgitation: Clinical and hemodynamic features. *Chest.* 1980;78:436-441.

19. Sutton GC, Craige E. Clinical signs of severe acute mitral regurgitation. *Am J Cardiol.* 1967;20:141-144.

20. Cohen LS, Mason DT, Braunwald E. Significance of an atrial gallop sound in mitral regurgitation: A clue to the diagnosis of rupture chordae tendineae. *Circulation.* 1967;35:112-118.

21. Maisel AS, Gilpin EA, Klein L, et al. The murmur of papillary muscle dysfunction in acute myocardial infarction: Clinical features and prognostic implications. *Am Heart J.* 1986;112:705-711.

22. Barlow JB, Bosman CK, Pocock WA, Marchand P. Late systolic murmurs and non-ejection ("mid-late") systolic clicks: An analysis of 90 patients. *Br Heart J.* 1968; 30:203-218.

23. Devereux RB, Perloff JK, Reichek N, Josephson ME. Mitral valve prolapse. *Circulation.* 1976;54:3-14.

24. Fontana ME, Wooley CF, Leighton RF, Lewis RP. Postural changes in left ventricular and mitral valvular dynamics in systolic click: Late systolic murmur syndrome. *Circulation.* 1975;51:165-173.

25. Barlow JB, Pocock WA, Marchand P, Denny M. The significance of late systolic murmurs. *Am Heart J.* 1963;66:443-452.

26. Ronan JA. Cardiac auscultation: Opening snaps, systolic clicks, and ejection sounds. *Heart Dis Stroke.* 1993;2:188-191.

27. Perloff JK, Child JS. Clinical and epidemiologic issues in mitral valve prolapse: Overview and perspective. *Am Heart J.* 1987;113:1324-1332.

28. Perloff JK, Child JS, Edwards JE. New guidelines for the clinical diagnosis of mitral valve prolapse. *Am J Cardiol.* 1986;57:1124-1129.

29. Tofler OB, H. TG. Use of auscultation to follow patients with mitral systolic clicks and murmurs. *Am J Cardiol.* 1990;66:1355-1358.

30. Müller O, Shillingford J. Tricuspid incompetence. *Br Heart J.* 1954;16:195-207.

31. Gooch AS, Cha SD, Maranhao V. The use of the hepatic pressure maneuver to identify the murmur of tricuspid regurgitation. *Clin Cardiol.* 1983;6:277-280.

32. Salazar E, Levine HD. Rheumatic tricuspid regurgitation: The clinical spectrum. *Am J Med.* 1962;33:111-129.

33. Maisel AS, Atwood JE, Goldberger AL. Hepatojugular reflux: Useful in the bedside diagnosis of tricuspid regurgitation. *Ann Intern Med.* 1984;101:781-782.

34. Lingamneni R, Cha SD, Maranhao V, et al. Tricuspid regurgitation: Clinical and angiographic assessment. *Cath Cardiovasc Diag.* 1979;5:7-17.

35. Vitums VC, Gooch AS, Evans JM. Bedside maneuvers to augment the murmur of tricuspid regurgitation. *Med Ann DC.* 1969;38:533-542.

36. Schilder DP, Harvey WP. Confusion of tricuspid incompetence with mitral insufficiency: A pitfall in the selection of patients for mitral surgery. *Am Heart J.* 1957; 54:352-367.

37. Perloff JK. The physiologic mechanisms of cardiac and vascular physical signs. *J Am Coll Cardiol.* 1983;1:184-198.

38. Pitts WR, Lange RA, Cigarroa JE, Hillis LD. Predictive value of prominent right atrial V waves in assessing the presence and severity of tricuspid regurgitation. *Am J Cardiol.* 1999;83:617-618.

39. Perloff JK. Auscultatory and phonocardiographic manifestations of pulmonary hypertension. *Prog Cardiovasc Dis.* 1967;9:303-340.

40. Willius FA, Keys TE. *Classics of cardiology: A collection of classic works on the heart and circulation with comprehensive biographic accounts of the authors,* Vol 2. New York: Henry Schuman, Inc; 1941.

41. Perez JE, Smith CA, Meltzer VN. Pulmonic valve insufficiency: A common cause of transient diastolic murmurs in renal failure. *Ann Intern Med.* 1985;103:497-502.

42. Fortuin NJ, Craige E. Echocardiographic studies of genesis of mitral diastolic murmurs. *Br Heart J.* 1973;35:75-81.

43. Toutouzas P, Koidakis A, Velimezis A, Avgoustakis D. Mechanism of diastolic rumble and presystolic murmur in mitral stenosis. *Br Heart J.* 1974;36:1096-1105.

44. Criley JM, Hermer AJ. The crescendo presystolic murmur of mitral stenosis with atrial fibrillation. *N Engl J Med.* 1971;285:1284-1287.

45. Constant J. *Bedside cardiology.* Boston: Little, Brown and Company; 1985.

46. Aronow WS, Schwartz KS, Koenigsberg M. Correlation of murmurs of mitral stenosis and mitral regurgitation with presence or absence of mitral anular calcium in persons older than 62 years in a long-term health care facility. *Am J Cardiol.* 1987; 59:181-182.

47. Whitaker W. Clinical diagnosis of pulmonary hypertension in patients with mitral stenosis. *Q J Med.* 1954;23:105-112.

48. Rault R. Transmitted murmurs in patients undergoing hemodialysis. *Arch Intern Med.* 1989;149:1392-1393.

43

Disorders of the Pericardium

PERICARDITIS AND THE PERICARDIAL RUB

I. INTRODUCTION

The pericardial rub is a physical sign of pericarditis, or inflammation of the pericardium, which is caused by a wide variety of disorders, including infections, connective tissue diseases, myocardial infarction, neoplasia, uremia, and trauma.

In the 1820s, shortly after the introduction of the stethoscope, Collin first described the pericardial rub as a sound "similar to that of the crackling of new leather."[1]

II. THE FINDING

Pericardial rubs are grating, scratching, or creaking sounds that are loudest near the left sternal border and are most apparent when the patient is sitting upright,

510

leaning forward, and holding his or her breath in deep expiration.[2,3] They resemble the sound of two pieces of sandpaper being rubbed together. Compared with heart murmurs, the pericardial rub has more high-frequency energy and sounds closer to the ear.[2] Rubs often become louder during inspiration, and up to one fourth are palpable.[3]

In about 50% of patients, the rub has three components per cardiac cycle—one during ventricular systole and two during diastole (middiastole and atrial systole).* In about one third of patients, only two components are heard (usually the atrial and ventricular systolic rub), and in the remaining 15%, only a single-component ventricular systolic rub is heard.[3]

III. CLINICAL SIGNIFICANCE

A. THE RUB AND PERICARDITIS

Because the diagnosis of pericarditis relies on bedside criteria, one of which is the rub, the diagnostic accuracy of the rub cannot be assessed. The other two criteria for pericarditis are the characteristic pericardial chest pain (precordial pleuritic pain radiating to the trapezius ridge, which is relieved by sitting up) and the characteristic electrocardiographic changes (diffuse concave ST elevation, PR segment depression, absence of Q waves).[4,5] Most clinical studies of pericarditis require two of these three criteria. Echocardiography is not a criteria for pericarditis, because only half of patients with pericarditis have detectable pericardial effusions.[4,5]

B. THE RUB AND PERICARDIAL EFFUSION

Although the pericardial rub suggests the rubbing together of contiguous pericardial surfaces, the sound often persists after accumulation of significant pericardial effusions.[3,6] The rub is heard, for example, in up to one fourth of patients with cardiac tamponade (see later). Therefore, the *presence* of the rub cannot be used to argue *against* the development of pericardial effusion.

C. THE RUB AND NEOPLASTIC DISEASE

In patients with known cancer, who subsequently develop pericardial disease, the presence of a rub argues that the pericarditis is idiopathic or radiation-induced, not neoplastic pericarditis [sensitivity 62%, specificity 89%, positive likelihood ratio (LR) = 5.5, negative LR = 0.4].[7]

---

*These three components represent the three moments in the cardiac cycle when the ventricle is moving the most.

D. THE RUB AND MYOCARDIAL INFARCTION

A pericardial rub is found in 5–20% of patients with acute myocardial infarction, usually appearing between hospital days 1 and 3.[8-12] The incidence is lowest (i.e., 5–7%) in patients receiving immediate thrombolytic medications or angioplasty.[10,12] Compared with patients who do not develop rubs, patients with rubs have significantly larger myocardial infarctions, lower ejection fractions, more extensive coronary artery disease, and more complications, including congestive heart failure and atrial arrhythmias.[8,10,11] In these patients, however, tamponade is rare, even if they receive thrombolytic medications.[10]

CARDIAC TAMPONADE

I. INTRODUCTION

Cardiac tamponade is present when a pericardial effusion has become so large and tense that intrapericardial pressures exceed the normal filling (i.e., diastolic) pressures of the heart, thus impairing diastolic filling of the heart and reducing cardiac output.

The history of diagnosing tamponade illustrates well the tension that sometimes exists between older diagnostic standards, based on physical signs, and newer ones, based on clinical imaging. For example, early descriptions of tamponade, which were based on catastrophic acute intrapericardial hemorrhage, emphasized hypotension, elevated neck veins, and the small, quiet heart as diagnostic findings ("Beck's triad").[13,14] Later, after it became obvious that many medical patients with tamponade had normal blood pressure and loud heart tones, the definition of tamponade shifted to emphasize large pericardial effusions, elevated neck veins, pulsus paradoxus, and relief of symptoms and signs after pericardiocentesis.[15] Finally, in the 1980s, several echocardiographic criteria for tamponade were introduced,[14,16] although studies have subsequently shown that relying solely on these criteria sometimes identifies patients who fail to improve symptomatically or physiologically after pericardiocentesis.[17-19]

Therefore, the diagnosis of tamponade should not rely solely on the echocardiographic report but requires synthesis of all the findings, emphasizing especially the ones from physical diagnosis—elevated neck veins, tachycardia, and pulsus paradoxus.[20]

II. THE FINDINGS

Table 43-1 presents the physical signs observed in several studies of patients with proven cardiac tamponade, most of whom presented with shortness of

Table 43-1	Cardiac Tamponade*	
Physical Finding†		**Frequency (%)‡**
Neck veins		
Elevated neck veins		100
Kussmaul's sign		0
Arterial pulse		
Tachycardia (>100 beats/min)		81–100
Blood pressure		
Systolic blood pressure greater than 100 mm Hg		58–100
Pulsus paradoxus >10 mm Hg		98
Pulsus paradoxus >20 mm Hg		78
Pulsus paradoxus >30 mm Hg		49
Pulsus paradoxus >40 mm Hg		38
Total paradox		23
Auscultation of heart		
Diminished heart tones		36–84
Pericardial rub		27
Other		
Hepatomegaly		58
Edema		27

Data from 121 patients from references 15, 21–24.
Diagnostic standard: For tamponade, cardiac output that improved after drainage of pericardial effusion.
†*Definition of finding: For total paradox, palpable pulse disappears completely during inspiration.*
‡*Results are overall mean frequency or, if statistically heterogeneous, the range of values.*

breath.[15,24] The definition and pathogenesis of pulsus paradoxus and elevated neck veins are discussed in Chapters 13 and 32.

The three key findings of tamponade are elevated neck veins (100% of patients), tachycardia (81%–100% of patients), and pulsus paradoxus greater than 10 mm Hg (98% of patients). In patients with pericardial effusions, the finding of pulsus paradoxus greater than 12 mm Hg detects tamponade with a sensitivity of 98%, specificity of 83%, positive LR of 5.9, and negative LR of 0.03 (see Chapter 13).[25]

Cardiac tamponade is one of the few causes of elevated neck veins with absent *y* descent (see Chapter 32). This finding contrasts sharply with the exaggerated *y* descent of constrictive pericarditis (see later).

CONSTRICTIVE PERICARDITIS

I. INTRODUCTION

Constrictive pericarditis is present when calcification or fibrosis of the pericardium impairs diastolic filling, which then elevates venous pressure and reduces cardiac output.

II. THE FINDINGS

Table 43-2 presents the physical signs of patients with constrictive pericarditis, most of whom presented with edema, abdominal swelling, and dyspnea.[30,31,33] The key physical findings are elevated neck veins (98%), prominent y descent in venous waveform (57%–94%), pericardial knock (28%–94%), and hepatomegaly (87%–100%).

Table 43-2 Constrictive Pericarditis*

Physical Finding	Frequency (%)†
Neck veins	
Elevated neck veins	98
Prominent y descent (Friedrich's sign)	57–94
Kussmaul's sign	50
Arterial pulse	
Irregularly irregular (atrial fibrillation)	36–70
Blood pressure	
Pulsus paradoxus >10 mm Hg	17–43
Auscultation of heart	
Pericardial knock	28–94
Pericardial rub	4
Other	
Hepatomegaly	87–100
Edema	63
Ascites	53–89

Data from 181 patients from references 21, 26–32.
Diagnostic standard: For constrictive pericarditis, surgical and postmortem findings,[21,26,27,30] sometimes in combination with hemodynamic findings.[28,29,31,32]
†*Results are overall mean frequency or, if statistically heterogeneous, the range of values.*

A. NECK VEINS (SEE ALSO CHAPTER 32)

In addition to the elevated venous pressure, the venous waveform displays a unusually prominent *y* descent, which, combined with an exaggerated *x´* descent, creates two conspicuous dips per cardiac cycle, making the waveform appear to trace an "M" or "W" with each arterial pulse ("Friedrich's sign," see Chapter 32). Sometimes these movements are transmitted to the liver, causing it to pulsate inward twice with each cardiac cycle.[34]

The prominent *y* descent occurs because diastolic filling is only impaired during the last two thirds of diastole. At the moment the tricuspid valve opens (beginning of diastole and beginning of *y* descent), the right atrium empties rapidly and with no resistance (causing a prominent *y* descent), although eventually the relaxing ventricle meets the limits of the rigid pericardial shell and pressures again rise.[35] This finding contrasts with that observed in tamponade, which impairs diastolic filling throughout diastole and thus eliminates the *y* descent.

B. KUSSMAUL'S SIGN

Kussmaul's sign is the paradoxical increase in venous pressure during inspiration. This sign, present in 50% of patients with constriction, is discussed in Chapter 32.

C. PERICARDIAL KNOCK

The pericardial knock is a loud, high-frequency early diastolic sound heard between the apex and left lower sternal border. It is discussed in Chapter 38.

D. OTHER FINDINGS

Up to 90% of patients with constrictive pericarditis have systolic retraction of the apical impulse (see Chapter 34).[32,36]

According to traditional teachings, pulsus paradoxus is a not a finding of constrictive pericarditis, yet the studies reviewed in Table 43-2 show that pulsus paradoxus is present in 17%–43% of patients with constrictive pericarditis.[21,26,31,33] This seeming contradiction probably reflects different definitions for pulsus paradoxus. If pulsus paradoxus is defined as greater than 10 mm Hg inspiratory fall in systolic blood pressure (i.e., the usual definition), 17%–43% of patients in these studies had the finding[21,33]; however, if it is instead defined as greater than 20 mm Hg inspiratory fall, then no patient had the finding.[21] In contrast, the usual pulsus paradoxus in patients with tamponade is 20–50 mm Hg (see Table 43-1).[15]

Therefore, mild degrees of pulsus paradoxus (10–20 mm Hg) are commonly observed in patients with constrictive pericarditis, but larger degrees (>20 mm Hg) are not and suggest tamponade or another cause of the finding (see Chapter 13).

REFERENCES

1. Stokes W. *An introduction to the use of the stethoscope* (facsimile edition by the Classics of Cardiology Library). Edinburgh: Maclachlin and Stewart; 1825.

2. Harvey WP. Auscultatory findings in diseases of the pericardium. *Am J Cardiol.* 1961;7:15–20.

3. Spodick DH. Pericardial rub: Prospective, multiple observer investigation of pericardial friction in 100 patients. *Am J Cardiol.* 1975;35:357–362.

4. Permanyer-Miralda G, Sagrista-Sauleda J, Soler-Soler J. Primary acute pericardial disease: A prospective series of 231 consecutive patients. *Am J Cardiol.* 1985;56:623–630.

5. Zayas R, Anguita M, Torres F, et al. Incidence of specific etiology and role of methods for specific etiologic diagnosis of primary acute pericarditis. *Am J Cardiol.* 1995;75:378–382.

6. Markiewicz W, Brik A, Brook G, et al. Pericardial rub in pericardial effusion: Lack of correlation with amount of fluid. *Chest.* 1980;77:643–646.

7. Posner MR, Cohen GI, Skarin AT. Pericardial disease in patients with cancer: The differentiation of malignant from idiopathic and radiation-induced pericarditis. *Am J Med.* 1981;71:407–413.

8. Tofler GH, Muller JE, Stone PH, et al. Pericarditis in acute myocardial infarction: Characterization and clinical significance. *Am Heart J.* 1989;117:86–91.

9. Lichstein E, Liu HM, Gupta P. Pericarditis complication acute myocardial infarction: Incidence of complications and significance of electrocardiogram on admission. *Am Heart J.* 1974;87:246–252.

10. Wall TC, Califf RM, Harrelson-Woodlief L, et al. Usefulness of a pericardial friction rub after thrombolytic therapy during acute myocardial infarction in predicting amount of myocardial damage. *Am J Cardiol.* 1990;66:1418–1421.

11. Dubois C, Smeets JP, Demoulin JC, et al. Frequency and clinical significance of pericardial friction rubs in the acute phase of myocardial infarction. *Eur Heart J.* 1985;6:766–768.

12. Sugiura T, Nakamura S, Kudo Y, et al. Clinical factors associated with persistent pericardial effusion after successful primary coronary angioplasty. *Chest.* 2005;128:798–803.

13. Beck CS. Two cardiac compression triads. *JAMA.* 1935;104:714–716.

14. Fowler NO. Cardiac tamponade: A clinical or an echocardiographic diagnosis? *Circulation.* 1993;87:1738–1741.

15. Guberman BA, Fowler NO, Engel PJ, et al. Cardiac tamponade in medical patients. *Circulation.* 1981;64:633–640.

16. Himelman RB, Kircher B, Rockey DC, Schiller NB. Inferior vena cava plethora with blunted respiratory response: A sensitive echocardiographic sign of cardiac tamponade. *J Am Coll Cardiol.* 1988;12:1470–1477.

17. Levine MJ, Lorell BH, Diver DJ, Come PC. Implications of echocardiographically assisted diagnosis of pericardial tamponade in contemporary medical

patients: Detection before hemodynamic embarrassment. *J Am Coll Cardiol.* 1991;17:59–65.

18. Materazzo C, Piotti P, Meazza R, et al. Respiratory changes in transvalvular flow velocities versus two-dimensional echocardiographic findings in the diagnosis of cardiac tamponade. *Ital Heart J.* 2003;4:186–192.

19. Merce J, Sagrista-Sauleda J, Permanyer-Miralda G, et al. Correlation between clinical and Doppler echocardiographic findings in patients with moderate and large pericardial effusion: Implications for the diagnosis of cardiac tamponade. *Am Heart J.* 1999;138:759–764.

20. Hancock EW. Cardiac tamponade. *Heart Dis Stroke.* 1994;3:155–158.

21. Lange RL, Botticelli JT, Tsagaris TJ, et al. Diagnostic signs in compressive cardiac disorders: Constrictive pericarditis, pericardial effusion, and tamponade. *Circulation.* 1966;33:763–777.

22. Reddy PS, Curtiss EI, O'Toole JD, Shaver JA. Cardiac tamponade: Hemodynamic observations in man. *Circulation.* 1978;58:265–272.

23. Brown J, MacKinnon D, King A, Vanderbush E. Elevated arterial blood pressure in cardiac tamponade. *N Engl J Med.* 1992;327:463–466.

24. Markiewicz W, Borovik R, Ecker S. Cardiac tamponade in medical patients: Treatment and prognosis in the echocardiographic era. *Am Heart J.* 1986;111:1138–1142.

25. Curtiss EI, Reddy PS, Uretsky BF, Cecchetti AA. Pulsus paradoxus: Definition and relation to the severity of cardiac tamponade. *Am Heart J.* 1988;115:391–398.

26. Paul O, Castleman B, White PD. Chronic constrictive pericarditis: A study of 53 cases. *Am J Med Sci.* 1948;216:361–377.

27. Mounsey P. The early diastolic sound of constrictive pericarditis. *Br Heart J.* 1955;17:143–152.

28. Tyberg TI, Goodyer AVN, Langou RA. Genesis of pericardial knock in constrictive pericarditis. *Am J Cardiol.* 1980;46:570–575.

29. Schiavone WA. The changing etiology of constrictive pericarditis in a large referral center. *Am J Cardiol.* 1986;58:373–375.

30. Evans W, Jackson F. Constrictive pericarditis. *Br Heart J.* 1952;14:53–69.

31. Wood P. Chronic constrictive pericarditis. *Am J Cardiol.* 1961;7:48–61.

32. El-Sherif A, El-Said G. Jugular, hepatic, and praecordial pulsations in constrictive pericarditis. *Br Heart J.* 1971;33:305–312.

33. Cameron J, Oesterle SN, Baldwin JC, Hancock EW. The etiologic spectrum of constrictive pericarditis. *Am Heart J.* 1987;113(2 Part 1):354–360.

34. Coralli RJ, Crawley IS. Hepatic pulsations in constrictive pericarditis. *Am J Cardiol.* 1986;58:370–373.

35. Shabetai R, Fowler NO, Guntheroth WG. The hemodynamics of cardiac tamponade and constrictive pericarditis. *Am J Cardiol.* 1970;26:480–489.

36. Boicourt OW, Nagle RE, Mounsey JPD. The clinical significance of systolic retraction of the apical impulse. *Br Heart J.* 1965;27:379–391.

Congestive Heart Failure

I. INTRODUCTION

Heart failure is a clinical syndrome characterized by impaired ventricular performance, elevated diastolic filling pressures, and diminished exercise capacity. Patients with heart failure and ventricular disease may have a low ventricular ejection fraction ("systolic dysfunction") or normal ejection fraction ("diastolic dysfunction").

Clear descriptions of the signs of heart failure date to the Middle Ages.[1] In the seventeenth century, just after Harvey published his discovery of the circulation of blood, clinicians began to correlate the pathologic observation of large heart chambers and congested lungs with the clinical observations of dyspnea and edema.[2]

II. THE FINDINGS

Many of the findings of heart failure are discussed fully in other chapters of the book, including pulsus alternans and the dicrotic pulse (see Chapter 13),

Cheyne-Stokes respirations (see Chapter 17), crackles (see Chapter 27), elevated neck veins (see Chapter 32), the abdominojugular test (see Chapter 32), displaced apical impulse (see Chapter 34), and third heart sound (see Chapter 37).

This chapter reviews one finding not discussed extensively elsewhere, the abnormal Valsalva response, and then presents the diagnostic accuracy of all findings of congestive heart failure.

III. THE VALSALVA RESPONSE

A. INTRODUCTION

The "Valsalva maneuver" consists of forced expiration against a closed glottis after a full inspiration.[3] The "Valsalva response" refers to the changes in blood pressure and pulse that occur during both the strain phase of the maneuver and the recovery period after the strain is released.

Valsalva introduced his maneuver in 1704 as a technique to expel pus from the middle ear.[3,4] The maneuver was forgotten, however, until 1859, when Weber showed he could use it to interrupt his arterial pulse at will (an experiment he stopped after he made himself faint and develop convulsions).[4] Beginning in the 1950s, many different investigators reported that the Valsalva response was distinctly abnormal in patients with congestive heart failure.[5-9]

B. TECHNIQUE

To perform the maneuver, the patient should take a deep breath in and bear down, as if straining to have a bowel movement. The clinician measures the Valsalva response by using a blood pressure cuff, as described later. In clinical studies, the straining phase is standardized by having the patient's mouthpiece connected to a pressure transducer, which should demonstrate an increment of 30–40 mm Hg for at least 10 seconds.

The Valsalva maneuver is contraindicated in patients with recent eye or central nervous system surgery or hemorrhage. It is also unwise to perform the maneuver in patients with acute coronary ischemia, because it may induce arrhythmias, although in patients with chronic ischemic heart disease the maneuver is safe and was once even used to terminate episodes of angina.[10]

C. THE NORMAL VALSALVA RESPONSE

The normal Valsalva response is divided into four phases (Fig. 44-1).[3] In phase 1, the arterial systolic blood pressure rises temporarily because the increased intrathoracic pressure is transmitted directly to the aorta. In phase 2, blood pressure falls because of reduced venous return with continuing straining.

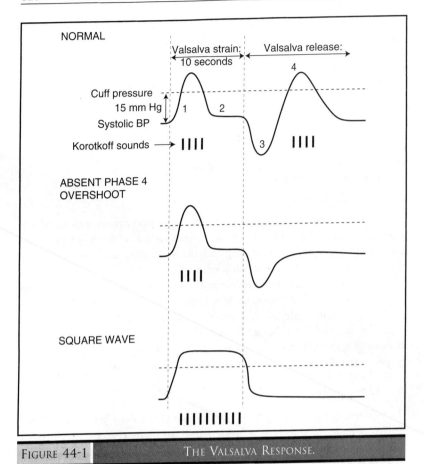

FIGURE 44-1   THE VALSALVA RESPONSE.

The *solid* line in each drawing depicts changes in systolic blood pressure over time during the Valsalva maneuver. The three types of Valsalva responses are normal (*top*), absent phase 4 overshoot (*middle*), and square wave (*bottom*). The clinician distinguishes these responses by inflating the blood pressure cuff 15 mm Hg above the patient's resting systolic blood pressure (horizontal dotted line) and listening for Korotkoff sounds. Korotkoff sounds appear in phase 1 and 4 in the normal response, in phase 1 only in the absent phase 4 overshoot response, and in phases 1 and 2 only in the square wave response. See text.

In phase 3, just after release of straining, pressure falls further because of temporary pooling of blood in the pulmonary veins. In phase 4, the arterial pressure overshoots to levels above the control values, primarily because of reflex sympathetic activity induced by previous hypotension. The changes in heart rate are exactly out of phase with the blood pressure: the heart rate increases during phases 2 and 3 and slows during phase 4.

The clinician identifies these four phases by inflating the blood pressure cuff on the patient's arm 15 mm Hg higher than the patient's resting systolic blood pressure and maintaining this cuff pressure during the straining phase and for 30 seconds afterward, at the same time listening for Korotkoff sounds just as if measuring blood pressure. Korotkoff sounds appear whenever the patient's systolic pressure exceeds the cuff pressure. Therefore, during the normal Valsalva response, Korotkoff sounds appear during phase 1 and phase 4 but are absent during phases 2 and 3.

D. THE ABNORMAL VALSALVA RESPONSE (SEE FIG. 44-1)

In patients with congestive heart failure, there are two abnormal Valsalva responses: (**1**) **absent phase 4 overshoot,** in which the arterial pressure fails to rise during phase 4 (Korotkoff sounds during phase 1 only), and (**2**) **square wave response,** in which the arterial pressure rises in parallel with intrathoracic pressure (Korotkoff sounds during phases 1 and 2 only).

In all three interpretable responses—normal, absent phase 4 overshoot, and square wave response—Korotkoff sounds appear during phase 1. If sounds do not appear during this phase, the intrathoracic pressure did not increase high enough during the maneuver, and the test is therefore *not* interpretable.

β-blocker medications may cause a false-positive response, primarily by eliminating the phase 4 overshoot.[11]

E. PATHOGENESIS OF THE ABNORMAL VALSALVA RESPONSE

In patients with congestive heart failure, Korotkoff sounds fail to appear during phase 4 because the weakened heart cannot increase cardiac output in response to hypotension (there is a direct relationship between the degree of overshoot and patient's ejection fraction, $r = 0.72$).[11] Although the cause of the square wave response is still debated, it probably represents the combined effect of neurohormonal activation, peripheral venoconstriction, and increased central blood volume.[7,8,12,13] Phase 2 hypotension may not occur because increased central venous blood volume maintains venous return to the right heart despite the Valsalva strain, and the congested lungs have an ample supply of blood for the left heart.*

---

*The same pathophysiology probably explains the finding of reversed pulsus paradoxus in some patients with congestive heart failure receiving positive pressure ventilation (see Chapter 13).

III. CLINICAL SIGNIFICANCE

EBM Boxes 44-1 and 44-2 present the diagnostic accuracy of physical signs for congestive heart failure. EBM Box 44-1 refers to the diagnosis of elevated left heart filling pressures and therefore applies to the diagnosis of systolic or diastolic dysfunction. The ability to accurately detect elevated left heart filling pressures is especially important in patients with dyspnea, because elevated pressures implicate the heart as the cause of the patient's symptoms. EBM

Box 44-1 Congestive Heart Failure—Elevated Left Heart Filling Pressures*

Finding (Ref)[†]	Sensitivity (%)	Specificity (%)	Likelihood Ratio if Finding Present	Absent
Vital signs				
Heart rate >100/min at rest[14]	6	99	**5.5**	NS
Abnormal Valsalva response[15]	95	88	**7.6**	**0.1**
Lung examination				
Crackles[11,14,16,17]	12–23	88–96	NS	NS
Heart examination				
Elevated jugular venous pressure[11,14,17]	10–58	96–97	**3.9**	NS
Positive abdominojugular test[17–19]	55–84	83–98	**8.0**	**0.3**
Supine apical impulse lateral to MCL[16]	42	93	**5.8**	NS
S_3 gallop[11,14,16]	12–32	95–96	**5.7**	NS
S_4 gallop[11]	71	50	NS	NS
Other findings				
Edema[11,14]	10	93–96	NS	NS

NS, not significant; MCL, midclavicular line; likelihood ratio (LR) if finding present = positive LR; LR if finding absent = negative LR.
Diagnostic standard: For elevated left heart filling pressures, pulmonary capillary wedge pressure >12 mm Hg[16] or >15 mm Hg,[15,17–19] or left ventricular end diastolic pressure >15 mm Hg.[11,14]
†*Definition of findings: For abnormal Valsalva response, absent phase 4 overshoot or square wave response (see text); for positive abdominojugular test, sustained rise in jugular venous pressure during 10–15 seconds of midabdominal pressure (see text).*

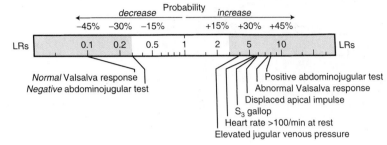

ELEVATED LEFT HEART FILLING PRESSURE

Probability
decrease → increase
−45% −30% −15%   +15% +30% +45%

LRs   0.1   0.2   0.5   1   2   5   10   LRs

Normal Valsalva response
Negative abdominojugular test

Positive abdominojugular test
Abnormal Valsalva response
Displaced apical impulse
S_3 gallop
Heart rate >100/min at rest
Elevated jugular venous pressure

Box 44-2   Congestive Heart Failure—Low Ejection Fraction*

Finding (Ref)†	Sensitivity (%)	Specificity (%)	Likelihood Ratio if Finding Present	Absent
Vital signs				
Heart rate >100 beats/min at rest[25]	22	92	2.8	NS
Abnormal Valsalva response[26,27]	69–88	90–91	**7.6**	**0.3**
Lung examination				
Crackles[25,28,29]	10–29	77–98	NS	NS
Heart examination				
Elevated neck veins[25,28]	7–18	98	**7.9**	NS
Supine apical impulse lateral to MCL[25,28,29]	24–66	93–98	**10.1**	0.6
S_3 gallop[28–31]	11–51	86–98	**3.4**	0.7
Murmur of mitral regurgitation[29]	25	89	NS	NS
Other				
Hepatomegaly[28]	3	97	NS	NS
Edema[28,31]	8–20	86–98	NS	NS

NS, not significant; MCL, midclavicular line; likelihood ratio (LR) if finding present = positive LR; LR if finding absent = negative LR.

*Diagnostic standards: For low ejection fraction, radionuclide left ventricular ejection fraction < 0.50[26,27,29,30] or < 0.53,[28] ejection fraction < 0.50 by echocardiography,[31] or left ventricular fractional shortening < 25% by echocardiography.[25]

†Definition of findings: For abnormal Valsalva response, absent phase 4 overshoot or square wave response (see text).

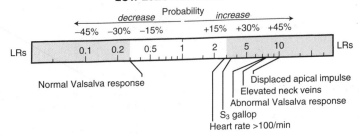

Box 44-2 refers to the diagnosis of depressed left ventricular ejection fraction and therefore applies only to the diagnosis of systolic dysfunction.

This information should only be used when evaluating patients similar to those enrolled in the studies cited in EBM Boxes 44-1 and 44-2. These patients were all adults who presented to the clinician primarily for evaluation of chest pain or dyspnea. Most had no prior history of congestive heart failure, and many had an alternative explanation for dyspnea, such as lung disease.

A. DETECTING ELEVATED LEFT HEART FILLING PRESSURES

In descending order of their likelihood ratios (LRs), the findings arguing most *for* the diagnosis of elevated filling pressures are a positive abdominojugular test (LR = 8.0, see EBM Box 44-1), abnormal Valsalva response (i.e., either absent phase 4 overshoot or square wave response, LR = 7.6), displaced apical impulse (LR = 5.8), third heart sound (LR = 5.7), tachycardia (LR = 5.5), and elevated venous pressure (LR = 3.9). The absence of any of these findings (except the abnormal Valsalva response and positive abdominojugular test) provides the clinician no useful diagnostic information because many patients with heart failure lack these findings.

The presence of crackles, fourth heart sound, or edema does not indicate elevated left heart filling pressures in these patients. Crackles are unhelpful because they are uncommon in chronic heart failure and because many other disorders causing dyspnea also produce crackles. If the finding of crackles is instead just applied to patients with known cardiomyopathy (e.g., those awaiting cardiac transplantation), they become a more accurate sign of elevated filling pressure, detecting pulmonary capillary wedge pressures ≥20 mm Hg with a sensitivity of 19% to 64%, specificity of 82% to 94%, and a positive LR of 3.4. The finding is probably more accurate in this setting because other diagnoses causing crackles have already been excluded.[17,20,21]

A small instrument similar to a digital pulse oximeter has been designed that measures and records the pulse pressure during the Valsalva maneuver.[22] This instrument calculates the "pulse-amplitude ratio," which is the ratio of the pulse pressure at the end of phase 2 divided by that at the beginning of phase 1. Patients with a normal Valsalva response have a low pulse-amplitude ratio (because pulse pressure at the end of phase 2 is much less than that at the beginning of phase 1), whereas those with the square wave response have a higher ratio (near the value of 1.0). Several studies have shown a direct relationship between the pulse-amplitude ratio and the pulmonary capillary wedge pressure ($r = 0.81-0.92$),[13,22-24] and in one study, a pulse amplitude ratio greater than 0.7 detected a measured pulmonary capillary wedge pressure greater than 15 mm Hg with a sensitivity of 91%, specificity of 95%, positive LR of 18.2, and negative LR of 0.1.[24]

B. DETECTING DEPRESSED LEFT VENTRICULAR EJECTION FRACTION

Some of the same signs that detect elevated filling pressures also indicate a depressed ejection fraction: displaced apical impulse (LR = 10.1; see EBM Box 44-2), elevated neck veins (LR = 7.9), abnormal Valsalva response (either absent phase 4 overshoot or square wave response, LR = 7.6; see EBM Box 44-2), and third heart sound (LR = 3.4). The *absence* of any of these findings (excepting Valsalva response) is not particularly compelling because many patients with ejection fractions less than 50% lack these findings. However, the absence of the third heart sound does argue against an ejection fraction less than 30% (LR = 0.3; see Chapter 37).[29,30]

Some investigators believe that the abnormal Valsalva response is primarily a sign of elevated filling pressure, not low ejection fraction, citing data correlating the degree of Valsalva abnormality with left atrial pressure ($r = 0.77, p = .005$) but not ejection fraction.[15,22,32] This apparent contradiction may reflect varying prevalence of diastolic dysfunction in different investigators' practices. Assuming that the sign is primarily one of elevated filling pressures, it will therefore also be a good sign of depressed ejection fraction if most patients with heart failure in the clinician's practice have systolic dysfunction (see EBM Box 44-2),[26,27] but it will not predict ejection fraction if there is a mixture of patients with systolic and diastolic dysfunction.[15,22,32]

Several findings provide no useful diagnostic information when assessing the patient's ejection fraction: crackles, murmur of mitral regurgitation, hepatomegaly, or edema (all LRs not significant; see EBM Box 44-2).

C. PROPORTIONAL PULSE PRESSURE

In patients with known dilated cardiomyopathy and severe left ventricular dysfunction, a proportional pulse pressure (i.e., arterial pulse pressure divided by the systolic blood pressure) less than 0.25 detects a low cardiac index (i.e., ≤ 2.2 L/min/m^2) with a sensitivity of 70% to 91%, specificity of 83% to 93%, positive LR of 6.9, and negative LR of 0.2.[21,33]

D. PHYSICAL SIGNS AND CONSENSUS DIAGNOSIS OF CONGESTIVE HEART FAILURE

Recent investigations[34-37] into the diagnostic accuracy of B-type natriuretic peptide in patients with acute dyspnea have further addressed the value of physical examination. In contrast to the studies in EBM Boxes 44-1 and 44-2, however, these studies used expert judgment as the diagnostic standard for heart failure, based on the retrospective review of patient's presenting findings, laboratory tests, and response to treatment. These studies confirm the value of the third heart sound (LR = 8.8) and elevated neck veins (LR = 4.3). Nonetheless, because it is possible that judgments about final diagnosis were influenced by the physical findings themselves, they are excluded from the tables.

E. PROGNOSIS IN HEART FAILURE

In patients with clinically suspected ischemic heart disease, the physical signs of heart failure are independent predictors of mortality, adding prognostic information to that already provided by the patient's age, exercise capacity, and measured ejection fraction.[38,39] One-year cardiac mortality is higher for those with a displaced apical impulse (39% vs. 12% without the finding, $p = .005$) or the third heart sound (57% vs. 14% without the finding, $p = .002$).[16]

REFERENCES

1. Lutz JE. A XII century description of congestive heart failure. *Am J Cardiol.* 1988; 61:494-495.
2. Nolan J. A historical review of heart failure. *Scot Med J.* 1993;38:53-57.
3. Nishimura RA, Tajik AJ. The Valsalva maneuver and response revisited. *Mayo Clin Proc.* 1986;61:211n217.
4. Dawson PM. An historical sketch of the Valsalva experiment. *Bull Hist Med.* 1943; 14:295-320.
5. Ard RW, Twining RH. Evaluation of Valsalva test in bedside diagnosis of dyspnea. *Am J Med Sci.* 1957;234:403-412.
6. Burroughs RW, Bruce RA. Significance of abnormal phase II response to Valsalva maneuver in cardiac patients. *Circulation.* 1956;14:72-76.
7. Gorlin R, Knowled JH, Storey CF. The Valsalva maneuver as a test of cardiac function. *Am J Med.* 1957;22:197-212.
8. Judson WE, Hatcher JD, Wilkins RW. Blood pressure responses to the Valsalva maneuver in cardiac patients with and without congestive failure. *Circulation.* 1955;11:889-899.

9. Irvin CW. Valsalva maneuver as a diagnostic aid. *JAMA*. 1959;170:787-791.

10. Levine HJ, McIntryre KM, Glovsky MM. Relief of angina pectoris by Valsalva maneuver. *N Engl J Med*. 1966;275:487-488.

11. Zema MJ, Restivo B, Sos T, et al. Left ventricular dysfunction: Bedside Valsalva manoeuvre. *Br Heart J*. 1980;44:560-569.

12. Brunner-LaRocca H, Weilenmann D, Rickli H, et al. Is blood pressure response to the Valsalva maneuver related to neurohormones, exercise capacity, and clinical findings in heart failure? *Chest*. 1999;116:861-867.

13. Uehara H, Takenaka I, Aoyama K, et al. A new method of predicting pulmonary capillary wedge pressure: The arterial pressure ratio. *Anaesthesia*. 2000;55:113-117.

14. Harlan WR, Oberman A, Grim R, Rosati RA. Chronic congestive heart failure in coronary artery disease: Clinical criteria. *Ann Intern Med*. 1977;86:133-138.

15. Schmidt DE, Shah PK. Accurate detection of elevated left ventricular filling pressure by a simplified bedside application of the Valsalva maneuver. *Am J Cardiol*. 1993;71:462-464.

16. Gadsboll N, Hoilund-Carlsen PF, Nielsen GG, et al. Symptoms and signs of heart failure in patients with myocardial infarction: Reproducibility and relationship to chest X-ray, radionuclide ventriculography and right heart catheterization. *Eur Heart J*. 1989;10:1017-1028.

17. Butman SM, Ewy GA, Standen JR, et al. Bedside cardiovascular examination in patients with severe chronic heart failure: Importance of rest or inducible jugular venous distension. *J Am Coll Cardiol*. 1993;22:968-974.

18. Sochowski RA, Dubbin JD, Naqvi SZ. Clinical and hemodynamic assessment of the hepatojugular reflux. *Am J Cardiol*. 1990;66:1002-1006.

19. Ewy GA. The abdominojugular test: Technique and hemodynamic correlates. *Ann Intern Med*. 1988;109:456-460.

20. Chakko S, Woska D, Martinez H, et al. Clinical, radiographic, and hemodynamic correlations in chronic congestive heart failure: Conflicting results may lead to inappropriate care. *Am J Med*. 1991;90:353-359.

21. Stevenson LW, Perloff JK. The limited reliability of physical signs for estimating hemodynamics in chronic heart failure. *JAMA*. 1989;261:884-888.

22. McIntyre KM, Vita JA, Lambrew CT, et al. A noninvasive method of predicting pulmonary-capillary wedge pressure. *N Engl J Med*. 1992;327:1715-1720.

23. Sharma GVRK, Woods PA, Lambrew CT, et al. Evaluation of a noninvasive system for determining left ventricular filling pressure. *Arch Intern Med*. 2002;162:2084-2088.

24. Weilenmann D, Rickli H, Follath F, et al. Noninvasive evaluation of pulmonary capillary wedge pressure by BP response to the Valsalva maneuver. *Chest*. 2002;122:140-145.

25. Davie AP, Caruana FL, Sutherland GR, McMurray JJV. Assessing diagnosis in heart failure: Which features are any use? *Q J Med*. 1997;90:335-339.

26. Zema MJ, Caccavano M, Kligfield P. Detection of left ventricular dysfunction in ambulatory subjects with the bedside Valsalva maneuver. *Am J Med.* 1983;75: 241-248.

27. Zema MJ, Masters AP, Margouleff D. Dyspnea: The heart or the lungs? Differentiation at bedside by use of the simple Valsalva maneuver. *Chest.* 1984;85:59-64.

28. Gadsboll N, Hoilund-Carlsen PF, Nielsen GG, et al. Interobserver agreement and accuracy of bedside estimation of right and left ventricular ejection fraction in acute myocardial infarction. *Am J Cardiol.* 1989;63:1301-1307.

29. Mattleman SJ, Hakki AH, Iskandrian AS, et al. Reliability of bedside evaluation in determining left ventricular function: Correlation with left ventricular ejection fraction determined by radionuclide ventriculography. *J Am Coll Cardiol.* 1983;1:417-420.

30. Patel R, Bushnell DL, Sobotka PA. Implications of an audible third heart sound in evaluating cardiac function. *West J Med.* 1993;158:606-609.

31. Tribouilloy CM, Enriquez-Sarano M, Mohty D, et al. Pathophysiologic determinants of third heart sounds: A prospective clinical and Doppler echocardiographic study. *Am J Med.* 2001;111:96-102.

32. Bernardi L, Saviolo R, Spodick DH. Do hemodynamic responses to the Valsalva maneuver reflect myocardial dysfunction? *Chest.* 1989;95:986-991.

33. Rohde LE, Beck-da-Silva L, Goldraich L, et al. Reliability and prognostic value of traditional signs and symptoms in outpatients with congestive heart failure. *Can J Cardiol.* 2004;20:697-702.

34. Dao Q, Krishnaswamy P, Kazanegra R, et al. Utility of B-type natriuretic peptide in the diagnosis of congestive heart failure in an urgent-care setting. *J Am Coll Cardiol.* 2001;37:379-385.

35. Knudsen CW, Omland T, Clopton P, et al. Diagnostic value of B-type natriuretic peptide and chest radiographic findings in patients with acute dyspnea. *Am J Med.* 2004;116:363-368.

36. Logeart D, Saudubray C, Beyne P, et al. Comparative value of Doppler echocardiography and B-type natriuretic peptide assay in the etiologic diagnosis of acute dyspnea. *J Am Coll Cardiol.* 2002;40:1794-1800.

37. Mueller T, Gegenhuber A, Poelz W, Haltmayer M. Diagnostic accuracy of B type natriuretic peptide and amino terminal proBNP in the emergency diagnosis of heart failure. *Heart.* 2005;91:606-612.

38. Marantz PR, Tobin JN, Wassertheil-Smoller S, et al. Prognosis in ischemic heart disease: Can you tell as much at the bedside as in the nuclear laboratory? *Arch Intern Med.* 1992;152:2433-2437.

39. Likoff MJ, Chandler SL, Kay HR. Clinical determinants of mortality in chronic congestive heart failure secondary to idiopathic dilated or to ischemic cardiomyopathy. *Am J Cardiol.* 1987;59:634-638.

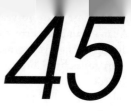

Coronary Artery Disease

I. INTRODUCTION

Coronary disease is the leading cause of heart disease and death in the United States,[1] and chest pain now accounts for 8%–10% of all new complaints of patients presenting to clinics or emergency departments.[2-4] The bedside diagnosis of chest pain is difficult and at times humbling, as illustrated by the fact that up to 1%–8% of patients with myocardial infarction (confirmed by cardiac biomarkers) are misdiagnosed and discharged home from emergency departments.[5-10] The focus of this chapter is to identify all aspects of the initial patient encounter—patient interview, physical examination, and the electrocardiogram—that help distinguish patients with angina and myocardial infarction from those with mimicking disorders.

The first clear description of angina pectoris was in 1768 by William Heberden, who coined the term* and provided a clinical description that has

---

*Heberden based the term *angina* on the Greek *agkhone*, which means "strangling." This Greek root also forms the basis for the English words "anxiety" and "anguish." Heberden's selection of "angina" was unfortunate, because the term had already been applied to other conditions of the throat, such as Vincent's *angina* or Ludwig's *angina*.

been unsurpassed. Just 8 years later, Edward Jenner linked angina to "ossification" of the coronary arteries and insufficient coronary blood flow,[11] and in 1878 (more than 50 years before the introduction of electrocardiography), Adam Hammer correctly diagnosed the first case of myocardial infarction during life in a young man with sudden collapse, bradycardia, and enfeebled heart tones.[12,13] Coronary disease was once considered to be an uncommon disorder—the great 19th century American cardiologist Austin Flint found only 7 cases of angina in his clinical records[14] and Osler personally observed only 40 cases during his career.[11]

II. THE FINDINGS

A. INTRODUCTION

Unlike other clinical problems in cardiology such as valvular disease and heart failure, patients with coronary artery disease have few or no physical findings. For more than 100 years, the most important aspect of diagnosing coronary disease has been the patient's description of chest pain, whereas the most important element in diagnosing myocardial infarction (at least since 1918) has been the electrocardiogram.

B. DESCRIPTION OF CHEST PAIN

Heberden wrote that angina is a "most disagreeable sensation in the breast" that seizes patients "while they are walking" yet vanishes "the moment they stand still."[15] Modern definitions of "typical angina" retain most of Heberden's essential features, by defining it as substernal discomfort with three characteristics: (1) it is precipitated by exertion, (2) it is improved by rest or nitroglycerin (or both), and (3) it lasts less than 10 minutes. (Many patients also describe radiation of the pain to the shoulders, jaw, or inner aspect of the arm). In contrast, "atypical angina" is substernal discomfort with atypical features (e.g., it is not always relieved by nitroglycerin, not always brought on by exertion, or relieved after 15 to 20 minutes of rest), and "nonanginal" chest pain lacks all features of typical angina (i.e., it is unrelated to activity, unrelieved by nitroglycerin, or otherwise not suggestive of angina).

C. PHYSICAL FINDINGS

Some of the findings that appear in EBM Boxes 45-1 and 45-2 are discussed in other chapters: crackles (Chapter 27), displaced precordial pulsation (Chapter 34), and the third heart sound (Chapter 37).

Box 45-1   Coronary Artery Disease*

Finding (Ref)[†]	Sensitivity (%)	Specificity (%)	Likelihood Ratio if Finding Present	Absent
PATIENT INTERVIEW				
Description of chest pain				
Classification of chest pain[29–36]				
Typical angina	50–91	78–94	**5.8**	...
Atypical angina	8–44	...	1.2	...
Non-anginal chest pain	4–22	14–50	**0.1**	...
Pain duration >30 minutes[37]	1	86	**0.1**	NS
Associated dysphagia[37]	5	80	**0.2**	NS
Other				
Male sex[18,20,34,35,38–41]	72–86	36–58	1.7	**0.3**
Age[20,35,38,39,41,42]				
<30 years	0–1	97–98	NS	...
30–49 years	16–38	...	0.6	...
50–70 years	62–73	...	1.3	...
>70 years	2–52	67–99	2.6	...
Prior myocardial infarction[34,36,39–41,43,44]	42–69	66–99	**3.8**	0.6
PHYSICAL EXAMINATION				
Ear lobe crease[16–20]	26–80	33–96	2.3	0.6
Arcus senilis[45]	40	86	**3.0**	0.7
Chest wall tenderness[37,46,47]	1–25	69–97	NS	NS
Ankle-to-arm pressure index < 0.9[48]	20	95	**4.1**	0.8
Laterally displaced apical impulse[49]	5	100	NS	NS
ELECTROCARDIOGRAM				
Normal[36,49,50]	15–33	50–69	NS	NS
ST/T wave abnormalities[29,36,44]	14–44	73–93	NS	NS

NS, not significant; likelihood ratio (LR) if finding present = positive LR; LR if finding absent = negative LR.

*Diagnostic standard: For coronary artery disease, coronary angiography reveals >50%,[6–20,30,32–34,36,38,42,43,45,47,48,50] > 60%,[49] or > 70-75%[29,31,35,37,39–41,44] stenosis of any epicardial vessel.

†Definition of findings: For classification of chest pain, earlobe crease, and arcus senilis, see text.

CORONARY ARTERY DISEASE

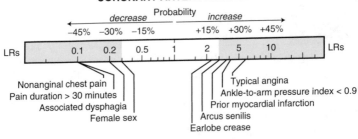

1.   Earlobe Crease

The earlobe crease is a diagonal crease across the earlobe, connecting the lowest point on the tragus to the outside of the earlobe (Fig. 45-1). Some investigators define the finding as a crease traversing at least one third the distance from tragus to posterior pinna,[16,17] whereas others require the crease to extend the total distance.[18-20] In a letter to the editor written in 1973,[21] Frank first presented the "positive ear-lobe sign" as a sign tightly associated with other cardiovascular risk factors. Although its association with coronary disease remains controversial and its pathogenesis a mystery, many investigators have shown that the earlobe crease is a modest risk factor for coronary artery disease, independent of other traditional risk factors such as hypertension, age, diabetes mellitus, family history, hyperlipidemia, obesity, and cigarette smoking.[16,18,19,22,23]

2.   Arcus Senilis

Arcus senilis is a white or grayish opaque ring about the circumference of the cornea. Since the 1830s, this sign has been associated with both older age (hence, "senilis") and vascular disease (Virchow considered it a definite sign of heart disease).[24] Modern investigators[25,26] continue to suggest arcus senilis is linked to coronary disease, independent of its association with hyperlipidemia, although others challenge this view.[24]

3.   Ankle-to-Arm Pressure Index

After positioning the patient supine, the clinician uses a hand-held Doppler stethoscope to measure the highest systolic blood pressure in the posterior tibial or dorsalis pedis artery (i.e., the "ankle" pressure). The "ankle-to-arm pressure index" represents this ankle pressure divided by the systolic pressure in the brachial artery (see Chapter 50).

D.   GASTROINTESTINAL (GI) COCKTAIL

For many years, clinicians working in emergency departments have mixed liquid antacids with other substances (most commonly viscous lidocaine, a topical

Box 45-2 — Myocardial Infarction*

Finding (Ref)[†]	Sensitivity (%)	Specificity (%)	Likelihood Ratio if Finding Present	Absent
Patient interview				
Male sex[53–59]	59–72	33–61	**1.3**	0.7
Age[53,58,59]				
< 40 years	4	81	**0.2**	...
40–59 years	34	...	NS	...
≥ 60 years	47–74	54–68	1.5	...
Sharp pain[58,60]	8–16	59–70	**0.3**	1.3
Pleuritic pain[58–60]	3–6	74–82	**0.2**	1.2
Positional pain[58,59]	3–11	75–87	**0.3**	1.1
Relief of pain with nitroglycerin[61,62]	19–70	28–77	NS	NS
Physical examination				
Chest wall tenderness[58–60]	3–15	64–83	**0.3**	1.3
Diaphoretic appearance[59,60]	28–53	73–94	2.9	0.7
Systolic blood pressure <100 mm Hg[55]	6	98	**3.6**	NS
Jugular venous distension[54]	10	96	2.4	NS
Pulmonary crackles[54,60]	20–38	82–91	2.1	NS
Third heart sound[60]	16	95	**3.2**	NS
Electrocardiogram				
Normal[53,55,58,60,63–65]	1–13	48–77	**0.2**	1.5
Nonspecific ST changes[58,65]	5–7	47–78	**0.2**	NS
ST elevation[55,58,60,64–66]	31–49	97–100	**22.0**	0.6
ST depression[55,60,64,65]	20–62	88–96	**4.5**	0.8
T wave inversion[55,60,64]	9–39	84–94	2.2	NS

NS, not significant; likelihood ratio (LR) if finding present = positive LR; LR if finding absent = negative LR.

*Diagnostic standard: For myocardial infarction, development of new electrocardiographic Q waves, elevations of cardiac biomarkers (CK-MB or troponin), or both; except for the studies of nitroglycerin effect, which used a broader definition of "active coronary disease" that combined myocardial infarction, positive stress test, or abnormal coronary arteriogram.[61,62]

[†]Definition of findings: For relief of pain with nitroglycerin, complete relief within 5 minutes[62] or within 10 minutes of administering nitroglycerin.[61] All electrocardiographic abnormalities refer to findings that are new or of unknown duration.

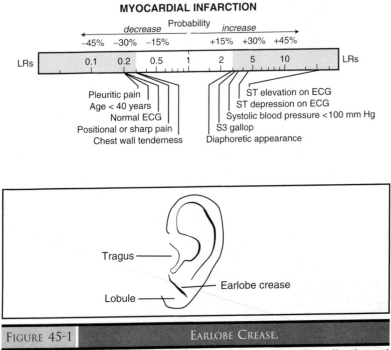

MYOCARDIAL INFARCTION

FIGURE 45-1	EARLOBE CREASE.

The earlobe crease is a diagonal crease extending from the lowest point on the tragus to the outside of the earlobe. See text.

anesthetic, and Donnatal, an antispasmodic) to create "GI cocktails," which are administered orally to patients presenting with chest or upper abdominal discomfort. Because a GI cocktail should act topically only on GI mucosa, prompt relief of a patient's discomfort is said to support a GI cause of pain (and, by inference, argue against a cardiac cause of the pain). Although antacid, lidocaine, and Donnatal are the standard ingredients of GI cocktail, some investigators have shown that antacid alone (without lidocaine or Donnatal) may relieve pain just as well.[27]

III. CLINICAL SIGNIFICANCE

A. DIAGNOSING CORONARY ARTERY DISEASE

EBM Box 45-1 summarizes the accuracy of bedside findings in diagnosing coronary artery disease (based on study of more than 10,000 patients).[28] Almost all of the patients in these studies presented to outpatient clinics with intermittent chest pain, and the diagnosis of coronary artery disease was based on subsequent cardiac catheterization revealing a significant stenosis (>50%–70% luminal narrowing) in any major epicardial vessel (i.e., single-vessel disease or worse).

According to the likelihood ratios (LRs) in EBM Box 45-1 the strongest arguments *for* coronary artery disease in a patient with intermittent chest pain are "typical angina" (LR = 5.8), ankle-to-arm pressure index less than 0.9 (LR = 4.1), prior myocardial infarction (LR = 3.8), arcus senilis (LR = 3.0), age older than 70 years (LR = 2.6), and a positive ear lobe crease (LR = 2.3).

These studies confirm Heberden's original impression that the key diagnostic finding in patients with chest pain is the patient's actual description of pain. Many investigators have attempted to improve on Heberden's definition of "typical angina" by dissecting apart the individual components of the patient's description (e.g., response to nitroglycerin or the pain's quality) or by creating complicated angina scoring schemes, but each of these attempts to improve diagnosis is less accurate than the clinician's global perception of whether the patient's pain is "typical angina" or not.[28]

The findings that argue *against* coronary artery disease in these studies are chest pain that is "nonanginal" (i.e., pain unrelated to activity, unrelieved by nitroglycerin, or otherwise not suggestive of angina, LR = 0.1), pain duration greater than 30 minutes (LR = 0.1), and associated dysphagia (LR = 0.2).

Unhelpful findings include "atypical angina," chest wall tenderness, and a displaced apical impulse. Additional descriptors of the pain, such as burning pain, pain made worse by food or emotion, and radiation of the pain to the arms, are also unhelpful (i.e., they appear just as often in patients with coronary disease as in patients with noncardiac chest pain, and the LRs are not different from the value of 1.0).[28] Interestingly, electrocardiographic findings (i.e., normal vs. abnormal, presence or absence of nonspecific ST changes) also are diagnostically unhelpful in these studies (LR not significant, see EBM Box 45-1).

Assessment of the patient's traditional risk factors—hypertension, diabetes mellitus, cigarette smoking, family history, or combinations of these—carry much less diagnostic weight than the patient's description of pain. Each of these risk factors—except for cholesterol level greater than 300 mg/dL (LR = 4.0) and cholesterol less than 200 mg/dL (LR = 0.3)—has an LR between the values of 1.2 and 2.3, thus changing probability of disease little, if at all.[28,51,52] Even combinations of three or more risk factors change probability of coronary disease relatively little (LR = 2.2, a value similar to the LR for the earlobe crease).[28]

B.   DIAGNOSING MYOCARDIAL INFARCTION

EBM Box 45-2 summarizes the findings in thousands of patients presenting to emergency departments with sustained acute chest pain unrelated to trauma and unexplained by the chest radiograph. The diagnosis of myocardial infarction was confirmed by the development of new q waves on the electrocardiogram, elevations of cardiac biomarkers (CK-MB or troponin), or both.

According to the LRs in EBM Box 45-2, the most compelling argument *for* myocardial infarction is new electrocardiographic ST elevation (LR = 22) or ST depression (LR = 4.5). Several additional physical findings have modest value in diagnosing myocardial infarction: systolic blood pressure less than 100 mm Hg (LR = 3.6), a third heart sound (LR = 3.2), diaphoretic appearance (LR = 2.9), jugular venous distension (LR = 2.4), and pulmonary crackles (LR = 2.1). Radiation of pain to the right arm (LR = 4.7) increases probability of myocardial infarction more than radiation to the left arm (LR = 1.8),[28,53,54,60] although fewer patients with infarction have radiation to the right arm (15%-41% of patients) than the left arm (34% to 55%). The only findings arguing *against* myocardial infarction in these studies are pain that is pleuritic (LR = 0.2), positional (LR = 0.3), or sharp (LR = 0.3); a normal electrocardiogram (LR = 0.2); chest wall tenderness (LR = 0.3); and age younger than 40 years (LR = 0.2).

The response to nitroglycerin fails to discriminate between cardiac and noncardiac causes of chest pain evaluated (LR not significant, see EBM Box 45-2). This may reflect the temporary nature of most chest pain or perhaps the noncardiac effects of nitroglycerin. Nonetheless, even though the response to nitroglycerin lacks diagnostic value in patients with sustained chest pain, it remains a key element in the definition of "typical angina."

One interesting contrast between the diagnosis of coronary disease (see EBM Box 45-1) and myocardial infarction (see EBM Box 45-2) is that chest wall tenderness argues against myocardial infarction (LR = 0.3, see EBM Box 45-2) but lacks diagnostic value when considering coronary artery disease (LR not significant, see EBM Box 45-1). This difference may reflect a higher prevalence of chest wall disorders in patients without disease in the acute chest pain studies.

C. RISK FACTORS AND CORONARY DISEASE

In patients with sustained chest pain, the presence or absence of traditional cardiovascular risk factors again carries little or no diagnostic weight (positive LRs = 1.2 to 1.7).[28] There are two important reasons why risk factors fail to discriminate well in diagnostic studies. One, traditional cardiovascular risk factors are mostly derived from study of middle-aged white residents of Framingham, Massachusetts.[67] They may thus overestimate the risk in other populations, something that has been demonstrated in British men,[68] elderly Americans,[69] and Japanese-American, Native American, and Hispanic populations.[70] A second reason is the fundamental difference between risk factors and diagnostic signs. Risk factors precede disease, presumably play a role in causing the disease, and become apparent only after study of large groups of *asymptomatic* individuals. Diagnostic signs, in contrast, appear first after the onset of disease, are *caused by* the disease, and become evident only after study of a relatively smaller group of *symptomatic* individuals. It is possible, for example, that certain risk factors associated with coronary disease are also associated with noncardiac causes of pain, which would neutralize any diagnostic value (e.g., cigarette smoking may also increase the risk of chest wall pain, making it appear just as often in patients with noncardiac pain as those with cardiac pain. The resulting LR would therefore have a value near 1.0).

D. GI COCKTAIL

The existing literature suggests that the GI cocktail has questionable diagnostic value. One problem is that clinicians usually administer the GI cocktail just minutes away from other active medications, such as narcotics, nitroglycerin, antiemetics, histamine blockers, or ketorolac, thus clouding interpretation of the test's results.[71] Another problem is that the viscous lidocaine is absorbed, and even though most patients have levels less than 1 μg/mL (usual therapeutic levels are 2 to 5 μg/mL), instances of toxicity and seizures have occurred.[71-73] A final and most troubling problem is the many documented examples of GI cocktail relieving the discomfort of disorders distant from the gastroesophageal mucosa, such as myocardial infarction,[72,74] hepatitis, pancreatitis, or cholecystitis.[75]

E. PROGNOSIS AND ACUTE CHEST PAIN

In patients with acute chest pain, clinicians are interested in diagnosing more than just myocardial infarction, because many acute coronary syndromes *without* infarction are also associated with life-threatening complications that require intensive monitoring and treatment. To identify all patients at risk for such complications, Goldman has developed a rule that assesses the patient's electrocardiogram and the presence or absence of three additional bedside findings: (1) systolic blood pressure less than 110 mm Hg, (2) crackles heard above the bases bilaterally, and (3) chest pain that is either worse than prior angina, the same as prior myocardial infarction, or occurs in the post-infarction or post-revascularization setting.[76] According to this rule, patients have a "high risk" of life-threatening complications in the first 24 hours of hospitalization if there is either (1) electrocardiograph ST elevation or Q waves (not known to be old), OR (2) electrocardiographic ST depression or T wave inversion (not known to be old) AND two or more of the three bedside findings. Patients are classified as "very low risk" if their electrocardiogram reveals no ST/T wave changes or Q waves and they lack all three bedside findings.

EBM Box 45-3 indicates that in patients with acute chest pain a "high risk" classification increases the likelihood of life-threatening complications in the subsequent 24 hours (LR = 8.7, see EBM Box 45-3), whereas a "very low" classification indicates a favorable prognosis (LR = 0.1, see EBM Box 45-3). This

Box
45-3

Predicting Life-Threatening
Complications in Patients with Acute
Chest Pain

Finding (Ref)[†]	Sensitivity (%)	Specificity (%)	Likelihood Ratio if Finding	
			Present	Absent
Goldman classification				
"High" risk[76,77]	51–88	92–93	**8.7**	...
"Very low" risk[76–78]	7–13	42–53	**0.1**	...

*Diagnostic standard: For life-threatening complications, *any of the following during the first 24 hours of hospitalization: arrhythmias (ventricular fibrillation, cardiac arrest, new complete heart block, insertion of temporary pacemaker, emergency cardioversion), pump failure (cardiogenic shock, use of intra-aortic balloon pump, intubation), or ischemia (recurrent ischemic chest pain requiring bypass surgery or percutaneous intervention).*[76]
[†]*Definition of findings: For high risk and very low risk, see text.*

LIFE-THREATENING COMPLICATIONS (IF CHEST PAIN)

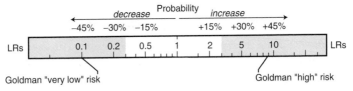

rule compares favorably to the diagnostic accuracy of elevated troponin T levels, drawn at least 6 hours after the onset of chest pain in patients without ST elevation, in predicting cardiac events in the subsequent 30 days (positive LR = 6.1, negative LR = 0.2).[79]

REFERENCES

1. *National Vital Statistics Report.* 2002;50:8.
2. Kroenke K, Mangelsdorf AD. Common symptoms in ambulatory care: Incidence, evaluation, therapy, and outcome. *Am J Med.* 1989;86:262-266.
3. Qamar A, McPherson C, Babb J, et al. The Goldman algorithm revisited: Prospective evaluation of a computer-derived algorithm versus unaided physician judgment in suspected acute myocardial infarction. *Am Heart J.* 1999;138:705-709.
4. Burt CW. Summary statistics for acute cardiac ischemia and chest pain visits to United States EDs, 1995-1996. *Am J Emerg Med.* 1999;17:552-559.

5. Lee TH, Rouan GW, Weisberg MC. Clinical characteristics and natural history of patients with acute myocardial infarction sent home from the emergency room. *Am J Cardiol.* 1987;60:219-224.

6. Goldman L, Weinberg M, Weisberg M, et al. A computer-derived protocol to aid the diagnosis of emergency room patients with acute chest pain. *N Engl J Med.* 1982;307:588-596.

7. Pozen MW, D'Agostino RB, Selker HP, et al. A predictive instrument to improve coronary-care-unit admission practices in acute ischemic heart disease: A prospective multicenter clinical trial. *N Engl J Med.* 1984;310:1273-1278.

8. Pope JH, Aufderheide TP, Ruthazer R, et al. Missed diagnoses of acute cardiac ischemia in the emergency department. *N Engl J Med.* 2000;342:1163-1170.

9. McCarthy BD, Beshansky JR, D'Agostino RB, Selker HP. Missed diagnoses of acute myocardial infarction in the emergency department: Results from a multicenter study. *Ann Emerg Med.* 1993;22:579-582.

10. Schor S, Behar S, Modan B, et al. Disposition of presumed coronary patients from an emergency room: A follow-up study. *JAMA.* 1976;236:941-943.

11. Osler W. *Lectures on angina pectoris and allied states*, 1st ed. New York: D. Appleton and Company; 1897.

12. Major R. *Classic descriptions of disease: With biographical sketches of the authors.* Springfield: Charles C Thomas; 1932.

13. Burch GE, DePasquale NP. *A history of electrocardiography*. Chicago: Year Book Medical Publishers, Inc; 1964.

14. Flint A. *A practical treatise on the diagnosis, pathology, and treatment of diseases of the heart.* Philadelphia: Blanchard and Lea; 1859:260.

15. Eslick GD. Chest pain: A historical perspective. *Int J Cardiol.* 2001;77:5-11.

16. Elliott WJ, Powell LH. Diagonal earlobe creases and prognosis in patients with suspected coronary artery disease. *Am J Med.* 1996;100:205-211.

17. Brady PM, Zive MA, Goldberg RJ, et al. A new wrinkle to the earlobe crease. *Arch Intern Med.* 1987;147:65-66.

18. Haft JI, Gonnella GR, Kirtane JS, Anastasiades A. Correlation of ear crease sign with coronary arteriographic findings. *Cardiovasc Med.* 1979;4:861-867.

19. Kaukola S, Manninen V, Valle M, Halonen PI. Ear-lobe crease and coronary atherosclerosis. *Lancet.* 1979;2:1377.

20. Toyosaki N, Tsuchiya M, Hashimoto T, et al. Earlobe crease and coronary heart disease in Japanese. *Heart Vessels.* 1986;2:161-165.

21. Frank ST. Aural sign of coronary-artery disease. *N Engl J Med.* 1973;289: 327-328.

22. Elliott WJ, Karrison T. Increased all-cause and cardiac morbidity and mortality associated with the diagonal earlobe crease: A prospective cohort study. *Am J Med.* 1991;91:247-254.

23. Ishii T, Asuwa N, Masuda S, et al. Earlobe crease and atherosclerosis: An autopsy study. *J Am Geriatr Soc.* 1990;38:871-876.

24. McAndrew GM, Ogston D. Arcus senilis and coronary artery disease. *Am Heart J.* 1965;70:838-840.

25. Chambless LE, Fuchs FD, Linn S, et al. The association of corneal arcus with coronary heart disease and cardiovascular disease mortality in the Lipid Research Clinics mortality follow-up study. *Am J Public Health.* 1990;80:1200-1204.

26. Rosenman RH, Brand RJ, Sholtz RI, Jenkins CD. Relation of corneal arcus to cardiovascular risk factors and the incidence of coronary disease. *N Engl J Med.* 1974;291:1322-1324.

27. Berman D, Graber M, Clark P, et al. The GI cocktail in the treatment of dyspepsia: A randomized, double-blind clinical trial. *Acad Emerg Med.* 2001;8:446.

28. Chun AA, McGee SR. Bedside diagnosis of coronary artery disease: A systematic review. *Am J Med.* 2004;117:334-343.

29. Weiner DA, Ryan TJ, McCabe CH, et al. Exercise stress testing: Correlations among history of angina, ST-segment response and prevalence of coronary-artery disease in the coronary artery surgery study (CASS). *N Engl J Med.* 1979;301:230-235.

30. Proudfit WL, Shirey EK. Selective cine coronary arteriography: Correlation with clinical findings in 1000 patients. *Circulation.* 1966;33:901-910.

31. Peissens J, van Mieghem W, Kesteloot H, de Geest H. Diagnostic value of clinical history, exercise testing and atrial pacing in patients with chest pain. *Am J Cardiol.* 1974;33:351-356.

32. McConahay DR, McCallister BD, Smith RE. Postexercise electrocardiography: Correlations with coronary arteriography and left ventricular hemodynamics. *Am J Cardiol.* 1971;28:1-9.

33. Mason RE, Likar I, Biern RO, Ross RS. Multiple-lead exercise electrocardiography: Experience in 107 normal subjects and 67 patients with angina pectoris, and comparison with coronary cinearteriography in 84 patients. *Circulation.* 1967;34: 517-525.

34. Detry JMR, Kapita BM, Cosyns J, et al. Diagnostic value of history and maximal exercise electrocardiography in men and women suspected of coronary heart disease. *Circulation.* 1977;56:756-769.

35. Chaitman BR, Bourassa MG, Davis K, et al. Angiographic prevalence of high-risk coronary artery disease in patient subsets (CASS). *Circulation.* 1981;64:360-367.

36. Campeau L, Bouraussa MG, Bois MA, et al. Clinical significance of selective coronary cinearteriography. *Can Med Assoc J.* 1968;99:1063-1068.

37. Cooke RA, Smeeton N, Chambers JB. Comparative study of chest pain characteristics in patients with normal and abnormal coronary angiograms. *Heart.* 1997;78:142-146.

38. Pearson TA, Bulkley BH, Achuff SC, et al. The association of low levels of HDL cholesterol and arteriographically defined coronary artery disease. *Am J Epidemiol.* 1979;109:285-295.

39. Holmes DR, Elveback LR, Frye RL, et al. Association of risk factor variables and coronary artery disease documented with angiography. *Circulation.* 1981;63:293-299.

40. Hartz A, Grubb B, Wild R, et al. The association of waist hip ratio and angiographically determined coronary artery disease. *Intern J Obes.* 1990;14:657-665.

41. Pryor DB, Shaw L, Harrell FE, et al. Estimating the likelihood of severe coronary artery disease. *Am J Med.* 1991;80:553-562.

42. Elder AT, Shaw TRD, Turnbull CM, Starkey IR. Elderly and younger patients selected to undergo coronary angiography. *Br Med J.* 1991;303:950-953.

43. Gurevitz O, Janos M, Boyko V, et al. Clinical profile and long-term prognosis of women <50 years of age referred for coronary angiography for evaluation of chest pain. *Am J Cardiol.* 2000;85:806-809.

44. Miranda CP, Lehmann KG, Froelicher VF. Correlation between resting ST segment depression, exercise testing, coronary angiography, and long-term prognosis. *Am Heart J.* 1991;122:1617-1628.

45. Hoogerbrugge N, Happee C, va Domburg R, et al. Corneal arcus: Indicator for severity of coronary atherosclerosis? *Neth J Med.* 1999;55:184-187.

46. Levine PR, Mascette AM. Musculoskeletal chest pain in patients with "angina": A prospective study. *South Med J.* 1989;82:580-585.

47. Wu EB, Smeeton N, Chambers JB. A chest pain score for stratifying the risk of coronary artery disease in patients having day case coronary angiography. *Int J Cardiol.* 2001;78:257-264.

48. Papamichael CM, Lekakis JP, Stametelopoulos KS, et al. Ankle-brachial index as a predictor of the extent of coronary atherosclerosis and cardiovascular events in patients with coronary artery disease. *Am J Cardiol.* 2000;86:615-618.

49. Mukerji V, Alpert MA, Hewett JE, Parker BM. Can patients with chest pain and normal coronary arteries be discriminated from those with coronary artery disease prior to coronary angiography? *Angiology.* 1989;40:276-282.

50. Linhart JW, Turnoff HB. Maximum treadmill exercise test in patients with abnormal control electrocardiograms. *Circulation.* 1974;49:667-672.

51. Welch CC, Proudfit WL, Sheldon WC. Coronary arteriographic findings in 1000 women under age 50. *Am J Cardiol.* 1975;35:211-215.

52. Welch CC, Proudfit WL, Sones FM, et al. Cinecoronary arteriography in young men. *Circulation.* 1970;42:647-652.

53. Berger JP, Buclin T, Haller E, et al. Right arm involvement and pain extension can help to differentiate coronary diseases from chest pain of other origin: A prospective emergency ward study of 278 consecutive patients admitted for chest pain. *J Intern Med.* 1990;227:165-172.

54. Baxt WG. Use of an artificial neural network for the diagnosis of myocardial infarction. *Ann Intern Med.* 1991;115:843-848.

55. Herlitz J, Karlson BW, Karlsson T, et al. A description of the characteristics and outcome of patients hospitalized for acute chest pain in relation to whether they were admitted to the coronary care unit or not in the thrombolytic era. *Int J Cardiol.* 2002;82:279-287.

56. Herlitz J, Starke M, Hansson E, et al. Early identification of patients with an acute coronary syndrome as assessed by dispatchers and the ambulance crew. *Am J Emerg Med.* 2002;20:196-201.

57. Herlitz J, Bang A, Isaksson L, Karlsson T. Ambulance dispatchers' estimation of intensity of pain and presence of associated symptoms in relation to outcome in patients who call for an ambulance because of acute chest pain. *Eur Heart J.* 1995; 16:1789-1794.

58. Lee TH, Cook EF, Weisberg M, et al. Acute chest pain in the emergency room: Identification and examination of low-risk patients. *Arch Intern Med.* 1985;145:65-69.

59. Solomon CG, Lee TH, Cook EF, et al. Comparison of clinical presentation of acute myocardial infarction in patients older than 65 years of age to younger patients: The multicenter chest pain study experience. *Am J Cardiol.* 1989;63:772-776.

60. Tierney WM, Fitzgerald J, McHenry R, et al. Physicians' estimates of the probability of myocardial infarction in emergency room patients with chest pain. *Med Decis Making.* 1986;6:12-17.

61. Shry EA, Dacus J, Van de Graaff E, et al. Usefulness of the response to sublingual nitroglycerin as a predictor of ischemic chest pain in the emergency department. *Am J Cardiol.* 2002;90:1264-1266.

62. Henrikson CA, Howell EE, Bush DE, et al. Chest pain relief by nitroglycerin does not predict active coronary artery disease. *Ann Intern Med.* 2003;139:979-986.

63. Brush JE, Brand DA, Acampora D, Chalmer B, Wackers FJ. Use of the initial electrocardiogram to predict in-hospital complications of acute myocardial infarction. *N Engl J Med.* 1985;312:1137-1141.

64. Karlson BW, Herlitz J, Wiklund O, et al. Early prediction of acute myocardial infarction from clinical history, examination and electrocardiogram in the emergency room. *Am J Cardiol.* 1991;68:171-175.

65. Rouan GW, Lee TH, F CE, et al. Clinical characteristics and outcome of acute myocardial infarction in patients with initially normal or nonspecific electrocardiograms (A report from the Multicenter Chest Pain Study). *Am J Cardiol.* 1989;64:1087-1092.

66. Aufderheide TP, Hendley GE, Woo J, et al. A prospective evaluation of prehospital 12-lead ECG application in chest pain patients. *J Electrocardiol.* 1992;24(Suppl):8-13.

67. Truett J, Cornfield J, Kannel W. A multivariate analysis of the risk of coronary heart disease in Framingham. *J Chron Dis.* 1967;20:511-524.

68. Prindle P, Emberson J, Lampe F, et al. Predictive accuracy of the Framingham coronary risk score in British men: Prospective cohort study. *BMJ.* 2003;327:1267-1270.

69. Psaty BM, Anderson M, Kronmal RA, et al. The association between lipid levels and the risks of incident myocardial infarction, stroke, and total mortality: The Cardiovascular Health study. *J Am Geriatr Soc.* 2004;52:1639-1647.

70. D'Agostino RB, Grundy S, Sullivan LM, Wilson P. Validation of the Framingham coronary heart disease prediction scores: Results of a multiple ethnic groups investigation. *JAMA.* 2001;286:180-187.

71. Wrenn K, Slovis CM, Gongaware J. Using the "GI cocktail": A descriptive study. *Ann Emerg Med*. 1995;26:687-690.

72. Schwartz GR. Xylocaine viscous as an aid in the differential diagnosis of chest pain. *JACEP*. 1976;5:981-983.

73. Hess GP, Walson PD. Seizures secondary to oral viscous lidocaine. *Ann Emerg Med*. 1988;17:725-727.

74. Dickinson MW. The "GI cocktail in the evaluation of chest pain in the emergency department. *J Emerg Med*. 1996;14:245-246.

75. Welling LR, A WW. The emergency department treatment of dyspepsia with antacids and oral lidocaine. *Ann Emerg Med*. 1990;19:785-788.

76. Goldman L, Cook EF, Johnson PA, et al. Prediction of the need for intensive care in patients who come to emergency departments with acute chest pain. *N Engl J Med*. 1996;334:1498-1504.

77. Reilly B, Durairaj L, Husain S, et al. Performance and potential impact of a chest pain prediction rule in a large public hospital. *Am J Med*. 1999;106:285-291.

78. Durairaj L, Reilly B, Das K, et al. Emergency department admissions to inpatient cardiac telemetry beds: A prospective cohort study of risk stratification and outcomes. *Am J Med*. 2001;110:7-11.

79. Hamm CW, Goldmann BU, Heeschen C, et al. Emergency room triage of patients with acute chest pain by means of rapid testing for cardiac troponin T or troponin I. *N Engl J Med*. 1997;337:1648-1653.

ABDOMEN

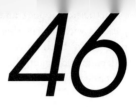

Inspection of the Abdomen

This chapter reviews two physical signs, ecchymosis of the abdominal wall and Sister Mary Joseph's nodule. Jaundice and dilated abdominal veins are discussed in Chapter 6, the signs of malnutrition in Chapter 10, and abnormal respiratory movements of the abdominal wall in Chapter 17.

ECCHYMOSIS OF THE ABDOMINAL WALL

I. THE FINDINGS

Ecchymosis of the abdominal wall is an important sign of retroperitoneal or intraperitoneal hemorrhage. Periumbilical ecchymosis is called "Cullen's sign," after the American pathologist and clinician who first described the finding in a patient with ectopic pregnancy in 1918.* Flank ecchymosis is often called "Grey

---

*Cullen was well versed in the anatomy of the umbilicus, having just 2 years before his report published the book *Embryology, Anatomy, and Diseases of the Umbilicus, Together with the Urachus,* which contained 27 chapters on the umbilicus.[1,2]

Turner's sign" or "Turner's sign," after the British surgeon Gilbert Grey Turner who described the sign in a patient with hemorrhagic pancreatitis in 1920.[3] Nonetheless, Cullen's and Turner's signs are rare, occurring in less than 3% of patients with pancreatitis[4] and less than 1% of patients with ruptured ectopic pregnancy.[5] Both signs have since been described in a wide variety of other disorders, including intrahepatic hemorrhage from tumor,[6–8] amebic liver abscess,[9] ischemic bowel,[10] splenic rupture,[11] rectus sheath hematoma,[12] perforated duodenal ulcer,[13] ruptured abdominal aortic aneurysm,[14] percutaneous liver biopsy,[15] and coronary angiography.[16]

II. PATHOGENESIS

The discoloration of the skin is actually due to the collection of blood in the subcutaneous fascial planes not the dispersion of red cells within lymphatics as has been sometimes surmised.[17] In patients with pancreatitis, computed tomography often reveals collections of fluid within the fascial planes behind the kidney, which at some point may reach the lateral border of the quadratus lumborum muscle, from where they may pass to the subcutaneous tissues of the lateral abdominal wall.[18] Presumably, the mechanism of Grey Turner's sign in other causes of retroperitoneal hemorrhage is the same. In most patients with Cullen's signs, blood travels to the periumbilical area through the falciform ligament, which connects to the retroperitoneum via the lesser omentum and transverse mesocolon (the falciform ligament and lesser omentum are the embryologic remnants of the ventral mesentery, into which the liver has grown).

In patients with ectopic pregnancy, however, the falciform ligament is probably not responsible for Cullen's sign, because the ecchymosis of these patients is often located on the abdominal wall below the umbilicus, yet the falciform ligament attaches to the abdominal wall above the umbilicus. Some investigators have hypothesized that fascial planes connecting the broad ligament and the lower abdominal wall are responsible for Cullen's sign in ectopic pregnancy,[18] although this does not explain why the sign sometimes appears in patients with free rupture into the peritoneal cavity outside of the broad ligament.[5]

SISTER MARY JOSEPH'S NODULE

I. THE FINDING

Sister Mary Joseph's nodule is metastatic carcinoma of the umbilicus. It usually presents as a hard dermal or subcutaneous nodule, and in about 20% of patients with the lesion, it represents the initial sign of malignancy.[19] Most patients have metastatic adenocarcinoma, usually from the stomach, large bowel, pancreas, or ovary.[19-23] It is an ominous sign, the average survival after discovery being only 10 to 11 months.[19,20]

The finding is named after Sister Mary Joseph, who, as first surgical assistant to William J. Mayo, noted the association between the umbilical nodule and intra-abdominal malignancy. Sister Mary Joseph was born Julia Dempsey in 1856; before Vatican II in 1965, all Franciscan nuns took the name of Mary as a prefix to an additional name.[24-26] Dr. Mayo discussed the sign as early as 1928, calling it the "pants-button umbilicus,"[27] and it was not until Sir Hamilton Bailey's 1949 edition of *Physical Signs in Clinical Surgery* (10 years after Sister Mary Joseph's death) that the term "Sister Joseph's nodule" was used.[28]

A mimic of the Sister Mary Joseph nodule is an omphalith, which is the hardened concretion of keratin and sebum in the umbilicus from inadequate hygiene.[29] Careful examination of these patients, however, manages to extract the debris.

II. PATHOGENESIS

There are many potential avenues of spread to the umbilicus: vascular and lymphatic connections to the retroperitoneum, axilla, and inguinal regions, and embryologic remnants that connect the umbilicus to the bladder and retroperitoneum.[30] Nonetheless, the umbilicus and periumbilical tissues represent the thinnest part of the abdominal wall, and in one series of patients, direct spread from peritoneal tumor implants through the abdominal wall was the most common cause of the umbilical nodule.[19]

REFERENCES

1. Young RH. History of gynecological pathology. I. Dr. Thomas S. Cullen. *Int J Gynecol Pathol*. 1996;15:181-186.
2. Cullen TS. *Embryology, anatomy, and diseases of the umbilicus, together with the urachus*. Philadelphia: W.B. Saunders; 1916.
3. Turner GG. Local discoloration of the abdominal wall as a sign of acute pancreatitis. *Br J Surg*. 1920;7:394-395.
4. Dickson AP, Imrie CW. The incidence and prognosis of body wall ecchymosis in acute pancreatitis. *Surg Gynecol Obstet*. 1984;159:343-347.
5. Merrill JA. Cullen's sign: A historical review and report of histologic observations. *Obstet Gynecol*. 1958;12:317-324.

6. Mabin TA, Gelfand M. Cullen's signs, a feature in liver disease. *Br Med J.* 1974;1:493-494.

7. Marinella MA. Cullen's sign associated with metastatic thyroid cancer. *N Engl J Med.* 1999;340:149-150.

8. Sevastianos VA, Deutsch M, Dourakis SP. Grey-Turner's sign as the first indication of a ruptured hepatocellular carcinoma. *J Clin Oncol.* 2004;22:1156-1157.

9. Misra A, Agrahari D, Gupta R. Cullen's sign in amoebic liver abscess. *Postgrad Med J.* 2002;78:427-428.

10. Kelley ML. Discolorations of flanks and abdominal wall. *Arch Intern Med.* 1961;108:132-135.

11. Chung MA, Oung C, Szilagyi A. Cullen's sign: It doesn't always mean hemorrhagic pancreatitis. *Am J Gastroenterol.* 1992;87:1026-1028.

12. Guthrie CM, Stanfey HA. Rectus sheath haematoma presenting with Cullen's sign and Grey-Turner's sign. *Scot Med J.* 1996;41:54-55.

13. Evans DM. Cullen's sign in perforated duodenal ulcer. *Br Med J.* 1971;1:154.

14. Armour RH, Clifton MA, Marsh CH. Balloon catheter control of a rupture abdominal aortic aneurysm in a patient with Cullen's sign. *Br J Surg.* 1978;65:350.

15. Capron JP, Chivrac D, Delamarre J, et al. Cullen's sign after percutaneous liver biopsy. *Gastroenterol.* 1977;73:1185-1191.

16. Spence MS, Webb SW. Cullen's sign after coronary angiography. *Heart.* 2000; 83:640.

17. Bem J, Bradley EL. Subcutaneous manifestations of severe acute pancreatitis. *Pancreas.* 1998;16:551-555.

18. Meyers MA, Feldberg MAM, Oliphant M. Grey Turner's sign and Cullen's sign in acute pancreatitis. *Gastrointest Radiol.* 1989;14:31-37.

19. Powell FC, Cooper AJ, Massa MC, et al. Sister Mary Joseph's nodule: A clinical and histologic study. *J Am Acad Dermatol.* 1984;10:610-615.

20. Dubreuil A, Dompmartin A, Barjot P, et al. Umbilical metastasis or Sister Mary Joseph's nodule. *Int J Dermatol.* 1998;37:7-13.

21. Urbano FL. Sister Joseph's nodule. *Hosp Physician.* 2001:33-35, 44.

22. Schiffer JT, Park C, Jefferson BK. Cases from the Osler Medical Service at Johns Hopkins University. Sister Mary Joseph nodule. *Am J Med.* 2003;114:68-70.

23. Barrow MV. Metastatic tumors of the umbilicus. *J Chronic Dis.* 1966;19: 1113-1117.

24. Nelson CW. Historical profiles of Mayo: 100th anniversary of Sister Mary Joseph Dempsey. *Mayo Clin Proc.* 1992;67:512.

25. O'Neill TW, O'Brien AAJ. Sister (Mary) Joseph's nodule. *Ir Med J.* 1987; 80:296.

26. Steensma DP. Sister (Mary) Joseph's nodule. *Ann Intern Med.* 2000;133:237.

27. Key JD, Shephard DAE, Walters W. Sister Mary Joseph's nodule and its relationship to diagnosis of carcinoma of the umbilicus. *Minn Med.* 1976;59:561-566.

28. Bailey H. *Demonstrations of physical signs in clinical surgery*, 11th ed. Baltimore: Williams and Wilkins; 1949.

29. Amaro R, Goldstein JA, Cely CM, Rogers AI. Pseudo Sister Mary Joseph's nodule. *Am J Gastroenterol*. 1999;94:1949-1950.

30. Coll DM, Meyer JM, Mader M, Smith RC. Imaging appearances of Sister Mary Joseph's nodule. *Br J Radiol*. 1999;72:1230-1233.

47

Palpation and Percussion of the Abdomen

I. INTRODUCTORY COMMENTS ON TECHNIQUE

Palpation of the abdomen may reveal abnormal tenderness, tumors, hernias, aneurysms, or organomegaly (i.e., of the liver, spleen, or gallbladder). To help the patient relax and to minimize pain during palpation, experienced clinicians all recommend that the clinician's hands should be warm, the technique soft and gentle, and the expected tender areas palpated last. Other maneuvers designed to help the patient relax include drawing up the patient's knees, encouraging deep breathing, or engaging the patient in conversation.

In the days before clinical imaging, palpation of a relaxed abdomen was so essential that patients with tense abdominal muscles were often reexamined after immersion in a hot bath or after anesthesia had been induced with ether or chloroform, to determine whether an abnormality was present or not.[1]

II. LIVER

A. LIVER SPAN
1. The Finding

The liver span is the distance in centimeters between the upper border of the liver in the right midclavicular line, as determined by percussion (i.e., where lung resonance changes to liver dullness), and the lower border, as determined by either percussion or palpation. Clinicians have been measuring the liver span ever since Piorry introduced topographic percussion in 1828.[2-4] After introduction of the x-ray, however, it became apparent that the estimated span often differed from the actual span, and most clinicians instead adopted the view that the percussed liver span was just an index of liver size, not a precise measurement.[5]

2. Clinical Significance

The clinician's assessment of liver span almost always underestimates the actual value. Clinicians place the upper border too low (2–5 cm)[6,7] and lower border too high (>2 cm in about half of patients),[6,8] except in patients with chronic obstructive lung disease, in whom the error with the top border is less.[6] The liver span is the same whether the patient is percussed during quiet respirations or full-held expiration.[9]

Nonetheless, most studies of liver percussion make two important points: First, the estimated span does correlate modestly with actual span, as determined by ultrasonography or scintigraphy ($r = 0.6$–0.7).[5,7,8,10] This correlation is much better in patients with diseased livers than with healthy livers.[7,10] And second, the percussed liver span is dependent on the clinician's technique, and consequently, one clinician's "normal liver span" is not the same as another's. The heavier the clinician's percussion stroke, the smaller the measured span and the greater the error in underestimating the actual liver size (see also Chapter 26).[6,9] This explains why published estimates of the "normal liver span" range from as low as 6 cm to as high as 15 cm*[8,12-14] and why experienced clinicians, each examining the same patient, differ in their estimate of the patient's span, *on average*, by 8 cm.[15]

These comments would imply that each clinician could determine his or her own "normal liver span," based on examination of hundreds of healthy persons, and then use this span as a benchmark to indicate whether a patient's span is abnormally large or not. Nonetheless, two studies applying a standardized percussion technique failed to accurately detect hepatomegaly (likelihood ratio [LR] not significant, EBM Box 47-1).

---

*The normal upper limit for the cephalocaudad dimension of the liver on ultrasonography is 13 cm.[11]

Box 47-1 Detection of Enlarged Liver and Spleen*

Finding (Ref)[†]	Sensitivity (%)	Specificity (%)	Likelihood Ratio if Finding	
			Present	Absent
LIVER				
Percussion span ≥10 cm in MCL				
Detecting enlarged liver[8,16]	61–92	30–43	NS	NS
Palpable liver				
Detecting liver edge below costal margin[17]	48	100	**233.7**	0.5
Detecting enlarged liver[16,18–20]	39–71	56–85	1.8	0.6
SPLEEN				
Palpable spleen				
Detecting enlarged spleen[18,19,21–28]	18–78	89–99	**8.5**	0.5
Splenic percussion signs				
Detecting enlarged spleen[22,23,27–29]				
Spleen percussion sign	25–85	32–94	1.7	0.7
Nixon method	25–66	68–95	2.0	0.7
Traube's space dullness	11–76	63–95	2.1	0.8

NS, not significant; likelihood ratio (LR) if finding present = positive LR; LR if finding absent = negative LR; MCL, midclavicular line.
*Diagnostic standard: For enlarged liver, liver enlarged by scintigraphy,[18,20] craniocaudal span >13 cm by ultrasonography,[8,16] or postmortem weight of liver >2000 g[19]; for enlarged spleen, spleen enlarged by ultrasonography,[22,23,26–28] scintigraphy,[18,21,24,29] or postmortem weight >200 g[19] or >250 g.[25]
†Definition of findings: For percussed liver span, using light percussion technique; for splenic percussion signs, see text.

DETECTION OF ENLARGED LIVER AND SPLEEN

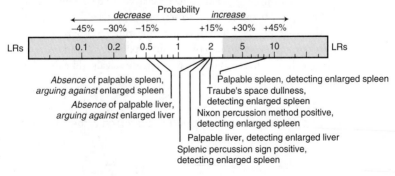

B. PALPABLE LIVER EDGE

1. The Finding

To palpate the liver edge, the clinician begins by gently palpating the patient's right *lower* quadrant. As the patient breathes in and out, the clinician moves the palpating hand upward 1 to 2 cm at a time, at each location searching for a liver edge that moves down during inspiration and strikes the clinician's fingers. Once the edge is located, the clinician should note its consistency (a cirrhotic liver is firmer than a healthy one)[10] and whether the edge has any irregularities or masses.[30]

Anatomically, the normal liver extends on average 5 cm below the right costal margin at the midclavicular line.[7]

2. Clinical Significance

a. Detection of Hepatomegaly

If clinicians palpate what they believe is the patient's liver edge extending below the costal margin, they are virtually always correct (LR = 233.7; see EBM Box 47-1). Nonetheless, the distance between the liver edge and costal margin has little to do with the overall liver size, and the finding of a palpable liver edge is an unreliable sign of hepatomegaly (LR only 1.8; see EBM Box 47-1). Moreover, about half of livers that extend below the costal margin are not palpable.[10,17] The *consistency* of the liver parenchyma probably determines in part whether a liver is palpable, because in patients with cirrhosis, whose livers are smaller but firmer than normal, the liver's edge is palpable 95% of the time.[10]

b. Palpable Liver and Other Disorders

In patients with chronic liver disease, the finding of an enlarged, palpable liver edge is a modest argument for cirrhosis (LR = 2.0; EBM Box 47-2), more so if the liver is felt in the epigastrium (LR = 2.6) or if its edge is unusually firm (LR = 2.7). In patients with jaundice, the findings of a palpable liver and liver tenderness are unhelpful, both appearing equally often in patients with hepatocellular disease (i.e., nonobstructive jaundice) as in those with obstructive jaundice (LR not significant, see Chapter 6). In patients with lymphadenopathy, the finding of palpable liver fails to distinguish those with serious infections and malignancies from those with benign, self-limited disorders (LR not significant; see Chapter 24).

C. AUSCULTATORY PERCUSSION—"SCRATCH TEST"

1. The Finding

Auscultatory percussion (see also Chapter 26) is often used to locate the lower border of the liver. According to traditional teachings, the moment the clinician's percussing digit crosses the border of the liver and begins to strike

Box 47-2 Palpation of Liver and Spleen in Various Disorders*

Finding (Ref)†	Sensitivity (%)	Specificity (%)	Likelihood Ratio if Finding Present	Absent
LIVER				
Enlarged palpable liver in patients with chronic liver disease, detecting cirrhosis[31-36]	31–96	20–96	2.0	0.6
Palpable liver in epigastrium in patients with chronic liver disease, detecting cirrhosis[36]	86	68	2.6	**0.2**
Liver edge firm to palpation in patients with chronic liver disease, detecting cirrhosis[32,35]	71–78	71–74	2.7	0.4
Palpable liver in patients with jaundice, detecting hepatocellular disease (nonobstructive jaundice)[37,38]	71–83	15–17	NS	NS
Liver tenderness in patients with jaundice, detecting hepatocellular disease (nonobstructive jaundice)[37,38]	37–38	70–78	NS	NS
Palpable liver in patients with lymphadenopathy, detecting serious disease[39,40]	14–16	86–89	NS	NS
SPLEEN				
Palpable spleen in returning travelers with fever, detecting malaria[41]	19	97	**6.6**	0.8
Palpable spleen in patients with jaundice, detecting hepatocellular disease (nonobstructive jaundice)[37,38]	29–47	83–90	2.9	0.7

(continued)

Box 47-2 — Palpation of Liver and Spleen in Various Disorders*—Cont'd

Finding (Ref)[†]	Sensitivity (%)	Specificity (%)	Likelihood Ratio if Finding Present	Likelihood Ratio if Finding Absent
Palpable spleen in patients with chronic liver disease, detecting cirrhosis[32–36,42–45]	5–85	35–98	2.3	0.8
Palpable spleen in patients with lymphadenopathy, detecting serious disease[39,40,46]	5–10	92–96	NS	NS

NS, not significant; likelihood ratio (LR) if finding present = positive LR; LR if finding absent = negative LR; MCL, midclavicular line.
*Diagnostic standard: For nonobstructive (vs. obstructive) jaundice, needle biopsy of liver, surgical exploration, or autopsy; for cirrhosis, needle biopsy of liver (see Chapter 6); for serious disease (in patients with lymphadenopathy), see Chapter 24.

PALPATION OF LIVER AND SPLEEN IN VARIOUS DISORDERS

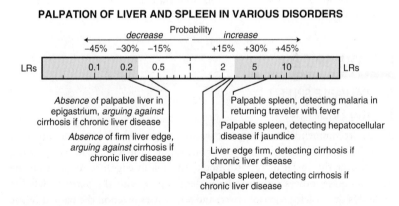

abdominal wall over the liver, the sound heard through the stethoscope becomes louder.

Nonetheless, the lack of consensus on the proper technique of locating the liver will quickly discourage the serious student of auscultatory percussion. Various experts recommend placing the stethoscope on the xiphoid,[6,47] near the umbilicus,[48] superior to[49] or at the costal margin,[50] at four separate positions over the liver,[51] or above the suspected center.[52] According to various authorities, the clinician should percuss with a finger and pleximeter, [52] a finger alone,[49] a bristle brush,[51] or a corrugated rod.[51] The direction of the stroke should be circular,[1] centripetal,[52] centrifugal,[51] left to right,[50] or always in a longitudinal axis and toward the liver.[6,49]

2. Clinical Significance

The evidence supporting auscultatory percussion of the liver is mixed and meager. Only one study supports the technique, showing that 78% of estimates of the lower border are within 2 cm of the actual border (by ultrasonography), compared with 44% for conventional percussion and palpation.[49] Another study showed that palpation of the liver was more accurate than auscultatory percussion.[6] A third study showed that there was no correlation whatsoever between the distance of the liver edge below the costal margin, located by auscultatory percussion, and the actual distance (by ultrasonography) for any of 11 different examiners.[47]

D. PULSATILE LIVER

The finding of a pulsatile liver has been described in tricuspid regurgitation with high pulmonary pressures (30% to 91% of patients, see Chapter 42)[53–57] and constrictive pericarditis (55% of patients in one study).[58,59] In patients with the holosystolic murmur of tricuspid regurgitation, the finding of a pulsatile liver argues that the regurgitation is moderate to severe (LR = 3.9; see Chapter 42).[57]

III. THE SPLEEN

A. PALPABLE SPLEEN

1. The Finding

Experts recommend many different ways to palpate the spleen: some palpate from the patient's right side and others from the patient's left side (curling the fingers over the costal margin to "hook" the spleen edge); some position the patient supine, others position the patient supine with the patient's left fist under his or her left posterior chest, and still others position the patient in the right lateral decubitus position. One study comparing the three different positions found all to be equivalent,[23] and the approach the clinician uses probably depends most on personal preference.

2. Clinical Significance
a. Detection of Splenomegaly

EBM Box 47-1 indicates that the finding of a palpable spleen argues strongly *for* splenomegaly (LR = 8.5; see EBM Box 47-1). Although many enlarged spleens are not palpable (sensitivity is only 18% to 78%), virtually all massively enlarged spleens (i.e., weight >1 kg or scintigraphic span >22 cm) are detectable by palpation.[25,60]

b. Etiology of Splenomegaly

The common causes of splenomegaly are hepatic disease (i.e., portal hypertension), hematologic disorders (e.g., leukemias, lymphomas, myelofibrosis), infectious disease (e.g., HIV infection), and primary splenic disorders (e.g., splenic infarction or hematoma).[61,62] The presence of left upper quadrant tenderness and pain argues *for* a primary splenic disorder or hematologic disorder.[62] Associated lymphadenopathy practically excludes hepatic disease and points to one of the other disorders (LR = 0.04).[62] The finding of a palpable liver argues *for* hepatic disease (LR = 2.7), and the finding of massive splenomegaly (i.e., spleen extends to level of umbilicus) argues modestly for hematologic disease (LR = 2.1).[62]

c. Palpable Spleen and Other Disorders

In returning travelers from tropical countries who are febrile, the finding of a palpable spleen argues significantly for the diagnosis of malaria (LR = 6.6; see EBM Box 47-2). In patients with jaundice, the palpable spleen argues modestly for hepatocellular disease (i.e., nonobstructive jaundice, LR = 2.9; see Chapter 6), and in patients with chronic liver disease it argues modestly for cirrhosis (LR = 2.3). In patients with lymphadenopathy, a palpable spleen is found just as often in patients with serious infections and malignancies as in those with benign, self-limited disorders (LR not significant, see Chapter 24).

B. SPLENIC PERCUSSION SIGNS

1. The Findings

There are three commonly used splenic percussion signs.

a. Spleen Percussion Sign

Castell described this sign in 1967,[13] finding it a useful way to measure splenic size in patients with infectious mononucleosis. The clinician percusses the lowest left intercostal space in the anterior axillary line (usually the eighth or ninth); if the percussion note in this location, usually resonant, becomes dull with a full inspiration, the test is positive. Since Castell's original description, other investigators have regarded any dullness at this location as a positive response (i.e., whether during inspiration or expiration).

b. Nixon's Method

Nixon described this sign in 1954,[63] finding it accurate in his experience of 60 splenic aspiration biopsies. The patient is positioned in the right lateral decubitus position, and the clinician percusses from the lower level of pulmonary resonance in the posterior axillary line downward obliquely to the lower midanterior costal margin. The test is positive if the border of dullness on this line lies more than 8 cm from the costal margin.

c. Traube's Space Dullness

Traube's space is the triangular space, normally tympanic, that is over the left lower anterior part of the chest. Its upper border is marked by the limits of cardiac dullness (usually the sixth rib), its lower border is the costal margin, and its lateral border is the anterior axillary line. Although Traube suggested that dullness in this space was a sign of pleural effusion,[64] Parrino (in 1987) suggested that it could be a sign of splenic enlargement.[65]

2. Clinical Significance

Positive percussion signs are much less convincing than palpation (positive LRs = 1.7-2.1; see EBM Box 47-1). Traube's space dullness becomes even less accurate in overweight patients or those who have recently eaten.[66]

IV. GALLBLADDER: COURVOISIER'S SIGN

A. THE FINDING

Courvoisier's sign is a *palpable nontender* gallbladder in a patient with *jaundice*, a finding that has been traditionally associated with malignant obstruction of the biliary system. Many textbooks call the sign "Courvoisier's law," as if the positive result were pathognomonic of malignancy, although the Swiss surgeon Courvoisier originally presented the finding in 1890 as only an interesting observation.[67] Writing in a monograph on biliary tract disorders, he stated that, among 187 patients with jaundice and common duct obstruction, a dilated gallbladder was found in only 20% of patients with stones, compared with 92% of patients having other disorders, mostly malignancy.[68,69]

B. CLINICAL SIGNIFICANCE

Summarizing the information about Courvoisier's sign is difficult because various authors define the sign differently. Some apply it to patients without jaundice (clearly not what Courvoisier intended)[70]; others define the positive sign as any palpable gallbladder, tender or nontender (some patients with cholecystitis have tender enlarged gallbladders)[71-73]; and still others expand the positive sign to include a dilated gallbladder discovered during surgery, clinical imaging, or even autopsy.[74]

Restricting analysis to those studies defining the positive sign as a palpable gallbladder in a jaundice patient, EBM Box 47-3 indicates that Courvoisier's

Box 47-3　Palpation of Gallbladder, Bladder, and Aorta*

Finding (Ref)[†]	Sensitivity (%)	Specificity (%)	Likelihood Ratio if Finding	
			Present	Absent
GALLBLADDER				
Palpable gallbladder				
Detecting obstructed bile ducts in patients with jaundice[37]	31	99	**26.0**	0.7
Detecting malignant obstruction in patients with obstructive jaundice[37,70, 72,75]	26–55	83–90	2.6	0.7
BLADDER				
Palpable bladder				
Detecting ≥400 mL urine in bladder[76]	82	56	1.9	**0.3**
AORTA				
Expansile pulsating epigastric mass				
Detecting abdominal aortic aneurysm[77–84]	22–68	75–99	**8.0**	0.6

Likelihood ratio (LR) if finding present = positive LR; LR if finding absent = negative LR.
*Diagnostic standard: For obstructive jaundice and malignant obstruction, needle biopsy of liver, surgical exploration, or autopsy; for ≥400 mL urine in bladder, bladder ultrasound[76]; for abdominal aortic aneurysm, ultrasonography revealing focal dilation of infrarenal aorta >3 cm in diameter,[78,79,81–84] > 4 cm in diameter,[80] or >1.5 cm larger than proximal aorta.[77]

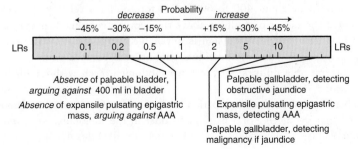

PALPATION OF GALLBLADDER, BLADDER, AND AORTA

Absence of palpable bladder, *arguing against* 400 ml in bladder

Absence of expansile pulsating epigastric mass, *arguing against* AAA

Palpable gallbladder, detecting obstructive jaundice

Expansile pulsating epigastric mass, detecting AAA

Palpable gallbladder, detecting malignancy if jaundice

sign is a compelling argument for extrahepatic obstruction of the biliary system (i.e., stones or malignancy, but not hepatocellular disease, LR = 26.0). Among patients with biliary obstruction, however, the sign argues only modestly for malignancy and against stones (LR = 2.6). Consequently, if there is a "law" to Courvoisier's sign, it is that the palpable gallbladder in a jaundiced patient indicates extrahepatic obstruction, not that the obstruction is caused by malignancy.

C. PATHOGENESIS

Courvoisier's original hypothesis—that the gallbladder of choledocholithiasis fails to dilate because its walls are fibrotic from chronic cholecystitis—is probably incorrect, because experiments with gallbladders of jaundiced patients show that the wall stiffness of dilated and nondilated gallbladders is similar.[85] Instead, patients with dilated gallbladders have (1) much higher operative intraductal pressures and (2) longer duration of jaundice than those with normal-sized gallbladders.

The relationship between duration of jaundice and dilation of gallbladder explains why Courvoisier's original findings are different from the studies in EBM Box 47-3. When analysis is restricted to just those patients with extrahepatic obstruction, the sensitivity of the dilated gallbladder in malignant obstruction today (25% to 55%) is lower than it was for Courvoisier (i.e., 92%) (although the specificity is similar, 80% to 90%). The reduced sensitivity may simply reflect the fact that patients with malignant obstruction today, compared with those from a century ago, are diagnosed sooner with clinical imaging, before pressures rise enough to enlarge the gallbladder greatly.

V.   BLADDER VOLUME

For more than a century, clinicians have investigated percussing the suprapubic area to detect bladder volume; most studies reveal that the bladder volume must be about 400 to 600 mL before dullness reliably appears.[86] Although the extent of dullness above the symphysis pubis does correlate with bladder volume,[86,87] the sign is unreliable overall because the results vary tremendously among individual patients and because many patients have inexplicable dullness of the lower abdomen, even without bladder distention.[4,86]

There are few studies of palpation of the bladder. One study has demonstrated that the *absence* of a palpable bladder in the suprapubic area argues *against* bladder volumes ≥400 mL[76] (LR = 0.3; see EBM Box 47-3).

VI. ASCITES

A. THE FINDINGS

In patients with ascites lying supine, peritoneal fluid gravitates to the flanks, and the air-filled intestines float up to occupy the periumbilical space. This distribution of fluid and air causes four characteristic signs of ascites: (1) **bulging flanks.** (2) **Flank dullness.** Flank dullness is positive if there is a *horizontal* border between dullness in the flank area and resonance or tympany in the periumbilical area. (3) **Shifting dullness.** Shifting dullness describes flank dullness whose position shifts as the patient changes position, usually by rolling on to one side. The sign is based on the principle that the air-filled loops of intestine, floating on peritoneal fluid, move to the uppermost position in the abdomen. In a patient with a positive response, the border between resonance and dullness shifts away from the side that is most dependent. To be positive, the shifting border should remain horizontal. (4) **Fluid wave.** To elicit the fluid wave, the clinician places one hand against the lateral wall of the abdomen and uses the other hand to tap firmly on the opposite lateral wall. In the positive response, the tap generates a wave that is transmitted through the abdomen and felt as a sudden shock by the other hand. Because a false-positive response may result from waves traveling through the subcutaneous tissue of the anterior abdominal wall, the clinician should always use the patient's hand or that of an assistant to apply firm pressure against the anterior abdominal wall.

In addition to these four signs, most patients with ascites also have edema, both from hypoalbuminemia and from the weight of the peritoneal fluid compressing the veins to the legs.[88]

B. PATHOGENESIS

In experiments with cadavers performed a century ago, Müller showed that 1000 mL of fluid injected into the peritoneal space was undetectable by physical examination (i.e., flank or shifting dullness), 1500 mL resulted in some flank dullness, and 2000 mL was the smallest volume to cause shifting dullness.[86] The living abdominal wall is probably more elastic than the cadaver's, and it is likely that the careful clinician can detect smaller amounts of ascites in patients. However, one small study of healthy volunteers still showed that injection of 500–1100 mL of fluid was necessary before shifting dullness appeared.[89] A significant cause of false-positive flank dullness or shifting dullness is accumulation of fluid within loops of the colon.[89,90] This condition, called "pseudoascites" in the days before clinical imaging,[90] typically occurred in patients with diarrheal illnesses.

C. CLINICAL SIGNIFICANCE

In patients with abdominal distention, the findings arguing the most *for* ascites are the positive fluid wave (LR = 5.0; EBM Box 47-4) and presence of edema

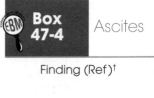

Box 47-4   Ascites

Finding (Ref)†	Sensitivity (%)	Specificity (%)	Likelihood Ratio if Finding	
			Present	Absent
INSPECTION				
Bulging flanks[91–93]	73–93	44–70	1.9	0.4
Edema[92]	87	77	**3.8**	**0.2**
PALPATION AND PERCUSSION				
Flank dullness[91,92]	80–94	29–69	NS	**0.3**
Shifting dullness[91–93]	60–87	56–90	2.3	0.4
Fluid wave[91–93]	50–80	82–92	**5.0**	0.5

NS, not significant; likelihood ratio (LR) if finding present = positive LR; LR if finding absent = negative LR.

*Diagnostic standard: For ascites, peritoneal fluid by ultrasonography.

†Definition of findings: For shifting dullness, border between resonance and dullness "shifts" when patient rolls from supine to left lateral decubitus position or right lateral decubitus position; Cattau required a shift in both positions,[91] Simel in only 1 of 2 positions,[92] and Cummings used only the right lateral decubitus position at 45 degrees and required a shift >1 cm.[93]

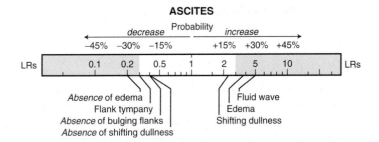

(LR = 3.8). The strongest arguments *against* the presence of ascites are the absence of edema (LR = 0.2) and the absence of flank dullness (LR = 0.3). Shifting dullness shifts the probability of ascites modestly upward when present (LR = 2.3) and modestly downward when absent (LR = 0.4). Findings having relatively little diagnostic value are positive flank dullness, positive bulging flanks, and negative fluid wave. The finding of a flat or everted umbilicus was also diagnostically unhelpful in one study.[92]

Auscultatory percussion also has been recommended to detect ascites,[94–96] although only the puddle sign (auscultatory percussion of the prone patient) has been formally tested,[91,92] proving to be diagnostically unhelpful.

VII. ABDOMINAL AORTIC ANEURYSM

A. INTRODUCTION

Abdominal aortic aneurysm is a focal ballooning of the infrarenal abdominal aorta, traditionally defined as a diameter greater than 3 to 4 cm. It is a disorder of elderly patients, affecting 1% to 2% of patients older than the age of 50 years.[97,98] Abdominal aortic aneurysms tend to enlarge slowly, but some rupture catastrophically with an overall mortality of up to 90%.[99]

B. THE FINDING

Because the normal aorta bifurcates at the level of the umbilicus, palpable aortic aneurysms usually are found in the epigastrium. The clinician should place one hand on each side of the aorta and measure its diameter, subtracting the estimated thickness of two layers of skin and subcutaneous tissue. Most studies do not specifically define the positive finding (instead stating simply the positive finding is "aortic aneurysm present by palpation"), although others define it as an estimated diameter greater than 3 cm using the previously described method.[78]

Importantly, an aortic aneurysm pushes the two hands *apart*, a finding called *expansile* pulsation.[100] Other prominent epigastric pulsations sometimes occur in patients with thin abdomens or in those with epigastric masses overlying the normal aorta, but unless these pulsations are expansile, they do not indicate an aneurysm.

C. CLINICAL SIGNIFICANCE

According to EBM Box 47-3, the finding of a palpable epigastric pulsation suggestive of aneurysm argues strongly that one is present (LR = 8.0; see EBM Box 47-3). In contrast, the absence of this finding is much less helpful (the LR is only 0.6), simply because the sensitivity for the finding is as low as 22% (i.e., up to 78% of patients with aneurysms lack a prominent pulsation).

The two most important variables governing whether an aneurysm is palpable are (1) the size of the aneurysm and (2) the girth of the patient's abdomen. Aneurysms between 3–5 cm in diameter are the most difficult ones to detect, and if "aneurysm" is instead defined as a focal bulging greater than 5 cm in diameter—the diameter usually indicating surgical repair—the sensitivity of bedside examination increases to more than 80% in almost all series.[78,98,101] Aneurysms are also more difficult to detect in patients with larger abdominal girths.[77,78,101,102] After restricting the analysis to just those patients with an abdominal girth less than 100 cm (measured at the umbilicus)[77,78] or to patients in whom the clinician can palpate the aorta,[78,102,103] the sensitivity of the examination exceeds 88% in all studies. These results indicate that the negative examination argues strongly against an aneurysm greater than 5 cm in diameter, especially if the patient has a girth less than 100 cm or has a palpable aorta.

The most common cause for a false-positive examination is an abnormally tortuous aorta.[104,105] Rare causes are a horseshoe kidney, intra-abdominal tumor, or paraaortic adenopathy.[104,105]

REFERENCES

1. Cabot RC. *Physical diagnosis*. New York: William Wood and Co; 1926.
2. Risse GB. Pierre A. Piorry (1794-1879): The French "master of percussion". *Chest*. 1971;60:484-488.
3. Sakula A. Pierre Adolphe Piorry (1794-1879): Pioneer of percussion and pleximetry. *Thorax*. 1979;34:575-581.
4. McGee S. Percussion and physical diagnosis: Separating myth from science. *Disease-a-Month*. 1995;41:643-692.
5. Zelman S, Pickard CM. Roentgen and autopsy evaluation of percussion of the liver and spleen. *Gastroenterology*. 1955;29:1037-1045.
6. Sullivan S, Krasner N, Williams R. The clinical estimation of liver size: A comparison of techniques and an analysis of the source of error. *Br Med J*. 1976;2:1042-1043.
7. Peternel WW, Schaefer JW, Schiff L. Clinical evaluation of liver size and hepatic scintiscan. *Am J Dig Dis*. 1966;11:346-350.
8. Sapira JD, Williamson DL. How big is the normal liver? *Arch Intern Med*. 1979;139:971-973.
9. Castell DO, O'Brien KD, Muench H, Chalmers TC. Estimation of liver size by percussion in normal individuals. *Ann Intern Med*. 1969;70:1183-1189.
10. Zoli M, Magalotti D, Grimaldi M, et al. Physical examination of the liver: Is it still worth it? *Am J Gastroenterol*. 1995;90:1428-1432.
11. Niederau C, Sonnenberg A, Mueller JE, et al. Sonographic measurements of the normal liver, spleen, pancreas, and portal vein. *Radiology*. 1983;149:537-540.
12. Goodman JL. The enlarged liver in diabetes mellitus: Its determination by percussion. *Am J Digest Dis*. 1950;18:181-185.
13. Castell DO. The spleen percussion sign: A useful diagnostic technique. *Ann Intern Med*. 1967;67:1265-1267.
14. Naftalis J, Leevy CM. Clinical estimation of liver size. *Am J Dig Dis*. 1963;8:236-243.
15. Blendis LM, McNeilly WJ, Sheppard L, et al. Observer variation in the clinical and radiological assessment of hepatosplenomegaly. *Br Med J*. 1970;1:727-730.
16. Rajnish J, Amandeep S, Namita J, et al. Accuracy and reliability of palpation and percussion for detecting hepatomegaly: A rural hospital-based study. *Indian J Gastroenterol*. 2004;23:171-174.
17. Ariel IM, Briceno M. The disparity of the size of the liver as determined by physical examination and by hepatic gammascanning in 504 patients. *Med Ped Oncol*. 1976;2:69-73.

18. Halpern S, Coel M, Ashburn W, et al. Correlation of liver and spleen size: Determinations by nuclear medicine studies and physical examination. *Arch Intern Med.* 1974;134:123-124.

19. Riemenschneider PA, Whalen JP. The relative accuracy of estimation of enlargement of the liver and spleen by radiologic and clinical methods. *Am J Roentgen Rad Ther Nuc Med.* 1965;94:462-468.

20. Rosenfield AT, Laufer I, Schneider PB. The significance of a palpable liver: A correlation of clinical and radioisotope studies. *Am J Roent Rad Ther Nuc Med.* 1974; 122:313-317.

21. Westin J, Lanner L, Larsson A, Weinfeld A. Spleen size in polycythemia: A clinical and scintigraphic study. *Acta Med Scand.* 1972;191:263-271.

22. Tamayo SG, Rickman LS, Mathews WC, et al. Examiner dependence on physical diagnostic tests for the detection of splenomegaly: A prospective study with multiple observers. *J Gen Intern Med.* 1993;8:69-75.

23. Barkun AN, Camus M, Green L, et al. The bedside assessment of splenic enlargement. *Am J Med.* 1991;91:512-518.

24. Holzbach RT, Clark RE, Shipley RA, Kent WB, Lindsay GE. Evaluation of spleen size by radioactive scanning. *J Lab Clin Med.* 1962;60:902-913.

25. Ingeberg S, Stockel M, Sorensen PJ. Prediction of spleen size by routine radioisotope scintigraphy. *Acta Haemat.* 1983;69:243-248.

26. Gerspacher-Lara R, Pinto-Silva RA, Serufo JC, et al. Splenic palpation for the evaluation of morbidity due to *Schistosomiasis mansoni. Mem Inst Oswaldo Cruz.* 1998;93(Suppl 1):245-248.

27. Dubey S, Swaroop A, Jain R, et al. Percussion of Traube's space: A useful index of splenic enlargement. *JAPI.* 2000;48:326-328.

28. Chongtham DS, Singh MM, Kalantri SP, Pathak S. Accuracy of palpation and percussion manoeuvres in the diagnosis of splenomegaly. *Indian J Med Sci.* 1997; 51:409-416.

29. Sullivan S, Williams R. Reliability of clinical techniques for detecting splenic enlargement. *Br Med J.* 1976;2:1043-1044.

30. Fenster F, Klatskin G. Manifestations of metastatic tumors of the liver: A study of eighty-one patients subjected to needle biopsy. *Am J Med.* 1961;31:238-248.

31. Hamberg KJ, Carstenesen B, Sorensen TIA, Eghoje K. Accuracy of clinical diagnosis of cirrhosis among alcohol-abusing men. *J Clin Epidemiol.* 1996;49:1295-1301.

32. Marmo R, Romano M, Peduto A, et al. Decision-making model for a non-invasive diagnosis of compensated liver cirrhosis. *Ital J Gastroenterol.* 1993;25:1-8.

33. Nakamura T, Nakamura S, Aikawa T, et al. Clinical studies of alcoholic hepatic diseases. *Tohoku J Exp Med.* 1967;93:179-189.

34. Rankin JGD, Orrego-Matte H, Deschenes J, et al. Alcoholic liver disease: The problem of diagnosis. *Alcohol Clin Exp Res.* 1978;2:327-338.

35. Tine F, Caltagirone M, Camma C, et al. Clinical indicants of compensated cirrhosis: a prospective study. In: Dianzani MU, Gentilini P, eds. *Chronic liver damage:*

Proceedings of the Annual Meeting of the Italian national programme on liver cirrhosis, San Miniato, Italy 11-13 January 1990. Amsterdam: Excerpta Medica; 1990: 187-198.

36. McCormick PA, Nolan N. Palpable epigastric liver as a physical sign of cirrhosis: A prospective study. *Eur J Gastroenterol Hepatol.* 2004;16:1331-1334.

37. Schenker S, Balint J, Schiff L. Differential diagnosis of jaundice: Report of a prospective study of 61 proved cases. *Am J Dig Dis.* 1962;7:449-463.

38. Burbank F. A computer diagnostic system for the diagnosis of prolonged undifferentiating liver disease. *Am J Med.* 1969;46:401-415.

39. Vassilakopoulos TP, Pangalis GA. Application of a prediction rule to select which patients presenting with lymphadenopathy should undergo a lymph node biopsy. *Medicine.* 2000;79:338-347.

40. Slap GB, Brooks JSJ, Schwartz JS. When to perform biopsies of enlarged peripheral lymph nodes in young patients. *JAMA.* 1984;252:1321-1326.

41. O'Brien D, Tobin S, Brown GV, Torresi J. Fever in returned travelers: Review of hospital admissions for a 3-year period. *Clin Infect Dis.* 2001;33:603-609.

42. Cozzolino G, Lonardo A, Francica G, et al. Differential diagnosis between hepatic cirrhosis and chronic active hepatitis: Specificity and sensitivity of physical and laboratory findings in a series from the Mediterranean area. *Am J Gastroenterol.* 1983;78:442-445.

43. Czaja AJ, Wolf AM, Baggenstoss AH. Clinical assessment of cirrhosis in severe chronic active liver disease: Specificity and sensitivity of physical and laboratory findings. *Mayo Clin Proc.* 1980;55:360-364.

44. Hay CRM, Preston FE, Triger DR, et al. Predictive markers of chronic liver disease in hemophilia. *Blood.* 1987;69:1595-1599.

45. Lashner BA, Jonas RB, Tang HS, et al. Chronic hepatitis: Disease factors at diagnosis predictive of mortality. *Am J Med.* 1988;85:609-614.

46. Tokuda Y, Kishaba Y, Kato J, Nakazato N. Assessing the validity of a model to identify patients for lymph node biopsy. *Medicine.* 2003;82:414-418.

47. Tucker WN, Saab S, Rickman LS, Mathews WC. The scratch test is unreliable for detecting the liver edge. *J Clin Gastroenterol.* 1997;25:410-414.

48. Kukowka A. Auskultatorische Methode zur bestimmung der Lebergroesse—ein einfaches, probates Schnellverfahren. *Z Allgemeinmedizin.* 1972;48:1645-1646.

49. Fuller GN, Hargreaves MR, King DM. Scratch test in clinical examination of liver. *Lancet.* 1988;1:181.

50. Rinzler SH. Re-emphasis of the auscultatory method for ascertaining the size of the liver. *N Y State J Med.* 1950;50:300.

51. Sehrwald. Ueber die Brauchbarkeit des Phonoendosckopes. *Dtsch Arch Klin Med.* 1904;79:450-467.

52. Camman GP, Clark A. A new mode of ascertaining the dimensions, form, and condition of internal organs by percussion. *N Y J Med Surg.* 1840;3:62-96.

53. Terry RB. Coupled hepatic pulsations in tricuspid incompetence (a new physical sign). *Am Heart J.* 1959;57:158-159.

54. Salazar E, Levine HD. Rheumatic tricuspid regurgitation: The clinical spectrum. *Am J Med.* 1962;33:111-129.

55. Lingamneni R, Cha SD, Maranhao V, et al. Tricuspid regurgitation: Clinical and angiographic assessment. *Cath Cardiovasc Diag.* 1979;5:7-17.

56. Müller O, Shillingford J. Tricuspid incompetence. *Br Heart J.* 1954;16:195–207.

57. Cha SD, Gooch AS. Diagnosis of tricuspid regurgitation. *Arch Intern Med.* 1983; 143:1763-1768.

58. El-Sherif A, El-Said G. Jugular, hepatic, and praecordial pulsations in constrictive pericarditis. *Br Heart J.* 1971;33:305-312.

59. Coralli RJ, Crawley IS. Hepatic pulsations in constrictive pericarditis. *Am J Cardiol.* 1986;58:370-373.

60. Arkles LB, Gill GD, Molan MP. A palpable spleen is not necessarily enlarged or pathological. *Med J Austral.* 1986;145:15-17.

61. Lipp WF, Eckstein EH, Aaron AH. The clinical significance of the palpable spleen. *Gastroenterology.* 1944;3:287–291.

62. O'Reilly RA. Splenomegaly at a United States County hospital: Diagnostic evaluation of 170 patients. *Am J Med Sci.* 1996; 312:160-165.

63. Nixon RK. The detection of splenomegaly by percussion. *N Engl J Med.* 1954; 250:166-167.

64. Verghese A, Krish G, Karnad A. Ludwig Traube: The man and his space. *Arch Intern Med.* 1992;152:701-703.

65. Parrino TA. The art and science of percussion. *Hosp Pract.* 1987;99:25-36.

66. Barkun AN, Camus M, Meagher T, et al. Splenic enlargement and Traube's space: How useful is percussion? *Am J Med.* 1989;87:562-566.

67. Ludwig Courvoisier (1843-1918): Courvoisier's sign. *JAMA.* 1968;204:165.

68. Verghese A, Dison C, Berk SL. Courvoisier's "Law": An eponym in evolution. *Am J Gastroenterol.* 1987;8:248-250.

69. Delpre G, Kadish U. Courvoisier's gallbladder: "Render unto Caesar that which is Caesar's." *Dig Dis Sci.* 1987;32:446.

70. Viteri AL. Courvoisier's law and evaluation of the jaundiced patient. *Tex Med.* 1980;76:60-61.

71. Gunn A, Keddie N. Some clinical observations on patients with gallstones. *Lancet.* 1972;2:239-241.

72. Chen JJ, Changchien CS, Tai DI, Kuo CH. Gallbladder volume in patients with common hepatic duct dilatation: An evaluation of Courvoisier's sign using ultrasonography. *Scand J Gastroenterol.* 1994;29:284-288.

73. Fournier AM, Michel J. Courvoisier's sign revisited: Two patients with palpable gallbladder. *South Med J.* 1992;85:548-550.

74. Mikal S, Campbell AJA. Carcinoma of the pancreas: Diagnostic and operative criteria based on one hundred consecutive autopsies. *Surgery.* 1950;28:963-969.

75. Zollinger R, Kevorkian AY. Surgical aspects of obstructive jaundice. *N Engl J Med.* 1939;221:486-488.

76. Weatherall M, Harwood M. The accuracy of clinical assessment of bladder volume. *Arch Phys Med Rehabil.* 2002;83:1300-1302.

77. Lederle FA, Walker JM, Reinke DB. Selective screening for abdominal aortic aneurysms with physical examination and ultrasound. *Arch Intern Med.* 1988;148:1753-1756.

78. Fink HA, Lederle FA, Roth CS, et al. The accuracy of physical examination to detect abdominal aortic aneurysm. *Arch Intern Med.* 2000;160:833-836.

79. Twomey A, Twomey E, Wilkins RA, Lewis JD. Unrecognised aneurysmal disease in male hypertensive patients. *Int Angiol.* 1986;5:269-273.

80. Collin J, Walton J, Araujo L, Lindsell D. Oxford screening programme for abdominal aortic aneurysm in men aged 65 to 74 years. *Lancet.* 1988;2:613-615.

81. Allen PIM, Gourevitch D, McKinley J, et al. Population screening for aortic aneurysms. *Lancet.* 1987;2:736.

82. Al Zahrani HA, Rawas M, Maimani A, et al. Screening for abdominal aortic aneurysm in the Jeddah area, western Saudi Arabia. *Cardiovasc Surg.* 1996;4:87-92.

83. Andersson AP, ellitsgaard N, Jorgensen B, et al. Screening for abdominal aortic aneurysm in 295 outpatients with intermittent claudication. *Vasc Surg.* 1991;25:516-520.

84. MacSweeney STR, O'Meara M, Alexander C, et al. High prevalence of unsuspected abdominal aortic aneurysm in patients with confirmed symptomatic peripheral or cerebral arterial disease. *Br J Surg.* 1993;80:582-584.

85. Chung RS. Pathogenesis of the "Courvoisier gallbladder." *Dig Dis Sci.* 1983;28:33-38.

86. Müller F. Einige Beobachtungen aus dem Percussionscurs. *Berl Klin Wochenschr.* 1895;32:278-280.

87. Guarino JR. Auscultatory percussion of the urinary bladder. *Arch Intern Med.* 1985;145:1823-1825.

88. Hussey HH, Jeghers H. Practical considerations of venous pressure. *N Engl J Med.* 1947;237:776-782; 812-778.

89. Moses WR. Shifting dullness in the abdomen. *South Med J.* 1946;39:985-987.

90. Sahli H. *A treatise on diagnostic methods of examination.* Philadelphia: WB Saunders; 1911.

91. Cattau EL, Benjamin SB, Knuff TE, Castell DO. The accuracy of the physical examination in the diagnosis of suspected ascites. *JAMA.* 1982;247:1164-1166.

92. Simel DL, Halvorsen RA, Feussner JR. Quantitating bedside diagnosis: Clinical evaluation of ascites. *J Gen Intern Med.* 1988;3:423-428.

93. Cummings S, Papadakis M, Melnick J, et al. The predictive value of physical examination for ascites. *West J Med.* 1985;142:633-636.

94. Guarino JR. Auscultatory percussion to detect ascites. *N Engl J Med.* 1986;315:1555-1556.

95. McLean ACJ. Diagnosis of ascites by auscultatory percussion and hand-held ultrasound unit. *Lancet.* 1987;2:1526-1527.

96. Lawson JD, Weissbein AS. The puddle sign: An aid in the diagnosis of minimal ascites. *N Engl J Med.* 1959;260:652-654.

97. Lederle FA, Johnson GR, Wilson SE, et al. Prevalence and associations of abdominal aortic aneurysm detected through screening. *Ann Intern Med.* 1997;126:441-449.

98. Lederle FA, Simel DL. Does this patient have abdominal aortic aneurysm? *JAMA.* 1999;281:77-82.

99. Ernst CB. Abdominal aortic aneurysm. *N Engl J Med.* 1993;328:1167-1172.

100. Osler W. Aneurysm of the abdominal aorta. *Lancet.* 1905;2:1089-1096.

101. Chervu A, Clagett P, Valentine J, et al. Role of physical examination in detection of abdominal aortic aneurysms. *Surgery.* 1995;117:454-457.

102. Arnell TD, de Virgilio C, Donayre C, et al. Abdominal aortic aneurysm screening in elderly males with atherosclerosis: The value of the physical exam. *Am Surg.* 1996;62:861-864.

103. Cabellon S, Moncrief CL, Pierre DR, Cavanaugh DG. Incidence of abdominal aortic aneurysms in patients with atheromatous arterial disease. *Am J Surg.* 1983;146:575-576.

104. Nusbaum JW, Freimanis AK, Thomford NR. Echography in the diagnosis of abdominal aortic aneurysm. *Arch Surg.* 1971;102:385-388.

105. Robicsek F, Daugherty HK, Mullen DC, et al. The value of angiography in the diagnosis of unruptured aneurysms of the abdominal aorta. *Ann Thor Surg.* 1971; 11:538-550.

48

Abdominal Pain and Tenderness

ACUTE ABDOMINAL PAIN

I. INTRODUCTION

Among patients presenting with acute abdominal pain and tenderness (i.e., pain lasting < 7 days), the most common diagnoses are nonspecific abdominal pain (43% of patients), acute appendicitis (4% to 20%), acute cholecystitis (3% to 9%), small bowel obstruction (4%), and ureterolithiasis (4%).[1-4] The term "acute abdomen" usually refers to those conditions causing abrupt abdominal pain and tenderness and requiring urgent diagnosis and surgical intervention, such as appendicitis, bowel obstruction, and perforated intra-abdominal organs.

In patients with the acute abdomen, clinicians often order computed tomography of the abdomen because it accurately distinguishes appendicitis from alternative diagnoses and because it detects perforation and abscess formation.[5] Nonetheless, bedside diagnosis remains the fundamental diagnostic tool in all patients with the acute abdomen.[6] After the clinician analyzes the bedside findings, some patients can be safely discharged home without further imaging, because the probability of peritonitis is so low. Other patients should proceed directly to the operating room, because the probability of peritonitis is so high. Those patients whose bedside findings are equivocal or suggest abscess formation benefit the most from further imaging with computed tomography.[5]

II. THE FINDINGS

The two most common causes of the acute abdomen are (1) peritonitis, from inflammation (appendicitis, cholecystitis) or perforation of a viscus (appendix, peptic ulcer of stomach or duodenum, diverticulum) and (2) bowel obstruction. Both peritonitis and obstruction cause abdominal tenderness. Additional findings are discussed later.

A. PERITONITIS

The additional findings of peritonitis are guarding and rigidity, rebound tenderness, percussion tenderness, a positive cough test, and a *negative* abdominal wall tenderness test.

1. Guarding and Rigidity

Guarding refers to *voluntary contraction* of the abdominal wall musculature, usually the result of fear, anxiety, or the laying on of cold hands.[7] Rigidity refers to *involuntary contraction* of the abdominal musculature in response to peritoneal inflammation, a reflex that the patient cannot control.[7] Experienced surgeons distinguish guarding from rigidity in two ways. First, they attempt to distract the patient during examination, often by engaging the patient in conversation or using the stethoscope to gently palpate the abdomen.[8,9] Second, they examine the patient repeatedly over time. Guarding, but not rigidity, diminishes as the patient is distracted and fluctuates in intensity over time, sometimes even disappearing.

The first clinician to clearly describe rigidity was the Roman physician Celsus, writing in 30 AD.[10]

2. Rebound Tenderness

To elicit rebound tenderness, the clinician maintains pressure over an area of tenderness and then withdraws the hand abruptly. If the patient winces with pain on withdrawal of the hand, the test is positive. Many expert surgeons discourage using the rebound tenderness test, regarding it "unnecessary,"[7,11] "cruel,"[6] or a "popular and somewhat unkind way of emphasizing what is already obvious."[12]

Rebound tenderness was originally described by J. Moritz Blumberg (1873–1955), a German surgeon and gynecologist, who believed that pain in the lower abdomen after abrupt withdrawal of the hand from the *left* lower abdominal quadrant was a sign of appendicitis (i.e., Blumberg's sign).[13]

3. Percussion Tenderness

In patients with peritonitis, sudden movements of the abdominal wall cause pain, such as those produced during abdominal percussion. Percussion tenderness is present if light percussion strokes cause pain.

4. Cough Test

The cough test is based on the same principle as percussion tenderness (i.e., jarring movements of the abdominal wall cause pain in patients with peritonitis). The cough test is positive if the patient, in response to a cough, shows signs of pain, such as flinching, grimacing, or moving hands toward the abdomen.[14]

5. Abdominal Wall Tenderness Test

In 1926 Carnett introduced the abdominal wall tenderness test[15] as a way to diagnose lesions in the abdominal wall that cause abdominal pain and tenderness and sometimes mimic peritonitis. In this test, the clinician locates the area of maximal tenderness by gentle palpation and then applies enough pressure to elicit moderate tenderness. The patient is then asked to fold the arms on the chest and lift the head and shoulders, as if performing a partial sit-up. If this maneuver causes increased tenderness at the site of palpation, the test is positive,[16] which traditionally argues against peritonitis because tense abdominal wall muscles should protect the peritoneum from the clinician's hands.

One well-recognized cause of acute abdominal wall tenderness is diabetic neuropathy (i.e., "thoraco-abdominal neuropathy" involving nerve roots T7 to T11; lesions of T1 to T6 cause chest pain).[17-22] In addition to a positive abdominal wall tenderness test, characteristic signs of this disorder are cutaneous hypersensitivity, often of contiguous dermatomes, and weakness of the abdominal muscles, causing ipsilateral bulging of the abdominal wall that sometimes resembles a hernia.[18,19,21]

B. APPENDICITIS

1. McBurney's Point Tenderness

In a paper read before the New York Surgical Society in 1889 that cited the advantages of early operation in appendicitis, Charles McBurney stated that all patients with appendicitis have maximal pain and tenderness "determined by the pressure of the finger (at a point) very exactly between an inch and a half and two inches from the anterior superior spinous process of the ilium on a straight line drawn from that process to the umbilicus."[23,24]

2.   Rovsing's Sign

Rovsing's sign (Neils T. Rovsing, 1862–1927, Danish surgeon) is positive when pressure over the patient's *left* lower quadrant causes pain in the right lower quadrant.[7] This sign is sometimes called indirect tenderness.

3.   Rectal Tenderness

In patients with appendicitis whose inflammation is confined to the pelvis, rectal examination may reveal tenderness, especially on the right side, and some patients with perforation may have a rectal mass (i.e., pelvic abscess).

4.   Psoas Sign

The inflamed appendix may lie against the right psoas muscle, causing the patient to shorten that muscle by drawing up the right knee. To elicit the psoas sign, the patient lies down on the left side and the clinician hyperextends the right hip. Painful hip extension is the positive response.[7,11]

5.   Obturator Sign

The obturator sign is based on the same principle as the psoas sign, that stretching a pelvic muscle irritated by an inflamed appendix causes pain. To stretch the right obturator internus muscle and elicit the sign, the clinician flexes the patient's right hip and knee and then internally rotates the right hip.[7,11]

C.   CHOLECYSTITIS AND MURPHY'S SIGN

Patients with acute cholecystitis present with continuous epigastric or right upper quadrant pain, nausea, and vomiting. The traditional physical signs are fever, right upper quadrant tenderness, and a positive Murphy's sign. In 1903, the American surgeon Charles Murphy stated that the hypersensitive gallbladder of cholecystitis prevents the patient from taking in a "full, deep inspiration when the clinician's fingers are hooked up beneath the right costal arch below the hepatic margin. The diaphragm forces the liver down until the sensitive gallbladder reaches the examining fingers, when the inspiration suddenly ceases as though it had been shut off."[25]

Most clinicians elicit Murphy's sign by palpating the right upper quadrant of the supine patient. In his original description, Murphy proposed other methods, such as the "deep grip palpation" technique, in which the clinician examines the seated patient from behind and curls the fingertips of his or her right hand under the right costal margin, and the "hammer stroke percussion" technique, in which the clinician strikes a finger pointed into the right upper quadrant with the ulnar aspect of the other hand.[25]

D.   SMALL BOWEL OBSTRUCTION

Small bowel obstruction presents with abdominal pain and vomiting. The traditional physical signs are abdominal distension and tenderness, visible peristalsis, and abnormal bowel sounds (initially, high-pitched tinkling sounds followed by diminished or absent bowel sounds).[7,11] Signs of peritonitis (e.g., rigidity, rebound) may appear if portions of the bowel become ischemic.

III. CLINICAL SIGNIFICANCE

EBM Box 48-1, EBM Box 48-2, EBM Box 48-3, and EBM Box 48-4 present the physical findings of the acute abdomen. EBM Boxes 48-1 and 48-4 apply to all patients with acute abdominal pain and tenderness and address how well physical signs identify peritonitis (see EBM Box 48-1) and small bowel

 Box 48-1   Acute Abdominal Pain, Signs Detecting Peritonitis*

Finding (Ref)[†]	Sensitivity (%)	Specificity (%)	Likelihood Ratio if Finding Present	Absent
Abdominal examination				
Guarding[2,26–33]	13–76	56–97	2.6	0.6
Rigidity[2,30–32,34]	6–40	86–100	**3.9**	NS
Rebound tenderness[2,26–40]	40–95	20–89	2.1	0.5
Percussion tenderness[33]	65	73	2.4	0.5
Abnormal bowel sounds[2,32]	25–61	44–95	NS	0.8
Rectal examination				
Rectal tenderness[2,29,30,32,33,35,36,41]	20–53	41–96	NS	NS
Other tests				
Positive abdominal wall tenderness test[16,42]	1–5	32–72	**0.1**	NS
Positive cough test[14,26,34,40]	73–84	44–79	1.8	0.4

NS, not significant; likelihood ratio (LR) if finding present = positive LR; LR if finding absent = negative LR.
*Diagnostic standard: For peritonitis, surgical exploration and follow-up of patients not operated on; causes of peritonitis included appendicitis (most common), cholecystitis, and perforated ulcer. One study also included patients with pancreatitis.[32]
†Definition of findings: For abnormal bowel sounds, absent, diminished, or hyperactive; for abdominal wall tenderness test, see text; for positive cough test, the patient is asked to cough, and during the cough shows signs of pain or clearly reduces the intensity of the cough to avoid pain.[26]

PERITONITIS

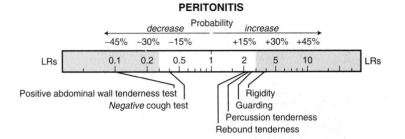

 Box 48-2 Acute Right Lower Quadrant Tenderness, Signs Detecting Appendicitis*

Finding (Ref)[†]	Sensitivity (%)	Specificity (%)	Likelihood Ratio if Finding	
			Present	Absent
Vital signs				
Fever[26,36,39,44]	47–81	40–70	1.5	0.6
Abdominal examination				
Severe right lower quadrant tenderness[26,27]	87–99	8–65	NS	**0.2**
McBurney's point tenderness[26,27,45]	50–94	75–86	**3.4**	0.4
Rovsing's sign[27,28,31,41]	22–68	58–96	2.5	0.7
Rectal examination				
Rectal tenderness[29,30,33,35,36,41]	38–53	41–62	NS	NS
Other signs				
Psoas sign[28,29,33]	13–42	79–97	2.0	NS
Obturator sign[29]	8	94	NS	NS

NS, not significant; likelihood ratio (LR) if finding present = positive LR; LR if finding absent = negative LR.

*Diagnostic standard: For appendicitis, surgical findings, histology, and follow-up of patients not operated on.

[†]Definition of findings: For fever, temperature > 37.3° C[36,39,44] or not defined[26]; for positive cough test, see EBM Box 48-1.

APPENDICITIS

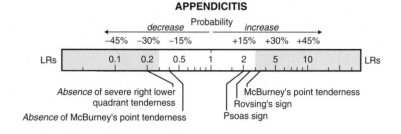

CHOLECYSTITIS

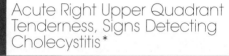

Box 48-3 — Acute Right Upper Quadrant Tenderness, Signs Detecting Cholecystitis*

Finding (Ref)†	Sensitivity (%)	Specificity (%)	Likelihood Ratio if Finding Present	Likelihood Ratio if Finding Absent
Fever[60–63]	29–44	37–83	NS	NS
Murphy's sign[64–66]	48–97	48–79	1.9	0.6
Back tenderness[67]	27	36	0.4	2.0
Right upper quadrant mass[60,62,63,67]	2–23	70–99	NS	NS

NS, not significant; likelihood ratio (LR) if finding present = positive LR; LR if finding absent = negative LR.

*Diagnostic standard: For cholecystitis, positive hepatobiliary scintiscan[65] or surgical findings and histology.[60,62–64,66,67]

†Definition of findings: For fever, temperature >37.5°C,[63] >37.7°C,[61] >38°C,[62] or undefined.[60]

obstruction (see EBM Box 48-4) (these studies included almost 4000 patients). EBM Boxes 48-2 and 48-3 refer to only a subset of patients with abdominal pain: EBM Box 48-2 applies to patients with right lower quadrant tenderness and suspected appendicitis, and EBM Box 48-3 applies to patients with right upper quadrant pain and suspected cholecystitis.

Box 48-4 Acute Abdominal Pain, Signs Detecting Bowel Obstruction*

Finding (Ref)[†]	Sensitivity (%)	Specificity (%)	Likelihood Ratio if Finding	
			Present	Absent
Inspection of abdomen				
Visible peristalsis[3]	6	100	**18.8**	NS
Distended abdomen[1,3,32]	58–67	89–96	**9.6**	0.4
Palpation of abdomen				
Guarding[1,2,32]	20–63	47–78	NS	NS
Rigidity[1–3,32]	6–18	75–99	NS	NS
Rebound tenderness[1,2,32]	22–40	52–82	NS	NS
Auscultation of abdomen				
Hyperactive bowel sounds[3,32]	40–42	89–94	**5.0**	0.6
Abnormal bowel sounds[1–3,32]	63–93	43–88	**3.2**	0.4
Rectal examination				
Rectal tenderness[1,2,32]	4–26	72–94	NS	NS

NS, not significant; likelihood ratio (LR) if finding present = positive LR; LR if finding absent = negative LR.
**Diagnostic standard:* For small bowel obstruction, surgical findings, abdominal radiographs, and clinical follow-up.*
[†]Definition of findings: For abnormal bowel sounds, hyperactive, absent, or diminished bowel sounds.

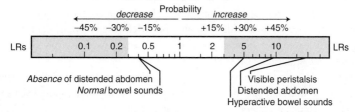

BOWEL OBSTRUCTION

A. PERITONITIS (SEE EBM BOX 48-1)

The primary cause of peritonitis in the studies of EBM Box 48-1 was appendicitis, although some patients had perforated ulcers, perforated diverticula, or cholecystitis. According to these studies, the most compelling findings arguing *for* peritonitis are rigidity [likelihood ratio (LR) = 3.9], guarding (LR = 2.6), and percussion tenderness (LR = 2.4). The findings arguing the most *against* peritonitis are a *positive* abdominal wall tenderness test (LR = 0.1) and a *negative* cough test (LR = 0.4). The presence or absence of rebound tenderness (positive LR = 2.1, negative LR = 0.5) shifts probability relatively little, confirming the long-held opinion of expert surgeons that rebound tenderness adds little to what clinicians already know from gentle palpation.

Unhelpful findings in the diagnosis of peritonitis are the character of the bowel sounds and the presence or absence of rectal tenderness.

B. APPENDICITIS

In patients with acute abdominal pain, the *absence* of right lower quadrant tenderness is a compelling argument *against* the diagnosis of appendicitis (sensitivity of right lower quadrant tenderness is 94% to 97%, negative LR = 0.1).[40,43]

1. Individual Findings (See EBM Box 48-2)

Just as rigidity and guarding argue for peritonitis in patients with acute abdominal pain (see EBM Box 48-1), these findings also argue for appendicitis in patients with right lower quadrant pain (the positive LR for rigidity is 3.2; for guarding, 2.3).[26–31,33,34] Other findings that argue *for* appendicitis are McBurney's point tenderness (LR = 3.4), a positive Rovsing's sign (LR = 2.5), and positive psoas sign (LR = 2.0). The absence of severe right lower quadrant tenderness (LR = 0.2), the absence of McBurney's point tenderness (LR = 0.4), and the negative cough test argue *against* appendicitis (LR = 0.4).[26,34] Again, rebound tenderness is one of the least discriminating of signs (positive LR = 1.9, negative LR = 0.5).*

McBurney's point tenderness may have even greater accuracy if every patient's appendix were precisely at McBurney's point, but radiologic investigation reveals that location of the normal appendix sometimes lies a short distance away.[46] In one study of patients with acute abdominal pain, clinicians first located the patient's appendix using hand-held ultrasound equipment. Maximal pinpoint tenderness over this "sonographic McBurney's point" had superior diagnostic accuracy for detecting appendicitis (sensitivity 87%, specificity 90%, positive LR 8.4, negative LR 0.1).[47]

In contrast to a long-held traditional teaching, giving analgesics to patients with acute abdominal pain does not change the accuracy of individual signs nor reduce the clinician's overall diagnostic accuracy.[48,49]

Findings having little or no diagnostic value in diagnosing appendicitis are rectal tenderness (whether the tenderness is generalized or confined to the right rectum) and the obturator sign (LRs not significant).[50] Nonetheless, a rectal

---

*The likelihood ratios for rigidity, guarding, rebound tenderness, and cough test do not appear in EBM Box 48-2, because they are similar to those already shown in EBM Box 48-1.

examination should still be performed to detect the rare patient (2% or less) with a pelvic abscess and rectal mass.[30,32]

2. Combination of Findings

Many scoring systems have been developed to improve diagnostic accuracy and reduce the negative appendectomy rate in patients with acute right lower quadrant tenderness.[27,28,36,41,43,51–56] Most of these scoring systems, however, are suboptimal because they are based on either simple conversion of individual LRs to "diagnostic weights," without first performing tests of independence,[28,36,41,51,52,54] or on arbitrary diagnostic weights based on traditional teachings.[53] The few studies available that looked at the independence of findings investigated relatively few physical signs.[27,40,43,56] When scoring systems are compared to usual clinical care, they fail to reduce the duration of hospital stay, frequency of nontherapeutic operations, or number of delayed surgeries resulting in perforations,[57] and in some studies, they are actually inferior to the clinical judgment of experienced surgeons.[4,56,58,59]

C. CHOLECYSTITIS (SEE EBM BOX 48-3)

In patients with right upper quadrant pain and suspected cholecystitis, a positive Murphy's sign argues modestly *for* cholecystitis (LR = 1.9). The presence of back tenderness argues somewhat *against* cholecystitis (LR = 0.4), probably because it is more commonly found in alternative diagnoses such as renal disease or pancreatitis.[67] The presence or absence of a right upper quadrant mass is unhelpful, probably because a palpable tender gallbladder is uncommon in cholecystitis (sensitivity <25%) and because the sensation of a right upper quadrant mass may occur in other diagnoses, such as liver disease or localized rigidity of the abdominal wall from other disorders.

There is also a "sonographic Murphy's sign," elicited during ultrasonography of the right upper quadrant, which is simply the finding of maximal tenderness over the gallbladder. Studies of this sign in patients with right upper quadrant pain reveal much better diagnostic accuracy than conventional palpation: sensitivity 63%, specificity 94%, positive LR = 9.9, and negative LR = 0.4.[68] The superior accuracy of this sign, which also relies on palpation of the abdominal wall, suggests that the poorer accuracy of conventional palpation is due to the difficulty precisely locating the position of the gallbladder.

Murphy's sign may be even less accurate in elderly patients, because up to 25% of patients older than 60 years of age with cholecystitis lack any abdominal tenderness whatsoever.[69] Although most of these patients have abdominal pain, some have altered mental status and lack this symptom as well.

In patients with a pyogenic liver abscess, the presence of Murphy's sign argues that the patient has associated biliary tract sepsis (sensitivity 32%, specificity 88%, positive LR 2.8, negative LR not significant).[70]

D. SMALL BOWEL OBSTRUCTION (SEE EBM BOX 48-4)

In patients with acute abdominal pain, the findings of visible peristalsis (LR = 18.8), abdominal distension (LR = 9.6), and hyperactive bowel sounds (LR = 5.0) all argue *for* bowel obstruction (though visible peristalsis is a rare finding, occurring in only 6% of patients). Diminished or absent bowel sounds also occur in obstruction, being found in 1 of 4 patients.[3,32]

The findings arguing somewhat *against* obstruction are normal bowel sounds (i.e., not hyperactive, absent, or diminished) and the absence of a distended abdomen (both LRs = 0.4). Nonetheless, 30% to 40% of patients with obstruction lack abdominal distension, especially early in the course or if the obstruction is high in the intestines. The findings of peritoneal irritation—rigidity and rebound tenderness—argue neither for nor against the diagnosis of obstruction.

E. RENAL COLIC

In one study of 1333 patients presenting with acute abdominal pain, two findings were accurate signs of ureterolithiasis (as diagnosed by imaging or follow-up): loin tenderness (sensitivity 15%, specificity 99%, positive LR = 27.7, negative LR = 0.9) and renal tenderness (sensitivity 86%, specificity 76%, positive LR = 3.6, negative LR = 0.2). As compelling as these findings are, they are less important than the finding of microscopic hematuria, which has a sensitivity of 75%, specificity of 99%, positive LR of 73.1, and negative LR of 0.3.[71]

CHRONIC ABDOMINAL PAIN

In one study of patients with chronic abdominal pain, the abdominal wall tenderness test (see "Abdominal Wall Tenderness Test") argued significantly *against* a visceral cause of the pain (LR = 0.1; EBM Box 48-5). In these patients, a positive abdominal wall tenderness test argued that the pain would respond to an injection of combined anesthetic/corticosteroid into the tender spot and that *no* serious pathology would be discovered during 3 or more months of follow-up (LR = 7.0).[72]

Beyond this finding, there is relatively little information on the accuracy of examination in diagnosing chronic abdominal pain. Most studies show that the finding of abdominal tenderness is common in many nonorganic disorders and has little diagnostic value. In patients with suspected biliary colic, right upper quadrant tenderness does not distinguish patients with cholelithiasis from

Box 48-5 Chronic Abdominal Pain*

Finding (Ref)[†]	Sensitivity (%)	Specificity (%)	Likelihood Ratio if Finding	
			Present	Absent
Positive abdominal wall tenderness test, detecting visceral pain[72]	11	21	**0.1**	**4.2**
Right upper quadrant tenderness, detecting cholelithiasis[73]	53	51	NS	NS
Lower abdominal tenderness, detecting cholelithiasis[73]	21	57	0.5	1.4
Epigastric tenderness, detecting positive upper endoscopy[74]	63	31	NS	NS

NS, not significant; likelihood ratio (LR) if finding present = positive LR; LR if finding absent = negative LR.
*Diagnostic standard: For cholelithiasis, ultrasonography or oral cholecystogram[73]; for positive upper endoscopy, findings on upper gastrointestinal endoscopy, most of which were peptic ulcers; for visceral pain, pain originating from an intraabdominal organ or structure (i.e., not abdominal wall).
†Definition of findings: For abdominal wall tenderness test, see text.

CHRONIC ABDOMINAL PAIN

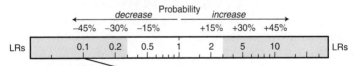

Positive abdominal wall tenderness test, *arguing against* visceral pain

those without, although lower abdominal tenderness argues modestly against cholelithiasis (LR = 0.5; see EBM Box 48-5). In patients with dyspepsia, epigastric tenderness does not help predict whether upper endoscopy will reveal an ulcer, some other abnormality, or normal findings.

Even if the finding of tenderness has little value, abdominal examination is still important in these patients, to detect masses, organomegaly, and signs of a surgical abdomen (see previous).

REFERENCES

1. Eskelinen M, Ikonen J, Lipponen P. Contributions of history-taking, physical examination, and computer assistance to diagnosis of acute small-bowel obstruction: A prospective study of 1333 patients with acute abdominal pain. *Scand J Gastroenterol.* 1994;29:715-721.

2. Brewer RJ, Golden GT, Hitch DC, et al. Abdominal pain: An analysis of 1000 consecutive cases in a University hospital emergency room. *Am J Surg.* 1976;131: 219-223.

3. Böhner H, Yang Z, Franke C, et al. Simple data from history and physical examination help to exclude bowel obstruction and to avoid radiographic studies in patients with acute abdominal pain. *Eur J Surg.* 1998;164:777-784.

4. Ohmann C, Yang Q, Franke C. Diagnostic scores for acute appendicitis. *Eur J Surg.* 1995;161:273-281.

5. Paulson EK, Kalady MF, Pappas TN. Suspected appendicitis. *N Engl J Med.* 2003; 348:236-242.

6. Silen W. Pitfalls to avoid when evaluating severe abdominal pain. *J Crit Ill.* 1992;7: 685-689.

7. Clain A, ed. *Hamilton Bailey's demonstrations of physical signs in clinical surgery.* Bristol: Wright; 1986.

8. Meyerowitz BR. Abdominal palpation by stethoscope. *Arch Surg.* 1976;111:831.

9. Mellinkoff SM. "Stethoscope sign." *N Engl J Med.* 1964;271:630.

10. Celsus. De Medicina. Spencer WG, trans. *De Medicina* (English translation of Latin edition written between A.D. 25 and 35, printed in 1478). Cambridge: Harvard University Press; 1953.

11. Cope Z. *The early diagnosis of the acute abdomen.* London: Oxford University Press; 1972.

12. Lawrie R. Acute peritonitis. *Practitioner.* 1964;192:759-765.

13. Bailey H. *Demonstrations of physical signs in clinical surgery,* 11th ed. Baltimore: Williams and Wilkins; 1949.

14. Bennett DH, Tambeur LJMT, Campbell WB. Use of coughing test to diagnose peritonitis. *Br Med J.* 1994;308:1336.

15. Carnett JB. Intercostal neuralgia as a cause of abdominal pain and tenderness. *Surg Gynecol Obstet.* 1926;42:625-632.

16. Gray DWR, G. S, Dixon JM, Collin J. Is abdominal wall tenderness a useful sign in the diagnosis of non-specific abdominal pain? *Ann R Coll Surg Engl.* 1988;70: 233-234.

17. Hershfield NB. The abdominal wall: A frequently overlooked source of abdominal pain. *J Clin Gastroenterol.* 1992;14:199-202.

18. Chaudhuri KR, Wren DR, Werring D, Watkins PJ. Unilateral abdominal muscle herniation with pain: A distinctive variant of diabetic radiculopathy. *Diab Med.* 1997;14:803-807.

19. Stewart JD. Diabetic truncal neuropathy: Topography of the sensory deficit. *Ann Neurol.* 1989;25:233-238.

20. Sun SF, Streib EW. Diabetic thoracoabdominal neuropathy: Clinical and electro-diagnostic features. *Ann Neurol.* 1981;9:75-79.

21. Parry GJ, Floberg J. Diabetic truncal neuropathy presenting as abdominal hernia. *Neurology.* 1989;39:1488-1490.

22. Kikta DG, Breuer AC, Wilbourn AJ. Thoracic root pain in diabetes: The spectrum of clinical and electromyographic findings. *Ann Neurol.* 1982;11:80-85.

23. McBurney C. Experience with early operative interference in cases of disease of the vermiform appendix (reprinted in classic articles in colonic and rectal surgery). *Dis Colon Rect.* 1998;26(4):291-303.

24. Cope Z. *A history of the acute abdomen.* London: Oxford University Press; 1965.

25. Aldea PA, Meehan JP, Sternbach G. The acute abdomen and Murphy's signs. *J Emerg Med.* 1986;4:57-63.

26. Golledge J, Toms AP, Franklin IJ, et al. Assessment of peritonism in appendicitis. *Ann R Coll Surg Engl.* 1996;78:11-14.

27. Andersson RE, Hugander AP, Ghazi SH, et al. Diagnostic value of disease history, clinical presentation, and inflammatory parameters of appendicitis. *World J Surg.* 1999;23:133-140.

28. Izbicki JR, Knoefel WT, Wilker DK, et al. Accurate diagnosis of acute appendicitis: A retrospective and prospective analysis of 686 patients. *Eur J Surg.* 1992;158:227-231.

29. Berry J, Malt RA. Appendicitis near its centenary. *Ann Surg.* 1984;200:567-575.

30. Dixon JM, Elton RA, Rainey JB, Macleod DAD. Rectal examination in patients with pain in the right lower quadrant of the abdomen. *Br Med J.* 1991;302:386-388.

31. Alshehri MY, Ibrahim A, Abuaisha N, et al. Value of rebound tenderness in acute appendicitis. *East Afr Med J.* 1995;72:504-507.

32. Staniland JR, Ditchburn J, De Dombal FT. Clinical presentation of acute abdomen: Study of 600 patients. *Br Med J.* 1972;3:393-398.

33. John H, Neff U, Kelemen M. Appendicitis diagnosis today: Clinical and ultrasonic deductions. *World J Surg.* 1993;17:243-249.

34. Fenyo G, Linberg G, Blind P, et al. Diagnostic decision support in suspected acute appendicitis: Validation of a simplified scoring system. *Eur J Surg.* 1997;163:831-838.

35. Nauta RJ, Magnant C. Observation versus operation for abdominal pain in the right lower quadrant: Roles of the clinical examination and the leukocyte count. *Am J Surg.* 1986;151:746-748.

36. Alvarado A. A practical score for the early diagnosis of acute appendicitis. *Ann Emerg Med.* 1986;15:557-564.

37. Liddington MI, Thomson WHF. Rebound tenderness test. *Br J Surg.* 1991;78:795-796.

38. Prout WG. The significance of rebound tenderness in the acute abdomen. *Br J Surg.* 1970;57:508-510.

39. Gwynn LK. The diagnosis of acute appendicitis: Clinical assessment versus computed tomography evaluation. *J Emerg Med.* 2001;21:119-123.

40. Hallan S, Asberg A, Edna TH. Estimating the probability of acute appendicitis using clinical criteria of a stuctured record sheet: The physician against the computer. *Eur J Surg.* 1997;163:427-432.

41. Jahn H, Mathiesen FK, Neckelmann K, et al. Comparison of clinical judgment and diagnostic ultrasonography in the diagnosis of acute appendicitis: Experience with a score-aided diagnosis. *Eur J Surg.* 1997;163:433-443.

42. Thomson H, Francis DMA. Abdominal-wall tenderness: A useful sign in the acute abdomen. *Lancet.* 1977;2:1053-1054.

43. Eskelinen M, Ikonen J, Lipponen P. The value of history-taking, physical examination, and computer assistance in the diagnosis of acute appendicitis in patients more than 50 years old. *Scand J Gastroenterol.* 1995;30:349-355.

44. Cardall T, Glasser J, Guss DA. Clinical value of the total white blood cell count and temperature in the evaluation of patients with suspected appendicitis. *Acad Emerg Med.* 2004;11:1021-1027.

45. Lane R, Grabham J. A useful sign for the diagnosis of peritoneal irritation in the right iliac fossa. *Ann R Coll Surg Engl.* 1997;79:128-129.

46. Ramsden WH, Mannion RAJ, Simpkins KC, DeDombal FT. Is the appendix where you think it is—And if not does it matter? *Clin Radiol.* 1993;47:100-103.

47. Soda K, Nemoto K, Yoshizawa S, et al. Detection of pinpoint tenderness on the appendix under ultrasonography is useful to confirm acute appendicitis. *Arch Surg.* 2001;136:1136-1140.

48. Mahadevan M, Graff L. Prospective randomized study of analgesic use for ED patients with right lower quadrant abndominal pain. *Am J Emerg Med.* 2000;18: 753-756.

49. Thomas SH, Silen W, Cheeman F, et al. Effects of morphine analgesia on diagnostic accuracy in emergency department patients with abdominal pain: A prospective, randomized trial. *J Am Coll Surg.* 2003;196:18-31.

50. Manimaran N, Galland RB. Significance of routine digital rectal examination in adults presenting with abdominal pain. *Ann R Coll Surg Engl.* 2004;86:292-295.

51. Arnbjörnsson E. Scoring system for computer-aided diagnosis of acute appendicitis: The value of prospective versus retrospective studies. *Ann Chir Gynaecol.* 1985;74:159-166.

52. Teicher I, Landa B, Cohen M, et al. Scoring system to aid in diagnoses of appendicitis. *Ann Surg.* 1982;198:753-759.

53. Christian F, Christian GP. A simple scoring system to reduce the negative appendicectomy rate. *Ann R Coll Surg Engl.* 1992;74:281-285.

54. Fenyo G. Routine use of a scoring system for decision-making in suspected acute appendicitis in adults. *Acta Chir Scand.* 1987;153:545-551.

55. Van Way CW, Murphy JR, Dunn EL, Elerding SC. A feasibility study of computer aided diagnosis in appendicitis. *Surg Gynecol Obstetr.* 1982;155:685-688.

56. Ohmann C, Franke C, Yang Q. Clinical benefit of a diagnostic score for appendicitis: Results of a prospective interventional study. *Arch Surg.* 1999;134:993-996.

57. Douglas CD, Macpherson NE, Davidson PM, Gani JS. Randomised controlled trial of ultrasonography in diagnosis of acute appendicitis, incorporating the Alvarado score. *BMJ.* 2000;321:919-922.

58. Pruekprasert P, Geater A, Ksuntigij P, et al. Accuracy in diagnosis of acute appendicitis by comparing serum C-reactive protein measurements, Alvarado score and clinical impression of surgeons. *J Med Assoc Thai.* 2004;87:296-302.

59. Zielke A, Sitter H, Rampp T, et al. Clinical decision-making, ultrasonography, and scores for evaluation of suspected acute appendicitis. *World J Surg.* 2001;25:578-584.

60. Bednarz GM, Kalff V, Kelly MJ. Hepatobiliary scintigraphy: Increasing the accuracy of the preoperative diagnosis of acute cholecystitis. *Med J Aust.* 1986;145:316-318.

61. Gruber PJ, Silverman RA, Gottesfeld S, Flaster E. Presence of fever and leukocytosis in acute cholecystitis. *Ann Emerg Med.* 1996;28:273-277.

62. Wegge C, Kjaergaaqrd J. Evaluation of symptoms and signs of gallstone disease in patients admitted with upper abdominal pain. *Scand J Gastroenterol.* 1985;20:933-936.

63. Schofield PF, Hulton NR, Baildam AD. Is it acute cholecystitis? *Ann R Coll Surg Engl.* 1986;68:14-16.

64. Adedeji OA, McAdam WAF. Murphy's sign, acute cholecystitis and elderly people. *J R Coll Surg Engl.* 1996;41:88-89.

65. Singer AJ, McCracken G, Henry MC, et al. Correlation among clinical, laboratory, and hepatobiliary scanning findings in patients with suspected acute cholecystitis. *Ann Emerg Med.* 1996;28:267-272.

66. Mills LD, Mills T, Foster B. Association of clinical and laboratory variables with ultrasound findings in right upper quadrant abdominal pain. *South Med J.* 2005; 98:155-161.

67. Halasz NA. Counterfeit cholecystitis: A common diagnostic dilemma. *Am J Surg.* 1975;130:189-193.

68. Ralls PW, Halls J, Lapin SA, et al. Prospective evaluation of the sonographic Murphy sign in suspected acute cholecystitis. *J Clin Ultrasound.* 1982;10:113-115.

69. Morrow DJ, Thompson J, Wilson SE. Acute cholecystitis in the elderly: A surgical emergency. *Arch Surg.* 1978;113:1149-1152.

70. Chen SC, Yen CH, Tsao SM, et al. Comparison of pyogenic liver abscesses of biliary and cryptogenic origin. *Swiss Med Wkly.* 2005;135:344-351.

71. Eskelinen M, Ikonen J, Lipponen P. Usefulness of history-taking, physical examination and diagnostic scoring in acute renal colic. *Eur Urol.* 1998;34:467-473.

72. Srinivasan R, Greenbaum DS. Chronic abdominal wall pain: A frequently overlooked problem. Practical approach to diagnosis and management. *Am J Gastroenterol.* 2002; 97:824-830.

73. Diehl AK, Sugarek NJ, Todd KH. Clinical evaluation for gallstone disease: Usefulness of symptoms and signs in diagnosis. *Am J Med.* 1990;89:29-33.

74. Priebe WM, DaCosta LR, Beck IT. Is epigastric tenderness a sign of peptic ulcer disease? *Gastroenterology.* 1982;82:16-19.

Auscultation of the Abdomen

ABDOMINAL BRUITS

I. THE FINDING

Abdominal bruits are murmurs heard during auscultation of the abdomen. Like any murmur generated outside the four heart chambers, abdominal bruits may extend beyond the confines of the first and second heart sounds from systole into diastole (i.e., they may be "continuous"; see Chapter 39). Most bruits are detected in the epigastrium or upper abdominal quadrants.

II. CLINICAL SIGNIFICANCE

A. BRUITS IN HEALTHY PERSONS

Bruits occur in 4% to 20% of healthy persons.[1-5] Abdominal bruits are more common in those younger than 40 years than in older persons.[1,4-6]

Characteristically, the abdominal bruit of a healthy individual is systolic, medium- to low-pitched, and audible between the xiphoid process and umbilicus.[1] Only rarely does it spread to the patient's sides, in contrast to abnormal bruits, which are often loudest away from the epigastrium (see later). Arteriograms reveal that the most common source for the normal abdominal bruit is the patient's celiac artery.[6]

B. RENOVASCULAR HYPERTENSION

In patients with renal artery stenosis and renovascular hypertension, an abdominal bruit may be heard in the epigastrium, although the sound some-times radiates to one side.[1] In one study of patients referred because of severe hypertension that was difficult to control—a setting suggesting reno-vascular hypertension—the finding of a *systolic/diastolic* abdominal bruit was virtually diagnostic for renovascular hypertension (likelihood ratio [LR] = 38.9, EBM Box 49-1). In contrast, the finding in similar patients of *any* abdominal bruit (i.e., one not necessarily extending into diastole) is less com-pelling (LR = 5.6), probably because they also occur in persons without ren-ovascular hypertension (see "Bruits in Healthy Persons").

The abdominal bruit of renovascular hypertension, however, does not always originate in the renal artery. In one study of patients undergoing surgery for renal artery stenosis, intraoperative auscultation localized the bruit to the

Box 49-1 Auscultation of Abdomen*

Finding (Ref)	Sensitivity (%)	Specificity (%)	Likelihood Ratio if Finding	
			Present	Absent
Abdominal bruit—any				
Detecting renovascular hypertension[2,3,7,8]	27–56	89–96	**5.6**	0.6
Detecting abdominal aortic aneurysm[9]	11	95	NS	NS
Abdominal bruit—systolic/diastolic				
Detecting renovascular hypertension[10]	39	99	**38.9**	0.6

NS, not significant; likelihood ratio (LR) if finding present = positive LR; LR if finding absent = negative LR.
Diagnostic standard: For renovascular hypertension, renal angiography,[2,3,7,8] sometimes combined with renal vein renin ratio >1.5[10] or cure of hypertension after surgery [7]; for abdominal aortic aneurysm, see EBM Box 47-2 in Chapter 47.

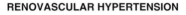

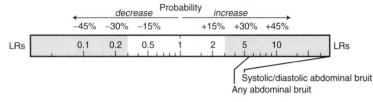

RENOVASCULAR HYPERTENSION

renal arteries as the sole source only about half the time.[1] In the remaining patients, other vessels alone or with the renal artery generated the sound. Possibly, bruits in these patients are general markers of vascular disease, just as the finding of a carotid bruit has been associated with disease in other distant vascular beds, such as the coronary vasculature.[11]

C.   OTHER DISORDERS

Harsh, epigastric or right upper quadrant bruits (systolic and continuous) have been repeatedly described in patients with hepatic malignancies[12,13] and hepatic cirrhosis.[12,14] In these patients, the sound may represent extrinsic compression of vessels by tumor or regenerating nodules, the hypervascular tumor, or portosystemic collateral vessels. Left upper quadrant bruits occur in patients with carcinoma of the body of the pancreas (8 of 21 patients in one study).[15] Other rare causes of abdominal bruits are renal artery aneurysms,[16] aortocaval fistulae,[17] ischemic bowel disease,[18] and celiac compression syndrome.[19] Although an abdominal bruit is traditionally associated with abdominal aortic aneurysm, the finding had no diagnostic value in one study (LR not significant, see EBM Box 49-1).[9]

HEPATIC RUB

In the absence of recent liver biopsy, the finding of a hepatic friction rub has been repeatedly associated with intrahepatic malignancy, either hepatoma or metastatic disease.[13,20] In one study of tumors metastatic to the liver, 10% of patients had a hepatic friction rub.[21]

BOWEL SOUNDS

I.   THE FINDING

Most clinicians have great difficulty making any sense out of a patient's bowel sounds, for two reasons: (1) Normal bowel sounds, from moment to moment, vary greatly in pitch, intensity, and frequency. One healthy person may have no bowel sounds for up to 4 minutes, but when examined later may have more than 30 discrete sounds per minute.[22] The activity of normal bowel sounds may cycle with peak-to-peak periods as long as 50 to 60 minutes,[23] meaning that any analysis based on even several minutes of bedside auscultation is a very incomplete sample. (2) Bowel sounds generated at one point of the intestinal tract radiate widely over the entire abdominal wall.[22,24] The sounds heard in the right lower quadrant, for example, may actually originate in the stomach. This dissemination of bowel sounds makes the practice of listening to them in all four quadrants fundamentally unsound, because, as an example, the left lower quadrant may be quieter than the left upper quadrant not because the descending colon is making less noise than the stomach, but instead because the entire abdomen has become quieter, at least for the moment the clinician is listening to the lower quadrant.

Most bowel sounds are generated in the stomach, followed by the large intestine and then the small bowel.[25] The overall frequency of bowel sounds increases after a meal.[26] The actual cause of bowel sounds is still debated; experiments with exteriorized loops of bowel in dogs show many intestinal contractions to be silent, although sound often occurs when contractions propel contents through a bowel segment that is not relaxed.[22]

II. CLINICAL SIGNIFICANCE

Analysis of the bowel sounds has modest value in diagnosing small bowel obstruction. After experimental complete bowel obstruction in animals, bowel sounds are hyperactive for about 30 minutes before becoming diminished or absent.[23] In patients with small bowel obstruction, clinical observation shows that about 40% have hyperactive bowel sounds and about 25% have diminished or absent bowel sounds.[27,28] Consequently, because most patients with small bowel obstruction have abnormal bowel sounds, the finding of *normal* bowel sounds in a patient with acute abdominal pain argues somewhat *against* the diagnosis of bowel obstruction (LR = 0.4, see EBM Box 48-4 in Chapter 48).

A traditional finding of peritonitis is diminished or absent bowel sounds, although studies of patients with acute abdominal pain show this finding to be unreliable (see Chapter 48).

REFERENCES

1. Julius S, Stewart BH. Diagnostic significance of abdominal murmurs. *N Engl J Med.* 1967;276:1175-1178.

2. Krijnen P, van Jaarsveld BC, Steyerberg EW, et al. A clinical prediction rule for renal artery stenosis. *Ann Intern Med.* 1998;129:705-711.

3. Carmichael DJS, Mathias CJ, Snell ME, Peart S. Detection and investigation of renal artery stenosis. *Lancet.* 1986;1:667-670.

4. McSherry JA. The prevalence of epigastric bruit. *J R Coll Gen Pract.* 1979;29:170-172.

5. Rivin AU. Abdominal vascular sounds. *JAMA.* 1972;221:688-690.

6. McLoughlin MJ, Colapinto RF, Hobbs BB. Abdominal bruits: Clinical and angiographic correlation. *JAMA.* 1975;232:1238-1242.

7. Simon N, Franklin SS, Bleifer KH, Maxwell MH. Clinical characteristics of renovascular hypertension. *JAMA.* 1972;220:1209-1218.

8. Svetsky LP, Helms MJ, Dunnick NR, Klotman PE. Clinical characteristics useful in screening for renovascular disease. *South Med J.* 1990;83:743-747.

9. Lederle FA, Walker JM, Reinke DB. Selective screening for abdominal aortic aneurysms with physical examination and ultrasound. *Arch Intern Med.* 1988;148:1753-1756.

10. Grim CE, Luft FC, Weinberger MH, Grim CM. Sensitivity and specificity of screening tests for renal vascular hypertension. *Ann Intern Med.* 1979;91:617-622.

11. Heymann A, Wilkerson WE, Heyden S, et al. Risk of stroke in asymptomatic persons with cervical arterial bruits: A population study in Evans County, Georgia. *N Engl J Med.* 1980;302:838-841.

12. Clain D, Wartnaby K, Sherlock S. Abdominal arterial murmurs in liver disease. *Lancet.* 1966;2:516-519.

13. Sherman HI, Hardison JE. The importance of a coexistent hepatic rub and bruit: A clue to the diagnosis of cancer of the liver. *JAMA.* 1979;241:1495.

14. McFadzean AJS, Gray J. Hepatic venous hum in cirrhosis of liver. *Lancet.* 1953;2:1128-1130.

15. Serebro H. A diagnostic sign of carcinoma of the body of the pancreas. *Lancet.* 1965;1:85-86.

16. Okamoto M, Hashimoto M, Sueda T, et al. Renal artery aneurysm: The significance of abdominal bruit and use of color Doppler. *Int Med.* 1992;31:1217-1219.

17. Potyk DK, Guthrie CR. Spontaneous aortocaval fistula. *Ann Emerg Med.* 1995;25:424-427.

18. Sarr MG, Dickson ER, Newcomer AD. Diastolic bruit in chronic intestinal ischemia: Recognition by abdominal phonoangiography. *Dig Dis Sci.* 1980;25:761-762.

19. Gutnik LM. Celiac artery compression syndrome. *Am J Med.* 1984;76:334-336.

20. Fred HL, Brown GR. The hepatic friction rub. *N Engl J Med.* 1962;266:554-555.

21. Fenster F, Klatskin G. Manifestations of metastatic tumors of the liver: A study of eighty-one patients subjected to needle biopsy. *Am J Med.* 1961;31:238-248.

22. Milton GW. Normal bowel sounds. *Med J Aust.* 1958;2:490-493.

23. Mynors JM. The bowel sounds. *S Afr J Surg.* 1969;7:87-91.

24. Watson WC, Knox EC. Phonoenterography: The recording and analysis of bowel sounds. *Gut.* 1967;8:88-94.

25. Politzer JP, Devroede G, Vasseur C, et al. The genesis of bowel sounds: Influence of viscus and gastrointestinal content. *Gastroenterology.* 1976;71:282-285.

26. Vasseur C, Devroede G, Dalle D, et al. Postprandial bowel sounds. *IEEE Trans Biomed Eng.* 1975;22:443-448.

27. Böhner H, Yang Z, Franke C, et al. Simple data from history and physical examination help to exclude bowel obstruction and to avoid radiographic studies in patients with acute abdominal pain. *Eur J Surg.* 1998;164:777-784.

28. Staniland JR, Ditchburn J, De Dombal FT. Clinical presentation of acute abdomen: Study of 600 patients. *Br Med J.* 1972;3:393-398.

EXTREMITIES

50

Peripheral Vascular Disease

I. INTRODUCTION

Chronic arterial disease usually affects three distinct segments in the lower limbs: (1) the aortoiliac (especially the infrarenal abdominal aorta and common iliac arteries), (2) the femoropopliteal (especially the superficial femoral artery in the adductor canal), and (3) the peroneotibial (below the knee).[1] Disease in each segment produces distinct patterns of claudication (Table 50-1). Most patients have aortoiliac disease, femoropopliteal disease, or both.[2] Disease below the knee is uncommon, except in diabetics and patients with thromboangiitis obliterans.

The diagnostic standard for chronic lower-extremity ischemia is the ankle-to-arm systolic pressure index (AAI), which is obtained by measuring the highest systolic blood pressure at the ankle (dorsalis pedis and posterior tibial arteries) with a hand-held Doppler flowmeter and dividing it by the blood pressure in the brachial artery. Values less than 0.97 are abnormal (i.e., the lower 2.5% of measurements from large numbers of young, nonsmoking, asymptomatic persons).[3–5] Most patients with claudication have AAIs between 0.5 and 0.8 and disease in

Table 50-1	Diagnosis of Peripheral Arterial Disease: Traditional Approach			
Anatomic Segment	Location of Claudication	Pulse Examination		
		Femoral*	Popliteal	Pedal
Aortoiliac	Buttock, thigh, calf†	Absent	Absent	Absent
Femoropopliteal*	Calf	Present	Absent	Absent
Peroneotibial	None or foot‡	Present	Present	Absent

Adapted from reference 1.

*"Femoro" of "femoropopliteal" indicates the superficial femoral artery; "Femoral" of "femoral pulse" indicates the common femoral artery.

†May cause erectile dysfunction if internal iliac arteries are involved.

‡Disease in this segment usually causes no claudication in patients with diabetes but causes foot pain in those with thromboangiitis obliterans (Buerger's disease).

only a single segment; those with limb-threatening ischemia (i.e., rest pain, gangrene) have AAIs less than 0.5 and disease in at least two segments.[4,5]

II. THE FINDINGS

A. APPEARANCE OF THE FOOT

In contrast to earlier writers on peripheral vascular disease, who emphasized the physical sign of gangrene, the American surgeon Leo Buerger wrote in his 1924 book *The Circulatory Disturbances of the Extremities* that there were various "prodromal" signs of vascular disease, including toe and foot ulcers, poor capillary refill, impaired nail growth, atrophic skin, foot pallor with elevation, and foot rubor in the lowered position.[6] Clinicians have since regarded these findings as characteristic of chronic lower limb ischemia, although some of them—especially poor capillary refill and dependent rubor—were controversial even in Buerger's time.[7,8]

B. PULSES

In studies of large numbers of healthy individuals, the dorsalis pedis pulse is not palpable 3% to 14% of the time and the posterior tibial pulse is not palpable 0% to 10% of the time.[9–14] Even so, when one of these arteries is congenitally small or absent, the other enlarges to make up the difference, explaining why only 0% to 2% of healthy individuals are missing both pedal pulses.[9,10,13]

The absence of both pedal pulses is common to disease of each of the three vascular segments and thus represents the best screening test for peripheral vascular disease (see Table 50-1).

C. BRUITS

A traditional finding of stenosis of a peripheral vessel is a limb bruit, either iliac (above the inguinal crease), femoral (in the thigh), or popliteal. Complete occlusion of a vessel should make the bruit disappear.

In patients who have undergone femoral artery puncture for cardiac catheterization, the presence of a continuous femoral bruit (i.e., one extending beyond the second heart sound and thus having both systolic and diastolic components) suggests an abnormal communication between an artery and vein (i.e., arteriovenous fistula, see Chapter 39).

D. ANCILLARY TESTS
1. Venous Filling Time

In patients with peripheral vascular disease, the veins of the feet fill abnormally slowly once they are emptied. After positioning the patient supine and identifying a prominent vein on the top of the foot, the clinician empties this vein by elevating the patient's leg to 45 degrees above the table surface for 1 minute. The patient then sits up and dangles the foot over the edge of the examining table, and the clinician records how long in seconds it takes for the vein to rise above the level of the skin surface. Measurements greater than 20 seconds are abnormal.[15]

2. Capillary Refill Time

To perform this test, the clinician applies firm pressure to the plantar skin of the distal great toe for 5 seconds and then times how long it takes for the normal skin color to return after releasing the pressure. In the great toe, measurements greater than 5 seconds are regarded as abnormal.[15]

3. Buerger's Test

In the Buerger test, the clinician observes the color of the patient's leg when it is elevated and then when it is lowered. Abnormal pallor with elevation and a deep rubor in the lowered position are features of vascular disease.[1,6] In Buerger's version of the test, the clinician elevated the leg to produce pallor and then simply recorded the angle at which the reddish hue returned as the limb was lowered (his "angle of circulatory sufficiency").[6] In the only investigated version of this test (EBM Box 50-1), the clinician elevated the leg 90 degrees from the table surface for 2 minutes and then dangled it perpendicular to the table edge for another 2 minutes. The positive response was abnormal pallor with elevation and the appearance of a dusky red flush spreading proximally from the toes in the dependent position.[16]

Box 50-1

Peripheral Vascular Disease*

Finding (Ref)[†]	Sensitivity (%)	Specificity (%)	Likelihood Ratio if Finding	
			Present	Absent
Inspection				
Wounds or sores on foot[17]	2	100	**7.0**	NS
Foot color abnormally pale, red, or blue[17]	35	87	2.8	0.7
Atrophic skin[15]	50	70	1.7	NS
Absent lower limb hair[15]	48	71	1.7	NS
Palpation				
Foot asymmetrically cooler[17]	10	98	**6.1**	0.9
Absent femoral pulse[17]	7	99	**6.1**	NS
Absent posterior tibial and dorsalis pedis pulses[17,18]	63–72	92–99	**14.9**	**0.3**
Auscultation				
Limb bruit present[17,19,20]	20–50	95–99	**7.3**	0.7
Ancillary tests				
Capillary refill time ≥ 5 seconds[15]	28	85	1.9	NS
Venous filling time > 20 seconds[15]	22	94	**3.6**	NS

NS, not significant; likelihood ratio (LR) if finding present = positive LR; LR if finding absent = negative LR.

Diagnostic standard: For peripheral vascular disease, ankle-arm index < 0.8–0.97 except for the study by Boyko[15] (i.e., atrophic skin, absent lower limb hair, capillary refill time, and venous filling time), which recruited diabetic patients exclusively and defined disease as AAI < 0.5.

[†]*Definition of findings: For limb bruit present, femoral artery bruit[17,20] or iliac, femoral, or popliteal bruit.[19]*

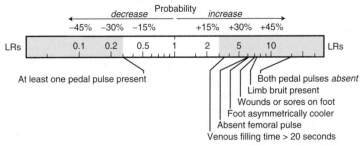

PERIPHERAL VASCULAR DISEASE

III. CLINICAL SIGNIFICANCE

A. DIAGNOSIS OF PERIPHERAL VASCULAR DISEASE

EBM Box 50-1 shows that the most compelling physical signs arguing *for* the presence of peripheral vascular disease in the symptomatic leg (i.e., AAI < 0.9) are the absence of both pedal pulses (likelihood ratio [LR] = 14.9), the presence of any limb bruit (LR = 7.3), the presence of wounds or sores on the foot (LR = 7.0), the absence of the femoral pulse (LR = 6.1), and the presence of asymmetric coolness of the foot (LR = 6.1). In another study,[15] the presence of a cool foot was not diagnostically helpful, although this study defined the abnormal finding as a foot cooler than the ipsilateral calf, which is actually a normal finding (i.e., in healthy individuals, the skin surface temperature diminishes toward the feet because of reduced cutaneous blood flow to conserve body heat).[1]

The only finding arguing *against* peripheral vascular disease is the presence of one or both pedal pulses (LR = 0.3), although studies show that up to 1 in 3 patients with disease have this finding. In these patients, however, the pulses often disappear during exercise (e.g., running in place, walking, toe-stands, or ankle flexion repeatedly against resistance), just as normal resting coronary blood flow in a patient with coronary artery disease may become abnormal after exercise.[21-23]

Findings that are unhelpful diagnostically are atrophic skin, hairless lower limbs,[24] and a prolonged capillary refill time. Writing soon after Buerger introduced the capillary refill time as a test of peripheral vascular disease (his "expression test"), Lewis[8] and Pickering[7] showed it was an unreliable sign, because prompt refill could occur from the veins of a limb rendered completely ischemic experimentally.*

B. DISTRIBUTION OF PERIPHERAL VASCULAR DISEASE

One study showed that vascular surgeons using traditional methods accurately localized the distribution of disease in 96% of 102 symptomatic patients, although the study omitted information about the relative value of specific findings.[25] Of the few studies available, one confirms the traditional teaching (see Table 50-1) that the finding of an absent or severely diminished femoral pulse in a symptomatic limb argues strongly *for* aortoiliac disease (sensitivity 39%, specificity 99%, positive LR = 31.0, negative LR = 0.6).[26] Also, in symptomatic limbs with a preserved popliteal pulse (i.e., a finding arguing against

---

*In adults, the capillary refill time is still used in looking for a disease. It has been proven unhelpful not only in peripheral vascular disease but also in the assessment of blood loss and hypovolemia (see Chapter 9).

occlusion of the aortoiliac or femoropopliteal segments), the presence of a limb bruit argues *for* the presence of stenoses on angiography, a finding of therapeutic importance because these patients may be candidates for angioplasty (sensitivity 80%, specificity 75%, positive LR = 3.2, negative LR = 0.3).[27] Finally, patients who have a positive Buerger's test have more extensive disease than those who are test negative, including more rest pain (60% vs. 8%) and gangrene (23% vs. 0%) and lower AAIs (mean ± SD, 0.37 ± 0.29 vs. 0.62 ± 0.23).[16]

C. COMPLICATIONS OF ARTERIAL PUNCTURE

Femoral artery puncture for cardiac catheterization may rarely be complicated by false aneurysm formation or the development of an arteriovenous fistula. In one study of patients with significant groin hematomas or new limb bruits after cardiac catheterization, two findings were diagnostic.[28] A continuous femoral bruit (i.e., one having both systolic and diastolic components) was diagnostic for arteriovenous fistula (sensitivity 96%, specificity 99%, positive LR 80.8, negative LR 0.04), and an expansile femoral pulsation (i.e., a dilated arterial pulsation whose walls expanded laterally with each beat) was diagnostic for false aneurysm formation (sensitivity 92%, specificity 93%, positive LR 13.8, negative LR 0.1). In this study, the diagnostic standard was duplex scanning, surgery, or both.

REFERENCES

1. McGee SR, Boyko EJ. Physical examination and chronic lower-extremity ischemia: A critical review. *Arch Intern Med.* 1998;158:1357-1364.
2. Mannick JA. Evaluation of chronic lower-extremity ischemia. *N Engl J Med.* 1983; 309:841-843.
3. Hiatt WR, Hoag S, Hamman RF. Effect of diagnostic criteria on the prevalence of peripheral arterial disease: The San Luis Valley diabetes study. *Circulation.* 1995;91: 1472-1479.
4. Carter SA. Indirect systolic pressures and pulse waves in arterial occlusive disease of the lower extremities. *Circulation.* 1968;37:624-637.
5. Ouriel K, McDonnell AE, Metz CE, Zarins CK. A critical evaluation of stress testing in the diagnosis of peripheral vascular disease. *Surgery.* 1982;91:686-693.
6. Buerger L. *The circulatory disturbances of the extremities: Including gangrene, vasomotor and trophic changes.* Philadelphia: WB Saunders; 1924.
7. Pickering GW. On the clinical recognition of structural disease of the peripheral vessels. *Br Med J.* 1933;2:1106-1110.
8. Lewis T. *Vascular disorders of the limbs.* New York: Macmillan; 1936.

9. Barnhorst DA, Barner HB. Prevalence of congenitally absent pedal pulses. *N Engl J Med.* 1968;278:264-265.

10. Morrison H. A study of the dorsalis pedis and posterior tibial pulses in one thousand individuals without symptoms of circulatory affections of the extremities. *N Engl J Med.* 1933;208:438-440.

11. Nuzzaci G, Giuliano G, Righi D, et al. A study of the semeiological reliability of dorsalis pedis artery and posterior tibial artery in the diagnosis of lower limb arterial occlusive disease. *Angiology.* 1984;35:767-772.

12. Robertson GSM, Ristic CD, Bullen BR. The incidence of congenitally absent foot pulses. *Ann R Coll Surg Eng.* 1990;72:99-100.

13. Silverman JJ. The incidence of palpable dorsalis pedis and posterior tibial pulsations in soldiers: An analysis of over 1000 infantry soldiers. *Am Heart J.* 1946;32:82-87.

14. Stephens GL. Palpable dorsalis pedis and posterior tibial pulses: Incidence in young men. *Arch Surg.* 1962;84:662-664.

15. Boyko EJ, Ahroni JH, Davignon D, et al. Diagnostic utility of the history and physical examination for peripheral vascular disease among patients with diabetes mellitus. *J Clin Epidemiol.* 1997;50:659-668.

16. Insall RL, Davies RJ, Prout WG. Significance of Buerger's test in the assessment of lower limb ischaemia. *J R Soc Med.* 1989;82:729-731.

17. Stoffers HEJH, Kester ADM, Kaiser V, et al. Diagnostic value of signs and symptoms associated with peripheral arterial occlusive disease seen in general practice: A multivariable approach. *Med Decis Making.* 1997;17:61-70.

18. Christensen JH, Freundlich M, Jacobsen BA, Falstie-Jensen N. Clinical relevance of pedal pulse palpation in patients suspected of peripheral arterial insufficiency. *J Intern Med.* 1989;226:95-99.

19. Carter SA. Arterial auscultation in peripheral vascular disease. *JAMA.* 1981;246:1682-1686.

20. Criqui MH, Fronek A, Klauber MRl, et al. The sensitivity, specificity, and predictive value of traditional clinical evaluation of peripheral arterial disease: Results from noninvasive testing in a defined population. *Circulation.* 1985;71:516-522.

21. Barner HB, Kaiser GC, Willman VL, Hanlon CR. Intermittent claudication with pedal pulses. *JAMA.* 1968;204:100-104.

22. Carter SA. Response of ankle systolic pressure to leg exercise in mild or questionable arterial disease. *N Engl J Med.* 1972;287:578-582.

23. DeWeese JA. Pedal pulses disappearing with exercise: A test for intermittent claudication. *N Engl J Med.* 1960;262:1214-1217.

24. Parfrey N, Ryan JF, Shanahan L, Brady MP. Hairless lower limbs and occlusive arterial disease. *Lancet.* 1976;1:276.

25. Baker WH, String ST, Hayes AC, Turner D. Diagnosis of peripheral occlusive disease: Comparison of clinical evaluation and noninvasive laboratory. *Arch Surg.* 1978;113:1308-1310.

26. Johnston KW, Demorais D, Colapinto RF. Difficulty in assessing the severity of aorto-iliac disease by clinical and arteriographic methods. *Angiology.* 1981;32:609-614.
27. Nicholson ML, Byrne RL, Steele GA, Callum KG. Predictive value of bruits and Doppler pressure measurements in detecting lower limb arterial stenosis. *Eur J Vasc Surg.* 1993;7:59-62.
28. Kent KC, McArdle CR, Kennedy B, et al. Accuracy of clinical examination in the evaluation of femoral false aneurysm and arteriovenous fistula. *Cardiovasc Surg.* 1993;1:504-506.

51

The Diabetic Foot

I. INTRODUCTION

The term "diabetic foot" refers to complications in a foot rendered hypesthetic from diabetic polyneuropathy. These include ulceration, Charcot arthropathy, and infection. Each year, 2.5% of diabetics develop a foot ulcer,[1] and the diabetic foot is the leading cause of hospitalization among diabetics and the overall leading cause of amputation in the United States.[2,3]

II. THE FINDINGS

A. FOOT ULCERATION

More than 75% of diabetic ulcers develop on the toes or on the plantar surface of the metatarsal heads.[4,5] Most of the remaining ulcers appear over the heel, plantar midfoot, or previous amputation sites. "Ulcer area" refers to the product of the maximum ulcer width and maximum ulcer length.

B. DIABETIC NEUROPATHY AND SEMMES-WEINSTEIN MONOFILAMENTS

Although neuropathy, ischemia, and infection all contribute to ulceration, the most important is neuropathy.[3,6] Conventional examination often fails to detect diabetic polyneuropathy, however, and about half of patients with diabetic ulceration lack complaints of numbness or pain[7] and can still detect the touch of a cotton wisp or pinprick.[4,8] Consequently, most diabetologists use a simple and more sensitive bedside tool, the Semmes-Weinstein monofilament, to identify which patients have sufficient neuropathy placing them at risk for ulceration.

According to traditional teachings, a foot that is able to sense the 5.07 monofilament* is protected from ulceration, whereas one that fails to perceive the 5.07 monofilament is predisposed to ulceration. To use the monofilament, the patient should be lying supine with eyes closed, and the monofilament should be applied perpendicular to the skin with enough force to buckle it for approximately 1 second.[10] The patient responds "yes" each time he or she senses the monofilament, as the clinician randomly tests each site on the foot multiple times.[11] In clinical studies, 1 to 10 different sites on the foot are tested,[12] but each study defines the abnormal result as inability to consistently sense the monofilament at *any* site. Testing the plantar surface of the first and fifth metatarsal heads may be the most efficient and overall accurate bedside maneuver.[12]

Monofilaments were first developed in 1898 by von Frey who glued thorns to hairs of various stiffness and calibrated them with a chemical balance ("von Frey hairs").[9] Nylon monofilaments were introduced in 1960 by Josephine Semmes and Sidney Weinstein, who used filaments of 20 different diameters (from 0.06 to 1.14 mm) to study sensation in patients with penetrating brain injuries.[13,14] Although the 5.07 monofilament is firmly entrenched as the standard for testing diabetic feet, this is based on an older study of patients with neuropathic foot ulcers from diabetes or leprosy, which used just 3 of the 20 monofilaments available.[10] The monofilaments studied were the 4.17 monofilament, which was selected because virtually all normal persons are able to sense it, and the stiffer 5.07 and 6.10 monofilaments. In the study, none of the patients with ulcers could sense the 4.17 or 5.07 monofilaments, although some could sense the 6.10 monofilament. These findings led the investigators to conclude that the ability to sense the 5.07 monofilament was protective

---

*The nominal value of a monofilament represents the common logarithm of 10 times the force in milligrams required to bow it (e.g., the 5.07 monofilament will buckle with 11.8 g of pressure, $\log_{10}(10 \times 11,800) = 5.07$).[9] Therefore, monofilaments with higher numbers are stiffer and more easily perceived than those with lower numbers.

(i.e., 6.10 was not protective and 4.17 was normal sensation). It is also possible, however, that a better indicator of protective sensation is one of the other seven monofilaments between 6.10 and 4.17 not used in the study, and in support of this hypothesis, one study has suggested that the 4.21 monofilament may be a better discriminatory threshold.[4]

C. CHARCOT JOINT

Charcot joint (neuro-arthropathy) refers to accelerated degenerative changes and ultimate joint destruction that follows repetitive trauma to insensitive, neuropathic joints. Although historically the most common causes were syphilis (affecting the larger joints of the lower extremity) and syringomyelia (affecting the larger joints of the upper extremity), the most common cause today is diabetes. In diabetic patients, Charcot joint characteristically affects the foot, including ankle, tarso-metatarsal, and metatarso-phalangeal (MTP) joints.[15,16]

Most patients present with a limp, difficulty putting on shoes, or soft tissue swelling suggesting fracture, acute arthritis, or sprain.[16] The characteristic physical findings are anesthetic or hypesthetic feet (100% of patients), bony deformities (69% of patients), and soft tissue swelling (17% of patients). Many patients also have ulceration and abnormal callus formation. The most common bony deformities are abnormal projections on the plantar arch ("rocker sole") or other unusual prominence of the dorsal or medial arches of the midfoot or the metatarso-phalangeal joint. Soft tissue swelling typically appears at the ankle and midfoot, sometimes with marked rubor and warmth that mimics arthritis.

Jean-Martin Charcot described Charcot neuro-arthropathy in 1868 in patients with tabes dorsalis,[17] although he credited the American Mitchell (1831) with the original description.[18]

D. OSTEOMYELITIS

In diabetic patients with foot ulceration and underlying radiographic abnormalities of the bone, it is very difficult to distinguish Charcot foot from osteomyelitis. One proposed test is the "probe test", in which the clinician gently probes the ulcer base with a sterile blunt 14.0-cm 5-Fr stainless steel eye probe. The test is positive, suggesting osteomyelitis, if the clinician detects a rock-hard, often gritty structure at the ulcer base without any intervening soft tissue.[5]

III. CLINICAL SIGNIFICANCE

A. THE SEMMES-WEINSTEIN MONOFILAMENT

According to the information presented in EBM Box 51-1, the *inability* to feel the 5.07 monofilament is a modest predictor of ulceration during 2 to 4 years

Box 51-1 The Diabetic Foot*

Finding (Ref)[†]	Sensitivity (%)	Specificity (%)	Likelihood Ratio if Finding	
			Present	Absent
Predictors of subsequent foot ulceration				
Unable to sense the 5.07 monofilament[19–22]	54–90	34–86	2.4	0.5
Predictors of osteomyelitis, in patients with foot ulcers				
Ulcer area >2 cm^2 [23]	56	92	**7.2**	0.5
Positive probe test[5]	66	85	**4.3**	0.4
Ulcer depth >3 mm or bone exposed[23]	82	77	**3.6**	**0.2**
Erythema, swelling, purulence[23]	36	77	NS	NS
Predictors of nonhealing wound at 20 weeks, in patients with foot ulcers[24]				
0 findings	14	70	0.5	...
1 finding	37	...	0.8	...
2 findings	35	...	1.8	...
3 findings	13	96	**3.5**	...

NS, not significant; likelihood ratio (LR) if finding present = positive LR; LR if finding absent = negative LR.
*Diagnostic standard: For foot ulceration, the appearance of an ulcer during 2 to 4 years of follow-up; for osteomyelitis, biopsy of the bone.
†Definition of findings: For positive probe test, ulcer area, and predictors of nonhealing wound, see text.

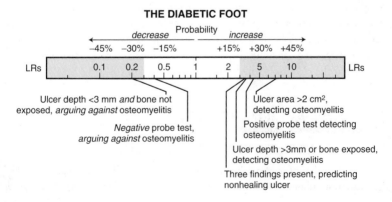

THE DIABETIC FOOT

of follow-up [likelihood ratio (LR) = 2.4, see EBM Box 51-1]. Another study has demonstrated that the *presence* of 5.07 monofilament sensation argues *against* subsequent amputation during 3 to 4 years of follow-up (LR = 0.3).[25] Monofilament sensation predicts complications better than other quantitative measures of sensation, including the 128-Hz tuning fork[26] and graded vibratory or thermal stimuli.[4,27]

B. OSTEOMYELITIS

In diabetic patients with foot ulceration, three findings argue *for* underlying osteomyelitis (defined by bone biopsy): ulcer area greater than 2 cm^2 (LR = 7.2), positive probe test (LR = 4.3), and ulcer depth greater than 3 mm or exposed bone (LR = 3.6). The findings of erythema, swelling, or purulence are unhelpful in diagnosing osteomyelitis.[23]

C. PREDICTORS OF NONHEALING WOUNDS

In one study of more than 27,000 diabetic foot ulcers treated with debridement, moist wound dressings, and measures to reduce pressure on the foot (e.g., special footwear, crutches, or wheelchairs), 53% failed to heal after 20 weeks[24]. This study identified three independent predictors of nonhealing ulcers: (1) wound age greater than 2 months, (2) wound size greater than 2 cm^2, and (3) full-thickness wound associated with exposed tendons, exposed joint, abscess, osteomyelitis, necrotic tissue, or limb gangrene.[24] The presence of all three of these predictors increases the likelihood that a diabetic foot ulcer will not heal by 20 weeks (LR = 3.5).

REFERENCES

1. Moss SE, Klein R, Klein BEK. The prevalence and incidence of lower extremity amputation in a diabetic population. *Arch Intern Med.* 1992;152:610-616.
2. Lipsky BA. Osteomyelitis of the foot in diabetic patients. *Clin Infect Dis.* 1997;25: 1318-1326.
3. Shaw JE, Boulton AJ. The pathogenesis of diabetic foot problems: An overview. *Diabetes.* 1997;46(Suppl 2):S58-61.
4. Sosenko JM, Kato M, Soto R, Bild DE. Comparison of quantitative sensory-threshold measures for their association with foot ulceration in diabetic patients. *Diab Care.* 1990;13:1057-1061.
5. Grayson ML, Gibbons GW, Balough K, et al. Probing to bone in infected pedal ulcers: A clinical sign of underlying osteomyelitis in diabetic patients. *JAMA.* 1995;273:721-723.
6. Caputo GM, Cavanagh PR, Ulbrecht JS, et al. Assessment and management of foot disease in patients with diabetes. *N Engl J Med.* 1994;331:854-860.

7. Kumar S, Ashe HA, Parnell LN, et al. The prevalence of foot ulceration and its correlates in type 2 diabetic patients: A population-based study. *Diabetic Med.* 1994;11: 480-484.

8. Valk GC, Nauta JJP, Strijers RLM, Bertelsmann FW. Clinical examination versus neurophysiological examination in the diagnosis of diabetic polyneuropathy. *Diab Med.* 1992;9:716-721.

9. Levin S, Pearsall G, Ruderman RJ. Von Frey's method of measuring pressure sensibility in the hand: An engineering analysis of the Weinstein-Semmes pressure aesthesiometer. *J Hand Surg Am.* 1978;3:211-216.

10. Birke JA, Sims DS. Plantar sensory threshold in the ulcerative foot. *Lepr Rev.* 1986;57:261-267.

11. Mueller MJ. Identifying patients with diabetes mellitus who are at risk for lower-extremity complications: Use of Semmes-Weinstein monofilaments. *Phys Ther.* 1996;76:68-71.

12. McGill M, Molyneaux L, Spencer R, et al. Possible sources of discrepancies in the use of the Semmes-Weinstein monofilament: Impact on prevalence of insensate foot and workload requirements. *Diabetes Care.* 1999;22:598-602.

13. Semmes J, Weinstein S, Ghent L, Teuber HL. *Somatosensory changes after penetrating brain wounds in man.* Cambridge: Harvard University Press; 1960.

14. Weinstein S, Sersen EA. Tactual sensitivity as a function of handedness and laterality. *J Compar Physiol Psychol.* 1961;54:665-669.

15. Gupta R. A short history of neuropathic arthropathy. *Clin Orthop.* 1993;296:43-49.

16. Sinha S, Munichoodappa CS, Kozak GP. Neuro-arthropathy (Charcot joints) in diabetes mellitus (clinical study of 101 cases). *Medicine (Baltimore).* 1972;51: 191-210.

17. Charcot JM. The classic: On arthropathies of cerebral or spinal origin. *Clin Orthop Relat Res.* 1993;296:4-7.

18. Kelly M. John Kearsley Mitchell (1793-1858) and the neurogenic theory of arthritis. *J History Med.* 1965;20:151-156.

19. Boyko EJ, Ahroni JH, Stensel V, et al. A prospective study of risk factors for diabetic foot ulcer. The Seattle Diabetic Foot study. *Diabetes Care.* 1999;22:1036-1042.

20. Rith-Najarian SJ, Stolusky T, Gohdes DM. Identifying diabetic patients at high risk for lower-extremity amputation in a primary health care setting: A prospective evaluation of simple screening criteria. *Diabetes Care.* 1992;15:1386-1389.

21. Pham H, Armstrong DG, Harvey C, et al. Screening techniques to identify people at high risk for diabetic foot ulceration. *Diabetes Care.* 2000;23:606-611.

22. Abbott CA, Carrington AL, Ashe H, et al. The North-West diabetes Foot Care Study: Incidence of, and risk factors for, new diabetic foot ulceration in a community-based patient cohort. *Diabetic Med.* 2002;19:377-384.

23. Newman LG, Waller J, Palestro J, et al. Unsuspected osteomyelitis in diabetic foot ulcers: Diagnosis and monitoring by leukocyte scanning with indium In 111 oxyquinoline. *JAMA.* 1991;266:1246-1251.

24. Margolis DJ, Allen-Taylor L, Hoffstad O, Berlin JA. Diabetic neuropathic foot ulcers: Predicting which ones will not heal. *Am J Med.* 2003;115:627-631.
25. Adler AI, Boyko EJ, Ahroni JH, Smith DG. Lower-extremity amputation in diabetes. The independent effects of peripheral vascular disease, sensory neuropathy, and foot ulcers. *Diabetes Care.* 1999;22:1029-1035.
26. McNeely MJ, Boyko EJ, Ahroni J, et al. The independent contributions of diabetic neuropathy and vasculopathy in foot ulceration. *Diabet Care.* 1995;18:216-219.
27. Litzelman DK, Marriott DJ, Vinicor F. Independent physiological predictors of foot lesions in patients with NIDDM. *Diabetes Care.* 1997;20:1273-1278.

52

Edema and Deep Vein Thrombosis

EDEMA

I. INTRODUCTION

Edema of a limb may occur because of increased venous pressure (e.g., venous insufficiency, congestive heart failure), increased vascular permeability (e.g., inflammation), decreased oncotic pressure (e.g., hypoalbuminemia), lymphatic obstruction (i.e., lymphedema), and deposition of additional tissue (e.g., lipedema). The most common causes of bilateral edema are congestive heart failure, chronic venous insufficiency, pulmonary hypertension without left heart failure, and drug-induced edema (e.g., nifedipine, nonsteroidal antiinflammatory medications).[1,2] The most common causes of unilateral swelling of the leg are deep vein thrombosis, Baker's cyst, and cellulitis (see later).[3-5]

II. THE FINDINGS

The pitting characteristics of edema reflect the viscosity of the edema fluid, which in turn depends largely on its protein concentration.[6–9] Edema fluid with low protein levels (e.g., hypoalbuminemia, congestive heart failure) pits easily and recovers relatively quickly compared with edema fluid that has higher protein levels (lymphedema, inflammatory edema).[7,8] A clue to "low protein edema" (i.e., edema associated with a serum albumin level <3.5 g/dL) is edema that pits easily with just 1 to 2 seconds of thumb pressure over the tibia, and then, after removal of the thumb, begins to recover within 2 to 3 seconds.[9]

Lymphedema is painless, firm edema that characteristically causes squaring of the toes and a dorsal hump on the foot. In contrast to venous edema, lymphedema varies little during the day and ulceration is uncommon unless there is secondary infection. Even though lymphedema has high protein levels, clinical experience shows that it does pit early in its course though it eventually becomes nonpitting, hard, and "woody" as a secondary fibrous reaction ensues.[6,10]

Lipedema consists of bilateral deposition of excess subcutaneous fatty tissue in the legs that does not pit with pressure and whose most characteristic feature is sparing of the feet.[11] Lipedema occurs exclusively in obese women.

III. CLINICAL SIGNIFICANCE

A. PITTING EDEMA

In patients with bilateral pitting edema of the legs, the most important diagnostic finding is the patient's venous pressure, estimated from examination of the neck veins. If the neck veins are abnormally distended, cardiac disease or pulmonary hypertension is at least partly responsible for the patient's edema; if they are normal, another cause is responsible, such as liver disease, nephrosis, chronic venous insufficiency, or one of the medications the patient is taking. Clinicians' estimates of venous pressure are accurate, with studies showing that the finding of elevated neck veins predicts an abnormally increased central venous pressure (i.e., > 8 cm H_2O) with a positive likelihood ratio (LR) of 9.0 (see Chapter 32).

In contrast, the finding of pitting edema by itself and without knowledge of the patient's venous pressure is an unreliable sign of cardiac disease. For example, in patients undergoing cardiac catheterization because of chest pain or dyspnea, the finding of edema (without knowledge of venous pressure) lacked any significant relationship with the patient's left heart pressures (see Chapter 44).[12,13]

B. LYMPHEDEMA

Lymphedema is classified as "primary" (i.e., congenital abnormality of the lymphatic systems) or "secondary" (damage to the lymphatics from previous radiation or surgery, malignant obstruction, or recurrent episodes of cellulitis). Primary lymphedema begins before the age of 40 years, may be bilateral (50% of cases), and affects women 10 times more often than men.[14] Secondary lymphedema from infection, radiation, or surgery affects men and women of all ages, is usually unilateral, and is preceded by the characteristic history. Malignant obstruction affects patients older than 40 years and is almost always unilateral (>95% of cases).[14] The most common cause of malignant lymphedema in the leg of men is metastatic prostate carcinoma; in women, it is lymphoma.[14] Lymphedema of the arm is almost always due to breast cancer, either the tumor itself, or combined treatment with surgery and radiation.[15]

DEEP VEIN THROMBOSIS

I. INTRODUCTION

Deep vein thrombosis is conventionally divided into *proximal* thrombosis (popliteal vein and above) and *distal* thrombosis (calf veins). Several studies have shown that only proximal thrombi are associated with clinically significant pulmonary emboli, and thus only these thrombi require treatment with anticoagulation.[16]

In patients with acutely painful and swollen calves, accurate diagnosis is essential, not only because untreated proximal thrombi may cause fatal pulmonary emboli but also because inappropriate administration of anticoagulation to persons without proximal thrombi risks unnecessarily life-threatening hemorrhage.

II. THE FINDINGS

A. INSPECTION AND PALPATION

The most important signs of vein thrombosis are tenderness and swelling. Calf asymmetry greater than 1.5 cm is abnormal, indicating significant edema of the larger limb or atrophy of the smaller one.[17]

Other traditional signs associated with deep vein thrombosis are a palpable cord, dilated superficial veins, Homans's sign, skin erythema, and altered skin temperature (both coolness and warmth have been proposed by different authorities). The basis for these signs, however, seems dubious. Because large muscles and dense fascial tissues encompass the deep veins of the legs, concealing them from the examiner's eyes and hands, it is difficult to conceive how a clinician could ever palpate the cord of a thrombosed deep vein. The increased collateral flow around an obstruction could make the superficial veins more conspicuous, but skin surface temperature and color reflect blood flow and vessel size of the minute vessels *of the dermis*,[18] which should not necessarily be different after venous obstruction.

B. HOMANS'S SIGN

In his extensive writings about venous thrombosis, the American surgeon John Homans contrasted two forms of the disease: bland thrombosis of the calf veins, which caused few symptoms other than mild swelling and pain, and iliofemoral thrombophlebitis ("phlegmasia alba dolens"), which caused generalized leg edema and cyanosis.[19–21] Homans believed that most pulmonary emboli originated in the bland calf thrombi and that, once diagnosed, the disorder should be treated by femoral vein ligation to prevent pulmonary emboli (anticoagulation was not yet being used). In 1941, Homans proposed that the "dorsiflexion sign"—"discomfort behind the knee on forced dorsiflexion of the foot"—was a sign of these difficult-to-diagnose calf thrombi.[20] Although contemporaries called the sign "Homans's sign,"[22] Homans never did and instead later credited another clinician for making the original description.[23]

Surgeons soon learned that there were many examples of a false positive Homans's sign (i.e., positive dorsiflexion sign but no clot found at surgery),[22,24] and in 1944, Homans redefined the positive response, stating that "discomfort need have no part in the reaction." Eventually, Homans became unenthusiastic about the sign[25,26] and has been quoted as saying "if you wanted to name a sign after me, why didn't you pick a good one?"[27]

C. PSEUDOTHROMBOPHLEBITIS

In a large series of patients presenting with suspected deep vein thrombosis, only one out of every four or five patients actually has the diagnosis.[28–32] An important mimic of deep vein thrombosis (i.e., "pseudothrombophlebitis") is Baker's cyst, which is a distended gastrocnemius-semimembranosus bursa that has dissected or ruptured into the calf or is compressing the popliteal vein.[33,34] A telltale sign of this disorder (and any other cause of calf hematoma) is crescent-shaped ecchymosis near either malleolus.[35,36]

III. CLINICAL SIGNIFICANCE

A. INDIVIDUAL FINDINGS

EBM Box 52-1 presents the diagnostic accuracy of physical signs for deep vein thrombosis, as applied to thousands of patients with acute calf pain, swelling, or both. Although some studies recruited outpatients[28,38,40–43,45–52] and

Box 52-1   Deep Vein Thrombosis*

Finding (Ref)[†]	Sensitivity (%)	Specificity (%)	Likelihood Ratio if Finding	
			Present	Absent
Inspection				
Any calf or ankle swelling[25,26,31,37–41]	41–90	8–74	1.2	0.7
Asymmetric calf swelling, ≥ 2 cm difference[30,42]	61–67	69–71	2.1	0.5
Swelling of entire leg[31,40,41,43]	34–57	58–80	1.5	0.8
Superficial venous dilation[26,40,41,43,44]	28–33	79–85	1.6	0.9
Erythema[37,38,44]	16–48	61–87	NS	NS
Superficial thrombophlebitis[39]	5	95	NS	NS
Palpation				
Tenderness[25,26,37–41,43,44]	19–85	10–80	NS	NS
Asymmetric skin coolness[26]	42	63	NS	NS
Asymmetric skin warmth[37,44]	29–71	51–77	1.4	NS
Palpable cord[31,44]	15–30	73–85	NS	NS
Other tests				
Homans's sign[25,26,31,37–39,44]	10–54	39–89	NS	NS

NS, not significant; likelihood ratio (LR) if finding present = positive LR; LR if finding absent = negative LR.

*Diagnostic standard: For deep venous thrombosis, positive contrast venography[25,26,31,37–39,44] or compression ultrasonography.[30,40–43]

†Definition of findings: All findings refer to the symptomatic leg.

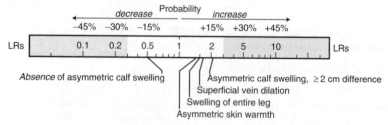

DEEP VENOUS THROMBOSIS

others both inpatients and outpatients,[30,31,44] the accuracy of individual signs is the same whether or not inpatients are included in the analysis. In almost all studies, "deep vein thrombosis" refers only to proximal thrombosis (popliteal vein or higher),[31,37,38,40–43,45–52] although a few studies included patients with proximal vein or isolated calf vein thrombosis (in these studies, however, only 15% to 29% had isolated calf thrombosis).[30,39,44] Most studies excluded patients with symptoms suggesting pulmonary embolism.

According to these studies, only the findings of asymmetric calf swelling (≥ 2 cm difference, LR = 2.1), superficial vein dilation (LR = 1.6), swelling of the entire leg (LR = 1.5), and asymmetric skin warmth (LR = 1.4) argue significantly *for* thrombosis, although the discriminatory value of all these signs is slight. The presence or absence of erythema, tenderness, skin coolness, palpable cord, and Homans's sign has no diagnostic value. As expected, the finding of superficial thrombophlebitis (i.e., visibly inflamed and tender subcutaneous veins) also lacks any relationship to pathology in the deep veins. No finding argues convincingly *against* the diagnosis of thrombosis (no LR <0.5).

Table 52-1	Wells Scoring Scheme for Pretest Probability of Deep Vein Thrombosis[28] *	
Clinical Feature		**Points**
RISK FACTORS		
Active cancer		1
Paralysis, paresis, or recent plaster immobilization of the lower extremities		1
Recently bedridden >3 days or major surgery, within 4 weeks		1
SIGNS		
Localized tenderness along the distribution of the deep venous system		1
Entire leg swollen		1
Asymmetric calf swelling (>3 cm difference, 10 cm below tibial tuberosity)		1
Asymmetric pitting edema		1
Collateral superficial veins (nonvaricose)		1
ALTERNATIVE DIAGNOSIS		
Alternative diagnosis as likely or more likely than deep venous thrombosis		−2

*Interpretation of score: High probability if 3 points or more, moderate probability if 1 or 2 points, and low probability if 0 points or less.

These same studies show that certain risk factors assist diagnosis, most importantly the presence of active cancer (sensitivity 7% to 39%, specificity 90% to 97%, positive LR = 2.9).[28,30,31,40–43,45,53] The findings of "recent immobilization" or "recent surgery" both increase the probability of deep venous thrombosis a smaller amount (positive LR for each finding is 1.6).

B. COMBINED FINDINGS

Given the meager accuracy of individual findings, Wells and others developed a simple scoring scheme (Table 52-1) that combines findings, stratifying patients into groups of "low," "moderate," or "high" probability for deep vein thrombosis.[28] The findings entering his model were all proven to be independent predictors in an earlier analysis.[29,54] This model has now been validated in several studies enrolling more than 5000 patients with suspected deep venous thrombosis: a low pretest probability (0 or fewer points by this model) argues against deep vein thrombosis (LR = 0.2, EBM Box 52-2), and a high pretest probability (3 or more points) significantly increases the probability of deep

Box 52-2 Wells Scoring Scheme for Deep Vein Thrombosis*

Pretest probability[28,32,46,48–52,55†]	Sensitivity (%)	Specificity (%)	Positive LR
Low pretest probability	2–21	36–77	**0.2**
Moderate pretest probability	13–39	...	NS
High pretest probability	38–87	71–96	**5.2**

NS, not significant.

*Diagnostic standard: For deep vein thrombosis, proximal vein clot by compression ultrasonography,[28,32,45,46,48–52] sometimes with contrast venography.[28] In some studies,[45,49,51] deep venous thrombosis was excluded without compression ultrasonography in patients with low clinical risk, normal D-dimer assay, and absence of venous thromboembolism during 3 months of follow-up.
†Definition of findings: For pretest probability, see Table 52-1.

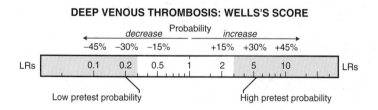

DEEP VENOUS THROMBOSIS: WELLS'S SCORE

vein thrombosis (LR = 5.0). The finding of a moderate pretest probability is diagnostically unhelpful.

If the clinical probability (using the Wells rule) is low and the D-dimer measurement is normal, the probability of deep vein thrombosis is so low (i.e., <1% in six of seven studies) that anticoagulants and further testing may safely be withheld.[45,49,50,53,56–58] Randomized studies show that this approach is as accurate and safe as performing compression ultrasonography in all patients.[59]

All other patients, especially those with high clinical probability, require compression ultrasonography to investigate further for deep vein thrombosis, even if their D-dimer test is normal. For example, in patients with high clinical probability but *normal* D-dimer measurements, compression ultrasonography reveals venous thromboembolism in up to 25%.[45,49,51,53]

REFERENCES

1. Ciocon JO, Galindo-Ciocon D, Galindo DJ. Raised leg exercises for leg edema in the elderly. *Angiology.* 1995;46:19-25.
2. Blankfield RP, Finkelhor RS, Alexander JJ, et al. Etiology and diagnosis of bilateral leg edema in primary care. *Am J Med.* 1998;105:192-197.
3. Belch JJF, McMillan NC, Fogelman I, et al. Combined phlebography and arthrography in patients with painful swollen calf. *Br Med J.* 1981;282:949.
4. Hall S, Littlejohn O, Brand C, et al. The painful swollen calf: A comparative evaluation of four investigative techniques. *Med J Austr.* 1986;144:356-358.
5. Simpson FG, Robinson PJ, Bark M, Losowsky MS. Prospective study of thrombophlebitis and "pseudothrombophlebitis." *Lancet.* 1980;1:331-333.
6. Bates DO, Levick JR, Mortimer PS. Quantification of rate and depth of pitting in human edema using an electronic tonometer. *Lymphology* 1994;27:159-172.
7. Berlyne GM, Kwan T, Li J, Caruso C. Oedema protein concentrations for differentiation of cellulitis and deep vein thrombosis. *Lancet.* 1989;2:728-729.
8. Crockett DJ. The protein levels of oedema fluids. *Lancet.* 1956;2:1179-1182.
9. Henry JA, Altmann P. Assessment of hypoproteinaemic oedema: A simple physical sign. *Br Med J.* 1978;1:890-891.
10. Tiwari A, Cheng KS, Button M, et al. Differential diagnosis, investigation, and current treatment of lower limb lymphedema. *Arch Surg.* 2003;138:152-161.
11. Allen EV, Hines EA. Lipedema of the legs: A syndrome characterized by fat legs and orthostatic edema. *Proc Staff Mayo Clin.* 1940;15:184-187.
12. Harlan WR, Oberman A, Grim R, Rosati RA. Chronic congestive heart failure in coronary artery disease: Clinical criteria. *Ann Intern Med.* 1977;86:133-138.
13. Zema MJ, Restivo B, Sos T, et al. Left ventricular dysfunction: Bedside Valsalva manoeuvre. *Br Heart J.* 1980;44:560-569.

14. Smith RD, Spittell JA, Schirger A. Secondary lymphedema of the leg: Its characteristics and diagnostic implications. *JAMA.* 1963;185:80-82.

15. Browse NL. Lymphoedema of the arm. *Br Med J.* 1987;295:3-4.

16. Huisman MV, Büller HR, ten Cate JW, Vreeken J. Serial impedance plethysmography for suspected deep venous thrombosis in outpatients: The Amsterdam general practitioner study. *N Engl J Med.* 1986;314:823-828.

17. Stein PD, Henry JW, Gopalakrishnan D, Relyea B. Asymmetry of calves in the assessment of patients with suspected acute pulmonary embolism. *Chest.* 1995;107: 936-939.

18. Lewis T. *The blood vessels of the human skin and their responses.* London: Shaw and Sons; 1927.

19. Homans J. Thrombosis of the deep veins of the lower leg, causing pulmonary embolism. *N Engl J Med.* 1934;211:993-997.

20. Homans J. Exploration and division of the femoral and iliac veins in the treatment of thrombophlebitis of the leg. *N Engl J Med.* 1941;224:179-186.

21. Homans J. Thrombosis as a complication of venography. *JAMA.* 1942;119:136.

22. Moses WR. The early diagnosis of phlebothrombosis. *N Engl J Med.* 1946;234: 288-291.

23. Homans J. Venous thrombosis and pulmonary embolism. *N Engl J Med.* 1947;236:196-201.

24. Allen AW, Linton RR, Donaldson GA. Thrombosis and embolism: Review of 202 patients treated by femoral vein interruption. *Ann Surg.* 1943;118:728-740.

25. Cranley JJ, Canos AJ, Sull WJ. The diagnosis of deep venous thrombosis: Fallibility of clinical signs. *Arch Surg.* 1976;111:34-36.

26. Haeger K. Problems of acute deep venous thrombosis. I. The interpretation of signs and symptoms. *Angiology.* 1969;20:219-223.

27. Barker WF. To the memory of John Homans, M.D., 1877–1954. *Maj Probl Clin Surg.* 1966;4:v-vii.

28. Wells PS, Anderson DR, Bormanis J, et al. Value of assessment of pretest probability of deep-vein thrombosis in clinical management. *Lancet.* 1997;350:1795-1798.

29. Wells PS, Hirsh J, Anderson DR, et al. Accuracy of clinical assessment of deep-vein thrombosis. *Lancet.* 1995;345:1326-1330.

30. Criado E, Burnham CB. Predictive value of clinical criteria for the diagnosis of deep vein thrombosis. *Surgery.* 1997;122:578-583.

31. Landefeld CS, McGuire E, Cohen AM. Clinical findings associated with acute proximal deep vein thrombosis: A basis for quantifying clinical judgment. *Am J Med.* 1990;88:382-388.

32. Miron MJ, Perrier A, Bounameaux H. Clinical assessment of suspected deep vein thrombosis: Comparison between a score and empirical assessment. *J Intern Med.* 2000;247:249-254.

33. Katz RS, Zizic TM, Arnold WP, Stevens MB. The pseudothrombophlebitis syndrome. *Medicine.* 1977;56:151-164.

34. Wigley RD. Popliteal cysts: Variations on a theme by Baker. *Semin Arthritis Rheum.* 1982;12:1-10.

35. Tibbutt DA, Gunning AJ. Calf haematoma: A new sign in differential diagnosis from deep vein thrombosis. *Br Med J.* 1974;4:204.

36. Kraag G, Thevathasan EM, Gordon DA, Walker IH. The hemorrhagic crescent sign of acute synovial rupture. *Ann Intern Med.* 1976;85:477-478.

37. Vaccaro P, Van Aman M, Miller S, et al. Shortcomings of physical examination and impedance plethysmography in the diagnosis of lower extremity deep venous thrombosis. *Angiology.* 1981;38:232-235.

38. O'Donnell TF, Abbott WM, Athanasoulis CA, et al. Diagnosis of deep venous thrombosis in the outpatient by venography. *Surg Gynecol Obstet.* 1980;150:69-74.

39. Molloy W, English J, O'Dwyer R, O'Connell. Clinical findings in the diagnosis of proximal deep vein thrombosis. *Ir Med J.* 1982;75:119-120.

40. Oudega R, Moons KGM, Hoes AW. Limited value of patient history and physical examination in diagnosing deep vein thrombosis in primary care. *Fam Pract.* 2005; 22:86-91.

41. Ruiz-Gimenez N, Friera A, Artieda P, et al. Rapid D-dimer test combined a clinical model for deep vein thrombosis: Validation with ultrasonography and clinical follow-up in 383 patients. *Thromb Haemost.* 2004;91:1237-1246.

42. Johanning JM, Franklin DP, Thomas DD, Elmore JR. D-dimer and calf circumference in the evaluation of outpatient deep venous thrombosis. *J Vasc Surg.* 2002;36: 877-880.

43. Oudega R, Moons KGM, Hoes AW. Ruling out deep venous thrombosis in primary care: A simple diagnostic algorithm including D-dimer testing. *Thromb Haemost.* 2005;94:200-205.

44. Kahn SR, Joseph L, Abenhaim L, Leclerc JR. Clinical prediction of deep vein thrombosis in patients with leg symptoms. *Thromb Haemost.* 1999;81:353-357.

45. Anderson DR, Kovasc MJ, Kovacs G, et al. Combined use of clinical assessment and D-dimer to improved the management of patients presenting to the emergency department with suspected deep vein thrombosis (the EDITED Study). *J Thromb Haemost.* 2003;1:645-651.

46. Anderson DR, Wells PS, MacLeod B, et al. Thrombosis in the emergency department. *Arch Intern Med.* 1999;159:477-482.

47. Bates SM, Kearon C, Crowther MA, et al. A diagnostic strategy involving a quantitative latex D-dimer assay reliably excludes deep venous thrombosis. *Ann Intern Med.* 2003;138:787-794.

48. Funfsinn N, Caliezi C, Baiasiutti FD, et al. Rapid D-dimer testing and pre-test clinical probability in the exclusion of deep venous thrombosis in symptomatic outpatients. *Blood Coagul Fibrinolysis.* 2001;12:165-170.

49. Kearon C, Ginsberg JS, Douketis J, et al. Management of suspected deep venous thrombosis in outpatients by using clinical assessment and D-dimer testing. *Ann Intern Med.* 2001;135:108-111.

50. Oudega R, Hoes AW, Moons KGM. The Wells rule does not adequately rule out deep venous thrombosis in primary care patients. *Ann Intern Med.* 2005;143:100-107.

51. Schutgens REG, Ackermark P, Haas FJLM, et al. Combination of a normal D-dimer concentration and a non-high pretest clinical probability score is a safe strategy to exclude deep venous thrombosis. *Circulation.* 2003;107:593-597.

52. Tick LW, Ton E, van Voorthuizen T, et al. Practical diagnostic management of patients with clinically suspected deep vein thrombosis by clinical probability test, compression ultrasonography, and D-dimer test. *Am J Med.* 2002;113:630-635.

53. Anderson DR, Wells PS, Stiell I, et al. Management of patients with suspected deep vein thrombosis in the emergency department: Combining use of a clinical diagnosis model with D-dimer testing. *J Emerg Med.* 2000;19:225-230.

54. Wells PS, Hirsh J, Anderson DR, et al. A simple clinical model for the diagnosis of deep-vein thrombosis combined with impedance plethysmography: Potential for an improvement in the diagnostic process. *J Intern Med.* 1998;243:15-23.

55. Aschwanden M, Labs KH, Jeanneret C, et al. The value of rapid D-dimer testing combined with structured clinical evaluation for the diagnosis of deep vein thrombosis. *J Vasc Surg.* 1999;30:929-935.

56. Cornuz J, Ghali WA, Hayoz D, et al. Clinical prediction of deep venous thrombosis using two risk assessment methods in combination with rapid quantitative D-dimer testing. *Am J Med.* 2002;112:198-203.

57. Ilkhanipour K, Wolfson AB, Walker H, et al. Combining clinical risk with D-dimer testing to rule out deep vein thrombosis. *J Emerg Med.* 2004;27:233-239.

58. Dryjski M, O'Brien-Irr MS, Harris LM, et al. Evaluation of a screening protocol to exclude the diagnosis of deep venous thrombosis among emergency department patients. *J Vasc Surg.* 2001;34:1010-1015.

59. Wells PS, Anderson DR, Rodger M, et al. Evaluation of D-dimer in the diagnosis of suspected deep-vein thrombosis. *N Engl J Med.* 2003;349:1227-1235.

53

Examination of the Musculoskeletal System

xamination of the musculoskeletal system includes *inspection* (for joint swelling, redness, and deformity), *palpation* (for joint warmth, tenderness, and crepitus*), and investigation of the joint's *range of motion*. Of these tests, range of motion is the most sensitive indicator of joint disease. The normal range of motion of joints is presented in Table 53-1.

Joint pain may originate in the joint itself (i.e., articular disease) or in extra-articular structures such as tendons, ligaments, or nerves. Articular disease characteristically causes swelling and tenderness that surrounds the entire joint and limits the entire repertoire of a joint's motion, during both active and passive movements. Extra-articular disease, in contrast, causes swelling and tenderness localized to only particular regions of the joint, affecting some aspects of the joint's range of motion while sparing others. Extra-articular disease also

---

*"Crepitus" is a vibratory sensation felt over joints during movement.

Table 53-1	Normal Range of Motion of Joints*		

Joint	Flexion/ Extension (degrees)	Abduction/ Adduction (degrees)	Rotation (degrees)
Shoulder	180	180 (abduction) 45 (adduction, across body)	90 (internal rotation) 90 (external rotation)
Elbow	150 (humero-ulnar)		180 (radio-humeral)
Wrist and carpal joints	70 (wrist extension) 80–90 (palmar flexion)	50 (ulnar deviation) 20–30 (radial deviation)	
Fingers (MCP, PIP, and DIP joints)	90 (MCP) 120 (PIP) 80 (DIP)	30–40 (MCP combined abduction/ adduction)	
Hip	10–20 (extension) 120 (flexion, knee flexed)	40 (abduction) 25 (adduction)	40 (internal rotation) 45 (external rotation)†
Knee	130		
Ankle and feet	45 (plantar flexion) 20 (dorsiflexion)		30 (inversion) 20 (eversion)

MCP, metacarpophalangeal; PIP, proximal interphalangeal; DIP, distal interphalangeal.
*From reference 1.
†Internal and external rotation if hip and knee flexed; less if hip and knee extended.

tends to limit active joint movements (i.e., voluntary movements) more than passive ones (i.e., movements with the muscles relaxed).

In joints lacking normal alignment, "dislocation" implies complete lack of contact between the two articular surfaces whereas "subluxation" implies residual contact but abnormal alignment. In a "valgus" deformity, the distal part of the limb is directed *away* from the body midline (e.g., "genu valgum" of knock-kneed individual; or "hallux valgus" of persons with bunions). In a "varus" deformity, the distal part is directed *toward* the body midline (e.g., "genu varum" of bow-legged individuals). A "recurvatum" deformity describes abnormal hyperextension of a joint (e.g., "genu recurvatum" of back-kneed individuals, common in patients with chronic quadriceps weakness, see Chapter 5).

An attentive physical examination is fundamental to musculoskeletal diagnosis because, in contrast to other organ systems, the bedside finding *is* the diagnostic standard for many musculoskeletal disorders (Table 53-2). For example, in patients with symmetric arthritis of the wrists and hands, ulnar deviation of the metacarpophalangeal joints, and Swan-neck deformities of the fingers, the diagnosis of rheumatoid arthritis is almost certain whether or not the serologic rheumatoid factor is present (if absent, the patient has "seronegative rheumatoid arthritis"). Instead of focusing on such syndrome-defining findings (for which calculating LRs is impossible), this chapter will focus on those disorders of the shoulder, knee, and ankle whose diagnosis still relies on clinical imaging or surgical findings (e.g., osteoarthritis and orthopedic injuries). Other chapters of this book review stance and gait (see Chapter 5), back pain (see Chapter 60), and hand pain (see Chapter 60).

Table 53-2	Abnormal Articular Findings and Implied Diagnosis*
Finding	**Diagnosis**
Shoulder	
Inspection	
Flattening of rounded lateral aspect of shoulder	Anterior dislocation
Swelling over anterior aspect	Glenohumeral synovitis; synovial cyst
Elbow	
Inspection	
Localized cystic swelling over olecranon	Olecranon bursitis
Swelling obscures para-olecranon grooves	Elbow synovitis
Nodules over extensor surface of ulna	Gouty tophi; rheumatoid nodules
Palpation	
Elbow pain and tenderness over lateral epicondyle	Lateral epicondylitis ("tennis elbow")
Elbow pain and tenderness over medial epicondyle	Medial epicondylitis ("golfer's elbow")
Wrists and carpal joints	
Inspection	
Firm, painless cystic swelling, often located over volar or dorsal wrist	Ganglion (synovial cyst)

continued

Table 53-2	Abnormal Articular Findings and Implied Diagnosis*—Cont'd

Finding	Diagnosis
Thickening of palmar aponeurosis, causing flexion deformity of MCP joints (4th finger > 5th finger > 3rd finger)	Dupuytren's contracture
Abnormal prominence of distal ulna	Subluxation of ulna (from chronic inflammatory arthritis, especially rheumatoid arthritis)
Nonpitting swelling proximal to wrist joint, sparing joint itself; associated clubbing of digits	Hypertrophic osteoarthropathy
Special tests	
Flexion and extension of digits causes snapping or catching sensation in palm	Trigger finger (flexor tenosynovitis)
Finkelstein's test: pain when patient makes fist with fingers over thumb and bends the wrist in an ulnar direction	Tenosynovitis of long abductor and short extensor of thumb, or "De Quervain's stenosing tenosynovitis")
Fingers	
Inspection	
Loss of normal knuckle wrinkles	PIP or DIP synovitis
Loss of "hills and valleys" between metacarpal heads	MCP synovitis
Ulnar deviation at metacarpophalangeal joints	Chronic inflammatory arthritis
Swan-neck deformity (flexion contracture at MCP joint, hyperextension of PIP joint, flexion of DIP joint)	Chronic inflammatory arthritis, especially rheumatoid arthritis
Boutonniere deformity (flexion of PIP, hyperextension of DIP)	Detachment of central slip of extensor tendon to PIP, common in rheumatoid arthritis
Osteophytes: Heberden's nodes at DIP, Bouchard's nodes at PIP	Osteoarthritis
Mallet finger: flexion deformity of DIP	Detachment of extensor tendon from base of distal phalanx or fracture
"Telescoping" or "opera glass hand": shortening of digits and destruction of IP joints	"Arthritis mutilans," in rheumatoid or psoriatic arthritis
Hip	
Inspection	
Trauma, hip externally rotated	Femoral neck fracture; anterior dislocation

| Table 53-2 | Abnormal Articular Findings and Implied Diagnosis*—Cont'd |

Finding	Diagnosis
Trauma, hip internally rotated	Posterior dislocation
Pelvic tilt (imaginary line through the anterior iliac spines is not horizontal)	Scoliosis; anatomic leg-length discrepancy; hip disease
Palpation	
Hip pain, tenderness localized over greater trochanter	Trochanteric bursitis
Hip pain, tenderness localized over middle third of inguinal ligament, lateral to femoral pulse	Iliopsoas bursitis
Hip pain and tenderness localized over ischial tuberosity	Ischiogluteal bursitis ("Weaver's bottom")
Knee	
Inspection	
Localized tenderness and swelling over patella	Prepatellar bursitis ("Housemaid's knees")
Generalized swelling of popliteal space	Baker's cyst (enlarged semimembranosus bursa, which communicates with knee joint)
Genu varum and genu valgum	See text
Palpation	
Knee pain and tenderness localized over medial aspect of upper tibia	Anserine bursitis
Distressed reaction if patella moved laterally ("apprehension test")	Recurrent patellar dislocation
Ankle and feet	
Inspection	
Flattening of longitudinal arch	Pes planus
Abnormal elevation of medial longitudinal arch	Pes cavus
Outward angulation of great toe with prominence over medial 1st MTP joint (bunion)	Hallux valgus
Hyperextension of MTP joints and flexion of PIP joints	Hammer toes
Palpation	
Nodules within Achilles tendon	Tendon xanthoma
Foot pain, localized tenderness over calcaneal origin of plantar fascia	Plantar fascitis
Foot pain, localized tenderness over plantar surface of MT heads	Metatarsalgia

continued

Table 53-2	Abnormal Articular Findings and Implied Diagnosis*—Cont'd

Finding	Diagnosis
Forefoot pain, tenderness between 2nd or 3rd toes or between 3rd and 4th toes	Morton's interdigital neuroma
Ankle pain, dysesthesias of sole, aggravated by forced dorsiflexion and eversion of foot	Tarsal tunnel syndrome

MCP, metacarpophalangeal; PIP, proximal interphalangeal; DIP, distal interphalangeal; MT, metatarsal; MTP, metatarsophalangeal.
*Special tests of the shoulder and knee are discussed in the text.

THE SHOULDER

I. INTRODUCTION

Shoulder pain is the third most common musculoskeletal complaint (the first two are back pain and knee pain).[2] The shoulder is vulnerable to pain because it is the only location in the human body where tendons (i.e., the rotator cuff tendons*) pass between moving bones (i.e., the acromion and humerus). This anatomy grants the shoulder great flexibility but also renders the rotator cuff tendons and accompanying bursa susceptible to inflammation, degeneration, and tears.

One popular method of classifying shoulder pain (Table 53-3), based on the work of the British orthopedic surgeon James Cyriax,[3,4] distinguishes the causes of shoulder pain by the location of pain, range of passive motion, strength of the rotator cuff muscles, and presence of "painful arc" (i.e., pain during arm elevation between the angles of 70 and 100 degrees, angles at which compression of the subacromial tissues is the greatest). Using this classification, 5% to 12% of patients with shoulder pain have capsular syndromes, 17% acute bursitis, 5% to 11% acromioclavicular syndromes, 47% to 65% subacromial syndromes, and 5% to 10% referred shoulder pain (e.g., cervical disc disease or myofascial pain).[5–8]

Nonetheless, some clinicians have questioned the utility and accuracy of this classification, for several reasons: (1) most shoulder syndromes are treated similarly with anti-inflammatory medications, injections, and physical therapy, no

---

*The tendons of the supraspinatus, infraspinatus, subscapularis, and teres minor muscles make up the rotator cuff.

Table 53-3	Shoulder Syndromes*			
Syndrome	Location of Pain	Range of Passive Motion	Other Findings
Capsular syndromes Adhesive capsulitis Glenohumeral arthritis	Outer arm	Limited[†] (all motions limited, especially external rotation and abduction)	
Acute bursitis[†]	Outer arm	Limited[†] (abduction especially limited)	
Acromioclavicular pain	Point of shoulder	Normal	Tenderness of acromioclavicular joint Pain worse during adduction of arm across body
Subacromial syndromes[‡] Rotator cuff tendonitis Rotator cuff tear	Outer arm	Normal	Painful arc Rotator cuff muscle strength: Normal in tendonitis Weak in rotator cuff tears

*From references 3–5.
[†]One way to test for limitation of passive motion is to ask the patient to bend over and try to touch his or her toes. In those with normal shoulder passive motion, the arms dangle toward the floor.
[‡]"Acute bursitis" and "subacromial disorders both represent disorders of the subacromial space, but "bursitis" causes inflammation and swelling that is more acute and severe, thus limiting motion.

matter what the diagnosis is[5]; (2) the different shoulder syndromes are indistinguishable from the patient's perspective, causing similar pain and disability over time[5,6]; (3) if the patient is examined a second time, the diagnosis changes 43% of the time[6]; and (4) more than 20 different bedside tests have been proposed to diagnose shoulder disorders, and new ones continue to appear,[9,10] suggesting that a comprehensive understanding of shoulder pain is still lacking.

Nonetheless, the bedside examination continues to play an important role in patients with shoulder pain, especially in distinguishing intrinsic shoulder syndromes from disorders causing referred pain, and in identifying rotator cuff tears, a condition sometimes requiring surgical repair. These subjects are the focus of this section.

II. THE FINDINGS

A. IMPINGEMENT SIGNS

Impingement signs reproduce subacromial pain by compressing the rotator cuff tendons between the head of the humerus and acromion. Of the many different impingement signs, the most popular are the "Neer impingement sign" and "Hawkins impingement sign" (Figs. 53-1 and 53-2). Both of these maneuvers

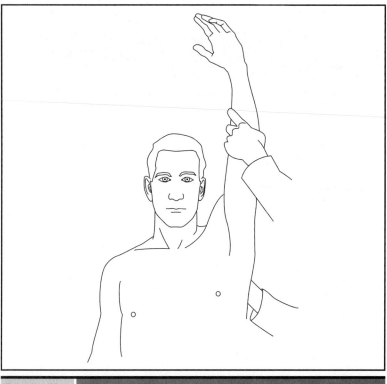

FIGURE 53-1	NEER IMPINGEMENT SIGN.[11]

The clinician prevents scapular motion with one hand and uses the other hand to raise the patient's arm in forward flexion, a position that presses the greater tuberosity of the humerus against the acromion.[11,12] Neer believed his sign was nonspecific (i.e., shoulder pains of all types worsened with this maneuver), but he taught that subacromial pain was the only shoulder syndrome whose positive impingement sign disappeared after injection of the subacromial space with lidocaine.

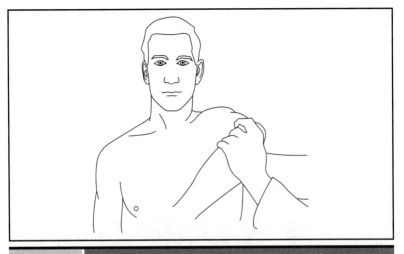

FIGURE 53-2	HAWKINS IMPINGEMENT SIGN.[13]

The clinician stands in front of the patient, flexes both the patient's shoulder and elbow to 90 degrees, and then internally rotates the patient's arm, a position that presses the greater tuberosity against the coracoacromial ligament.[12]

were originally introduced to select patients for specific surgical procedures. Neer's maneuver forces the humerus (and overlying rotator cuff tendons) against the *anterior* acromion, which Neer proposed resecting (i.e., anterior acromioplasty) in patients with persistent pain.[11] Hawkins' maneuver forces the greater tuberosity of the humerus against the coracoacromial ligament (the ligament forming the anterior roof over the rotator cuff). If patients develop pain during this maneuver and surgery is contemplated, Hawkins believed the coracoacromial ligament should be resected.[13]

B. YERGASON'S SIGN (FIG. 53-3)

Yergason's sign[14] has traditionally been associated with bicipital tendonitis, as if that were an isolated entity, but in fact most patients with inflammation of the biceps tendon also have disease of the rotator cuff. This occurs because progressive subacromial impingement causes wearing away of the supraspinatus tendon and underlying capsule, which then exposes the long head of the biceps tendon and subjects it to the same injurious forces. In fact, most tears of the biceps tendon are associated with advanced rotator cuff disease.[11,15,16]

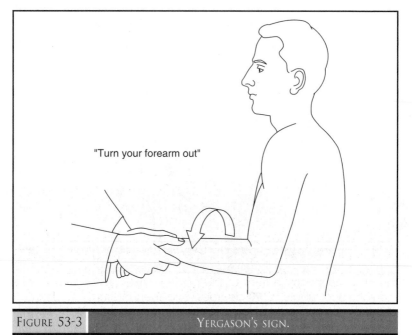

"Turn your forearm out"

FIGURE 53-3	YERGASON'S SIGN.

The clinician stands in front of the patient, flexes the patient's forearm 90 degrees at the elbow, and pronates the patient's wrist. The clinician then asks the patient to supinate the forearm against resistance (i.e., turn forearm in the direction of the arrow). Pain indicates a positive test, implying inflammation of the long head of the biceps tendon (the main supinator of the forearm).

C. MUSCLE ATROPHY

The clinician detects atrophy of the supraspinatus or infraspinatus muscles by inspecting the posterior scapula on the symptomatic side and noting any increased prominence of the scapular spine when compared with the contralateral side. Atrophy of these muscles may appear as soon as 2 to 3 weeks after a rotator cuff tear.

D. MUSCLE TESTING

The most important muscles to test in suspected tears of the rotator cuff are the supraspinatus muscle (involved in most rotator cuff tears) and the infraspinatus muscle (involved in 11% to 45% of tears).[16,17] The supraspinatus muscle abducts the shoulder, and the infraspinatus externally rotates it. Figures 53-4 and 53-5 describe how to test the strength of these muscles.

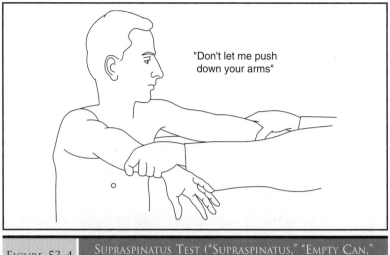

"Don't let me push down your arms"

FIGURE 53-4	SUPRASPINATUS TEST ("SUPRASPINATUS," "EMPTY CAN," OR "JOBE" TEST).

The clinician stands in front of the patient and elevates the patient's arms to 90 degrees in the plane of the scapula (i.e., "scaption," midway between forward flexion and sideways abduction). The patient's arms are internally rotated with thumbs pointing down (as if emptying a can). The patient is asked to hold this position and resist attempts to lower the arms to the side. Some investigators propose testing the supraspinatus muscle in a slightly different way, with the arms externally rotated and thumbs pointing up (i.e., "full can" test), because this position causes less pain than the "empty can" test. In clinical studies, both versions have similar diagnostic accuracy.[17]

E. DROPPED ARM TEST

The examiner lifts the patient's arm to abduct it as far as possible and releases it, asking the patient to lower the arm slowly back down to the side. In patients who have a positive test, indicating a torn rotator cuff, the patient can lower the arm smoothly until about 100 degrees, after which the smooth movements become irregular and the arm may fall suddenly to the side.[19,20]

The dropped arm test becomes positive at angles of less than 100 degrees, not because the supraspinatus is the most powerful abductor at this angle* but because the rotator cuff muscles must be intact to pull the humeral head tightly against the glenoid fossa, creating a fulcrum that allows the deltoid to smoothly lower the arm.

---

*The supraspinatus muscle is responsible for only the initial 30 degrees of abduction, whereas the deltoid muscle (uninvolved in rotator cuff disease) accounts for abduction between 30 and 180 degrees.

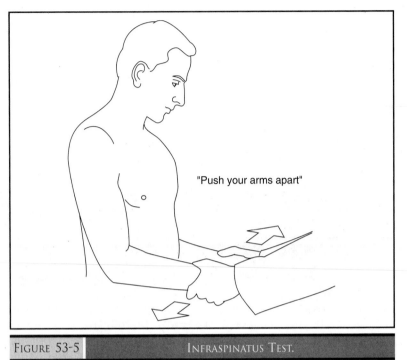

FIGURE 53-5 INFRASPINATUS TEST.

The clinician stands in front of the patient, and the patient's arms are at his or her side with elbows flexed 90 degrees and thumbs up. The examiner places his or her hands outside those of the patient's and directs the patient to move the arms out (i.e., direction of arrow), resisting the clinician's opposing inward pressure.[18]

F. PALPATING ROTATOR CUFF TEARS

Early descriptions of rotator cuff tears emphasized the importance of actually palpating the tear, just anterior to the acromial edge and through the deltoid muscle (Fig. 53-6).[21]

III. CLINICAL SIGNIFICANCE

A. ACROMIOCLAVICULAR JOINT PAIN

In patients who have pain at the shoulder joint suggesting acromioclavicular joint pain (see Table 53-3), neither acromioclavicular joint tenderness nor tenderness during acromioclavicular joint compression accurately identifies those

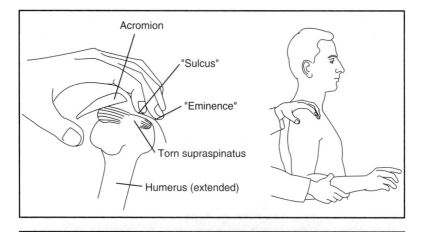

| FIGURE 53-6 | PALPATION OF ROTATOR CUFF TEARS. |

The clinician stands behind the patient, and the patient's arm is relaxed at the side with elbow flexed 90 degrees. The clinician palpates just below the patient's acromion with one hand and holds the patient's forearm with the other. The clinician then gently extends the patient's arm as far as possible and rotates the shoulder internally and externally to fully reveal the greater tuberosity and attached tissues. In patients with tears of the supraspinatus tendon (which normally inserts on the greater tuberosity), the clinician detects both an abnormal eminence and an abnormal sulcus posterior to this eminence. The abnormal eminence is the greater tuberosity with attached remnant of tendon, and the sulcus just behind it is the actual rent in the supraspinatus tendon. Comparison with the contralateral shoulder helps determine whether the suspected tear is real or not.

patients who experience relief after injection of acromioclavicular joint with lidocaine (likelihood ratios [LRs] not significant, EBM Box 53-1).

B. ROTATOR CUFF TENDONITIS

According to the LRs in EBM Box 53-1, the only finding arguing significantly for rotator cuff tendinitis in patients with shoulder pain is a positive Yergason's sign (LR = 2.8). This finding emphasizes once more the association between biceps tendon pain and rotator cuff disease.

Neither the presence of a positive Neer impingement sign nor the presence of a positive Hawkins sign significantly increases the probability of rotator cuff tendonitis (both LRs <1.5), simply because shoulder pains of all types worsen

Box 53-1 Shoulder Pain*

Finding (Ref)[†]	Sensitivity (%)	Specificity (%)	Likelihood Ratio if Finding	
			Present	Absent
DETECTING ACROMIOCLAVICULAR JOINT PAIN				
Acromioclavicular joint tenderness[8]	96	10	NS	NS
Tenderness with compression of acromioclavicular joint[8]	79	50	NS	NS
DETECTING ROTATOR CUFF TENDONITIS				
Hawkin's impingement sign[22,23]	92	26–44	1.4	**0.3**
Neer's impingement sign[22,23]	75–89	32–48	1.3	0.4
Hawkin's or Neer's impingement sign[23]	96	41	1.6	**0.1**
Yergason's sign[22]	37	87	2.8	0.7
Painful arc[22]	32	82	NS	NS
DETECTING ROTATOR CUFF TEAR–INDIVIDUAL FINDINGS				
Age[19]				
≤ 39 years	5	58	**0.1**	...
40–59 years	34	...	NS	...
≥ 60 years	62	81	**3.2**	...
Neer's impingement sign[23]	88	43	1.5	**0.3**
Hawkin's impingement sign[23]	83	51	1.7	**0.3**
Supraspinatus testing causes pain[16,17]	63–85	52–55	1.5	NS
Supraspinatus atrophy[18]	55	73	2.0	0.6
Infraspinatus atrophy[18]	55	73	2.0	0.6
Supraspinatus weakness[10,16–18,24]	41–84	58–70	2.0	0.5
Infraspinatus weakness[18]	76	57	1.8	0.4
Painful arc[18]	97	10	NS	**0.3**
Dropped arm test[19]	10	98	**5.0**	NS
Palpable tear[25,26]	91–96	75–97	**10.2**	**0.1**

(continued)

Box 53-1   Shoulder Pain*—Cont'd

Finding (Ref)[†]	Sensitivity (%)	Specificity (%)	Likelihood Ratio if Finding	
			Present	Absent

DETECTING ROTATOR CUFF TEAR – COMBINED FINDINGS[19]

3 findings	24	100	**48.0**	...
2 findings	37	...	**4.9**	...
1 finding	39	...	NS	...
0 findings	1	52	**0.02**	

NS, not significant; likelihood ratio (LR) if finding present = positive LR; LR if finding absent = negative LR.

*Diagnostic standard: For acromioclavicular joint pain, ≥50% reduction of pain within 10 minutes after injecting lidocaine into the acromioclavicular joint[8]; for rotator cuff tendonitis, relief of pain and full range of motion within 30 minutes after injecting lidocaine into subacromial space[22] or subacromial bursitis during arthroscopy[23]; for rotator cuff tear, presence of tear during arthrography,[18] magnetic resonance imaging,[17] or operation (arthroscopy or open repair).[10,16,19,23–26]

[†]Definition of findings: For tenderness with compression of the acromioclavicular joint, pain when the examiner compresses together his or her thumb (over the patient's posterolateral acromion) and index and middle fingers (over the patient's ipsilateral mid-clavicle)[8]; for combined findings, the clinician tallies how many of the following findings are present: (1) supraspinatus weakness, (2) weakness of external rotation (i.e., infraspinatus weakness), and (3) positive impingement sign (during external rotation, internal rotation, or both).[19]

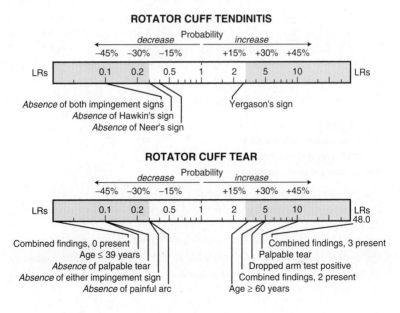

ROTATOR CUFF TENDINITIS

ROTATOR CUFF TEAR

during these maneuvers (i.e., specificity < 50%). In these clinical studies, however, the maneuvers were not repeated after lidocaine injection, as Neer originally proposed. A *negative* impingement sign, on the other hand, significantly decreases the probability of subacromial disease (negative LR for Hawkin's sign = 0.3, for Neer's sign = 0.4, see EBM Box 53-1). The absence of both impingement signs argues strongly against subacromial disease (LR = 0.1).

C.   ROTATOR CUFF TEARS
1.   Individual Findings

The most important bedside findings arguing for the presence of a rotator cuff tear in patients with shoulder pain are a positive dropped arm test (LR = 5.0, see EBM Box 53-1) and age ≥60 years (LR = 3.2). Findings that argue *against* the presence of rotator cuff tear are age ≤39 years (LR = 0.1), absence of painful arc (LR = 0.3), and negative impingement signs (LR = 0.3).

Although the reported diagnostic accuracy of palpating actual rents in the supraspinatus tendon is impressive (positive LR = 10.2, negative LR = 0.1, see EBM Box 53-1), these LRs derive from examinations by orthopedic surgeons who had a comprehensive understanding of the anatomy of the shoulder and considerable experience treating shoulder pain.[25,26] Whether other practitioners can duplicate this accuracy is unknown.

2.   Combined Findings

In a study of 400 patients with shoulder pain undergoing arthroscopy, Murrell and Walton identified three predictors of rotator cuff tear: supraspinatus weakness, weakness in external rotation (i.e., infraspinatus weakness), and a positive impingement sign.[19] According to the LRs in EBM Box 53-1, the presence of all three of these signs is a compelling argument for rotator cuff tear (LR = 48.0), whereas the absence of all three practically excludes the diagnosis (LR = 0.02).

THE KNEE

I.   INTRODUCTION

Knee pain affects up to 13% of the adult population and is second only to back pain among musculoskeletal complaints.[27] Common causes of knee pain include arthritis (osteoarthritis, rheumatoid arthritis, gout, and pseudogout), bursitis (prepatellar and anserine bursitis), and injuries to ligaments or menisci. Among patients presenting with knee trauma, 6% to 12% have significant fractures on knee radiographs,[28–33] and the most frequently injured internal structures are the medial collateral ligament, anterior cruciate ligament, and menisci (injuries of the medial meniscus outnumber lateral ones at least 3 to 1).[34-39]

II. THE FINDINGS

A. OTTAWA RULES FOR KNEE FRACTURE

Based on study of more than 1000 patients with acute blunt injury to the knee, Stiell and others have identified five independent predictors of clinically significant knee trauma (Table 53-4).[31] In this study, the "knee" was broadly considered to include the patella, the head and neck of the fibula, the proximal 8 cm of the tibia, and the distal 8 cm of the femur; "significant" trauma implied an injury requiring orthopedic consultation, splinting, or surgery.

B. TESTS OF LIGAMENT INJURIES

The stability of the knee depends on the joint capsule and two pairs of ligaments: the medial and lateral collateral ligaments, and the anterior and posterior cruciate ligaments (ACL and PCL).* The clinician tests each of these four ligaments by stressing the knee in a direction that the intact ligament would normally resist (specific tests appear later). If no movement occurs during stress

---

*The crossed cruciate ligaments are named for their attachment to the *tibial* surface, that is, the *anterior* cruciate ligament (ACL) crosses from the posterior femur to the *anterior* tibia; the *posterior* cruciate ligament (PCL) crosses from the anterior femur to the *posterior* tibia. "Cruciate" derives from Latin cruciatus, meaning "cross-shaped."

Table 53-4	Ottawa Rule for Knee Fracture[31,32]

A knee radiograph is indicated (and the rule is positive) if *any* of the following are present:
    Aged 55 years or older
    Tenderness at head of fibula
    Isolated tenderness of patella*
    Inability to flex to 90 degrees
    Inability to bear weight both immediately and in the emergency department (4 steps)†

---

*No bone tenderness of knee other than patella.
†Unable to transfer weight twice onto each lower limb regardless of limping.

testing or if small movements occur but abruptly end with a firm stop (i.e., a "hard" endpoint), the ligament is intact. If there is excessive laxity of movement or a "soft" or "mushy" endpoint, the ligament is damaged.

Blunt trauma to the outside of the knee often is associated with injury of the medial collateral ligament; trauma to the inside of the knee suggests injury of the lateral collateral ligament. Twisting of the knee after planting the foot is the characteristic mechanism of ACL injury, whereas deceleration of the flexed knee on a hard surface (e.g., striking the knee against the dashboard in an automobile accident) often precedes PCL injury. The mechanism of meniscal injuries resembles that of ACL injuries—twisting the knee after planting the foot—but unlike ACL injuries which are associated with immediate knee swelling, meniscal injuries are associated with swelling that appears only after a several hour delay (because the menisci are relatively avascular).[40,41]

1. Anterior Cruciate Ligament (ACL)

The ACL prevents anterior subluxation of the tibia on the femoral head. There are three common tests for this ligament: the anterior drawer sign, Lachman's sign, and the pivot shift sign (Figs. 53-7, 53-8, and 53-9).[42]

The pivot shift sign refers to the tendency of the tibia to sublux anteriorly in ACL-deficient knees when the knee is between 0 and 30 degrees of flexion, and the *spontaneous reduction* of the subluxed tibia as the knee is flexed past 40 degrees.[44,45] Patients with ACL injuries notice the pivot-shift phenomenon themselves when they plant their foot with extended knee in front of them (e.g., stopping suddenly from a run causes the tibia to shift forward, producing the sensation of the knee "giving way").[43] Figure 53-10 explains the mechanism of the pivot shift phenomenon. What specifically is responsible for the sudden reduction at 40 to 50 degrees is controversial, but most experts believe it is the pull of the iliotibial tract (whose action abruptly changes from a knee extensor to knee flexor beyond 40 degrees flexion)[44,46–49] and the geometric peculiarities of the convex tibial surface.[45,50]

Descriptions of the anterior drawer sign have been found in writings dating to the 1870s.[51] Lachman's test was attributed to the American orthopedic surgeon John Lachman by one of his students in 1976,[52] although the same sign was described a century earlier by European clinicians.[51] Photographs of patients demonstrating their own pivot shift phenomenon were published in 1920,[53] but the "pivot shift" test was formerly described in 1972.[54] The term itself is confusing, but according to Liorzou[47] it originated from an interview with a hockey player who stated "when I pivot, my knee shifts."

2. Posterior Cruciate Ligament

The PCL is the least likely internal structure of the knee to be injured.[34–36] Because this ligament resists posterior subluxation of the tibia on the femur, the conventional test is the "posterior drawer sign" (Fig. 53-11).

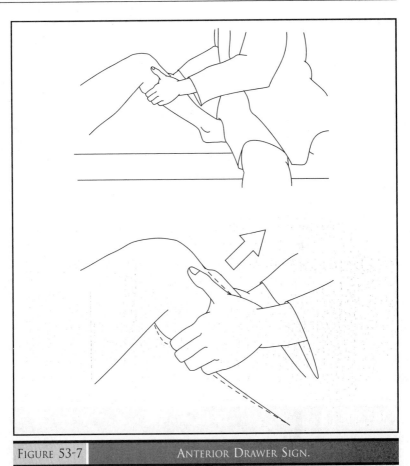

FIGURE 53-7	ANTERIOR DRAWER SIGN.

The patient lies supine with hip flexed at 45 degrees, knee flexed at 90 degrees, and foot flat on the table. The clinician sits on top of the patient's foot to stabilize it and stresses the ACL ligament by grasping the patient's upper calf and pulling forward. Abnormal anterior sub-luxation of the tibia (*arrow*) with a soft endpoint is a positive test.

3. Collateral Ligaments

Injury to either collateral ligament is identified by applying a varus or valgus stress to the knee and noting abnormal movement when compared with the contralateral side. Testing is performed with the knee straight and at 20 degrees flexion. Excessive movement during valgus stress indicates injury to the medial collateral ligament; excessive movement during varus stress indicates injury to the lateral collateral ligament.

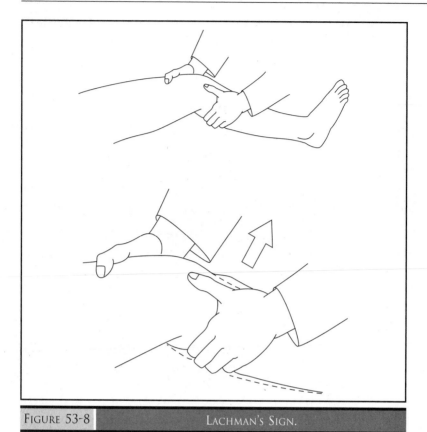

FIGURE 53-8 **FIGURE 53-8** **LACHMAN'S SIGN.**

Lachman's sign differs from the anterior drawer sign (see Fig. 53-7) by the position of the knee during testing. In Lachman's test, the hip is extended and the knee flexed at only 20 degrees. The clinician grasps the lower thigh with one hand and the upper calf with the other, pulling forward on the tibia to stress the ligament and reveal the abnormal anterior subluxation of the tibia (*arrow*).

C. TESTS OF MENISCAL INJURIES: THE MCMURRAY TEST

Tears of the *anterior* meniscus or large bucket-handle tears often displace tissue between the articular surfaces of the anterior tibia and femur, thus preventing full extension of the knee (or "locking"), a characteristic sign of meniscal injury.

Because tears of the posterior half of the meniscus are unlikely to cause locking and are therefore more difficult to detect, the British orthopedic surgeon McMurray proposed in 1949 additional diagnostic tests, one of which is now called the McMurray test (Fig. 53-12).[39,55-57]

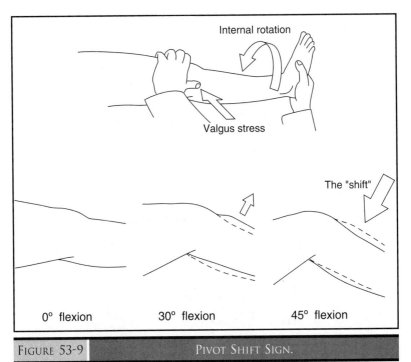

Internal rotation

Valgus stress

The "shift"

0° flexion   30° flexion   45° flexion

FIGURE 53-9   PIVOT SHIFT SIGN.

Many variations of this test have been published,[42] but the most common version begins with the patient supine, hip and knee extended. The clinician lifts the patient's leg, one hand over the fibula and the other at the ankle, pushing medially on the fibula (i.e., providing a valgus stress) and rotating internally the ankle and foot (and thus tibia). While maintaining these valgus and rotational stresses, the examiner slowly flexes the patient's knee. In the ACL-deficient knee, the tibia subluxes anteriorly, almost imperceptibly, during the initial 0 to 30 degrees flexion with these applied forces (*small arrow*). At 40 to 50 degrees, however, the tibia suddenly subluxes posteriorly ("the shift"), which constitutes a positive pivot shift test (and recalls for many patients the sensation of their "knee giving way").[43]

III. CLINICAL SIGNIFICANCE

A. DETECTING OSTEOARTHRITIS

In a study of 237 patients with various forms of chronic knee pain (i.e., osteoarthritis, rheumatoid arthritis, meniscal or ligament injuries, osteonecrosis, gout, septic arthritis, and other assorted connective tissue disorders),[58] the following findings

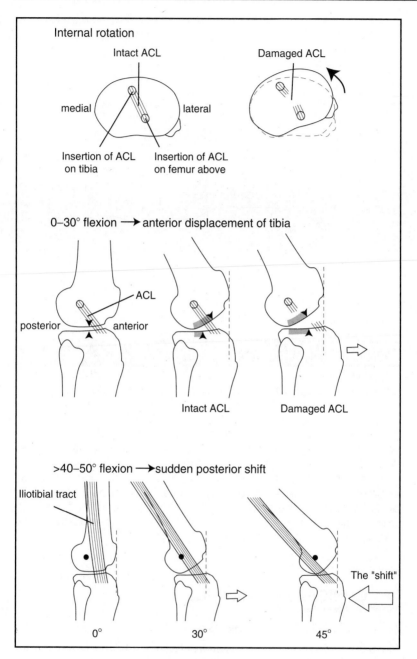

Internal rotation

Intact ACL

Damaged ACL

medial lateral

Insertion of ACL on tibia

Insertion of ACL on femur above

0–30° flexion → anterior displacement of tibia

ACL

posterior anterior

Intact ACL

Damaged ACL

>40–50° flexion → sudden posterior shift

Iliotibial tract

The "shift"

0°   30°   45°

argued *for* the diagnosis of osteoarthritis of the knee: palpable bony enlargement (LR = 11.8, EBM Box 53-2), genu varum deformity (LR = 3.4), stiffness lasting less than 30 minutes (LR = 3.0), or the presence of at least three of six characteristic findings listed in EBM Box 53-2 (LR = 3.1). The most compelling arguments *against* the diagnosis of osteoarthritis are two or fewer of the characteristic findings (LR = 0.1), morning stiffness lasting greater than 30 minutes (LR = 0.2), and absence of crepitus (LR = 0.2). The presence of valgus deformity is unhelpful (LR

FIGURE 53-10	MECHANISM OF THE PIVOT SHIFT.

The pivot shift phenomenon (i.e., positive test) refers to anterior displacement of the tibia with respect to the distal femur during the first 30 degrees of flexion and the sudden backward return of the tibia to its normal position after about 40 to 50 degrees flexion (see Fig. 53-9). This figure depicts what happens during internal rotation (*top row*), 0 to 30 degrees flexion (*middle row*), and beyond 40 to 50 degrees flexion (*bottom row*) in the anterior cruciate ligament (ACL)-deficient knee. *Top row* (view of the tibial plateau from above): Because of its oblique orientation (*left*), the ACL is the key ligament resisting internal rotation of the tibia (this also explains why many ACL injuries occur after the athlete plants the foot and then rotates the knee). If the ACL is torn (*right*), internal rotation causes excessive anterior movement of the tibia (with respect to the femur). (2) *Middle row* (0 to 30 degrees flexion): The *left* figure shows the orientation of the ACL, and the black arrowheads mark contiguous points on the femur and tibia when the knee is fully extended. During flexion of the knee when the ACL is intact (*middle* figure), the femur glides on the tibia, which results in a large surface area of the femur (gray shading) contacting a relatively small area on the tibia. If the ACL is damaged (*right* figure), such gliding does not occur and instead the femur rolls back on the tibia, which displaces the tibia anteriorly (see vertical dotted line). A valgus stress is applied during the pivot shift test because it ensures contact between the lateral femoral condyle and lateral tibial plateau, as occurs during normal weight-bearing. (3) *Bottom row:* When the knee is extended (*left*), the iliotibial tract is relaxed and lies in front of the axis of flexion (dark circle). At 30 degrees flexion (*middle*), the iliotibial tract is still in front of the axis of flexion, but it becomes taut in the ACL-deficient knee as the tibia is displaced anteriorly. At 45 degrees flexion (*right*), the iliotibial tract suddenly falls behind the axis of flexion, thus shifting from an extensor to a flexor of the knee and pulling the tibia backward into its normal alignment (the "shift").

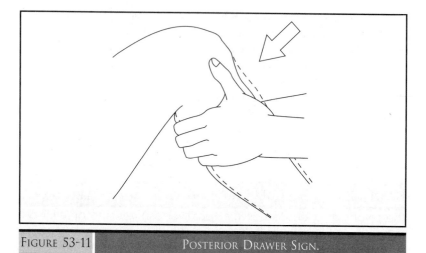

FIGURE 53-11   POSTERIOR DRAWER SIGN.

With the patient positioned as for the anterior drawer sign (see Fig. 53-7), the clinician pushes posteriorly on the patient's upper calf. In the PCL-deficient knee, this force reveals an abnormal posterior tibial movement (*arrow*) with a soft endpoint.

not significant), occurring just as often in patients with osteoarthritis as alternative diagnoses.

B. DETECTING KNEE FRACTURE

In patients presenting to emergency departments with knee trauma, the most compelling arguments *for* a clinically significant knee fracture are inability to flex the knee beyond 60 degrees (LR = 4.7, EBM Box 53-3)[29,31,32,59] inability to bear weight immediately after the injury and in the emergency department (LR = 3.6), tenderness at the head of the fibula (LR = 3.4), and age of 55 years or more (LR = 3.0). The most compelling argument *against* knee fracture is a negative Ottawa knee rule (LR = 0.1, i.e., lacking all five predictors from Table 53-4).

C. DETECTING LIGAMENT AND MENISCAL INJURIES

Most studies of soft tissue injuries of the knee are vulnerable to both *selection bias* (i.e., only patients scheduled for surgery are enrolled) and *verification bias* (i.e., the surgeons who operated on the patients are also the clinicians who examined the patients). Nonetheless, these biases may be less important that expected because other studies using independent diagnostic standards (e.g., magnetic resonance imaging [MRI])[60,61] reveal similar diagnostic accuracy for these clinical signs.

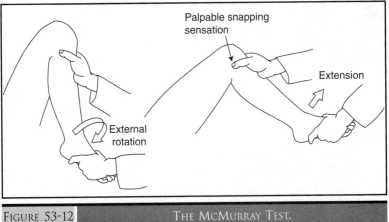

| FIGURE 53-12 | THE MCMURRAY TEST. |

The clinician flexes the patient's knee fully against the buttock and rotates the tibia (by grasping the patient's foot and ankle). The purpose of rotation is to bring the torn meniscal fragment, located on the posterior half of the meniscus, *anterior* to the curved surface of the femoral condyle: *external* rotation brings forward the *medial* meniscus; *internal* rotation, the *lateral* meniscus. This figure, therefore, depicts testing of the medial meniscus: the clinician places a free hand over the medial joint line, fully flexes the patient's knee, and then rotates the tibia externally. The clinician slowly extends the knee while maintaining this rotational force, thereby forcing the medial femoral condyle to glide forward on the tibia and *over* any torn fragment of meniscus. When the femur passes over the torn fragment, a palpable snapping sensation may be detected at the medial joint line (a positive test). To test the lateral meniscus, the clinician repeats the test while internally rotating the knee and palpating the lateral joint line. Popular orthopedic textbooks[55] and review articles[41,56,57] add varus and valgus stresses to their definitions of the McMurray test, although McMurray did not include this in his original description nor were they used in clinical studies testing the sign's accuracy (see Section III.B).[37,38]

1. Anterior Cruciate Ligament Injury

Any of the three physical tests of ACL injury, when positive, are compelling arguments *for* ACL injury: Lachman's sign (LR = 17.0, EBM Box 53-4), anterior drawer sign (LR = 11.5), and pivot shift sign (LR = 8.0). When these signs are absent, however, only the absence of Lachman's sign argues significantly against the probability of ACL injury (LR = 0.2).

Box 53-2 Diagnosis of Osteoarthritis, in Patients with Chronic Knee Pain

Finding (Ref)[†]	Sensitivity (%)	Specificity (%)	Likelihood Ratio if Finding Present	Absent
Individual findings				
Stiffness <30 minutes	85	72	**3.0**	**0.2**
Crepitus, passive motion	89	58	2.1	**0.2**
Bony enlargement	55	95	**11.8**	0.5
Palpable increase in temperature	14	52	**0.3**	1.6
Valgus deformity	24	83	NS	NS
Varus deformity	22	93	**3.4**	0.8
Combined findings				
At least 3 out of 6:	95	69	**3.1**	**0.1**
Age >50 years				
Stiffness <30 minutes				
Crepitus				
Bony tenderness along margins of joint				
Bone enlargement				
No palpable warmth				

NS, not significant; likelihood ratio (LR) if finding present = positive LR; LR if finding absent = negative LR.
*Diagnostic standard: For diagnosis of osteoarthritis, consensus of experts after review of patient's course, laboratory tests, and radiographs.
†Definition of findings: For morning stiffness < 30 minutes, when applied only to patients complaining of morning stiffness and knee pain.

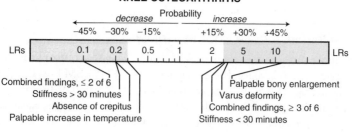

Box 53-3   Clinically Significant Knee Fracture*

Finding (Ref)[†]	Sensitivity (%)	Specificity (%)	Likelihood Ratio if Finding Present	Absent[†]
Individual findings				
Age ≥55 years[29,32]	23–48	87–88	**3.0**	NS
Joint effusion[29,31,32,59]	54–79	71–81	2.5	0.5
Ecchymosis[29]	19	91	NS	NS
Limitation of knee flexion[29,31,32]				
Not able to flex beyond 90 degrees	42–65	78–80	2.9	0.5
Not able to flex beyond 60 degrees	46–49	90	**4.7**	0.6
Isolated tenderness of patella[29,31,32]	25–31	85–89	2.2	0.8
Tenderness at head of fibula[29,31,32]	12–32	92–95	**3.4**	NS
Inability to bear weight, immediately and in emergency department[29,31,32]	46–58	81–89	**3.6**	0.6
Combined findings				
Ottawa knee rule positive[28–33]	83–99	19–54	1.7	**0.1**

NS, not significant; likelihood ratio (LR) if finding present = positive LR; LR if finding absent = negative LR.
*Diagnostic standard: For clinically significant knee fracture, one requiring orthopedic consultation, splinting, or surgery (i.e., one >5 mm in breadth or one associated with complete tendon or ligament disruption).
†Definition of findings: For isolated tenderness of the patella, no bony tenderness elsewhere on the knee[32]; for inability to bear weight immediately and in emergency department, unable to transfer weight twice onto each lower limb regardless of limping; for Ottawa rule positive, see Table 53-4.

Lachman's sign is more sensitive than the anterior drawer sign for three reasons[52]: (1) hemarthrosis from acute ACL injury may impair knee flexion and thus prevent testing of the anterior drawer test; (2) tense hamstring muscles, irritated from pain, directly oppose forward subluxation of the tibia during the anterior drawer sign (knee at 90 degrees) but do not interfere with anterior subluxation when the knee is at 20 degrees (because at this angle the hamstring pull is almost perpendicular to anterior subluxation of the tibia); and (3) the thick posterior edge of the medial meniscus acts as a wedge against the curved

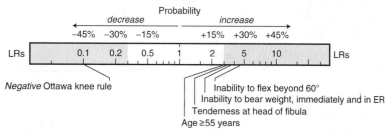

CLINICALLY SIGNIFICANT KNEE FRACTURE

femoral condyles and prevents anterior subluxation of the tibia when the knee is at 90 degrees (i.e., anterior drawer sign) but not when it is at 20 degrees (i.e., Lachman's sign). In support of this last hypothesis, the sensitivity of the anterior drawer sign in one study increased from 50% to 100% after medial meniscectomy.[52]

2. Meniscal Injury

Both the positive McMurray sign (LR = 8.2) and block to full extension of the knee (LR = 3.2) argue *for* the diagnosis of meniscal tear. No finding, however, argues compellingly *against* meniscal injury. Joint line tenderness, once felt to be a characteristic sign of meniscal injury, was unhelpful diagnostically in two studies.[38,64] It is possible that joint line tenderness reflects accompanying injury of the joint capsule or collateral ligaments, rather than injury to the meniscus per se.

3. Other Ligament Injuries

In one study of patients with knee injuries, valgus laxity during testing at both 0 and 20 degrees flexion was a pathognomonic sign of medial collateral ligament injury (sensitivity 79%, specificity 99%, positive LR = 146.5, negative LR = 0.2).[36] One study has confirmed the accuracy of bedside examination for tears of the PCL (sensitivity 90%, specificity 99%, positive LR = 91.8, negative LR = NS),[35] although this study unfortunately failed to define the specific technique used (although it almost certainly included the posterior drawer sign).

4. Variables Affecting Sensitivity of Signs

Signs of ligament injury are more likely to be positive if (1) the ligament tear is complete and not partial,[56] (2) the injury is chronic and not acute,[65,66] and (3) multiple ligaments are injured (e.g., in ACL-deficient knees, the anterior drawer sign is more likely to be positive if the medial collateral ligament is also injured).[67] Also, the degree to which the patient is relaxed influences the sensi-

Box 53-4   Ligament and Meniscal Injuries*

Finding (Ref)†	Sensitivity (%)	Specificity (%)	Likelihood Ratio if Finding	
			Present	Absent
DETECTING ANTERIOR CRUCIATE LIGAMENT TEAR				
Anterior drawer sign[36,52,60–63]	27–88	91–99	**11.5**	0.5
Lachman's sign[36,52,60–62]	48–96	90–99	**17.0**	**0.2**
Pivot shift sign[36,60,62]	6–32	96–99	**8.0**	NS
DETECTING MENISCAL INJURY				
McMurray sign[37,38]	17–29	96–98	**8.2**	0.8
Joint line tenderness[38,64]	58–85	30–53	NS	NS
Block to full extension[38]	44	86	**3.2**	0.7

NS, not significant; likelihood ratio (LR) if finding present = positive LR; LR if finding absent = negative LR.
*Diagnostic standard: For anterior cruciate tear, tear demonstrated by MRI imaging,[60,61] arthroscopy,[36,62] or surgery[52,63]; for meniscal tear, arthroscopy.[37,38,64]
†Definition of findings: see text.

LIGAMENT AND MENISCAL INJURIES

decrease   Probability   increase

	-45%	-30%	-15%		+15%	+30%	+45%	
LRs	0.1	0.2	0.5	1	2	5	10	LRs

Negative Lachman's sign,
arguing against ACL tear

Negative anterior drawer sign,
arguing against ACL tear

Lachman's sign, detecting ACL tear
Anterior drawer sign,
detecting ACL tear

McMurray sign, detecting meniscal injury
Pivot shift sign, detecting ACL tear

Block to full extension,
detecting meniscal injury

tivity of these signs, as illustrated by the observation that the sensitivity of most of these tests increases when patients are examined under anesthesia.[36,56,62,65,67]

5.   Predicting the Need for Knee Surgery

If all knee injuries were managed conservatively (e.g., by rest, bracing, and physical therapy), the detailed bedside examination described previously would have limited clinical utility. One study, however, enrolled patients with knee pain and demonstrated that many of these physical signs—limited knee flexion (<120 degrees) or extension, medial or lateral joint line tenderness, a positive McMurray test, a positive Lachman test, and a positive anterior drawer sign—independently predicted whether an experienced orthopedic surgeon would recommend nonarthroplasty knee surgery to the patient.[68]

THE ANKLE

I.   INTRODUCTION

In patients presenting with ankle or foot injuries to emergency departments, 8% to 14% are found to have a clinically significant fractures.[69–75]

II.   THE FINDING

Stiell and others have developed a prediction rule for clinically significant injuries, called the Ottawa ankle rule.[76,77] This rule focuses on the presence of tenderness at four locations and whether the patient is able to bear weight both immediately after the accident and later in the emergency department (Fig. 53-13). Importantly, it applies only to patients with injury of the ankle (i.e., distal 6 cm of tibia and fibula and talus) and midfoot (i.e., navicular bone, cuboid, cuneiforms, anterior process of the calcaneus, and base of the fifth metatarsal) and *not* to injury of the body and tuberosities of the calcaneus or injury more than 10 days old.

III.   CLINICAL SIGNIFICANCE

In patients with ankle injury, the most compelling argument for significant fracture is tenderness of the posterior medial malleolus (LR = 4.8, EBM Box 53-5). The strongest arguments against fracture are a negative Ottawa ankle rule (LR = 0.1) and ability to bear weight four steps in the emergency room (LR = 0.3).

In patients with midfoot pain, tenderness at the base of the fifth metatarsal bone increases the probability of fracture a small amount (LR = 2.9). A negative Ottawa foot rule argues strongly against midfoot fracture (LR = 0.1), though much of this argument rests on the absence of tenderness at the base of the fifth metatarsal (LR = 0.1).

Other studies combining the ankle and foot rules have confirmed their accuracy[69–75] and shown they reduce the need for radiographs by 14% to 34% and decrease medical costs and patient waiting times.[70,72–74,76,78,82–85]

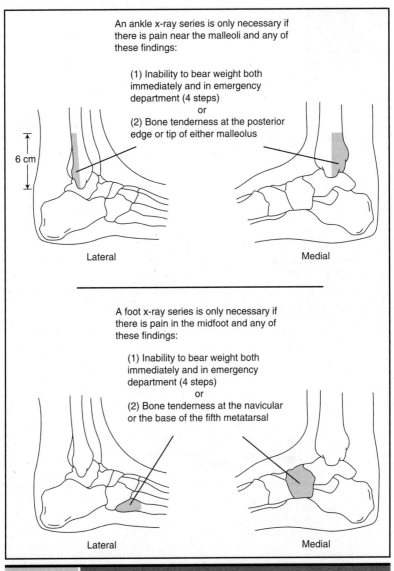

An ankle x-ray series is only necessary if there is pain near the malleoli and any of these findings:

(1) Inability to bear weight both immediately and in emergency department (4 steps)
or
(2) Bone tenderness at the posterior edge or tip of either malleolus

6 cm

Lateral   Medial

A foot x-ray series is only necessary if there is pain in the midfoot and any of these findings:

(1) Inability to bear weight both immediately and in emergency department (4 steps)
or
(2) Bone tenderness at the navicular or the base of the fifth metatarsal

Lateral   Medial

FIGURE 53-13   OTTAWA RULE FOR ANKLE OR MIDFOOT FRACTURE.

The rule for ankle pain is the top figure; the rule for midfoot pain is the bottom figure. The rule is positive if any indication for radiography is met. "Inability to take 4 steps" means the patient is unable to transfer weight twice onto each lower limb regardless of limping. Importantly, these rules apply *only* to patients with injury of the ankle or midfoot, and they exclude patients with injury to the body or tuberosities of the calcaneus. (Adapted from Stiell IG, Greenberg GH, McKnight RD, et al. Decision rules for the use of radiography in acute ankle injuries: Refinement and prospective validation. *JAMA.* 1993;269:1127-1132 with permission).

Box 53-5 Ankle and Midfoot Fracture*

Finding (Ref)†	Sensitivity (%)	Specificity (%)	Likelihood Ratio if Finding	
			Present	Absent
DETECTING ANKLE FRACTURE				
Tenderness over posterior lateral malleolus[76,77]	69–76	65–74	2.4	0.4
Tenderness over posterior medial malleolus[76,77]	34–47	87–95	**4.8**	0.6
Inability to bear weight immediately after injury[76,77]	61–68	72–79	2.6	0.5
Inability to bear weight 4 steps in the emergency room[76,77]	80–85	64–70	2.5	**0.3**
Ottawa ankle rule[70,72,76,78–80]	94–99	16–44	1.5	**0.1**
DETECTING MIDFOOT FRACTURE				
Tenderness at the base of the 5th metatarsal[76,77]	92–94	66–69	2.9	**0.1**
Tenderness of navicular bone[76,77]	3–12	74–90	0.4	NS
Inability to bear weight immediately[76,77]	18–28	74–82	NS	NS
Inability to bear weight 4 steps in the emergency room[76,77]	38–45	58–67	NS	NS
Ottawa foot rule[72,76,78–81]	88–99	21–79	2.1	**0.1**

NS, not significant; likelihood ratio (LR) if finding present = positive LR; LR if finding absent = negative LR.
*Diagnostic standard: For clinically significant ankle or midfoot fracture, bone fragments >3 mm in breadth (i.e., a size that might require plaster immobilization).
†Definition of findings: For Ottawa ankle and foot rules, see Fig. 53-13.

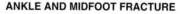

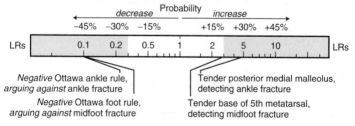

ANKLE AND MIDFOOT FRACTURE

REFERENCES

1. Beetham WP, Polley HF, Slocumb CH, Weaver WF. *Physical examination of the joints*. Philadelphia: WB Saunders; 1965.

2. Urwin M, Symmons D, Allison T, et al. Estimating the burden of musculoskeletal disorders in the community: The comparative prevalence of symptoms at different anatomical sites, and the relation to social deprivation. *Ann Rheum Dis*. 1998;57: 649-655.

3. Cyriax J. The shoulder. *Br J Hosp Med*. 1975:185-192.

4. Cyriax J. *Textbook of orthopedic medicine. Vol 1. Diagnosis of soft tissue disorders*, 8th ed. London: Bailliere Tindall; 1982.

5. van der Windt DAWM, Koes BW, de Jong BA, Bouter LM. Shoulder disorders in general practice: Incidence, patient characteristics, and management. *Ann Rheum Dis*. 1995;54:959-964.

6. van der Windt DAWM, Koes BW, Boeke AJP, et al. Shoulder disorders in general practice: Prognostic indicators of outcome. *Br J Gen Pract*. 1996;46:519-523.

7. Vecchio P, Kavanagh R, Hazleman BL, King RH. Shoulder pain in a community-based rheumatology clinic. *Br J Rheumatol*. 1995;34:440-442.

8. Walton J, Mahajan S, Paxinos A, et al. Diagnostic values of tests for acromioclavicular joint pain. *J Bone Joint Surg*. 2004;86-A:807-812.

9. Zaslav KR. Internal rotation resistance strength test: A new diagnostic test to differentiate intra-articular pathology from outlet (Neer) impingement syndrome in the shoulder. *J Shoulder Elbow Surg*. 2001;10:23-27.

10. Hertel R, Lambert SM, Gerber C. Lag signs in the diagnosis of rotator cuff rupture. *J Shoulder Elbow Surg*. 1996;5:307-313.

11. Neer CS. Impingement lesions. *Clin Orthop*. 1983;173:70-77.

12. Valadie AL, Jobe CM, Pink MM, et al. Anatomy of provocative tests for impingement syndrome of the shoulder. *J Shoulder Elbow Surg*. 2000;9:36-46.

13. Hawkins RJ, Kennedy JC. Impingement syndrome in athletes. *Am J Sports Med*. 1980;8:151-158.

14. Yergason RM. Supination sign. *J Bone Joint Surg Am*. 1931;13:160.

15. Beall DP, Williamson EE, Ly JQ, et al. Association of biceps tendon tears with rotatory cuff abnormalities: Degree of correlation with tears of the anterior and superior portions of the rotator cuff. *AJR*. 2003;180:633-639.

16. Leroux JL, Thomas E, Bonnel F, Blotman F. Diagnostic value of clinical tests for shoulder impingement syndrome. *Rev Rheum (Engl Ed)*. 1995;62:423-428.

17. Itoi E, Kido T, Sano A, Urayamana M, Sato K. Which is more useful, the "full can test" or the "empty can test", in detecting the torn supraspinatus tendon? *Am J Sports Med*. 1999;27:65-68.

18. Litaker D, Pioro M, El Bilbeisi H, Brems J. Returning to the bedside: Using the history and physical examination to identify rotatory cuff tears. *J Am Geriatr Soc*. 2000;48:1633-1637.

19. Murrell GAC, Walton JR. Diagnosis of rotator cuff tears. *Lancet.* 2001;357: 769-770.

20. Reider B. *The orthopaedic physical examination,* 2nd ed. Philadelphia: WB Saunders; 2005.

21. Codman EA. The classic: Rupture of the supraspinatus tendon. *Clin Orthoped.* 1990;254:3-26.

22. Calis M, Akgun K, Birtane M, et al. Diagnostic values of clinical diagnostic tests in subacromial impingement syndrome. *Ann Rheum Dis.* 2000;59:44-47.

23. MacDonald PB, Clark P, Sutherland K. An analysis of the diagnostic accuracy of the Hawkings and Neer subacromial impingement signs. *J Shoulder Elbow Surg.* 2000;9:299-301.

24. Holtby R, Razmjou H. Validity of the supraspinatus test as a single clinical test in diagnosing patients with rotator cuff pathology. *J Orthop Sports Phys Ther.* 2004;34: 194-200.

25. Lyons AR, Tomlinson JE. Clinical diagnosis of tears of the rotator cuff. *J Bone Joint Surg Br.* 1992;74B:414-415.

26. Wolf EM, Agrawal V. Transdeltoid palpation (the rent test) in the diagnosis of rotator cuff tears. *J Shoulder Elbow Surg.* 2001;10:470-473.

27. Cunningham LS, Kelsey JL. Epidemiology of musculoskeletal impairments and associated disability. *Am J Public Health.* 1984;74:574-579.

28. Emparanza JI, Aginaga JR. Validation of the Ottawa knee rules. *Ann Emerg Med.* 2001;38:364-368.

29. Richman PB, McCuskey CF, Nashed A, et al. Performance of two clinical decision rules for knee radiography. *J Emerg Med.* 1997;15:459-463.

30. Seaberg DC, Yealy DM, Lukens T, et al. Multicenter comparison of two clinical decision rules for the use of radiography in acute, high-risk injuries. *Ann Emerg Med.* 1998;32:8-13.

31. Stiell IG, Greenberg GH, Wells GA, et al. Derivation of a decision rule for the use of radiography in acute knee injuries. *Ann Emerg Med.* 1995;26:405-413.

32. Stiell IG, Greenberg GH, Wells GA, et al. Prospective validation of a decision rule for the use of radiography in acute knee injuries. *JAMA.* 1996;275:611-615.

33. Tigges S, Pitts S, Mukundan S, et al. External validation of the Ottawa knee rules in an urban trauma center in the United States. *AJR.* 1999;172:1069-1071.

34. Simonsen O, Jensen J, Mouritsen P, Lauritzen J. The accuracy of clinical examination of injury of the knee joint. *Injury.* 1984;16:96-101.

35. O'Shea KJ, Murphy KP, Heekin RD, Herzwurm PJ. The diagnostic accuracy of history, physical examination, and radiographs in the evaluation of traumatic knee disorders. *Am J Sports Med.* 1996;24:164-167.

36. Sandberg R, Balkfors B, Henricson A, Westlin N. Stability tests in knee ligament injuries. *Arch Orthop Traum Surg.* 1986;106:5-7.

37. Evans PJ, Bell GD, Frank C. Prospective evaluation of the McMurray test. *Am J Sports Med.* 1993;21:604-608.

38. Fowler PJ, Lubliner JA. The predictive value of five clinical signs in the evaluation of meniscal pathology. *Arthroscopy*. 1989;5:184-186.
39. McMurray TP. The semilunar cartilages. *Br J Surg*. 1949;29:407-414.
40. Smith CC. Evaluating the painful knee: A hands-on approach to acute ligamentous and meniscal injuries. *Adv Stud Med*. 2004;4:362-370.
41. Jackson JL, O'Malley PG, Kroenke K. Evaluation of acute knee pain in primary care. *Ann Intern Med*. 2003;139:575-588.
42. Larson RL. Physical examination in the diagnosis of rotatory instability. *Clin Orthoped*. 1983;172:38-44.
43. Malanga GA, Andrus S, Nadler SF, McLean J. Physical examination of the knee: A review of the original test description and scientific validity of common orthopedic tests. *Arch Phys Med Rehabil*. 2003;84:592-603.
44. Galway HR, MacIntosh DL. The lateral pivot shift: A symptom and sign of anterior cruciate ligament insufficiency. *Clin Orthoped*. 1980;147:45-50.
45. Matsumoto H. Mechanism of the pivot shift. *J Bone Joint Surg Br*. 1990;72B:816-821.
46. Kanamori A, Woo SLY, Ma CB, et al. The forces in the anterior cruciate ligament and knee kinematics during a simulated pivot shift test: A human cadaveric study using robotic technology. *Arthroscopy*. 2000;16:633-639.
47. Liorzou. *Knee ligaments: Clinical examination*. Berlin: Springer-Verlag; 1991.
48. Muller W. *The knee: Form, function, and ligament reconstruction*. Berlin: Springer-Verlag; 1983.
49. Losee RE. Concepts of pivot shift. *Clin Orthoped*. 1983;172:45-51.
50. Kujala UM, Nelimarkka O, Koskinen SK. Relationship between the pivot shift and the configuration of the lateral tibial plateau. *Arch Orthop Trauma Surg*. 1992;111:228-229.
51. Paessler HH, Michel D. How new if the Lachman test? *Am J Sports Med*. 1992;20:95-97.
52. Torg JS, Conrad W, Kalen V. Clinical diagnosis of anterior cruciate ligament instability in the athlete. *Am J Sports Med*. 1976;4:84-93.
53. Groves WEH. The crucial ligaments of the knee-joint: Their function, rupture, and the operative treatment of the same. *Br J Surg*. 1920;7:505-515.
54. Galway RD, Beaupre A, MacIntosh DL. Pivot shift: A clinical sign of symptomatic anterior cruciate insufficiency. *J Bone Joint Surg Br*. 1972;54-B:763-764.
55. Hoppenfeld S. *Physical examination of the spine and extremities*. Norwalk: Appleton and Lange; 1976.
56. Noyes FR, Bassett RW, Grood ES, Butler DL. Arthroscopy in acute traumatic hemarthrosis of the knee. *J Bone Joint Surg Am*. 1980;62A:687-695.
57. Solomon DH, Simel DL, Bates DW, et al. Does this patient have a torn meniscus or ligament of the knee? Value of the physical examination. *JAMA*. 2001;286:1610-1620.

58. Altman R, Asch E, Block D, et al. Development of criteria for the classification and reporting of osteoarthritis: Classification of osteoarthritis of the knee. *Arthritis Rheum*. 1986;29:1039-1049.

59. Seaberg DC, Jackson R. Clinical decision rule for knee radiographs. *Am J Emerg Med*. 1994;12:541-543.

60. Boeree NR, Ackroyd CE. Assessment of the menisci and cruciate ligaments: An audit of clinical practice. *Injury*. 1991;22:291-294.

61. Lee JK, Yao L, Phelps CT, et al. Anterior cruciate ligament tears: MR imaging compared with arthroscopy and clinical tests. *Radiology*. 1988;166:861-864.

62. Tonino AJ, Huy J, Schaafsma J. The diagnostic accuracy of knee testing in the acute injured knee: Initial examination versus examination under anesthesia with arthroscopy. *Acta Ortho Belg*. 1986;52:479-487.

63. Braunstein EM. Anterior cruciate ligament injuries: A comparison of arthrographic and physical diagnosis. *AJR*. 1982;136:423-425.

64. Shelbourne KD, Martini DJ, McCarroll JR, VanMeter CD. Correlation of joint line tenderness and meniscal lesions in patients with acute anterior cruciate ligament tears. *Am J Sports Med*. 1995;23:166-169.

65. Mitsou A, Vallianatos P. Clinical diagnosis of ruptures of the anterior cruciate ligament: A comparison between the Lachman test and the anterior drawer sign. *Injury*. 1988;19:427-428.

66. Jonsson T, Althoff B, Peterson L, Renstrom P. Clinical diagnosis of ruptures of the anterior cruciate ligament: A comparative study of the Lachman test and the anterior drawer sign. *Am J Sports Med*. 1982;10:100-102.

67. Donaldson WF, Warren RF, Wickiewicz T. A comparison of acute anterior cruciate ligament examinations: Initial versus examination under anesthesia. *Am J Sports Med*. 1985;13:5-10.

68. Solomon DH, Avorn J, Warsi A, et al. Which patients with knee problems are likely to benefit from nonarthroplasty surgery? Development of a clinical prediction rule. *Arch Intern Med*. 2004;164:509-513.

69. Keogh SP, Shafi A, Wijetunge DB. Comparison of Ottawa ankle rules and current local guidelines for use of radiography in acute ankle injuries. *J R Coll Surg Edinb*. 1998;43:341-343.

70. Leddy JJ, Smolinski RJ, Lawrence J, et al. Prospective evaluation of the Ottawa ankle rules in a university sports medicine center: With a modification to increase specificity for identifying malleolar fractures. *Am J Sports Med*. 1998;26:158-165.

71. McBride KL. Validation of the Ottawa ankle rules: Experience at a community hospital. *Can Fam Physician*. 1997;43:459-465.

72. Papacostas E, Malliaropoulos N, Papadopoulos A, Liouliakis C. Validation of Ottawa ankle rules protocol in Greek athletes: Study in the emergency departments of a district general hospital and a sports injuries clinic. *Br J Sports Med*. 2001;35:445-447.

73. Pigman EC, Klug RK, Sanford S, Jolly BT. Evaluation of the Ottawa clinical decision rules for the use of radiography in acute ankle and midfoot injuries in the emergency department: An independent site assessment. *Ann Emerg Med.* 1994;24:41-45.

74. Pijnenburg ACM, Glas AS, de Roos MAJ, et al. Radiography in acute ankle injuries: The Ottawa ankle rules versus local diagnostic decision rules. *Ann Emerg Med.* 2002;39:599-604.

75. Tay SY, Thoo FL, Sitoh YY, et al. The Ottawa ankle rules in Asia: Validating a clinical decision rule for requesting X-rays in twisting ankle and foot injuries. *J Emerg Med.* 1999;17:945-947.

76. Stiell IG, Greenberg GH, McKnight RD, et al. Decision rules for the use of radiography in acute ankle injuries: Refinement and prospective validation. *JAMA.* 1993;269:1127-1132.

77. Stiell IG, Greenberg GH, McKnight RD, et al. A study to develop clinical decision rules for the use of radiography in acute ankle injuries. *Ann Emerg Med.* 1992;21:384-390.

78. Auleley GR, Kerboull L, Durieux P, et al. Validation of the Ottawa ankle rules in France: A study in the surgical emergency department of a teaching hospital. *Ann Emerg Med.* 1998;32:14-18.

79. Broomhead A, Stuart P. Validation of the Ottawa ankle rules in Australia. *Emerg Med.* 2003;15:126-132.

80. Yuen MC, Sim SW, Lam HS, Tung WK. Validation of the Ottawa ankle rules in a Hong Kong ED. *Am J Emerg Med.* 2001;19:429-432.

81. Springer BA, Arciero RA, Tenuta JJ, Taylor DC. A prospective study of modified Ottawa ankle rules in a military population: Interobserver agreement between physical therapists and orthopaedic surgeons. *Am J Sports Med.* 2000;28:864-868.

82. Anis AH, Stiell IG, Stewart DG, Laupacis A. Cost-effectiveness analysis of the Ottawa ankle rules. *Ann Emerg Med.* 1995;26:422-428.

83. Auleley GR, Ravaud P, Giraudeau B, et al. Implementation of the Ottawa ankle rules in France: A multicenter randomized controlled trial. *JAMA.* 1997;277:1935-1939.

84. Stiell IG, Laupacis A, Brison R, et al. Multicenter trial to introduce the Ottawa ankle rules for use of radiography in acute ankle injuries. *BMJ.* 1995;311:594-597.

85. Stiell IG, McKnight RD, Greenberg GH, et al. Implementation of the Ottawa ankle rules. *JAMA.* 1994;271:827-832.

NEUROLOGIC
EXAMINATION

11

Visual Field Testing

I. INTRODUCTION

Abnormalities of peripheral vision are called "visual field defects." These defects, many of which can be detected at the bedside, provide important clues to the diagnosis of lesions throughout the visual pathways—retina, optic nerve, optic chiasm, optic tracts, optic radiations (parietal and temporal lobes), and occipital cortex (Fig. 54-1).

II. DEFINITION

The term **hemianopia** describes visual defects that occupy about half of an eye's visual space. **Quadrantanopia** describes defects confined mostly to about one fourth of an eye's visual space. **Homonymous** describes defects that affect the same side of the vertical meridian (i.e., right or left side) of both eyes. For example, a right homonymous hemianopia affects the right visual space of both eyes (i.e., the temporal field of the right eye and the nasal field of the left eye). "Homonymous" implies the defect does not cross the vertical meridian.

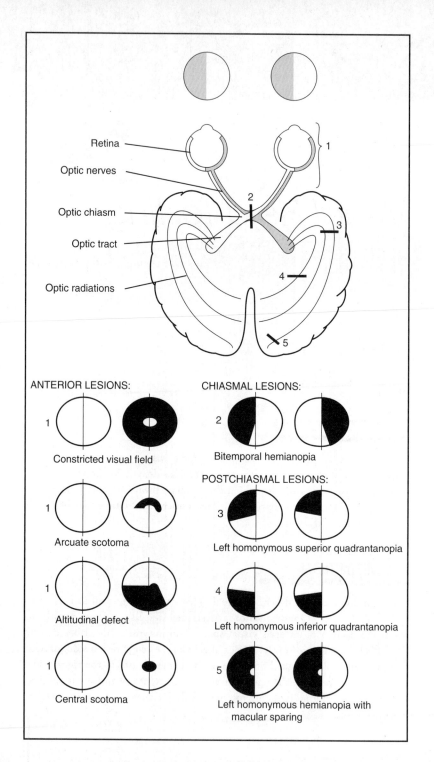

Retina

Optic nerves

Optic chiasm

Optic tract

Optic radiations

ANTERIOR LESIONS:

1
Constricted visual field

1
Arcuate scotoma

1
Altitudinal defect

1
Central scotoma

CHIASMAL LESIONS:

2
Bitemporal hemianopia

POSTCHIASMAL LESIONS:

3
Left homonymous superior quadrantanopia

4
Left homonymous inferior quadrantanopia

5
Left homonymous hemianopia with macular sparing

III.   THE ANATOMY OF THE VISUAL PATHWAYS

The key anatomic points in Fig. 54-1 are (1) Images from the visual fields are inverted throughout the retina and all neural pathways. Images from the temporal visual field fall on the nasal retina, and those from the nasal field on the temporal retina. Images from the *superior* visual fields are transmitted throughout the *inferior* visual pathways (inferior retina, inferior optic nerve and chiasm, and temporal lobe), and those from the *inferior* visual fields throughout the *superior* visual pathways (superior retina, superior optic nerve and chiasm, parietal lobe). (2) The nasal retinal fibers cross in the optic chiasm; therefore, disease of the optic chiasm causes defects in both temporal visual fields ("bitemporal hemianopia"). (3) The visual pathways posterior to the optic chiasm contain information from the same visual space of each eye: lesions in the *right* postchiasmal pathways cause defects in the *left* visual space of each eye (i.e., temporal field of left eye and nasal field of right eye), and those of the *left* postchiasmal pathways cause defects in the *right* visual space. Such defects, respecting the vertical meridian in each eye, are called "homonymous." (4) The visual pathways in the occipital cortex that contain information from the macula (point of fixation) are distant from those connected to the more peripheral fields.[1] Therefore, lesions of the occipital cortex may cause either homonymous defects sparing the macula or visual defects confined to just central vision.

IV.   TECHNIQUE

There are two traditional ways to test visual fields at the bedside: static confrontational testing and kinetic confrontational testing. In both techniques, the patient sits about 70 to 100 cm from the clinician and fixes on the clinician's

FIGURE 54-1	ANATOMY OF THE VISUAL PATHWAYS.

The anatomy of the visual pathways appears at the top of the figure; the light gray shading indicating how visual information from the left visual space eventually courses to the right brain. Visual field defects are at the bottom of the figure. Anterior defects (labeled 1, from disease of the optic nerve or retina) characteristically affect one eye and cause defects (the black shading) that may cross the vertical meridian (i.e., the vertical meridian is the vertical line bisecting each visual field). Chiasmal defects (labeled 2) and postchiasmal defects (labeled 3 for a lesion in the anterior temporal lobe, 4 for the parietal lobe, and 5 for the occipital cortex) characteristically affect both eyes and respect the vertical meridian.

own eye. Only one eye of the patient is tested at a time; the other is occluded with a card or the patient's hand.

A. STATIC TECHNIQUE

Using this technique, the clinician presents objects at a fixed point in the visual field, usually about 20 to 30 degrees from fixation. Typically, the clinician presents his or her hands to two visual quadrants simultaneously and asks the patient to count the number of fingers shown or indicate which index finger is wiggling.[2] Testing two quadrants simultaneously has the advantage of detecting some parietal lobe lesions that may allow patients to see an object in the contralateral field if it appears alone but not if another object is presented simultaneously to the healthy visual field.[3]

Throughout the examination, the clinician focuses on whether a defect respects the vertical or horizontal meridians of the visual field (see later). Defects crossing the vertical meridian are due to anterior disease (see later), whereas those respecting the vertical meridian are due to chiasmal disease (if the defect is bitemporal) or postchiasmal disease (if it is homonymous).

B. KINETIC TECHNIQUE

In this technique, the clinician tests one quadrant at a time by slowly moving an object (e.g., wiggling finger) from an extreme peripheral field toward fixation, the patient then indicating the moment he or she sees the object.

V. THE FINDINGS

Visual field defects are classified as "prechiasmal" (from disease in retina or optic nerves, often called "anterior defects"), "chiasmal," and "postchiasmal" (optic tracts, optic radiations, and occipital cortex).

A. ANTERIOR OR PRECHIASMAL DEFECTS

The characteristic features are the following:

1. One eye is affected (unless the retinal or optic nerve disorder is bilateral).
2. Visual acuity is poor. Most patients have diminished acuity or, if acuity is normal, other signs of anterior disease, such as an afferent pupillary defect (see Chapter 19), red color desaturation, abnormal retina examination, or an abnormal optic disc (drusen, cupping, or atrophy).
3. The defects may cross the vertical meridian. This occurs because retinal nerve fibers from the temporal retina arch across the vertical meridian to reach the optic disc and nerve (which lie on the nasal side of the retina). Damage to these fibers thus may cause a defect that crosses the vertical meridian. Small nerve

fiber defects may cause an "arcuate defect" (see Fig. 54-1), larger ones an "altitudinal defect" (having a sharp horizontal border in the nasal field). Damage to fibers from the macula may cause "central scotomas" and, to those preferentially affecting the most peripheral vision, "constricted visual fields."[4]

B. CHIASMAL DEFECTS

These defects are bitemporal hemianopias (see Fig. 54-1).

C. POSTCHIASMAL DEFECTS

The characteristics of these defects are the following:

1. Both eyes are affected, causing homonymous hemianopias or quadrantanopias.
2. Visual acuity is normal. This is true in more than 90% of cases. If visual acuity is abnormal, it is because of bilateral disease and thus the acuity in both eyes is the same.[5]
3. Pupil and retinal examination are normal. One important exception is the occasional finding of papilledema, caused by brain tumors affecting the optic radiations.

VI. CLINICAL SIGNIFICANCE

A. ETIOLOGY

Most anterior defects are caused by severe glaucoma, retinal emboli, and optic neuritis. Chiasmal defects are often due to a pituitary tumor just below the optic chiasm. More than 95% of postchiasmal defects are due to lesions of the temporal, parietal, and occipital lobes. Lesions of the optic tracts are rare.[5]

Although parietal and temporal lobe disease may cause inferior and superior quadrantanopias, respectively (see Fig. 54-1), lesions in these areas more often cause dense hemianopias or hemianopias that are denser inferiorly or superiorly, respectively.[5,6]

B. DIAGNOSTIC ACCURACY

EBM Box 54-1 summarizes the diagnostic accuracy of the confrontational technique for diagnosing visual field defects. Studies comparing static and kinetic techniques found both methods to be equivalent, although these studies were confined almost entirely to patients with anterior and chiasmal defects, not postchiasmal defects.[9,11]

EBM Box 54-1 reveals that, if the clinician finds a defect by confrontation, one is likely present by perimetry [likelihood ratios (LRs) = 6.1 to 6.8]. The absence of a defect, on the other hand, is less helpful, especially in patients with suspected anterior defects or those with chiasmal disease.

Box 54-1 Visual Field Defects*

Finding (Ref)	Sensitivity (%)	Specificity (%)	Likelihood Ratio if Finding	
			Present	Absent
Confrontation technique, detecting the following visual field defects[7–11]				
Anterior defects (retina and optic nerve)	11–58	93–99	**6.1**	0.7
Patchy defects	6			
Constriction of visual fields	58			
Arcuate defects	20–51			
Altitudinal defects	88			
Posterior defects (optic chiasm to occipital cortex)	43–86	86–95	**6.8**	0.4
Bitemporal hemianopia	45			
Homonymous hemianopia	80			
Patients with homonymous hemianopias, detecting parietal lobe disease				
Asymmetric optokinetic nystagmus[5]	93	84	**5.7**	**0.1**
Associated hemiparesis or aphasia[12]	90	95	**18.3**	**0.1**

Diagnostic standard: For visual field defects, conventional perimetry.

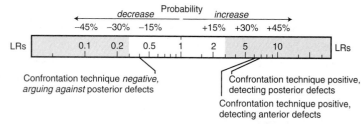

VISUAL FIELD DEFECTS

Confrontation technique *negative*, *arguing against* posterior defects

Confrontation technique positive, detecting posterior defects

Confrontation technique positive, detecting anterior defects

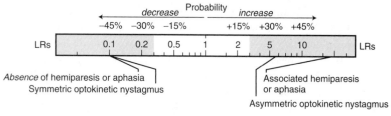

PARIETAL LOBE DISEASE (IF HOMONYMOUS HEMIANOPIA)

Absence of hemiparesis or aphasia
Symmetric optokinetic nystagmus

Associated hemiparesis or aphasia

Asymmetric optokinetic nystagmus

C. DIFFERENTIAL DIAGNOSIS OF POSTCHIASMAL DEFECTS

Homonymous hemianopias may be either an isolated finding or associated with other neurologic findings. The most common cause of an *isolated* homonymous hemianopia is an ischemic infarct of the occipital cortex.[12,13] In patients with associated hemiparesis, aphasia, or asymmetric optokinetic nystagmus, the most common diagnosis is parietal lobe disease.[5,12,14,15] Optokinetic nystagmus is a normal horizontal nystagmus that occurs when patients look at a vertically striped tape moving in front of them. The clinician moves the tape first to one side and then the other, comparing the amplitude of horizontal nystagmus produced, which should be equal in each direction. Parietal lobe lesions reduce or eliminate optokinetic nystagmus when the tape is moved toward the side with the lesion (Barany first made this observation in 1921).

In patients with homonymous defects, the presence of asymmetric optokinetic nystagmus, associated aphasia, or hemiparesis argues strongly *for* a parietal lobe lesion (LR = 5.7 for optokinetic nystagmus and LR = 18.3 for hemiparesis or aphasia), whereas the absence of these findings argues against a parietal lobe lesion (both LRs = 0.1) and makes an occipital or temporal lobe lesion more likely.

D. IMPROVING DETECTION OF VISUAL FIELD DEFECTS

Confrontation fails to detect some defects because they are too small, lack a sharp linear border (e.g., patchy defects of anterior disease), or are too peripheral (e.g., constricted visual fields; confrontation only tests the most central 20 to 30 degrees of visual space). To increase sensitivity of bedside examination, some experts have proposed the following techniques, each of which supplement routine confrontational testing:

1. Perform confrontational testing with red-colored squares or lights instead of fingers. In areas of early defects, patients may describe that the red light appears orange, pale yellow, or white.[16] In one study, this method detected chiasmal defects with an overall sensitivity of 79%.[9] Another study using a conventional red laser pointer projected in front of the patient detected anterior visual field defects with a sensitivity of 71%, specificity of 89%, positive LR of 6.3, and negative LR of 0.3.[10]
2. Repeat confrontational testing from 4 m away. Routine confrontational testing is performed from 1 m away; increasing the distance to 4 m may improve sensitivity for subtle arcuate scotomata (glaucoma or optic nerve disease) or macular sparing (some occipital cortex lesions).[17]
3. Examine the patient's perceptions of the clinician's face, positioned about 30 cm away. The clinician tests one eye at a time and asks whether any areas of the clinician's face are missing or distorted.[7,18] Nonetheless, the only study comparing this technique to others (primarily in patients with anterior visual field defects) found that the perception of the clinician's face had similar diagnostic accuracy to that of static or kinetic confrontational testing.[11]

REFERENCES

1. Trauzettel-Klosinski S, Reinhard J. The vertical field border in hemianopia and its significance for fixation and reading. *Invest Ophthalmol Vis Sci*. 1998;39: 2177-2186.

2. Welsh RC. Finger counting in the four quadrants as a method of visual field gross screening. *Arch Ophthalmol*. 1961;66:678-679.

3. Bender MB, Furlow LT. Phenomenon of visual extinction in homonymous fields and psychologic principles involved. *Arch Neurol Psychiatry*. 1945;53:29-45.

4. Kitazawa Y, Yamamoto T. Glaucomatous visual field defects: Their characteristics and how to detect them. *Clin Neurosci*. 1997;4:279-283.

5. Smith JL. Homonymous hemianopia: A review of one hundred cases. *Am J Ophthalmol*. 1962;54:616-623.

6. McFadzean RM, Hadley DM. Homonymous quadrantanopia respecting the horizontal meridian: A feature of striate and extrastriate cortical disease. *Neurology*. 1997;49:1741-1746.

7. Johnson LN, Baloh FG. The accuracy of confrontation visual field test in comparison with automated perimetry. *J Natl Med Assoc*. 1991;83:895-898.

8. Shahinfar S, Johnson LN, Madsen RW. Confrontation visual field loss as a function of decibel sensitivity loss on automated static perimetry: Implications on the accuracy of confrontation visual field testing. *Ophthalmology*. 1995;102:872-877.

9. Trobe JD, Acosta PC, Krischer JP, Trick GL. Confrontation visual field techniques in the detection of anterior visual pathway lesions. *Ann Neurol*. 1981;10:28-34.

10. Lee MS, Balcer LJ, Volpe NJ, et al. Laser pointer visual field screening. *J Neuro-Ophthalmol*. 2003;23:260-263.

11. Pandit RJ, Gales K, Griffiths PG. Effectiveness of testing visual fields by confrontation. *Lancet*. 2001;358:1339-1340.

12. Jacobsen DM. The localizing value of a quadrantanopia. *Arch Neurol*. 1997;54: 401-404.

13. Trobe JD, Lorber ML, Schlezinger NS. Isolated homonymous hemianopia. *Arch Ophthalmol*. 1973;89:377-381.

14. Smith JL, Cogan DG. Optokinetic nystagmus: A test for parietal lobe lesions (a study of 31 anatomically verified cases). *Am J Ophthalmol*. 1959;48:187-193.

15. Baloh RW, Yee RD, Honrubia V. Optokinetic nystagmus and parietal lobe lesions. *Ann Neurol*. 1980;7:269-276.

16. Frisen L. A versatile color confrontation test for the central visual field: A comparison with quantitative perimetry. *Arch Ophthalmol*. 1973;89:3-9.

17. Kodsi SR, Younge BR. The four-meter confrontation visual field test. *J Clin Neuroophthalmol*. 1993;13:40-43.

18. Reader AL, Harper DG. Confrontation visual-field testing. *JAMA*. 1976;236:250.

55

Nerves of the Eye Muscles (III, IV, and VI): Approach to Diplopia

DIPLOPIA

I. INTRODUCTION

Patients with lesions of cranial nerves III, IV, and VI have paralysis of one or more ocular muscles, which prevents the eyes from aligning properly and causes double vision, or diplopia. The most common mistake in analyzing diplopia, however, is to prematurely conclude that the patient must have neuropathy of one of these three nerves. Because less than half of the patients with diplopia actually have a cranial neuropathy, this chapter first emphasizes the general approach to *all* causes of diplopia.

II. DEFINITIONS

Diplopia may be **monocular** or **binocular.** Monocular diplopia persists after occluding one eye. Binocular diplopia depends on the visual axes of each eye being out of alignment and therefore disappears when one eye is occluded.

Several other terms are used to describe the findings of patients with *binocular diplopia.* **Heterotropia** is a general term for the finding of visual axes that are not parallel (synonyms are "squint" or "strabismus"). **Esotropia** means that one eye is converging or is deviated toward the nose (e.g., a left esotropia means that the left eye is deviated toward the nose). **Exotropia** means that one eye is diverging or is deviated toward the temple (e.g., a right exotropia means that the right eye is deviated out). **Hypertropia** means that one eye is deviated upward (e.g., a left hypertropia means that the left eye is elevated with respect to the right eye). Diplopia may be **horizontal**, with the two images side by side, or **vertical**, with one image higher than the other (the term "vertical diplopia" also encompasses diplopia with images separated both vertically and horizontally).

III. TECHNIQUE

A. GENERAL APPROACH

Figure 55-1 outlines the general approach to diplopia. The most important initial question is whether the diplopia is monocular or binocular, which can easily be addressed by covering one of the patient's eyes. Overall, 25% of all diplopia is monocular and 75% is binocular.[4]

In patients with binocular diplopia, the clinician can avoid misdiagnosing cranial neuropathy by first addressing the five questions listed in Fig. 55-1. Only after asking these questions should the clinician attempt to identify which eye muscle is weak.

B. IDENTIFYING THE WEAK MUSCLE

When examining the eye muscles, the clinician holds up his or her index finger or penlight and asks the patient to track it toward each of the six cardinal directions of gaze (i.e., left, left and up, left and down, right, right and up, right and down). These directions parallel the principal action of the six eye muscles, as described in Fig. 55-2.

There are two steps in identifying which eye muscle is weak. Step 1 reduces the number of possible weak eye muscles from 12 to 2. Step 2 then identifies which of these 2 muscles is causing the diplopia.

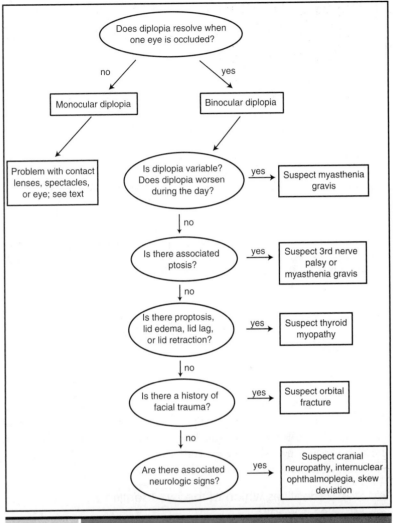

FIGURE 55-1

GENERAL APPROACH TO DIPLOPIA.

The clinician should first distinguish monocular from binocular diplopia and, in patients with binocular diplopia, address the five questions in the center column of the figure. Only then should the clinician identify which muscle is weak, although this is unnecessary if the clinician already suspects myasthenia (from fatigability) or full third nerve palsy (from weakness of the medial rectus, superior rectus, inferior rectus, and inferior oblique muscles, with or without a dilated pupil). Uncommon causes of diplopia and associated *ptosis*, not presented in the figure, are botulism, the Fisher variant of Guillain-Barré syndrome, and aberrant regeneration of the third nerve.[1,2] Uncommon causes of diplopia and associated *orbital findings* (e.g., proptosis) are carotid-cavernous fistula (which causes an orbital bruit),[3] orbital tumor, and pseudotumor.

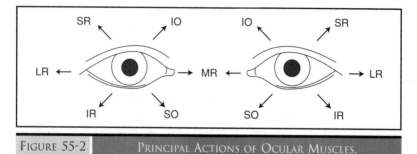

| FIGURE 55-2 | PRINCIPAL ACTIONS OF OCULAR MUSCLES. |

There are 12 ocular muscles, 6 in each eye. The actions of the medial rectus (MR) and lateral rectus (LR) are simple right and left lateral movements. Although the actions of the four vertical eye muscles—the superior rectus (SR), inferior rectus (IR), superior oblique (SO), and inferior oblique (IO)—are more complex, there is one direction of gaze, indicated in the figure, in which weakness is most apparent.

1. Step 1: The Worst Diplopia (and Heterotropia) Occurs When the Patient Looks in the Direction of the Weak Muscle

The clinician asks the patient which of the six cardinal directions aggravates the diplopia the most. According to this rule, the weak muscle is one of the two muscles responsible for this movement, one of which moves the right eye and the other the left eye. For example, diplopia that is worse on far right lateral gaze indicates weakness of the right lateral rectus or the left medial rectus. Diplopia that is worse when the patient looks to the left and down indicates a problem of the left inferior rectus or the right superior oblique.*

2. Step 2 Identifies Which of the Two Identified Muscles Is Weak

There are three techniques.

a. Simple Inspection of the Eyes

In patients with diplopia on far right lateral gaze, the weak muscle is the right lateral rectus if there is an esotropia, but the left medial rectus is weak if there

---

*Because the actions of the four vertical muscles are sometimes difficult to recall, a mnemonic by Maddox (1907) may be helpful: the affected muscle is "either the same-named rectus muscle or the most crossed-named oblique muscle." For example, if diplopia is worse when the patient looks to the *left* in a *superior* direction, the affected muscles are either the *left superior* rectus or *right inferior* oblique.

is an exotropia. In patients with diplopia that is worse when looking up and to the right, the weak muscle is the right superior rectus if there is a left hypertropia but the left inferior oblique if there is a right hypertropia.

Often, however, the heterotropia is not obvious, either because the visual axes are only out of line by a degree or two (too small to observe) or because the patient can compensate and temporarily pull the visual axes back into line. In these patients, the following techniques are helpful.

b. The Affected Eye Is the One with the Most Peripheral Image

By placing a red glass over one eye (usually the right eye), the patient is less likely to fuse the images, and, when looking at a penlight in the direction of maximal diplopia, sees two images, one red and one white. The most peripheral image belongs to the weak eye.

For example, in a patient whose maximal diplopia is to the left and down (and who has the red glass over the right eye), the weak muscle is the right superior oblique if the red image is most peripheral but the left inferior rectus if the white image is most peripheral.

c. The Cover/Uncover Test

To perform this test the clinician covers one eye while the patient looks in the direction of maximal diplopia. Covering one eye prevents fusion of the images, and any heterotropia that exists will return, although it is now obscured by occlusion of the eye. The clinician then observes which way that eye moves to pick up the image after it is uncovered. If it moves out, there was an esotropia; if it moves in, there was an exotropia, and if it moves down, that eye had a hypertropia.

IV. CLINICAL SIGNIFICANCE

A. MONOCULAR DIPLOPIA

Almost all patients with monocular diplopia have "extraocular" or "ocular" causes.[4-7] Common extraocular causes are the patient's spectacles (e.g., reflections off one or both surfaces of the lenses) or contact lenses (e.g., air bubble in the pupillary area, abnormal curves, or uneven thicknesses). This diplopia resolves after removal of the lenses and, in patients with spectacles, varies as the spectacles are moved in and out or up and down. Common "ocular" causes include problems in the lens (e.g., fluid clefts, early cataracts), cornea (e.g., astigmatism, keratitis), and eyelids (e.g., chalazion, prolonged reading that may allow drooping lids to temporarily deform the cornea). The diplopia of these patients resolves when patients look through a pinhole or when a card is held over half of the pupillary aperture (it resolves because the diplopia depends on irregularities of the optic media acting as tiny prisms that divert some rays off the fovea; the pinhole or card blocks these wayward rays and thus eliminates the problem).

Rare patients with monocular diplopia have a cerebral disease.[8,9] Despite traditional teachings, hysteria is a rare cause of monocular diplopia.

B. BINOCULAR DIPLOPIA

1. Etiology

Among patients with binocular diplopia, common final diagnoses are cranial neuropathy (III, IV, or VI; 40% of patients), eye muscle disease (thyroid ophthalmopathy, myasthenia gravis; 15% of patients), trauma (14%), supranuclear causes (internuclear ophthalmoplegia, skew deviation, 7%), other causes (12%), and unknown (12%).[4]

2. Weak Muscles and Their Clinical Significance

Incomplete palsies of the third cranial nerve are rare (in one study of 579 third nerve palsies, < 1% were partial).[10,11] Therefore, if only one or two of the third nerve muscles (i.e., superior rectus, inferior rectus, medial rectus, and inferior oblique) are weak, the diagnosis is almost certainly *not* a partial third nerve palsy but instead one of the diagnoses listed in the following sections.

a. Weak Superior Rectus Muscle

The clinician should consider **myasthenia gravis** (Fig. 55-3). Sixty-five percent of patients with myasthenia gravis present with ocular symptoms, usually diplopia and ptosis.[12] Symptoms often have a fluctuating course, worsen at the end of the day, or even alternate between the eyes. The most common muscles affected are the superior rectus and medial rectus, whose weakness clinicians can often bring out by having the patient sustain an upward or far lateral gaze for 30 seconds or more.[13,14]

In myasthenia gravis, the pupils are always normal.

b. Weak Inferior Rectus Muscle

The clinician should consider thyroid myopathy and orbital floor fracture.

(1) Thyroid Myopathy   Patients may have associated proptosis, lid lag, lid retraction, chemosis, and hyperemia at the insertions of the recti muscles (see Chapter 22). These findings are sometimes subtle, and because many patients are also clinically euthyroid, the only finding of thyroid myopathy may be heterotropia. The cause of diplopia is mechanical restriction of the eye muscles, which ophthalmologists confirm using the "forced duction test" (i.e., after

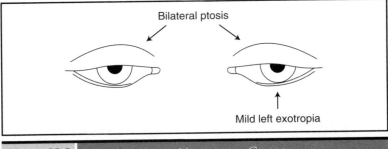

Bilateral ptosis

Mild left exotropia

FIGURE 55-3	MYASTHENIA GRAVIS.

Myasthenia gravis may mimic any ocular disorder causing diplopia, although most often it mimics weakness of the superior rectus muscle or medial rectus muscle (i.e., difficulty with sustained elevation or adduction of the eye, respectively). Clues to the diagnosis of myasthenia gravis are associated ptosis, fluctuating course, and *normal* pupils.

anesthetization of the conjunctiva, the ophthalmologist grasps the conjunctiva with toothed forceps and attempts to passively rotate the eye, detecting abnormal resistance in patients with thyroid myopathy).[10,15]

(2) Orbital Fracture   Diplopia is a complication of 58% of blowout fractures of the orbit and 20% of all midfacial fractures.[16] The heterotropia occurs because of swelling or entrapment of one of the eye muscles, most often the inferior rectus. In addition to the history of previous trauma, some patients have an additional clue, hypesthesia of the ipsilateral infraorbital area, which results from accompanying injury to the infraorbital branch of the trigeminal nerve. Diplopia may first become a problem for the patient days after the injury, when the swelling has had time to partially resolve.[10]

c. Weak Medial Rectus

The clinician should consider internuclear ophthalmoplegia and myasthenia gravis.

(1) Internuclear Ophthalmoplegia ("INO")[17-19]   Lesions in the medial longitudinal fasciculus (the periaqueductal pathway in the brainstem that links the nuclei of cranial nerves III, IV, and VI and coordinates conjugate eye movements) cause internuclear ophthalmoplegia (Fig. 55-4), whose features are (1) incomplete adduction of one eye on lateral gaze (i.e., the "weak" medial rectus) and (2) jerk nystagmus of the contralateral abducting eye. Many patients also have vertical nystagmus on upward gaze. The finding is named

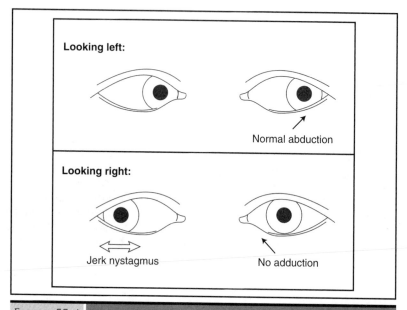

FIGURE 55-4	INTERNUCLEAR OPHTHALMOPLEGIA.

When the patient in the figure looks to the left (*top row*), both eyes move normally, but when the patient looks to the right (*bottom row*), the left eye fails to adduct ("weak" medial rectus) and the contralateral eye develops a jerk nystagmus. The finding is named for the side with weak adduction (i.e., in this example, a *left* internuclear ophthalmoplegia), and the lesion is in the *ipsilateral* medial longitudinal fasciculus (i.e., *left* medial longitudinal fasciculus in this example). See text.

according to the side with weak adduction. For example, in efforts to look to the far right, if the patient's left eye is unable to completely adduct and the right eye develops a jerk nystagmus, the patient has a left internuclear ophthalmoplegia (and a lesion in the left medial longitudinal fasciculus).

Ninety-seven percent of patients with *bilateral* INOs have multiple sclerosis, whereas *unilateral* INO has many causes, although the most common one is vertebral-basilar cerebrovascular disease.[18]

(2) Myasthenia Gravis (See "Weak Superior Rectus Muscle")
Myasthenia gravis sometimes causes medial rectus weakness. In contrast to the finding in patients with internuclear ophthalmoplegia, there is no jerk nystagmus of the abducting eye.

d. Weak Lateral Rectus

Weakness of this muscle almost always indicates damage to the **sixth cranial nerve** (see later), although mimics include myasthenia gravis and thyroid myopathy.[20]

e. Weak superior oblique

Weak superior oblique muscle indicates damage to the **fourth cranial nerve** (see later).

f. Weak inferior oblique

Weak inferior oblique usually indicates **Brown's syndrome.**[21,22] These patients appear to have a weak inferior oblique muscle, but the problem actually is in the superior oblique muscle and tendon, which are unable to move freely through their pulley (i.e., the trochlea). In some patients, Brown's syndrome is congenital. Acquired Brown's syndrome is a complication of orbital inflammation, surgery, and metastases.

3. Skew Deviation

Skew deviation has the following diagnostic features: (1) there is an acquired hypertropia, (2) there is associated cerebellar or brainstem disease, and (3) no other cause is apparent. The disease is usually ipsilateral to the lower eye, but otherwise the finding has minimal localizing value. Skew deviation mimics a weak inferior rectus 40% of the time, a weak inferior oblique 25% of the time, a weak superior rectus 17% of the time, and a weak superior oblique 17% of the time (although the head tilt test, described later, is negative).[10,23]

DISORDERS OF CRANIAL NERVES III, IV, AND VI

I. INTRODUCTION

Table 55-1 reviews the causes of *isolated* palsies of these three cranial nerves, based on analysis of more than 3500 patients reported in the literature.[24–32] Major causes are ischemic infarcts (all three nerves), intracranial aneurysms (especially the third cranial nerve), head trauma (especially the fourth cranial nerve), and tumors (especially when more than one of these nerves are affected). At least one fourth of isolated cranial neuropathies affecting these nerves remain idiopathic, even in the modern era of clinical imaging.[32]

	Oculomotor Nerve	Trochlear Nerve	Abducens Nerve	Mixed*
Proportion (%)†	31	10	45	14
Etiology (%)				
Head trauma	13	34	11	18
Neoplasm	11	5	19	29
Ischemic	25	22	17	7
Aneurysm	17	1	3	11
Other	13	9	22	19
Idiopathic	21	29	28	16

Table 55-1 Etiology of Isolated Palsies of Cranial Nerves III, IV, and VI

Based upon references 24–32.
*"Mixed" refers to combinations of cranial nerves III, IV, or VI
†"Proportion" is ratio of palsies affecting designated cranial nerve to total number of palsies affecting cranial nerve III, IV, and VI.

II. RULES FOR DIAGNOSING ISCHEMIC INFARCTS

One of the most common causes of *isolated* palsies of cranial nerves III, IV, or VI is ischemic infarction, a diagnosis made at the bedside based on the following criteria: (1) the palsy is isolated (i.e., no other neurologic or ophthalmologic findings); (2) the onset is abrupt; (3) the patient has risk factors for cerebrovascular disease, that is, is older than 50 years, has hypertension or diabetes; (4) no other cause is apparent; and (5) the palsy is self-limited, that is, resolves over several months. Seventy-five percent of ischemic mononeuropathies resolve within 4 months; persistence beyond this should prompt evaluation for other causes.

III. OCULOMOTOR NERVE (CRANIAL NERVE III)

A. THE FINDING

Complete weakness causes downward and outward deviation of the affected eye and ptosis (Fig. 55-5). The pupil may or may not be dilated, depending on the etiology of the patient's neuropathy.

B. CLINICAL SIGNIFICANCE

1. Pupil-Sparing Rule[33,34]

The most common causes of *isolated* third nerve paralysis are posterior communicating artery aneurysm (which must be managed aggressively) and ischemic

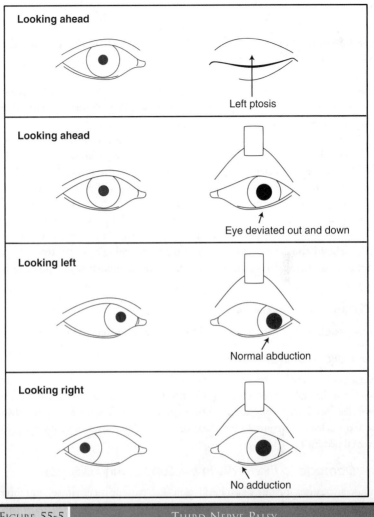

Looking ahead

Left ptosis

Looking ahead

Eye deviated out and down

Looking left

Normal abduction

Looking right

No adduction

FIGURE 55-5   THIRD NERVE PALSY.

Complete third nerve palsy (of the left eye in this example) causes
ptosis that obscures the position of the eye (*first row*). When the lid is
held open (by a piece of tape in this example) the eye appears deviated outward and slightly downward (*second row*), because of
unopposed action of the lateral rectus muscle (abducting the eye)
and superior oblique muscle (depressing the eye). In this example of
third nerve palsy, the pupil is dilated because the cause is an intracranial aneurysm; many ischemic third nerve palsies spare the pupil (see
"Pupil-Sparing Rule" in text). When the patient looks to the left (*third
row*), the intact lateral rectus abducts the eye normally. When the
patient looks to the right (*fourth row*), the left eye fails to adduct past
the midline. Further tests would also demonstrate that the left eye
cannot look up or down.

infarction of the third nerve (which is managed conservatively). In more than 95% of aneurysmal palsies, the pupil reacts sluggishly to light or is fixed and dilated, but in 73% of ischemic palsies, the pupil is spared.[26,27,29,35–39] These observations have led to the "pupil-sparing rule," which states that patients who have third nerve palsies that spare the pupil do not have aneurysms and can be safely managed expectantly.

Before applying this rule, however, there are three important caveats: (1) The rule applies only to patients with *complete* paralysis of the ocular muscles of the third nerve and *complete* sparing of the pupil. Up to 4% of patients with aneurysms do have sparing of the pupil although the third nerve muscles are only partially paralyzed.[27,29,36,38,40–45] (2) The rule should be applied very cautiously to patients aged 20 to 50 years, an age group in which ischemic infarcts are uncommon. (3) The rule only applies to patients with isolated third nerve palsies. Any other neurologic or ophthalmologic finding (e.g., hemiparesis, proptosis, other cranial neuropathy) disqualifies the rule.

2. Clinical Syndromes

Associated findings distinguish the different causes of third nerve palsy.[46]

a. Ipsilateral Brainstem

Damage to the third nerve fascicle as it exits the ipsilateral brain stem causes accompanying ipsilateral cerebellar signs (Nothnagel's syndrome, involving the superior cerebellar peduncle), contralateral hemitremor (Benedikt's syndrome, involving the red nucleus), or contralateral hemiparesis (Weber's syndrome, involving the cerebral peduncle).

b. Damage to the Nerve in the Subarachnoid Space

Important causes include uncal herniation (i.e., patient is comatose) and internal carotid-posterior communicating artery aneurysm (i.e., the third nerve palsy is isolated).

c. Ipsilateral Cavernous Sinus or Orbit

Lesions of the cavernous sinus or orbit cause simultaneous injury to cranial nerves III, IV, and VI (which causes total ophthalmoplegia), to the sympathetic nerves of the iris (contributing to a pupil that is small and unreactive), and to the ophthalmic distribution of the trigeminal nerve (causing hypesthesia of upper third of face). Orbital disease also causes early, prominent proptosis.

d. Ischemic Infarcts

Ischemic infarction causes an isolated third nerve palsy (see "Rules for Diagnosing Ischemic Infarcts" and "Pupil Sparing Rule").

IV. TROCHLEAR NERVE (CRANIAL NERVE IV)

A. THE FINDING

Paralysis of cranial nerve IV causes vertical diplopia and hypertropia of the affected eye. The hypertropia may not be evident on examination, however, and often the clinician will have to tilt the patient's head toward the affected side to bring out the finding (Fig. 55-6). Tilting the head aggravates the diplopia because it requires the ipsilateral eye to intort, which calls on simultaneous contraction of the superior oblique and superior rectus muscles. These two muscles work together, and the tendency of the superior oblique to depress the eye is normally balanced by that of the superior rectus to elevate the eye. If the superior oblique is weak, however, attempts to intort the eye (e.g., during tilting of the head) instead bring about unopposed action of the superior rectus, which elevates the eye and aggravates the vertical diplopia and hypertropia.

B. CLINICAL SIGNIFICANCE

1. Head Position

In studies of patients with isolated fourth nerve palsies, 45% actually habitually tilt their head away from the side of the lesion (to minimize any need for intorsion in the affected eye).[31,47,48] This habitual head tilting is often apparent in old photographs of patients with chronic fourth nerve palsies. As expected, when the head is tilted toward the affected side, the diplopia and hypertropia worsen in 96% of patients.[31,48]

2. Clinical Syndromes

The trochlear nerve has the longest intracranial course of any cranial nerve, in part explaining why trauma is the most common explanation for isolated lesions. Associated findings distinguish the different clinical syndromes.

a. *Contralateral Midbrain*

Associated findings are contralateral Horner's syndrome, contralateral dysmetria, and contralateral internuclear ophthalmoplegia. In all of these syndromes, the associated findings are contralateral because the trochlear nerves cross on their way to the eyes (i.e., the fourth cranial nerve innervating the right eye originates in the left brainstem).[49,50]

b. *Ipsilateral Cavernous Sinus or Orbit*

These lesions cause combinations of findings discussed previously in "Ipsilateral Cavernous Sinus or Orbit."

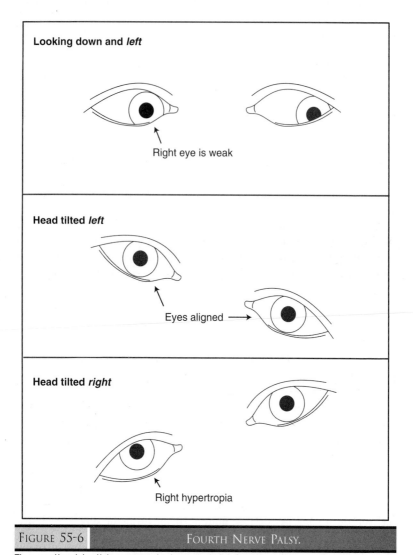

Looking down and *left*

Right eye is weak

Head tilted *left*

Eyes aligned →

Head tilted *right*

Right hypertropia

FIGURE 55-6   FOURTH NERVE PALSY.

The patient in this example has a right fourth nerve palsy. Diplopia is worst when looking down and to the left, indicating that the weak muscle is either the left inferior rectus muscle or right superior oblique muscle (see Fig. 55-2 for principal actions of eye muscles). Simple inspection (*first row*) reveals that the right eye lags behind the left eye, indicating that the weak muscle is indeed on the right side (i.e., right superior oblique). Tilting the head *away* from the affected side (i.e., to the *left* side, away from the weak *right* superior oblique, *second row*) aligns the eyes normally, but tilting the head toward the *affected* side (i.e., to the right side, *third row*) brings out a prominent right hypertropia (i.e., right eye is higher than the left eye). See text.

c. Ischemic Infarcts

Ischemic infarction causes an isolated fourth nerve palsy (see "Rules for Diagnosing Ischemic Infarcts").

V. ABDUCENS NERVE (CRANIAL NERVE VI)

A. THE FINDING

Paralysis of the sixth cranial nerve causes esotropia and an inability to fully abduct the affected eye (Fig. 55-7).

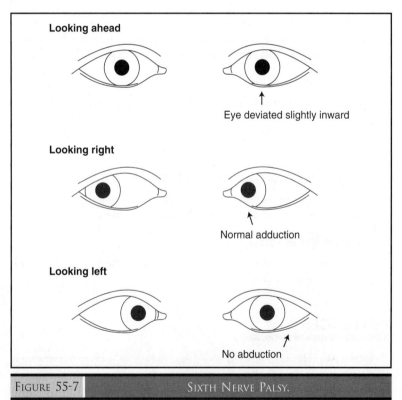

FIGURE 55-7	SIXTH NERVE PALSY.

When the patient in this example (who has a *left* sixth nerve palsy) looks ahead, there is a mild left esotropia (i.e., left eye is deviated toward the nose, *first row*). When looking to the right, the affected eye adducts normally (*second row*). When looking to the left, the left eye fails to abduct (*third row*).

B. CLINICAL SIGNIFICANCE

The various clinical syndromes are distinguished by their associated findings.

1. Ipsilateral Pons

Associated findings are contralateral hemiparesis (Raymond's syndrome), ipsilateral seventh nerve palsy and contralateral hemiparesis (Millard-Gubler syndrome), or ipsilateral Horner's syndrome, ipsilateral horizontal gaze palsy, and ipsilateral involvement of cranial nerves V, VII, and VIII (Foville's syndrome).

2. Damage to the Nerve in the Subarachnoid Space

Damage to the nerve in the subarachnoid space often causes an isolated sixth nerve palsy. Examples are meningitis, recent lumbar puncture (with subsequent leak of cerebrospinal fluid that leads to stretching of the nerve),[51] and pseudo-tumor cerebri (also from stretching of the nerve, brought on by elevated intracranial pressure; these patients may have associated papilledema).

3. At the Petrous Apex

Examples are complicated otitis media (Gradenigo's syndrome: associated ipsilateral decreased hearing, facial pain from involvement of the fifth cranial nerve, and ipsilateral seventh nerve palsy), petrous bone fracture (associated hemotympanum and Battle's sign), and nasopharyngeal carcinoma.[52]

4. Ipsilateral Cavernous Sinus or Orbit

These lesions cause combinations of findings discussed in "Ipsilateral Cavernous Sinus or Orbit (Section III. Oculomotor Nerve)."

5. Ischemic Infarcts

Ischemic infarction causes an isolated sixth nerve palsy (see "Rules for Diagnosing Ischemic Infarcts").

REFERENCES

1. Forster RK, Schatz NJ, Smith JL. A subtle eyelid sign in aberrant regeneration of the third nerve. *Am J Ophthalmol.* 1969;67:696-698.
2. Fisher M. An unusual variant of acute idiopathic polyneuritis (syndrome of ophthalmoplegia, ataxia, and areflexia). *N Engl J Med.* 1956;255:57-65.
3. Henderson JW, Schneider RC. The ocular findings in carotid-cavernous fistula in a series of 17 cases. *Am J Ophthalmol.* 1959;48:585-597.
4. Morris RJ. Double vision as a presenting symptom in an ophthalmic casualty department. *Eye.* 1991;5:124-129.

5. Coffeen P, Guyton DL. Monocular diplopia accompanying ordinary refractive errors. *Am J Ophthalmol.* 1988;105:451-459.

6. Amos JF. Diagnosis and management of monocular diplopia. *J Am Optometric Assoc.* 1982;53:101-115.

7. Records RE. Monocular diplopia. *Surv Ophthalmol.* 1980;24:303-306.

8. Bender MB. Polyopia and monocular diplopia of cerebral origin. *Arch Neurol Psychiatry.* 1945;54:323-328.

9. Meadows JC. Observations on a case of monocular diplopia of cerebral origin. *J Neurol Sci.* 1973;18:249-253.

10. Keane JR. Vertical diplopia. *Semin Neurol.* 1986;6:147-154.

11. Trobe JD. Isolated third nerve palsies. *Semin Neurol.* 1986;6:135-141.

12. Oosterhuis HJGH. The ocular signs and symptoms of myasthenia gravis. *Doc Ophthalmol.* 1982;52:363-378.

13. Osher RH. Myasthenic "oculomotor" palsy. *Arch Ophthalmol.* 1979;11:31-34.

14. Glaser JS. Myasthenic pseudo-internuclear ophthalmoplegia. *Arch Ophthalmol.* 1966;75:363-366.

15. Appen RE, Wendelborn D, Nolten WE. Diplopia in autoimmune thyroid disease. *Arch Intern Med.* 1982;142:898-901.

16. Al-Qurainy IA, Stassesn LFA, Dutton GN, Moos KF, El-Attar A. Diplopia following midfacial fractures. *Br J Oral Maxillofac Surg.* 1991;29:302-307.

17. Cogan DG. Internuclear ophthalmoplegia. *Arch Ophthalmol.* 1970;84:583-589.

18. Smith JL, Cogan DG. Internuclear ophthalmoplegia: A review of 58 cases. *Arch Ophthalmol.* 1959;61:687-694.

19. Keane JR. Internuclear ophthalmoplegia. *Arch Neurol.* 2005;62:714-717.

20. Galetta SL, Smith JL. Chronic isolated sixth nerve palsies. *Arch Neurol.* 1989;46:79-82.

21. Wilson ME, Eustis HS, Parks MM. Brown's syndrome. *Surv Ophthalmol.* 1989;34:153-172.

22. Brown HW. True and simulated superior oblique tendon sheath syndromes. *Doc Ophthalmol.* 1973;34:123-136.

23. Keane JR. Ocular skew deviation: Analysis of 100 cases. *Arch Neurol.* 1975;32:185-190.

24. Tiffin PAC, MacEwen CJ, Craig EA, Clayton G. Acquired palsy of the oculomotor, trochlear and abducens nerves. *Eye.* 1996;10:377-384.

25. Rush JA, Younge BR. Paralysis of cranial nerves III, IV, and VI. *Arch Ophthalmol.* 1981;99:76-79.

26. Rucker CW. Paralysis of the third, fourth and sixth cranial nerves. *Am J Ophthalmol.* 1958;46:787-794.

27. Rucker CW. The causes of paralysis of the third, fourth and sixth cranial nerves. *Am J Ophthalmol.* 1966;61:1293-1298.

28. Berlit P. Isolated and combined pareses of cranial nerves III, IV, and VI: A retrospective study of 412 patients. *J Neurol Sci.* 1991;103:10-15.

29. Green WR, Hackett ER, Schlezinger NS. Neuro-ophthalmologic evaluation of oculomotor nerve paralysis. *Arch Ophthalmol.* 1964;72:154-167.
30. Burger LJ, Kalvin NH, Smith JL. Acquired lesions of the fourth cranial nerve. *Brain.* 1970;93:567-574.
31. Khawam E, Scott AB, Jamplosky A. Acquired superior oblique palsy. *Arch Ophthalmol.* 1967;77:761-768.
32. Richards BW, Jones FR, Younge BR. Causes and prognosis in 4278 cases of paralysis of the oculomotor, trochlear, and abducens cranial nerves. *Am J Ophthalmol.* 1992;113:489-496.
33. Trobe JD. Third nerve palsy and the pupil. *Arch Ophthalmol.* 1988;106:601-602.
34. Trobe JD. Isolated pupil-sparing third nerve palsy. *Ophthalmology.* 1985;92:58-61.
35. Zorrilla E, Kozak GP. Ophthalmoplegia in diabetes mellitus. *Ann Intern Med.* 1967;67:968-976.
36. Capo H, Warren F, Kupersmith MJ. Evolution of oculomotor nerve palsies. *J Clin Neuroophthalmol.* 1992;12(1):12-15.
37. Hopf HC, Gutmann L. Diabetic 3rd nerve palsy: Evidence for a mesencephalic lesion. *Neurol.* 1990;40:1041-1045.
38. Cogan DG, Mount HTJ. Intracranial aneurysms causing ophthalmoplegia. *Arch Ophthalmol.* 1963;70:757-771.
39. Sanders S, Kawasaki A, Purvin VA. Patterns of extraocular muscle weakness in vasculopathic pupil-sparing, incomplete third nerve palsy. *J Neuro-Ophthalmol.* 2001;21:256-259.
40. Fujiwara S, Fujii K, Nishio S, et al. Oculomotor nerve palsy in patients with cerebral aneurysms. *Neurosurg Rev.* 1989;12:123-132.
41. Kissel JT, Burde RM, Klingele TG, Zeiger HE. Pupil-sparing oculomotor palsies with internal carotid-posterior communicating artery aneurysms. *Ann Neurol.* 1983;13:149-154.
42. Raja IA. Aneurysm-induced third nerve palsy. *J Neurosurg.* 1972;36:548-551.
43. Keane JR. Aneurysms and third nerve palsies. *Ann Neurol.* 1983;14:696-697.
44. Botterell EH, Lloyd LA, Hoffman HJ. Oculomotor palsy due to supraclinoid internal carotid artery berry aneurysm. *Am J Ophthalmol.* 1962;54:609-616.
45. Jacobson DM. Relative pupil-sparing third nerve palsy: Etiology and clinical variables predictive of a mass. *Neurology.* 2001;56:797-798.
46. Brazis PW. Localization of lesions of the oculomotor nerve: Recent concepts. *Mayo Clin Proc.* 1991;66:1029-1035.
47. Urist MJ. Head tilt in vertical muscle paresis. *Am J Ophthalmol.* 1970;69:440-442.
48. Younge BR, Sutula F. Analysis of trochlear nerve palsies: Diagnosis, etiology, and treatment. *Mayo Clin Proc.* 1977;52:11-18.
49. Brazis PW. Palsies of the trochlear nerve: Diagnosis and localization: Recent concepts. *Mayo Clin Proc.* 1993;68:501-509.

50. Guy J, Day AL, Mickle JP, Schatz NJ. Contralateral trochlear nerve paresis and ipsi-lateral Horner's syndrome. *Am J Ophthalmol*. 1989;107:73-76.
51. Bryce-Smith R, Macintosh RR. Sixth-nerve palsy after lumbar puncture and spinal analgesia. *Br Med J*. 1951;1:275-276.
52. Smith JL, Wheliss JA. Ocular manifestations of nasopharyngeal tumors. *Trans Am Acad Ophthalmol Otol*. 1962;66:659-664.

56

Miscellaneous Cranial Nerves

T able 56-1 reviews the physical examination of the 12 cranial nerves. Only cranial nerves I, V, VII, and IX through XII are discussed in this chapter. Cranial nerve II is discussed in Chapters 19 and 54; cranial nerve VIII, in Chapter 21, and cranial nerves III, IV, and VI, in Chapter 55.

OLFACTORY NERVE (I)

I. TECHNIQUE

The usual test for the sense of smell is placing a nonirritative substance, such as wintergreen or cloves, under one nostril at a time. One simple method uses the standard 70% isopropyl alcohol pad available in most clinics and wards.[1] Pungent substances such as ammonia should be avoided because they stimulate trigeminal nerve endings (i.e., cranial nerve V).

Table 56-1 The 12 Cranial Nerves

Cranial Nerve	Motor Examination	Sensory Examination	Reflex Examination
Olfactory nerve (I)		Detection of nonirritating odors	
Optic nerve (II)		Visual acuity Retinal examination	Afferent pupillary defect ("swinging flashlight test") Pupillary constriction (III only)
Nerves of the eye muscles: Oculomotor nerve (III) Trochlear nerve (IV) Abducens nerve (VI)	Extraocular movements (III, IV, and VI) Lid elevation (III only)		
Trigeminal nerve (V)	Masseter muscle Lateral pterygoid muscle	Pain, temperature, and touch sensation of the ipsilateral face	Corneal reflex (afferent limb) Jaw jerk (afferent and efferent limb) Glabellar reflex (afferent limb)
Facial nerve (VII)	All facial movements except lid elevation	Taste sensation to anterior 2/3 of the tongue	Corneal reflex (efferent limb) Glabellar reflex (efferent limb)
Vestibulocochlear nerve (VIII)		Tests of hearing (cochlear component)	Vestibulo-ocular reflex (vestibular component)
Glossopharyngeal nerve (IX)	Ipsilateral palate elevation (with X)	Sensation posterior pharynx Taste sensation to posterior 2/3 of tongue	Gag reflex (afferent limb and, with X, efferent limb)
Vagus nerve (X)	Ipsilateral palate elevation (with IX)		Gag reflex (efferent limb with IX)
Spinal accessory nerve (XI)	Trapezius muscle Sternocleidomastoid muscle		
Hypoglossal nerve (XII)	Genioglossus muscle		

II. CLINICAL SIGNIFICANCE

A. ANOSMIA

Anosmia is the complete absence of smell. The most common causes are upper respiratory infection and sinus disease (which obstructs the nasal passages) and previous head trauma (which damages the olfactory fibers).[2,3] Less common causes are Kallmann's syndrome (hypogonadotropic hypogonadism) and sphenoid ridge masses (e.g., meningioma, which causes the Foster-Kennedy syndrome, i.e., ipsilateral anosmia, ipsilateral optic atrophy, and contralateral papilledema).[2,4]

B. OLFACTORY DYSFUNCTION

Patients with olfactory dysfunction are able to detect odors but often misidentify them. Olfactory dysfunction is common in patients with Parkinson's disease[5,6] or after frontal or temporal lobectomies.[7] Patients with Parkinson's disease are much more likely to have olfactory dysfunction than patients with other parkinsonian syndromes such as vascular parkinsonism and progressive supranuclear palsy (see Chapter 57).[8–10]

TRIGEMINAL NERVE (V)

I. INTRODUCTION

The trigeminal sensory and motor nuclei are located in the pons, although the sensory nucleus extends through the medulla into the cervical spinal cord. The sensory branches of the trigeminal nerve innervate the upper face (V_1, ophthalmic division), mid-face (V_2, maxillary division), and lower face (V_3, mandibular division). The motor fibers to the masseter and lateral pterygoid muscles travel with the mandibular division (V_3).

II. THE FINDING

A. MOTOR WEAKNESS

Lesions of the motor component of the trigeminal nerve affect the masseter muscle (causing difficulty clenching that side of the jaw, sometimes with atrophy that flattens the contour of the cheek) and lateral pterygoid muscle (causing difficulty deviating the jaw to the opposite side; at rest the jaw may deviate toward the weak side).

B. SENSORY LOSS

Lesions of the sensory component cause diminished pain, temperature, and touch sensation in any or all of the three divisions on one side of the face. Sensation to most of the external ear (excluding the tragus) and the angle of the jaw is preserved in trigeminal lesions, because these areas are supplied by cervical sensory roots (see Fig. 58-1 in Chapter 58).

C. CORNEAL REFLEX

Unilateral gentle stimulation of the cornea normally causes bilateral blinking. The afferent limb of this reflex is the ipsilateral trigeminal nerve (only V_1 and V_2) and the efferent limb is both facial nerves (i.e., both eyes blink after stimulation of one cornea).

III. CLINICAL SIGNIFICANCE

A. MOTOR WEAKNESS

Unilateral weakness of the trigeminal muscles indicates disease of the proximal mandibular division (e.g., skull metastases) or a lesion in the ipsilateral pons (patients with pontine lesions have other associated neurologic findings, such as abnormalities of cranial nerves VI or VII, or contralateral hemiparesis). Unilateral weakness of the trigeminal muscles does not occur with cerebral hemispheric lesions because each trigeminal nucleus receives bilateral cortical innervation.[11] *Bilateral* weakness, however, may occur in bilateral cerebral hemispheric disease and cause great difficulty chewing (see "Pseudobulbar Palsy" later).

B. SENSORY LOSS

Sensory loss of the face may be part of a broader neurologic syndrome affecting sensation of the whole body and other neurologic functions (lesions of the cerebral hemisphere, thalamus, or brainstem) or may be isolated to the face (lesions of the peripheral nerve and its branches).

1. Sensory Loss of Face and Body

In thalamic and cerebral hemispheric lesions, sensation of the face and body is abnormal on the *same* side, contralateral to the lesion. There is often associated hemiparesis, aphasia, or both.[12-14] In brainstem lesions, the sensory abnormalities of the face and body are on *opposite* sides: sensation is diminished on the *ipsilateral* face but *contralateral* body (see Fig. 58-2 and Table 58-2 in Chapter 58).[15-19] Pontine lesions affect intraoral more than facial sensation, whereas medullary lesions affect facial more than intraoral sensation.[20]

2. Sensory Loss Isolated to the Face

Sensory loss isolated to the face is part of syndromes affecting the apex of the temporal bone (see Chapter 55, cranial nerve VI), the cavernous sinus syndrome (V_1 division only, see Chapter 55), and "numb chin syndrome." The numb chin syndrome, which describes the loss of sensation on the lower lip and chin, has an ominous prognosis in cancer patients and suggests the presence of metastatic disease to the ipsilateral mandible, base of skull, or leptomeninges.[21-23] These patients sometimes have abnormalities of other cranial nerves.

C. ABNORMAL CORNEAL REFLEX

The two limbs of the corneal reflex are cranial nerves V and VII. According to traditional teachings, unilateral trigeminal nerve dysfunction (i.e., in the ipsilateral brainstem, V_1, or V_2 divisions) prevents both eyes from blinking after stimulation of the ipsilateral cornea, whereas unilateral facial nerve dysfunction prevents the ipsilateral eye from blinking when its cornea is stimulated, although the contralateral eye blinks normally. The absent corneal reflex is felt to be particularly important in patients with unilateral sensorineural hearing loss, in whom it raises the possibility of cerebellopontine angle tumors, such as acoustic neuroma.

Nonetheless, the clinical utility of the asymmetric corneal reflex is limited. The reflex is inexplicable absent unilaterally in 8% of healthy elderly patients,[24] and the sensitivity of the absent reflex for acoustic neuroma is only 33%, the finding usually indicating the tumor has already grown to a large size (>2 cm in diameter).[25]

D. HERPES ZOSTER INFECTION AND THE NASOCILIARY BRANCH OF THE TRIGEMINAL NERVE ("HUTCHINSON'S SIGN")

About half of patients with *Herpes zoster* infection of the ophthalmic division of the trigeminal nerve ("herpes zoster ophthalmicus") develop vision-threatening complications such as uveitis and keratitis within 1 to 4 weeks of the onset of the rash (mean onset = 1.8 weeks).[26,27] In 1865, Hutchinson noted that the tip of the nose, cornea, and iris all share the same branch of the trigeminal nerve (the nasociliary nerve) and that if a patient with herpes zoster ophthalmicus developed vesicles on the tip of the nose (i.e., "Hutchinson's sign"), there was an increased risk of ocular complications.[28] The clinical utility of this sign, however, is limited: its accuracy is only modest [sensitivity 57% to 87%, specificity 77% to 82%, positive likelihood ratio (LR) = 3.5, negative LR = 0.3],[26,27] and today all patients with herpes zoster ophthalmicus, whether or not the tip of the nose or the eye is involved, should receive antiviral medications.[29]

FACIAL NERVE (VII)

I. THE FINDING

Lesions of the facial nerve may cause facial asymmetry (diminished ipsilateral nasolabial fold and widened ipsilateral palpebral fissure) and weakness of most ipsilateral facial muscles (muscles used during speaking, blinking, raising eyebrows, smiling, wrinkling the forehead, closing the eyes, showing teeth, and retracting the chin). There may be abnormalities of ipsilateral tearing (lacrimal gland), hearing (stapedius muscle), taste (anterior two third of the tongue), and the corneal and glabellar reflexes.

Facial nerve lesions do not cause ptosis, because the lid muscles are not innervated by the facial nerve but rather by sympathetic nerves and cranial nerve III.

II. CLINICAL SIGNIFICANCE

A. CENTRAL VERSUS PERIPHERAL FACIAL WEAKNESS

Unilateral facial weakness may be "central" (i.e., in upper motor neurons, from lesions in the contralateral motor cortex or descending pyramidal tracts) or "peripheral" (i.e., in lower motor neurons, from lesions in the peripheral nerve or facial nucleus in the ipsilateral pons).* These lesions are distinguished by the following two features.

1. Distribution of Weakness

Peripheral lesions affect both upper and lower facial muscles, whereas central lesions affect predominately the lower facial muscles. Wrinkling of the forehead is relatively spared in central lesions because the facial nuclei innervating these muscles receive bilateral cortical innervation.

2. Movements Affected

Peripheral lesions paralyze all facial movements on the side affected, whereas central lesions affect voluntary movements but spare emotional ones. The patient with central weakness (e.g., cerebral hemispheric stroke) may be unable to wrinkle one corner of the mouth volitionally yet can move it normally during laughter or crying. This occurs because emotional input to the facial nuclei does not come from the motor cortex.†[30,31]

---

*Chapter 57 defines "upper" and "lower" motor neurons.
†The opposite clinical finding, emotional paralysis without volitional paralysis, occurs with lesions of the thalamus or frontal lobe.[30,31]

B. PERIPHERAL NERVE LESIONS

1. Etiology

The causes of isolated peripheral facial palsies are idiopathic (50%–87%), surgical or accidental trauma (5%–22%), herpes zoster infections (Ramsey Hunt syndrome, 7%–13%), tumors (e.g., cholesteatoma, parotid tumors, 1%–6%), and miscellaneous disorders (8%–11%) (These figures originate in specialty referral centers and may over-represent unusual etiologies).[32–37] "Bell's palsy" refers to the idiopathic disorders, although evidence is mounting that it represents response to viral infection.[38]

2. Associated Findings

In patients with Bell's palsy, associated findings are diminished taste (52%), hyperacusis (8%–30%), increased tearing (19%–34%), and decreased tearing (2%–17%).[33–36,39–41] Increased tear production occurs because the weak orbicularis oculi muscle cannot contain and direct the tears down the nasolacrimal duct; decreased tearing reflects lacrimal gland dysfunction. Although 23% of patients also have sensory complaints, the finding of hypesthesia of the face (i.e., cranial nerve V) is variable: some investigators, arguing that Bell's palsy is part of a multiple cranial neuropathy, have found hypesthesia in as many as 48% of patients,[35,39] whereas other investigators have never found associated hypesthesia of the face.[33]

3. Topographic Diagnosis

The branches of the facial nerve diverge from the main trunk in predictable order: they are, proximally to distally, branches to the lacrimal gland, stapedius muscle, tongue (taste), and facial muscles.[35] Therefore, tests of tearing (Schirmer's tear test), stapedius function (stapedius reflex during audiometry), and taste should pinpoint the location of the lesion, although this is only accurate when the nerve is completely severed. In patients with patchy lesions (Bell's palsy or partial injuries), topographic diagnosis is often nonsensical (e.g., tearing reduced but taste and stapedius function preserved) and has minimal clinical value.[35,39,42]

4. Complications of Bell's Palsy[34,36,40,41]

Three complications occur after recovery from Bell's palsy.

a. Associated Movements ("Synkinesis", 55%–94% of Patients)

These are unexpected movements that probably result from aberrant regeneration. Examples are narrowing of the palpebral fissure when the patient smiles, or motion of the corner of the mouth when the patient closes the eyes tightly.

b.   Contracture (3%–36%)

Despite the name, this is increased muscle tone, not a fibrotic scar, which often restores facial symmetry even though some weakness persists.

c.   Crocodile Tears (2%–6%)

Crocodile tears occur from aberrant regeneration of salivary gland fibers to the lacrimal gland. When affected patients eat, tears form and run down the cheek or collect in the nose.

GLOSSOPHARYNGEAL (IX) AND VAGUS (X) NERVES

I.   FINDING

These nerves are considered together because their function is difficult to separate at the bedside and because clinical disorders usually affect both nerves simultaneously. There are three abnormal findings: (**1**) **Absent pharyngeal sensation,** which is usually tested with a cotton applicator stick touching the posterior oropharynx. (**2**) **Diminished velar movement.** The posterior edge of the soft palate is called the "velum" and its elevation, "velar movement," The soft palate should elevate as the patient vocalizes a prolonged "ah." (**3**) **Abnormal gag reflex.** During stimulation of the posterior tongue, pharynx, or soft palate, there is reflex elevation of the tongue and soft palate and constriction of the pharyngeal muscles. The gag reflex is labeled abnormal when it is diminished, absent, hyperactive, or asymmetric.

II.   CLINICAL SIGNIFICANCE

Abnormalities of these nerves may occur because of *bilateral* cerebral hemispheric disease or because of disease in the *ipsilateral* medulla or peripheral nerves (i.e., cranial nerves IX and X). *Unilateral* cerebral hemispheric disease does not ordinarily cause palatal weakness because each nucleus of these nerves receives bilateral corticobulbar innervation.

A.   BILATERAL CEREBRAL HEMISPHERIC LESIONS: PSEUDOBULBAR PALSY

Bilateral lesions above the level of the pons that disrupt the descending pyramidal tracts innervating brainstem motor nuclei may cause significant paralysis of the palate and pharynx, along with paralysis of the tongue, face, and muscles of chewing. This syndrome, "pseudobulbar palsy," affects about 4% of patients with cerebrovascular disease, who mostly have lacunar infarcts in both internal capsules.[43,44] The main clinical features are dysarthria, dysphagia, and paralysis of voluntary movements of the face.[45,46] Other findings are hyperactive jaw jerk (70% of patients), absent gag reflex (70%), and hyperactive emotional reflexes that cause spasmodic and often inappropriate crying and laughing (24%).[43,44,47–49] The animated facial movements that appear while the patient laughs or cries uncontrollably contrast markedly with the lack of voluntary facial movement and the patient's inability to mimic gestures.

The term "pseudobulbar," coined by Lepine in 1877,[44] is used because the lesion is supranuclear, to distinguish this syndrome from similar motor paralysis that may occur after damage to the brainstem nuclei themselves (i.e. "bulbar" paralysis).[44,45] The term is a misnomer, however, because "bulbar" refers to the medulla and two motor nuclei prominently affected in pseudobulbar palsy—those of the facial muscles (VII) and of chewing (V)—reside in the pons.

B. BEDSIDE PREDICTORS OF RISK OF ASPIRATION AFTER STROKE

In patients who have suffered bilateral strokes, significant dysfunction of cranial nerves IX and X makes the airway vulnerable to aspiration during swallowing. EBM Box 56-1 presents the accuracy of several bedside signs as predictors of aspiration in patients with strokes. The most significant arguments *for* risk of aspiration are drowsiness (LR = 3.4), abnormal water swallow test (LR = 3.2), and oxygen desaturation $\geq 2\%$ after the patient swallows a liquid (LR = 3.1; see footnote to EBM Box 56-1 for definitions of findings). The most compelling arguments *against* the risk of aspiration are normal pharyngeal sensation (LR = 0.03), absence of oxygen desaturation following a swallow (LR = 0.3), a normal water swallow test (LR = 0.4), and absence of dysphonia (LR = 0.4). The accuracy of other findings, including the abnormal gag reflex, presence of dysphonia, and abnormal cough, is only modest (EBM Box 56-1). Findings with no predictive value are abnormal sensation of face and tongue, tongue weakness, bilateral cranial nerve findings, and abnormal chest radiograph.[50]

The poor predictive value of the absent gag reflex is not surprising because the pharyngeal muscles involved in this reflex are not necessarily the same ones activated during normal swallowing to protect the airway. Moreover, the gag reflex is often absent in normal individuals, especially elderly patients.[65,66] Pharyngeal sensation, on the other hand, is rarely absent in normal individuals.[65]

C. LESIONS OF IPSILATERAL BRAINSTEM OR PERIPHERAL NERVE

The lateral medullary syndrome causes ipsilateral absence of pharyngeal sensation and reduced velar elevation, associated with Horner's syndrome and other sensory and cerebellar signs (see Table 58-2 in Chapter 58). The jugular

Aspiration After Stroke*

Finding (Ref)[†]	Sensitivity (%)	Specificity (%)	Likelihood Ratio if Finding	
			Present	Absent
Voice and cough				
Abnormal voluntary cough[50–58]	48–89	36–94	1.9	0.6
Dysphonia[50–55,57,59]	59–98	13–67	1.3	0.4
Dysarthria[53,57,60]	60–77	53–57	1.6	0.5
Neurologic examination				
Drowsiness[58,61]	50–76	65–92	**3.4**	0.5
Abnormal sensation face and tongue[50]	22	52	NS	NS
Absent pharyngeal sensation[61]	98	60	2.4	**0.03**
Tongue weakness[58,59]	50–72	47–91	NS	0.6
Bilateral cranial nerve signs[50,55]	71–73	30–39	NS	NS
Abnormal gag reflex[50–55,57–60]	53–91	18–82	1.5	0.6
Other tests				
Water swallow test[56–59,61,62]	47–85	58–93	**3.2**	0.4
Oxygen desaturation 0–2 min after swallowing[56,63,64]	73–87	39–88	**3.1**	**0.3**

NS, not significant; likelihood ratio (LR) if finding present = positive LR; LR if finding absent = negative LR.

*Diagnostic standard: For aspiration, fiberoptic examination[56] or videofluoroscopy (all other studies).

[†]Definition of findings: For abnormal voluntary cough, the patient is asked to cough as hard as possible and the resulting cough is absent, weak, breathy, or sluggish; for dysphonia, the patient is asked to sing a prolonged "ah" and the voice is breathy, hoarse, wet, harsh, or strained; for absent pharyngeal sensation, the patient cannot sense an applicator stick applied to the posterior oropharynx, on one or both sides; for abnormal gag reflex, the gag reflex is diminished, absent, hyperactive, or asymmetric; for water swallow test, drinking 5–90 mL of water in 5- to 10-mL sips causes coughing, choking, or alteration of the voice; for oxygen desaturation after swallowing, oxygen saturation decreases ≥2% 0–2 min after swallowing 10 mL of water[56] or 20 mL[64]–150 mL[63] of liquid barium.

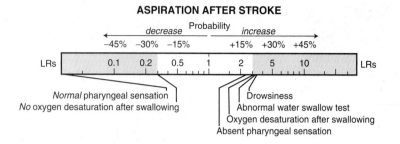

ASPIRATION AFTER STROKE

foramen syndrome (e.g., basilar skull fracture or glomus jugulare tumors) simultaneously disrupts cranial nerves IX, X, and XI, causing ipsilateral paralysis of the palate, vocal cords (hoarseness), and trapezius and sternocleidomastoid muscles.

SPINAL ACCESSORY NERVE (XI)

I. FINDING

The primary findings are a weakness or atrophy, or both, of the sternocleidomastoid muscle (which turns the head to the opposite side) and trapezius muscle (which elevates the ipsilateral shoulder).

II. CLINICAL SIGNIFICANCE

Unilateral weakness of these muscles may represent disease of the cerebral hemispheres, brainstem, spinal cord, or peripheral nerve. Atrophy indicates that the lesion is in the nucleus (i.e., brainstem or high cervical spinal cord) or peripheral nerve (i.e., the lesion is *not* in the cerebral hemispheres).

A. CEREBRAL HEMISPHERE

Lesions of the cerebral hemispheres affect the trapezius and sternocleidomastoid muscles differently: Lesions in one cerebral hemisphere weaken the *contralateral* trapezius but the *ipsilateral* sternocleidomastoid muscle.*[67] Therefore,

---

*Descending corticobulbar fibers to the sternocleidomastoid muscle are believed to cross twice to innervate the ipsilateral side. This innervation makes teleologic sense, because the sternocleidomastoid muscle turns the head to the opposite side, and the cerebral hemisphere is interested in turning the head to same side whose visual fields, eye movements, and motor function it control.[67]

in a hemispheric stroke, the patient may demonstrate weakness turning the head toward the hemiparetic side.[68] In a focal seizure, the head often deviates toward the seizing limbs.

B. BRAINSTEM OR HIGH CERVICAL SPINAL CORD

Lesions of the accessory nucleus, located in the medulla and high cervical spinal cord, may cause atrophy and weakness of the *ipsilateral* trapezius and sternocleidomastoid muscle (e.g., syringomyelia).

C. PERIPHERAL NERVE

Injuries to the peripheral nerve, which occur from trauma to the posterior triangle of the neck (e.g., surgical excision of lymph nodes, blunt trauma), may paralyze the *ipsilateral* trapezius or sternocleidomastoid muscles, although the sternocleidomastoid muscle is often spared because its branches diverge early from the main trunk of the nerve.[69] The jugular foramen syndrome, discussed above under the glossopharyngeal nerve, also affects cranial nerve XI along with cranial nerves IX and X.

HYPOGLOSSAL NERVE (XII)

I. FINDING

During protrusion of the tongue, each genioglossus muscle acts to push the tongue out and toward the opposite side. Normally these laterally directed forces balance each other, and the tongue remains in the midline. With unilateral hypoglossal weakness, however, the intact genioglossus muscle acts to deviate the tongue toward the opposite, or weak, side.

II. CLINICAL SIGNIFICANCE

Weakness of the genioglossus may represent disease in the cerebral hemisphere, brainstem, or peripheral nerve. Atrophy or fasciculations of the tongue indicate the lesion is either in the hypoglossal nucleus (brainstem) or hypoglossal nerve (i.e., *not* cerebral hemispheres).

A. CEREBRAL HEMISPHERE

Lesions of the cerebral hemisphere may cause weakness of the contralateral genioglossus. Therefore, the tongue deviates toward the side of the weak arm and leg.[70]

B. BRAINSTEM

The medial medullary syndrome causes ipsilateral hypoglossal paralysis, contralateral hemiparesis, and contralateral loss of proprioceptive and vibratory sensation (preserving pain and temperature sensation). Therefore, the tongue deviates away from the side of the weak arm and leg.

C. PERIPHERAL NERVE

The most common causes of lesions of the hypoglossal nerve are metastatic cancer (to base of skull, subarachnoid space, or neck) and trauma (e.g., gunshot wounds to the neck, radical neck surgery, carotid endarterectomy).[71]

Hypoglossal palsy in association with other cranial nerve findings occurs with both brainstem and peripheral nerve disorders, and therefore has little localizing value.[71]

REFERENCES

1. Davidson TM, Murphy C. Rapid clinical evaluation of anosmia: The alcohol sniff test. *Arch Otolaryngol Head Neck Surg.* 1997;123:591-594.
2. Deems DA, Doty RL, Settle G, et al. Smell and taste disorders: A study of 750 patients from the University of Pennsylvania smell and taste center. *Arch Otolaryngol Head Neck Surg.* 1991;117:519-528.
3. Holbrook EH, Leopold DA. Anosmia: Diagnosis and management. *Curr Opin Otolaryngol Head Neck Surg.* 2003;11:54-60.
4. Shiffman SS. Taste and smell in disease. *N Engl J Med.* 1983;308:1275-1279; 1337-1243.
5. Doty RL, Deems DA, Stellar S. Olfactory dysfunction in parkinsonism: A general deficit unrelated to neurologic signs, disease stage, or disease duration. *Neurology.* 1988;38:1237-1244.
6. Hawkes CH, Shephard BC, Daniel SE. Olfactory dysfunction in Parkinson's disease. *J Neurol Neurosurg Psychiatry.* 1997;62:436-446.
7. Zatorre RJ, Jones-Gotman M. Human olfactory discrimination after unilateral frontal or temporal lobectomy. *Brain.* 1991;114:71-84.
8. Khan NL, Katzenschlager R, Watt H, et al. Olfaction differentiates parkin disease from early-onset parkinsonism and Parkinson disease. *Neurology.* 2004;62:1224-1226.
9. Katzenschlager R, Zijlmans J, Evans A, et al. Olfactory function distinguishes vascular parkinsonism from Parkinson's disease. *J Neurol Neurosurg Psychiatry.* 2004;75:1749-1752.
10. Hawkes CH, Shephard BC, Daniel SE. Is Parkinson's disease a primary olfactory disorder? *Q J Med.* 1999;92:473-480.
11. Cruccu G, Fornarelli M, Manfredi M. Impairment of masticatory function in hemiplegia. *Neurol.* 1988;38:301-306.

12. Barraquer-Bordas L, Illa I, Escartin A, et al. Thalamic hemorrhage: A study of 23 patients with diagnosis by computed tomography. *Stroke.* 1981;12:524-527.

13. Kim JS. Pure sensory stroke: Clinical-radiological correlates of 21 cases. *Stroke.* 1992;23:983-987.

14. Walshe TM, Davis KR, Fisher CM. Thalamic hemorrhage: A computed tomographic-clinical correlation. *Neurology.* 1977;27:217-222.

15. Kim JS, Lee JH, Suh DC, Lee MC. Spectrum of lateral medullary syndrome: Correlation between clinical findings and magnetic resonance imaging in 33 subjects. *Stroke.* 1994;25:1405-1410.

16. Norrving B, Cronqvist S. Lateral medullary infarction: Prognosis in an unselected series. *Neurology* 1991;41:244-248.

17. Peterman AF, Siekert RG. The lateral medullary (Wallenberg) syndrome: Clinical features and prognosis. *Med Clin North Am.* 1960;44:887-895.

18. Sacco RL, Freddo L, Bellow JA, et al. Wallenberg's lateral medullary syndrome: Clinical-magnetic resonance imaging correlations. *Arch Neurol.* 1993;50:609-614.

19. Fisher CM, Karnes WE, Kubik CS. Lateral medullary infarction: The pattern of vascular occlusion. *J Neuropathol Exp Neurol.* 1961;20:323-379.

20. Graham SH, Sharp FR, Dillon W. Intraoral sensation in patients with brainstem lesions: Role of the rostral spinal trigeminal nuclei in pons. *Neurology.* 1988;38:1529-1533.

21. Lossos A, Siegal T. Numb chin syndrome in cancer patients: Etiology, response to treatment, and prognostic significance. *Neurology.* 1992;42:1181-1184.

22. Sweet JM. The numb chin syndrome: A critical sign for primary care physicians. *Arch Intern Med.* 2004;164:1347-1348.

23. Laurencet FM, Anchisi S, Tullen E, Dietrich PY. Mental neuropathy: Report of five cases and review of the literature. *Crit Rev Oncol Hematol.* 2000;34:71-79.

24. Rai GS, Elias-Jones A. The corneal reflex in elderly patients. *J Am Geriatr Soc.* 1979;27:317-318.

25. Harner SG, Laws ER. Clinical findings in patients with acoustic neuroma. *Mayo Clin Proc.* 1983;58:721-728.

26. Harding SP, Lipton JR, Wells JCD. Natural history of herpes zoster ophthalmicus: Predictors of postherpetic neuralgia and ocular involvement. *Br J Ophthalmol.* 1987;71:353-358.

27. Zaal MJW, Volker-Dieben HJ, D'Amaro J. Prognostic value of Hutchinson's sign in acute herpes zoster ophthalmicus. *Graefes Arch Clin Exp Ophthalmol.* 2003;241:187-191.

28. Tomkinson A, Doblin DG, Brown MJKM. Huchinson's sign and its importance in rhinology. *Rhinology.* 1995;33(3):180-182.

29. Pavan-Langston D. Herpes zoster ophthalmicus. *Neurology.* 1995;45 (suppl 8): S50-51.

30. Hopf HC, Mueller-Forell W, Hopf NJ. Localization of emotional and volitional facial paresis. *Neurology.* 1992;42:1918-1923.

31. Ross RT, Mathiesen R. Volitional and emotional supranuclear facial weakness. *N Engl J Med.* 1998;338:1515.

32. Mountain RE, Murray JAM, Quaba A, Maynard C. The Edinburgh facial palsy clinic: A review of three years' activity. *J R Coll Surg Edinb.* 1994;39: 275-279.

33. Hauser WA, Karnes WE, Annis J, Kurland LT. Incidence and prognosis of Bell's palsy in the population of Rochester, Minnesota. *Mayo Clin Proc.* 1971;46: 258-264.

34. Devriese PP, Schumacher T, Scheide A, et al. Incidence, prognosis and recovery of Bell's palsy: A survey of about 1000 patients (1974-1983). *Clin Otolaryngol.* 1990; 15:15-27.

35. Adour KK. Diagnosis and management of facial paralysis. *New Engl J Med.* 1982;307:348-351.

36. Park HW, Watkins AL. Facial paralysis: Analysis of 500 cases. *Arch Phys Med.* 1949;30:749-762.

37. May M, Klein SR. Differential diagnosis of facial nerve palsy. *Otolaryngol Clin North Am.* 1991;24:613-645.

38. Murakami S, Mizobuchi M, Nakashiro Y, et al. Bell palsy and Herpes simplex virus: Identification of viral DNA in endoneurial fluid and muscle. *Ann Intern Med.* 1996;124(1 part 1):27-30.

39. Adour KK, Byl FM, Hilsinger RL, et al. The true nature of Bell's palsy: Analysis of 1000 consecutive patients. *Laryngoscope.* 1978;88:787-801.

40. Katusic SK, Beard CM, Wiederholt WC, et al. Incidence, clinical features, and prognosis in Bell's palsy, Rochester, Minnesota, 1968-1982. *Ann Neurol.* 1986;20: 622-627.

41. Taverner D. Bell's palsy: A clinical and electromyographic study. *Brain.* 1955;78: 209-228.

42. Tonning FM. The reliability of level-diagnostic examinations in acute, peripheral facial palsy. *Acta Otolaryngol.* 1977;84:414-415.

43. Loeb C, Gandolfo C, Caponnetto C, Del Sette M. Pseudobulbar palsy: A clinical computed tomography study. *Eur Neurol.* 1990;30:42-46.

44. Besson G, Bogousslavsky J, Regli F, Maeder P. Acute pseudobulbar or suprabulbar palsy. *Arch Neurol.* 1991;48:501-507.

45. Flora GC. Pseudobulbar palsy. *Minn Med.* 1970;53:569-572.

46. Langworthy OR, Hesser FH. Syndrome of pseudobulbar palsy: An anatomic and physiologic analysis. *Arch Intern Med.* 1940;65:106-121.

47. Black DW. Pathological laughter. *J Nerv Ment Dis.* 1982;170:67-71.

48. Asfora WT, DeSalles AAF, Abe M, Kjellberg RN. Is the syndrome of pathological laughing and crying a manifestation of pseudobulbar palsy? *J Neurol Neurosurg Psychiatry.* 1989;52:523-525.

49. Lieberman A, Benson F. Control of emotional expression in pseudobulbar palsy: A personal experience. *Arch Neurol.* 1977;34:717-719.

50. Horner J, Massey EW, Riski JE, et al. Aspiration following stroke: Clinical correlates and outcome. *Neurology.* 1988;38:1359-1362.

51. Horner J, Massey EW, Brazer SR. Aspiration in bilateral stroke patients. *Neurology.* 1990;40:1686-1688.

52. Horner J, Brazer ST, Massey EW. Aspiration in bilateral stroke patients: A validation study. *Neurology.* 1993;43:430-433.

53. Daniels SK, Brailey K, Priestly DH, et al. Aspiration in patients with acute stroke. *Arch Phys Med Rehabil.* 1998;79:14-19.

54. Stanners AJ, Chapman AN, Bamford JM. Clinical predictors of aspiration soon after stroke. *Age Ageing.* 1993;22(Suppl 2):P17-P18.

55. Horner J, Massey EW. Silent aspiration following stroke. *Neurology.* 1988;38:317-319.

56. Lim SHB, Lieu PK, Phua SY, et al. Accuracy of bedside clinical methods compared with fiberoptic endoscopic examination of swallowing (FEES) in determining the risk of aspiration in acute stroke patients. *Dysphagia.* 2001;16:1-6.

57. McCullough GH, Wertz RT, Rosenbek JC. Sensitivity and specificity of clinica/bedside examination signs for detecting aspiration in adults subsequent to stroke. *J Commun Disorders.* 2001;34:55-72.

58. Smithard DG, O'Neill PA, England R, et al. Can bedside assessment reliably exclude aspiration following acute stroke? *Age Ageing.* 1998;27:99-106.

59. Nishiwaki K, Tsuji T, Liu M, et al. Identification of a simple screening tool for dysphagia in patients with stroke using factor analysis of multiple dysphagia variables. *J Rehabil Med.* 2005;37:247-251.

60. Horner J, Buoyer FG, Alberts MJ, Helms MJ. Dysphagia following brain-stem stroke: Clinical correlates and outcome. *Arch Neurol.* 1991;48:1170-1173.

61. Kidd K, Lawson J, Nesbitt R, MacMahon J. Aspiration in acute stroke: A clinical study with videofluoroscopy. *Q J Med.* 1993;86:825-829.

62. DePippo KL, Holas MA, Reding MJ. Validation of the 3-oz water swallow test for aspiration following stroke. *Arch Neurol.* 1992;49:1259-1261.

63. Collins MJ, Bakheit AMO. Does pulse oximetry reliably detect aspiration in dysphagic stroke patients? *Stroke.* 1997;28:1773-1775.

64. Smith HA, Lee SH, O'Neill PA, Connolly MJ. The combination of bedside swallowing assessment and oxygen saturation monitoring of swallowing in acute stroke: A safe and humane screening tool. *Age Ageing.* 2000;29:495-499.

65. Davies AE, Kidd K, Stone SP, MacMahon J. Pharyngeal sensation and gag reflex in healthy subjects. *Lancet.* 1995;345:487-488.

66. Leder SB. Gag reflex and dysphagia. *Head Neck.* 1996;18:138-140.

67. Manon-Espaillat R, Ruff RL. Dissociated weakness of sternocleidomastoid and trapezius muscles with lesions in the CNS. *Neurology.* 1988;38:796-797.

68. Mastaglia FL, Knezevic W, Thompson PD. Weakness of head turning in hemiplegia. *J Neurol Neurosurg Psychiatry.* 1986;49:195-197.

69. Berry H, MacDonald EA, Mrazek AC. Accessory nerve palsy: A review of 23 cases. *Can J Neurol Sci.* 1991;18:337-341.

70. Umapathi T, Venketasubramanian N, Leck KJ, et al. Tongue deviation in acute ischemic stroke: A study of supranuclear twelfth cranial nerve palsy in 30 stroke patients. *Cerebrovasc Dis.* 2000;10:462-465.

71. Keane JR. Twelfth-nerve palsy. *Arch Neurol.* 1996;53:561-566.

57

Examination of the Motor System: Approach to Weakness and Tremor

THE MOTOR EXAMINATION

Examination of the muscles includes inspection (for atrophy, hypertrophy, fasciculations, and tremor), percussion (for myotonia), palpation (for abnormal tone), full flexion and extension of the elbows and knees (to detect abnormal tone and nonneurologic restrictions to movement, such as contractures or joint disease), and tests of muscle strength.

I. MUSCLE STRENGTH

A. DEFINITIONS

Paralysis refers to loss of power of any degree, from mild weakness to complete loss. The suffixes **-plegia** and **-paresis** also indicate paralysis (e.g., "hemiplegia"), although "-paresis" is usually used to indicate incomplete paralysis. **Tetraparesis** indicates weakness of all four limbs (specialists in spinal cord disorders prefer this term over "quadriparesis"); **paraparesis**, weakness of both legs; **hemiparesis**, weakness of an arm and leg on one side of the body; and **monoparesis**, weakness of just one arm or leg.

B. THE FINDINGS

1. Technique

The clinician tests single muscles at a time by asking the patient to contract the muscle strongly while the clinician tries to resist any movement. Unilateral weakness is recognized by comparing the muscle to its companion on the opposite side; bilateral weakness, by comparing the strength to some standard recalled from clinical experience. The clinician grades the muscle's strength according to a 6-point system (0 through 5), as described later.

In patients with weakness, the clinician should systematically test all the muscles from head to foot, paying particular attention to which muscles are weak, whether proximal and distal muscles of a limb differ in strength, and whether the weakness of a monoparetic limb involves only muscles from a single spinal segment or peripheral nerve (see Chapter 60). An excellent, inexpensive handbook describes the proper technique for testing all of the important muscles of the arms and legs.[1]

Testing muscles by resisting their action, however, tends to overlook significant weakness at the hips and knees, where powerful antigravity muscles can easily overcome the physician's resistance even when significant weakness is present.[2] A better way to test these muscles is to use the patient's own body weight as the load the muscle must lift. For example, quadriceps weakness is more apparent by asking the patient to arise from a chair on the symptomatic leg than by manually resisting the patient's attempt to extend the knee.[3] Another method measures the time required by the patient to rise up from a chair and sit down 10 times. Patients without weakness accomplish this in 20 to 25 seconds (< 20 seconds if 50 years old and < 25 seconds if 75 years old). If patients require more time, proximal weakness of the legs is present unless an alternative explanation is present, such as joint or bone disease.[4]

2. Grading Muscle Strength

Muscle strength is graded using a conventional scale developed by the British Medical Research Council (MRC) during World War II (Table 57-1).[1] This scale, which is used universally, has one important drawback: it assigns a disproportionate

Table 57-1	Grading Muscle Strength

Grade	Finding
0	No contraction
1	Flicker or trace of contraction
2	Active movement with gravity eliminated
3	Active movement against gravity
4	Active movement against gravity and resistance
5	Normal power

From reference 1.

amount of a muscle's power to grade 4 strength. For example, the biceps muscle uses just 2% of its full power to overcome gravity (i.e., grade 3 strength), meaning almost 98% of the remaining range of power is grade 4.[5] Because of this drawback, many neurologists subdivide grade 4 into 3 more grades: "4 minus" (i.e., moves barely against resistance), "4," and "4 plus" (i.e., almost full power).

3. Special Tests for Unilateral Cerebral Lesions

In patients with cerebral lesions, measures of muscle power alone often underestimate the size of the lesion and the patient's functional disability. Three tests have been developed as more sensitive tests of motor function in these patients: upper limb drift ("pronator drift"), forearm rolling test,[6] and rapid finger tapping[7] (Fig. 57-1).

C. CLINICAL SIGNIFICANCE

See "Approach to Weakness" later.

II. ATROPHY AND HYPERTROPHY

A. ATROPHY

1. Definition

Atrophy describes muscles that are emaciated or wasted.

2. Technique

Atrophy is detected during inspection of the muscle. Examples are (1) a thenar eminence appearing abnormally flat when viewed from the side (e.g., cervical radiculopathy or carpal tunnel syndrome), (2) the anterior neck missing shadows because of atrophic sternocleidomastoid muscles (e.g., syringomyelia), or

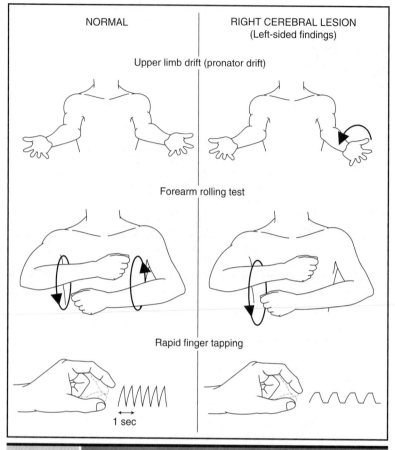

FIGURE 57-1 | SPECIAL TESTS FOR UNILATERAL CEREBRAL LESIONS.

The depicted patient has a right cerebral lesion with left-sided findings during three different tests: **(1) Upper limb drift ("pronator drift,"** *top row*). The patient stretches out both arms directly in front of him or her with palms upright (i.e., forearms supinated) and closes his or her eyes. This position is held for 45 seconds.[7] The arm contralateral to the hemispheric lesion drifts downward and pronates. **(2) Forearm rolling test (*middle row*).**[6] The patient bends each elbow and places both forearms parallel to each other. He or she then rotates the forearms about each other in a rapid rolling motion for 5 to 10 seconds in each direction. In the abnormal response, the forearm contralateral to the lesion is held still while the other arm "orbits" around it. **(3) Rapid finger tapping (*bottom row*).** The patient rapidly taps the thumb and index finger repeatedly at a speed of about two taps per second. In normal persons the movement has an even rhythm and large amplitude. Hemispheric lesions cause the contralateral finger and thumb to tap more slowly and with diminished amplitude, sometimes giving the appearance that the finger and thumb are sticking together.[7]

(3) metacarpal bones appearing unusually prominent on the back of the hand, from atrophic intrinsic muscles (e.g., polyneuropathy).

Significant asymmetry of the circumference of the arms or legs indicates atrophy of the smaller side (or edema of the other side). In normal persons, the difference in calf circumference between the right and left sides is less than 1 cm in 90% and less than 1.5 cm in 100% (measured 10 cm below the tibial tuberosity).[8] Measurements of thigh circumference correlate well with the muscle's cross-sectional area as measured by computed tomography ($r = 0.694$, $p < .01$).[9]

3. Clinical Significance

Atrophy is a feature of lower motor neuron disease* and muscle disuse (especially from adjacent joint disease or trauma).[12-14] In patients with sciatica, the finding of ipsilateral calf wasting (i.e., maximum circumference at least 1 cm less than contralateral side) accurately indicates lumbosacral nerve compression from disc herniation (likelihood ratio [LR] = 5.2, see Chapter 60).

B. HYPERTROPHY

Hypertrophy describes abnormal enlargement of a muscle. Bilateral calf hypertrophy is a typical feature of some muscular dystrophies, although it also is found in a wide variety of other neuromuscular diseases.[15]

III. FASCICULATIONS

A. DEFINITION

Fasciculations are involuntary rapid muscle twitches that are too weak to move a limb but are easily felt by patients and seen by clinicians. Most healthy people experience fasciculations at some time, especially in the muscles around their eyelids.

B. CLINICAL SIGNIFICANCE

Isolated fasciculations without other neurologic findings are benign.[16,17] When accompanied by weakness or atrophy, however, fasciculations indicate lower motor neuron disease, usually of the anterior horn cell or proximal peripheral nerve. Tongue fasciculations occur in up to one third of patients with amyotrophic lateral sclerosis (see "Approach to Weakness" later).[18]

---

*In the evaluation of weakness, a fundamental distinction is the separation of upper motor neuron lesions (i.e., located in the cerebral cortex, brainstem, or descending motor pathways of the spinal cord) from lower motor neuron lesions (i.e., located in the peripheral nerves and anterior horn cells of the spinal cord). William Gowers first distinguished the upper and lower motor segments in his 1888 *Manual of Diseases of the Nervous System*.[10,11] See Fig. 57-2 and "Approach to Weakness" later in this chapter.

IV. MUSCLE TONE

Muscle tone refers to involuntary muscle tension that clinicians perceive when repeatedly flexing and extending one of the patient's limbs. Assessing muscle tone assumes that the patient is relaxed and that any limitation is not due to bone or joint abnormalities. Muscle tone may be increased (e.g., spasticity, rigidity, or paratonia) or diminished (flaccidity).

A. INCREASED MUSCLE TONE

1. Spasticity

a. Definition

Spasticity is increased muscle tone that develops in patients with upper motor neuron lesions.[19-22] The increased muscle tone of spasticity has three characteristic features: (1) **Velocity-dependence.** The amount of muscle tone depends on the velocity of movement. There is more resistance with rapid movements and less resistance with slow ones. (2) **Flexor and extensor tone differ.** The tone in the flexors and extensors of a limb is not balanced, which commonly causes characteristic resting postures of that limb (see later). (3) **Associated weakness.** The muscle with spasticity is also weak. In addition, muscles shortened by spasticity eventually develop fixed contractures, unless the spasticity is treated.

b. Characteristic Postures

In spasticity, an imbalance in flexor and extensor tone commonly causes abnormal postures of the resting limb. In hemiplegia, for example, there is excess tone in the *flexors* of the arms and *extensors* of the legs, which causes the arm and hand to be fixed against the chest, flexed and internally rotated, and the leg to extend with the foot pointed (see Fig. 5-4 in Chapter 5).[23] In contrast, some patients with complete spinal cord lesions have excess tone in the *flexors* of the legs, which causes the legs to flex up on to the abdomen ("paraplegia-in-flexion").*[24]

---

*These hemiplegic and paraplegic postures recall the neurologic development of normal infants. Paraplegia-in-flexion resembles the initial posture of babies, their legs flexed against their chest. The infant eventually is able to extend the leg and stand (resembling extensor tone of hemiplegia), after descending pathways from the brain stem mature enough to overcome the spinal reflexes responsible for the flexed position. The infant eventually walks after cerebral connections mature enough to provide fine motor control. Damage to the cerebral hemispheres (e.g., stroke) disrupts this fine motor control and uncovers the extensor posture; damage to the spinal cord (e.g., severe multiple sclerosis or complete spinal cord transection) removes all supraspinal input, uncovering the original flexed posture of the legs.[20]

c. Clasp-Knife Phenomenon

Up to half of patients with spasticity have the "clasp-knife phenomenon," which is usually observed in the extensors of the knee, less often in the elbow flexors.[21,23] To elicit this phenomenon, the clinician extends the patient's knee using a constant velocity, but as the patient's knee nears full extension, the muscle tone of the quadriceps muscles increases dramatically and completes the movement, just as the blade of a pocket knife opens under the influence of its spring.[11] The clasp-knife phenomenon occurs because muscle tone is dependent on the muscle's length, the tone diminishing with stretching and increasing with shortening.

d. Relationship of Spasticity to Weakness

Although spasticity is a sign of upper motor neuron disease, its severity correlates poorly with the degree of weakness or hyperreflexia.[25,26] Patients with slowly developing cerebral hemisphere lesions usually develop spasticity and weakness in concert.[27] Patients with strokes or spinal cord injury, in contrast, develop immediate weakness and flaccidity, spasticity appearing only days to weeks later.[23] Some elderly patients with large strokes have persistent "flaccid hemiplegia," in which the paralyzed muscles never develop increased muscle tone despite being hyperreflexic.[27]

2. Rigidity
a. Definition

Rigidity is increased muscle tension that has three characteristic features: (**1**) **No velocity-dependence.** The resistance to movement is the same with slow and rapid movements. (**2**) **Flexor and extensor tone are the same.** (**3**) **No associated weakness.** Patients with rigidity lack the clasp-knife phenomenon.[20] "Cogwheel rigidity" refers to rigidity that gives way intermittently as if the patient's limb were the lever pulling over a ratchet.

b. Distinguishing Spasticity from Rigidity

Most clinicians distinguish spasticity from rigidity by repeatedly extending and flexing the patient's limbs and observing the characteristics noted above. In the 1950s, Wartenberg introduced a simple bedside test to assess motor tone and to distinguish spasticity from rigidity.*[28,29] In this test, the patient is seated on the edge of the examining table, which is open underneath

---

*Robert Wartenberg, who wrote many popular neurology textbooks in the 1950s, was an ardent opponent of eponyms and called his test the "test for pendulousness of the legs."

to allow the legs to swing unobstructed back and forth. The clinician lifts both feet to extend the knees, instructs the patient to relax, and then releases the legs. The normal lower limb swings back and forth six or seven times, smoothly and regularly in a perfect sagittal plane. In patients with spasticity, the limbs drop with normal velocity, but their movements are jerky and fall out of the sagittal plane, the great toe tracing zigzags or ellipses. In patients with rigidity, the swinging time and velocity are significantly reduced, resulting in a total of only one or two swings. Others have confirmed Wartenberg's findings.[28,30-34]

c. Clinical Significance

Rigidity is a common finding of extrapyramidal disease, the most common example of which is Parkinson's disease (see "Approach to Tremor" later).

3. Paratonia
a. Definition

Paratonia is excess muscle tension that is *not present at rest* but develops when the patient's limb *contacts* another object, as if such contact makes the patient unable to relax. There are two forms: oppositional paratonia ("**gegenhalten**") and facilitatory paratonia ("**mitgehen**"). In patients with oppositional paratonia, the clinician feels a stiffening of the limb with every applied movement, but unlike rigidity the stiffening depends entirely on contact and its force is proportional and opposite to the examiner's. Patients with facilitatory paratonia, in contrast, actively aid movements guided by the examiner.

b. Technique

One simple test of facilitatory paratonia is to take the arm of the seated patient and bend the elbow back and forth three times, from full flexion to 90 degrees extension. The clinician then releases the arm at the patient's lap and scores any further movement, 0 being no movement, 4 full flexion or more, and 1 to 3 intermediate movements.[35]

c. Clinical Significance

Both oppositional and facilitatory paratonia are associated with extensive frontal lobe disease and often appear in dementing illnesses.[35-39] Among patients with dementia, the severity of oppositional or facilitatory paratonia (including the score for the paratonia test described in Section b above) correlates inversely with the Folstein Mini-Mental Status Exam score ($r = -0.5$ to -0.7, $p < .05$).[35]

B. DECREASED MUSCLE TONE: HYPOTONIA ("FLACCIDITY")

1. Definition

Hypotonia refers to reduced or absent muscle tension.

2. Technique

There are many ways to detect the flaccid muscle: the limb feels like a "rag doll," the muscles feel soft and flabby, the outstretched arm when tapped demonstrates wider than normal excursions, or the knee jerks are abnormally pendular. The original definition of abnormally pendular knee jerks—more than three back-and-forth swings of the patient's leg during testing of the knee jerk—has to be revised, because many normal individuals have this finding.[40]

3. Clinical Significance

Hypotonia is a feature of lower motor neuron disease and cerebellar disease.

4. Pathogenesis

There is some evidence that "normal" muscle tone actually consists of tiny muscle contractions that assist the clinician in moving the extremity (even though the patient is trying to relax).[41] Clinicians perceive reduced muscle tension in hypotonic limbs because these contractions are absent.

V. MUSCLE PERCUSSION

Striking the muscle with a reflex hammer may elicit two abnormal findings, percussion myotonia and myoedema.

A. PERCUSSION MYOTONIA

1. The Finding

Percussion myotonia is a prolonged muscle contraction that lasts several seconds and causes a sustained dimple to appear on the skin. Percussion myotonia of the thenar eminence may actually draw the thumb into sustained opposition with the fingers.

2. Clinical Significance

Percussion myotonia is a feature of some myotonic syndromes, such as myotonia congenita and myotonic dystrophy.[42]

B. MYOEDEMA

1. The Finding

Myoedema is a focal mounding of muscle lasting seconds at the point of percussion. Unlike myotonia, myoedema causes a lump instead of a dimple, and the lump may be oriented crosswise or diagonal to the direction of muscle fibers.

Graves and Stokes originally described myoedema in 1830.

2. Clinical Significance

Myoedema is a normal physiologic response and does not indicate disease.[43] Its historical association with undernourished patients simply reflects the ease with which the response appears when there is no intervening subcutaneous fat.[43-45]

APPROACH TO WEAKNESS

I. CAUSE OF WEAKNESS

Neuromuscular weakness has four principal causes: (1) upper motor neuron disease ("pyramidal tract disease" or "central weakness"), (2) lower motor neuron disease ("denervation disease" or "peripheral weakness"), (3) neuromuscular junction disorders, and (4) muscle disease. Each disorder is associated with distinct physical signs (Table 57-2), neuroanatomy (Fig. 57-2), and etiologies (Table 57-3).

Most patients with weakness have disorders of the upper or lower motor neuron lesions. Clinicians should consider muscle disease in any patient with *symmetric* weakness of the *proximal* muscles of the arms and legs (sometimes associated with muscle pain, dysphagia, and weakness of the neck muscles). Disorders of the neuromuscular junction should be considered in patients whose weakness *varies* during the day or who have *ptosis* or *diplopia*. Associated abnormalities of sensation, tone, or reflexes of the weak limb exclude muscle or neuromuscular junction disease and argue for upper or lower motor neuron lesions.

II. THE FINDINGS

A. UPPER VERSUS LOWER MOTOR NEURON LESIONS

Both upper motor neuron weakness and lower motor neuron weakness tend to affect *distal* muscles in either a symmetric or asymmetric pattern.[46-48] The bedside findings that distinguish these two disorders are other neurologic findings in the weak limb, certain localizing signs of upper motor neuron disease, the Babinski sign, and the type of weakness produced.

Table 57-2 Differential Diagnosis of Weakness*

Location of Lesion	Motor Examination		Sensory Changes	Muscle Stretch Reflexes	Other Findings
	Muscle Tone	Atrophy or Fasciculations?			
Upper motor neuron	Spasticity	No	Sometimes	Increased	Babinski sign
Lower motor neuron	Hypotonia	Yes	Usually†	Decreased/absent	
Neuromuscular junction	Normal or hypotonia	No	No	Normal/decreased	Ptosis, diplopia
Muscle	Normal	No‡	No	Normal/decreased	Myotonia

*These characteristics are specific but not sensitive, and thus are helpful when present, not when absent. See section III.A.
†Sensory findings are in distribution of spinal segment, plexus, or peripheral nerve. See Chapter 60.
‡Atrophy may be a late finding.

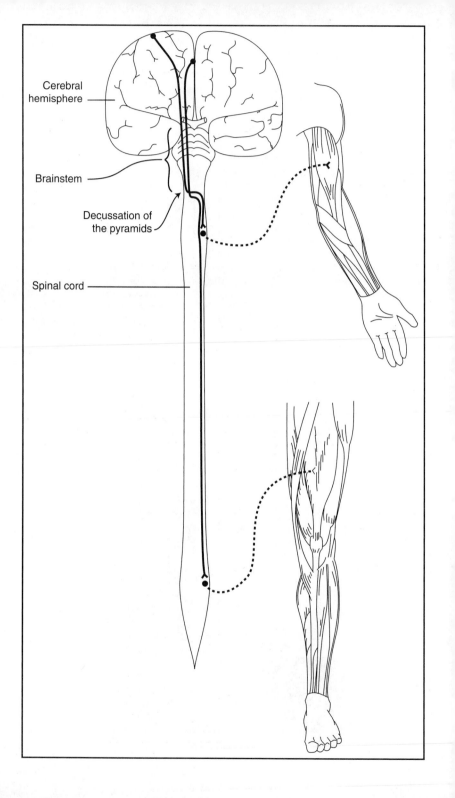

Cerebral hemisphere

Brainstem

Decussation of the pyramids

Spinal cord

Table 57-3	Common Etiologies of Neuromuscular Weakness

Location of Lesion	Common Etiology
Upper motor neuron	Cerebrovascular disease
	Multiple sclerosis
	Brain tumor
Lower motor neuron	Polyneuropathy (diabetes, alcoholism)
	Entrapment neuropathy
	Trauma
Neuromuscular junction	Myasthenia gravis
Muscle	Drug-induced myopathy
	Thyroid disease
	Polymyositis

1. Associated Findings in the Weak Limb (See Table 57-2)

Spasticity and hyperreflexia indicate central weakness; hypotonia, atrophy, fasciculations, and absent muscle stretch reflexes indicate peripheral weakness. In patients with central weakness, sensory abnormalities vary from the isolated loss of cortical sensations in the distal limb to dense loss of all sensation throughout the limb; if sensory abnormalities occur in peripheral weakness, they follow the distribution of spinal segments or peripheral nerves (see Chapter 60).

FIGURE 57-2	ANATOMY OF UPPER MOTOR AND LOWER MOTOR NEURONS.

The figure illustrates the entire pathway of nerves responsible for movement, from cerebral cortex to muscle. *Upper motor neurons (solid line)* extend from the cerebral cortex through the brainstem to the spinal cord. *Lower motor neurons (dotted line)* originate in the spinal cord and travel to muscles within peripheral nerves. Because the upper motor neurons cross to the contralateral side at the border between the brainstem and spinal cord ("decussation of the pyramids"), weakness of the upper motor neuron type may result from lesions in the *ipsilateral* spinal cord, *contralateral* brain stem, or *contralateral* cerebral hemisphere. Lesions of the spinal cord, where both upper and lower motor neurons reside, may cause weakness of both types: of the *lower motor neuron* type *at* the level of the lesion and of the *upper motor neuron* type in muscles whose peripheral nerves originate *below* the level of the lesion.

Table 57-4	Localizing Signs in Upper Motor Neuron Weakness

Anatomic Location	Associated Finding
Cerebral hemisphere	Seizures
	Hemianopia
	Aphasia (right hemiparesis)
	Inattention to left body, apraxia (left hemiparesis)
	Cortical sensory loss*
	Hyperactive jaw jerk
Brainstem	Crossed motor findings[†]
	Contralateral third nerve palsy (midbrain)
	Contralateral sixth nerve palsy (pons)
	Sensory loss on contralateral face*
Spinal cord	Sensory level*
	Pain and temperature sensory loss on contralateral arm and leg*
	No sensory or motor findings in face
	Additional lower motor neuron findings (atrophy, fasciculations)

*Chapter 58 describes the different sensory syndromes.
[†]Crossed motor findings refers to unilateral cranial nerve palsy opposite the side of limb weakness.

2.   Localizing Signs of Upper Motor Neuron Weakness

The upper motor neuron pathway extends from the cerebral cortex down through the spinal cord (see Fig. 57-2), traveling in tight quarters with central neurons innervating other structures. Consequently, in addition to producing central weakness, lesions along this pathway cause characteristic additional physical signs (Table 57-4) that confirm the weakness is of the central type and pinpoint its location.

3.   Babinski Sign

The Babinski sign (see Chapter 59) indicates central weakness. In the positive response, the great toe moves upward after a scratching stimulus to the sole of the patient's foot.

4.   Distribution of Weakness
a.   Limbs Affected

The findings of monoparesis, paraparesis, and tetraparesis are, by themselves, unhelpful because they may occur in either central or peripheral weakness. Only hemiparesis is specific, indicating a central lesion.

b. Movement Versus Muscle

Central lesions paralyze *movements*; peripheral lesions paralyze *muscles*. This occurs because neurons from a single area of the cerebral cortex connect to many different spinal cord segments and muscles to accomplish a particular movement. A single muscle has many movements and thus receives information from many different upper segments, all of which converge on the single peripheral nerve traveling to the muscle. A lesion in that nerve, therefore, obliterates a muscle's entire repertoire of movement; a lesion in an upper segment eliminates only one of many possible movements.[29]

One example of this is the contrast between peripheral facial weakness (Bell's palsy), which paralyzes all ipsilateral facial movements, and central facial weakness (e.g., strokes), which paralyzes voluntary movements but spares emotional ones (e.g., during laughing or crying; see Chapter 56).[49] Another example is the contrast between the peripheral paraparesis of Guillain-Barré syndrome, which paralyzes all leg movements, and the central paraparesis of spinal cord injury, which eliminates volitional movements of the legs but allows the powerful flexor spasms induced by a mild scratching of the patient's foot.[24]

B. THE DIAGNOSTIC PROCESS

1. Upper Motor Neuron Weakness

In patients with upper motor neuron weakness, associated neurologic findings indicate the *level* of the lesion (see Table 57-4); the distribution of weakness indicates the *side* of the lesion. For example, bilateral weakness (paraparesis or tetraparesis) indicates *bilateral* lesions (in the thoracic cord or higher if paraparesis, and in the cervical cord or higher if tetraparesis). Monoparesis or hemiparesis indicates a *unilateral* lesion, either in the *contralateral* cerebral hemisphere or brainstem or the *ipsilateral* spinal cord.*

Table 57-5 illustrates this diagnostic process in the analysis of central weakness. In the first column is the distribution of central weakness for hypothetical patients, which narrows the diagnostic possibilities to a smaller region of the central motor pathway (second column). The associated findings (third column) identify the level of the lesion within that region, thus pinpointing the lesion's location (fourth column).

2. Lower Motor Neuron Weakness

In patients with monoparesis of the lower motor neuron type, the clinician should determine whether the muscles affected are supplied by a single spinal

---

*It is the contralateral cerebral hemisphere and brainstem because the descending central motor pathways originate in the contralateral hemisphere, but it is the ipsilateral spinal cord because these pathways cross just below the brain stem (Fig. 57-2).

Table 57-5   Diagnostic Approach to Upper Motor Neuron Weakness

Distribution of Weakness	STEP ONE Diagnostic Possibilities	STEP TWO Additional Finding	STEP TWO Location of Lesion
Left monoparesis	Right cerebral hemisphere Right brainstem Left spinal cord	New seizures	Right cerebral hemisphere
Right hemiparesis	Left cerebral hemisphere Left brainstem Right spinal cord	Aphasia	Left cerebral hemisphere
		Right homonymous hemianopia	Left cerebral hemisphere
		Left sixth nerve palsy	Left brainstem
		Loss of sensation left arm and leg; face spared	Right spinal cord
Paraparesis	Bilateral lesion of thoracic cord or above	Sensory level at midchest; normal arm strength and reflexes; spine tenderness between scapulae	Bilateral lesion, thoracic cord
Tetraparesis	Bilateral lesion of cervical cord or above	Hyperactive jaw jerk; Dementia	Bilateral lesion, cerebral hemispheres
		Sensory level upper chest; absent biceps reflexes but hyperactive triceps reflexes	Bilateral lesion, cervical cord

segment (radiculopathy), peripheral nerve (peripheral neuropathy), or combination of the two (plexopathy). Further evaluation of these patients is discussed in Chapter 60.

In lower motor neuron weakness, the lesion is always *ipsilateral* to the side of the weakness.

3. Combined Upper and Lower Motor Neuron Weakness

Combined upper and lower motor neuron findings indicate disease in the spinal cord, the only anatomic location where both segments reside. Common causes are myelopathy and amyotrophic lateral sclerosis.

a. Myelopathy

Myelopathy is a term describing a spinal cord lesion confined to a discrete level (e.g., trauma, tumor, disc disease). The lesion causes motor, sensory, and reflex abnormalities *at* the level of the lesion and *below* it. The weakness is of the peripheral type *at* the level of the lesion (from damage to anterior horn cells and spinal roots),* and of the central type *below* the level of the lesion (from damage to the descending upper motor neuron paths).

---

*Exceptions to this are lesions at the foramen magnum and C3-4 level, which sometimes produce atrophy in the hands.[50]

Table 57-6	Segmental Innervation of Muscles*

Spinal Level	Muscles
Arm	
C5	Elbow flexors (biceps, brachialis)
C6	Wrist extensors (extensor carpi radialis longus and brevis)
C7	Elbow extensors (triceps)
C8	Finger flexors (flexor digitorum profundus of middle finger)
T1	Small finger abductors (abductor digiti minimi)
Leg	
L2	Hip flexors (iliopsoas)
L3	Knee extensors (quadriceps)
L4	Ankle dorsiflexors (tibialis anterior)
L5	Long toe extensors (extensor hallucis longus)
S1	Ankle plantarflexors (gastrocnemius, soleus)

Most muscles are innervated by nerves from more than one spinal root. This table, based on reference 51, simplifies this innervation to standardize the description of spinal cord injury. A more thorough description of segmental innervation of muscle appears in Tables 60-1 and 60-3 of Chapter 60.

Identifying the level of the lesion requires knowledge of which spinal segments innervate which muscle. Table 57-6 presents the standardized segmental innervation used internationally by spinal cord specialists (Chapter 60 discusses the derivation of this table). For example, in a patient with a lesion involving the C7 segment of the spinal cord, there is peripheral weakness in the C7 muscles (i.e., atrophy and weakness of the elbow extensors) but central weakness of all the muscles below this level (hyperreflexia and increased tone of the hands, legs, and feet, and a positive Babinski sign). The muscles from segments above C7, the biceps and wrist extensors, are normal.*

b. Amyotrophic Lateral Sclerosis

Amyotrophic lateral sclerosis is a degenerative disorder of descending motor tracts and motor nuclei of the spinal cord. The disorder causes both lower motor neuron findings (atrophy, fasciculations) and upper motor neuron findings (hyperreflexia). About half of patients have a Babinski response.[18] The disease may start in the arms (44%), legs (37%), or bulbar muscles (causing tongue fasciculations, change in voice, and difficulty swallowing, 19%).[18] There are no sensory findings.

Amyotrophic and cervical myelopathy are commonly confused at the bedside, even by experienced neurologists.[52] In patients with both upper and lower motor neuron signs, findings that argue in favor of amyotrophic lateral sclerosis are (1) prominent fasciculations, (2) absence of sensory findings, and (3) signs of lower motor neuron degeneration affecting more than one level of the spinal cord simultaneously†[53,54]

III. CLINICAL SIGNIFICANCE

The clinical significance of the motor examination cannot be tested in the conventional manner of this book, because bedside criteria alone are sufficient to diagnose many causes of weakness (e.g., cerebrovascular disease, amyotrophic lateral sclerosis, and peripheral nerve injuries are routinely diagnosed by bedside criteria).

Nonetheless, several investigations allow a few conclusions.

---

*By convention, the neurologic level in spinal cord injury refers to the most caudal level with *normal* function, rather than the first level with abnormal function.[51] The motor level for this hypothetical patient is C6.
†The four spinal cord "levels" are bulbar (jaw, face, tongue, larynx), cervical (neck, arm, hand, diaphragm), thoracic (back, abdomen), and lumbosacral (back, abdomen, leg, and foot).

A. CLINICAL SYNDROMES ARE OFTEN INCOMPLETE

Most studies show that the full lower motor or upper motor neuron syndromes, as depicted in Table 57-2, are often incomplete. In upper motor neuron weakness, up to 25% of patients lack exaggerated reflexes[47,55] and the absence of spasticity is common, especially in acute lesions (see previous). Similarly, in many examples of lower motor weakness, the nerve affected does not even innervate a clinical reflex (e.g., L5 radiculopathy, median or ulnar neuropathy), and therefore, the reflexes of the limbs are normal. Therefore, in the evaluation of weak patients, the *absence* of spasticity or hyperreflexia does *not* argue against the presence of upper motor neuron disease, nor does the *absence* of hypotonicity or hyporeflexia argue against the presence lower motor neuron disease.

On the other hand, the *presence* of abnormal reflexes is very helpful: In one study of patients with weakness, 87% had abnormal reflexes and in every case, areflexia correctly predicted lower motor neuron disease and hyperreflexia correctly predicted upper motor neuron disease.[47]

The fact that syndromes are often incomplete emphasizes the importance of the complete neurologic examination. For example, in a patient with weakness of the fingertips, in whom the absence of sensory or reflex changes prevents classifying the weakness as peripheral or central using the criteria of Table 57-2, the discovery of any additional neurologic finding from Table 57-4 indicates the lesion is central and pinpoints its location precisely.

B. PROXIMAL WEAKNESS INDICATES MUSCLE DISEASE

If "proximal weakness" is defined as strength of a limb's proximal muscles being one MRC grade less than the distal muscles, proximal weakness is seen in 92% of patients with muscle disease.[47] This means that the *absence* of proximal weakness is a strong argument against muscle disease.

C. FOR CEREBRAL HEMISPHERIC LESIONS, THE SPECIAL TESTS ARE VERY SENSITIVE

EBM Box 57-1 presents the diagnostic accuracy of various physical signs for detecting unilateral cerebral hemispheric lesions in patients undergoing computed tomography or magnetic resonance imaging of the head. In these patients, the most compelling arguments for disease in the *contralateral* cerebral hemisphere are a positive arm rolling test (LR = 21.7), Babinski response (LR = 19.0), pronator drift (LR = 10.3), positive finger tapping test (LR = 6.6), and hyperreflexia (LR = 5.8). The *absence* of pronator drift (LR = 0.1) and *negative* finger-tapping test (LR = 0.3) diminish significantly the probability of contralateral cerebral disease.

Some of the LRs on this table are spectacular compared with many of those in the general medicine section of this book, simply because, in the field of neurology,

Box 57-1 Unilateral Cerebral Hemispheric Disease*

Finding (Ref)[†]	Sensitivity (%)	Specificity (%)	Likelihood Ratio if Finding	
			Present	Absent
Arm rolling test[6,7]	45–87	98	**21.7**	NS
Pronator drift[6,7]	79–92	90–98	**10.3**	**0.1**
Finger tapping test[6,7]	73–79	88–93	**6.6**	**0.3**
Babinski response[6]	45	98	**19.0**	0.6
Hyperreflexia[7]	69	88	**5.8**	0.4
Hemianopia[6]	30	98	NS	0.7
Hemisensory disturbance[6]	29	98	NS	0.7

NS, not significant; likelihood ratio (LR) if finding present = positive LR; LR if finding absent = negative LR.

*Diagnostic standard: For unilateral cerebral hemispheric disease, magnetic resonance imaging or computed tomography.

[†]Definition of findings: For arm rolling test, pronator drift, and finger tapping test, see Fig. 57-1; and for hyperreflexia, reflex assessed to be 2 or more grades hyperreflexic than same reflex on opposite side (using the 0 to 4 scale, see Table 59-2 in Chapter 59).

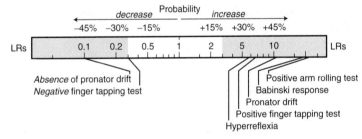

UNILATERAL CEREBRAL HEMISPHERIC DISEASE

the clinical signs still largely define the clinical problem. A cerebral lesion on imaging is "significant" (and therefore is called "disease") because it causes hemiparesis or some other neurologic sign. In contrast, we cannot say this about many signs from general medicine (e.g., aortic stenosis is not significant because it causes a heart murmur, but instead because it overloads the left ventricle and causes cardiac symptoms and death).

D. DIAGNOSIS OF PERIPHERAL NERVE DISORDERS

Chapter 60 discusses the clinical significance of muscle weakness and its localizing value to the diagnosis of peripheral nerve disorders.

TREMOR AND PARKINSON'S DISEASE

I. INTRODUCTION

In a remarkably concise essay written almost 200 years ago, the British physician James Parkinson described in nine pages most of the features we now associate with Parkinson's disease—insidious onset, asymmetric resting tremor, bradykinesia, postural instability, sialorrhea, flexed posture, shuffling steps, and festinating gait.[56] One sign Parkinson failed to describe was rigidity, which has led many historians to suggest that Parkinson based his conclusions solely on observation and never actually physically examined a patient.[57] In 1877, Charcot provided the first full account of Parkinson's disease that included rigidity.[57]

II. THE FINDING

The three cardinal findings in Parkinson's disease are resting tremor, bradykinesia, and cogwheel rigidity (rigidity is discussed previously in Section IV.A.2).

A. TREMOR

A tremor is a rhythmic involuntary oscillation of a body part. There are only two basic types: (1) **resting tremor** and (2) **action tremor.**[58,59] Resting tremors occur when muscles are inactive and the body part is completed supported against gravity. Action tremors occur during voluntary contraction of muscle and are further subdivided into *postural tremors* (e.g., when holding the arms outstretched), *intention tremors* (e.g., when a limb approaches a visually guided target such as finger-nose-finger testing), *task-related tremors* (e.g., when pouring water from cup to cup), and *isometric tremors* (e.g., when making a fist or gripping the examiner's fingers).* One confusing tremor is a postural tremor (i.e., action tremor) that continues after the examiner supports the outstretched arms (thus mimicking a resting tremor): If such patients are given a glass of water to drink, the

---

Intention tremor and *task-related tremor* are sometimes collectively referred to as *kinetic tremors,* that is, action tremors appearing during movement.

amplitude of true postural tremor increases or remains the same as the glass approaches the patient's mouth, whereas that of the genuine resting tremor diminishes in amplitude.

Movement disorder specialists have identified at least a dozen different types of tremor. The most common are essential tremor and Parkinsonian resting tremor.[58,59] Essential tremor is a 4- to 12-Hz* bilateral postural tremor that usually involves the hands or forearms. It may be asymmetric, and it may have an additional kinetic component (i.e., associated intention or task-related component). In contrast, the Parkinsonian resting tremor (which is only one of the different tremors that may appear in Parkinson's disease) is a 4- to 6-Hz "pill-rolling" tremor of the fingertips, hand, or forearm. It begins *asymmetrically*, initially in one hand, followed years later by involvement of the contralateral hand. Essential tremor may involve the jaw, tongue, or head (producing a characteristic rhythmic "nodding yes" or "shaking no" motion); the Parkinsonian tremor may involve jaw, lips, or tongue, but it spares the head.

B. BRADYKINESIA

Patients with bradykinesia have a reduced blink rate. Normal persons blink about 24 ± 15 times per minute, whereas patients with Parkinson's disease blink more slowly, about 12 ± 10 times per minute. Severely symptomatic patients blink only 5 to 6 times per minute.[60,61] The contrast between the reduced spontaneous blink rate but exaggerated reflex blink rate (during glabellar reflex testing, see Chapter 59) is striking in Parkinson's disease. During treatment with levodopa, the spontaneous blink rate increases as the reflex rate during glabellar testing diminishes.[62,63]

C. ATYPICAL FEATURES OF PARKINSON'S DISEASE

Confirming the diagnosis of Parkinson's disease during life is difficult because the disorder still lacks biochemical, genetic, or imaging diagnostic standards. In patients diagnosed during life with Parkinson's disease, 10% to 25% are discovered to have an alternative diagnosis at postmortem examination.[64-67] Many patients found to have an alternative diagnosis have one of a variety of neurodegenerative disorders collectively referred to as "Parkinson-plus" syndromes, which tend to progress more rapidly, present more symmetrically, and respond less well to levodopa than does Parkinson's disease.[68] Several clinical clues, called

---

*Hz indicates hertz, a unit of frequency equal to 1 cycle per second. A Parkinsonian tremor of 5 Hz, therefore, has 300 oscillations per minute (i.e., 5 × 60), which is why this tremor sometimes produces electrocardiographic artifacts that mimic tachyarrhythmias (e.g., atrial flutter or ventricular tachycardia).

Box 57-2 Suspected Parkinson's Disease*

Finding (Ref)[†]	Sensitivity (%)	Specificity (%)	Likelihood Ratio if Finding Present	Likelihood Ratio if Finding Absent
DIAGNOSING PARKINSON'S DISEASE				
Prominent rigidity on initial examination[69]	30	43	0.5	1.6
Tremor[69]	76	39	NS	NS
Tremor-dominant disease[64]	14	96	NS	NS
Signs are asymmetric[69]	55	66	NS	0.7
Bradykinesia [69]	90	3	NS	NS
Tremor, bradykinesia, rigidity[64]				
2 of 3 present	99	8	NS	NS
3 of 3 present	64	71	2.2	0.5
3 of 3 present, asymmetry, no atypical features	68	83	**4.1**	0.4
Good response to levodopa[69]	77	58	1.8	0.4
DIAGNOSING MULTIPLE SYSTEM ATROPHY				
Rapid progression[69,70]	54–64	78	2.5	0.6
Absence of tremor[69–71]	39–91	39–76	NS	NS
Speech and/or bulbar signs[69]	87	79	**4.1**	**0.2**
Autonomic dysfunction[69–71]	73–84	74–90	**4.3**	**0.3**
Cerebellar signs[69,71]	32–44	90–99	**9.5**	0.7
Pyramidal tract signs[69,71]	31–50	85–93	**4.0**	NS
Dementia[69,71]	17–25	36–45	**0.3**	1.9
DIAGNOSING PROGRESSIVE SUPRANUCLEAR PALSY				
Downgaze palsy AND postural instability within first year of symptoms[72]	50	99	**60.0**	0.5

NS, not significant; likelihood ratio (LR) if finding present = positive LR; LR if finding absent = negative LR.

*Diagnostic standard: For Parkinson's disease, careful clinical observation[73,74] or postmortem examination of brain revealing depletion of nigral pigmented neurons with Lewy bodies in remaining nerve cells (all other studies).

†Definition of findings: For atypical features, see text; for rapid progression, the appearance of unsteadiness and tendency to fall (i.e., Hoehn and Yahr score ≥3[75]) at initial visit[69] or within 3 years of onset of first symptom[70]; for speech or bulbar findings, dysarthria, dysphagia, and excessive sialorrhoea[69]; for autonomic dysfunction, symptomatic postural hypotension, urinary urge or fecal incontinence, or neurogenic bladder[69] or abnormalities on formal testing of cardiovascular reflexes[70]; for cerebellar findings, limb ataxia, intention tremor, gait ataxia, or nystagmus[69]; and for pyramidal tract findings, extensor plantar responses and hyperreflexia.[69] All LRs apply only to patients with suspected Parkinson's disease (i.e., some combination of tremor, bradykinesia, and rigidity).

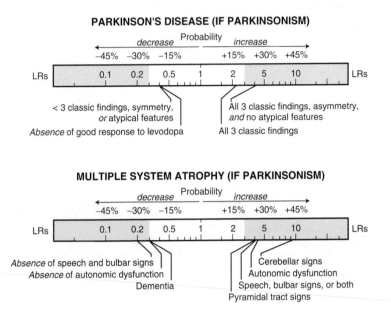

PARKINSON'S DISEASE (IF PARKINSONISM)

< 3 classic findings, symmetry, or atypical features
Absence of good response to levodopa

All 3 classic findings, asymmetry, *and* no atypical features
All 3 classic findings

MULTIPLE SYSTEM ATROPHY (IF PARKINSONISM)

Absence of speech and bulbar signs
Absence of autonomic dysfunction
Dementia

Cerebellar signs
Autonomic dysfunction
Speech, bulbar signs, or both
Pyramidal tract signs

"atypical features," suggest a diagnosis other than Parkinson's disease: (1) marked autonomic dysfunction (e.g., postural hypotension, neurogenic bladder or bowel), (2) early severe dementia, (3) pyramidal tract findings (i.e., upper motor neuron signs, see Table 57-2), (4) cerebellar findings, (5) supranuclear gaze palsy (i.e., difficulty looking down), (6) use of neuroleptic medications, (7) multiple prior strokes, and (7) encephalitis at the time of onset of symptoms.[64]

The two most common Parkinson-plus syndromes are multiple system atrophy* and progressive supranuclear palsy.

III. CLINICAL SIGNIFICANCE: DIAGNOSING PARKINSON'S DISEASE

In patients with combinations of tremor, bradykinesia, and rigidity, the most compelling additional argument that the patient has pathologic Parkinson's disease is the presence of all three of the following features (LR = 4.1, EBM Box

---

*Multiple system atrophy has three phenotypes: *Shy-Drager syndrome* (early autonomic insufficiency is prominent), *olivopontocerebellar atrophy* (cerebellar signs are prominent), and *striato-nigral degeneration* (both cerebellar and pyramidal tract signs are prominent).

57-2): (1) all three cardinal findings are present, (2) asymmetric onset, *and* (3) absence of atypical features (as defined previously). Three additional findings from the patient interview also support the diagnosis of Parkinson's disease: the complaint of feet suddenly freezing in doorways (LR = 4.4), the voice progressively becoming softer (LR = 3.2), or the handwriting becoming progressively smaller (i.e., micrographia, LR = 2.7).[73,74]

Multiple system atrophy is more likely if patients have cerebellar signs (LR = 9.5, see EBM Box 57-2), autonomic dysfunction (LR = 4.3), speech or bulbar signs (LR = 4.1), or pyramidal tract signs (LR = 4.0). Prominent dementia argues against the diagnosis of multiple system atrophy (LR = 0.3), as does the *absence* of autonomic dysfunction (LR = 0.3) and *absence* of speech and bulbar signs (LR = 0.2). Finally, the combination of a downgaze palsy and early postural instability from axial rigidity is pathognomic for the pathologic diagnosis of progressive supranuclear palsy (LR = 60).

REFERENCES

1. Medical Research Council. *Aids to the examination of the peripheral nervous system.* London: Bailliere Tindall; 1986.
2. Beasley WC. Quantitative muscle testing: Principles and applications to research and clinical services. *Arch Phys Med Rehabil.* 1961;42:398-425.
3. Rainville J, Jouve C, Finno M, Limke J. Comparison of four tests of quadriceps strength in L3 or L4 radiculopathies. *Spine.* 2003;28:2466-2471.
4. Csuka M, McCarty DJ. Simple method for measurement of lower extremity muscle strength. *Am J Med.* 1985;78:77-81.
5. van der Ploeg RJO, Oosterhuis HJGH, Reuvekamp J. Measuring muscle strength. *J Neurol.* 1984;231:200-203.
6. Sawyer RN, Hanna JP, Ruff RL, Leigh RJ. Asymmetry of forearm rolling as a sign of unilateral cerebral dysfunction. *Neurology.* 1993;43:1596-1598.
7. Teitelbaum JS, Eliasziw M, Garner M. Tests of motor function in patients suspected of having mild unilateral cerebral lesions. *Can J Neurol Sci.* 2002;29:337-344.
8. Stein PD, Henry JW, Gopalakrishnan D, Relyea B. Asymmetry of calves in the assessment of patients with suspected acute pulmonary embolism. *Chest.* 1995;107: 936-939.
9. Lorentzon R, Lars-Gunnar E, Sjostrom M, et al. Thigh musculature in relation to chronic anterior cruciate ligament tear: Muscle size, morphology, and mechanical output before reconstruction. *Am J Sport Med.* 1989;17:423-429.
10. York GK. Motor testing in neurology: An historical overview. *Semin Neurol.* 2002; 22:367-374.
11. Gowers WR. *A manual of diseases of the nervous system* (1981 facsimile by Classics of Medicine Library). Philadelphia: P. Blakiston, Son and Co; 1888.

12. Stokes M, Young A. The contribution of reflex inhibition to arthrogenous muscle weakness. *Clin Sci.* 1984;67:7-14.

13. Ross M, Worrell TW. Thigh and calf girth following knee injury and surgery. *J Occup Sport Phys Ther.* 1998;27:9-15.

14. Helliwell PS, Jackson S. Relationship between weakness and muscle wasting in rheumatoid arthritis. *Ann Rheum Dis.* 1994;53:726-728.

15. Reimers CD, Schlotter B, Eicke BM, Witt TN. Calf enlargement in neuromuscular diseases: A quantitative ultrasound study in 350 patients and review of the literature. *J Neurol Sci.* 1996;143:46-56.

16. Blexrud MD, Windebank AJ, Daube JR. Long-term follow-up of 121 patients with benign fasciculations. *Ann Neurol.* 1993;34:622-625.

17. Reed DM, Kurland LT. Muscle fasciculations in a healthy population. *Arch Neurol.* 1963;9:363-367.

18. Li TM, Alberman E, Swash M. Clinical features and associations of 560 cases of motor neuron disease. *J Neurol Neurosurg Psychiatry.* 1990;53:1043-1045.

19. Young RR. Spasticity: A review. *Neurology.* 1994;44(Suppl 9):S12-S20.

20. Lance JW. The control of muscle tone, reflexes, and movement: Robert Wartenberg lecture. *Neurology.* 1980;30:1303-1313.

21. Burke D, Gillies JD, Lance JW. The quadriceps stretch reflex in human spasticity. *J Neurol Neurosurg Psychiatry.* 1970;33:216-223.

22. Burke D, Gillies JD, Lance JW. Hamstrings stretch reflex in human spasticity. *J Neurol Neurosurg Psychiatry.* 1971;34:231-235.

23. Twitchell TE. The restoration of motor function following hemiplegia in man. *Brain.* 1951;74:443-480.

24. Marshall J. Observations on reflex changes in the lower limbs in spastic paraplegia in man. *Brain.* 1954;77:290-304.

25. Fellows SJ, Ross HF, Thilmann AF. The limitations of the tendon jerk as a marker of pathological stretch reflex activity in human spasticity. *J Neurol Neurosurg Psychiatry.* 1993;56:531-537.

26. Dohrmann GJ, Nowack WJ. Relationship between various clinical signs in lesions of the descending motor system. *Dis Nerv Sys.* 1974;35:375-377.

27. Landau WM. Spasticity: The fable of a neurological demon and the emperor's new therapy. *Arch Neurol.* 1974;31:217-219.

28. Wartenberg R. Pendulousness of the legs as a diagnostic test. *Neurology.* 1951;1:18-24.

29. Wartenberg R. *Diagnostic tests in neurology: A selection for office use.* Chicago: Year Book Publishers, Inc; 1953.

30. Brown RA, Lawson DA, Leslie GC, Part NJ. Observations on the applicability of the Wartenberg pendulum test to healthy, elderly subjects. *J Neurol Neurosurg Psychiatry.* 1988;51:1171-1177.

31. Bajd T, Vodovnik L. Pendulum testing of spasticity. *J Biomed Eng.* 1984;6:9-16.

32. Boczko M, Mumenthaler M. Modified pendulousness test to assess tonus of thigh muscles in spasticity. *Neurology.* 1958;8:846-851.

33. Brown RA, Lawson DA, Leslie GC, et al. Does the Wartenberg pendulum test differentiate quantitatively between spasticity and rigidity? A study in elderly stroke and Parkinson's patients. *J Neurol Neurosurg Psychiatry.* 1988;51: 1178-1186.

34. Nordmark E, Andersson G. Wartenberg pendulum test: Objective quantification of muscle tone in children with spastic diplegia undergoing selective dorsal rhizotomy. *Dev Med Child Neurol.* 2002;44:26-33.

35. Beversdorf DQ, Heilman KM. Facilitory paratonic and frontal lobe functioning. *Neurology.* 1998;51:968-971.

36. Tyrrell P, Rossor M. The association of gegenhalten in the upper limbs with dyspraxia. *J Neurol Neurosurg Psychiatry.* 1988;51:995-997.

37. O'Keefe ST, Kazeem H, Philpott RM, et al. Gait disturbance in Alzheimer's disease: A clinical study. *Age Ageing.* 1996;25:313-316.

38. Denny-Brown D. The nature of apraxia. *J Nerv Ment Dis.* 1958;126:9-32.

39. Chatterjee A. Feeling frontal dysfunction: Facilitory paratonia and the regulation of motor behavior. *Neurology.* 1998;51:937-939.

40. Pickett JB, Tatum EJ. Pendular knee reflexes: A reliable sign of hypotonia? *Lancet.* 1984;2:236-237.

41. van der Meche FGA, van Gijn J. Hypotonia: An erroneous clinical concept? *Brain.* 1986;109:1169-1178.

42. Barchi RL. Myotonia. *Neurol Clin.* 1988;6:473-484.

43. Hornung K, Nix WA. Myoedema: A clinical and electrophysiological evaluation. *Eur Neurol.* 1992;32:130-133.

44. Conn RD, Smith RH. Malnutrition, myoedema, and Muehrcke's lines. *Arch Intern Med.* 1965;116:875-878.

45. Jones MP, Parkes WE. Myoidema. *Clin Sci.* 1955;14:97-100.

46. Adams RW, Gandevia SC, Skuse NF. The distribution of muscle weakness in upper motoneuron lesions affecting the lower limb. *Brain.* 1990;113:1459-1476.

47. Thijs RD, Notermans NC, Wokke JHJ, et al. Distribution of muscle weakness of central and peripheral origin. *J Neurol Neurosurg Psychiatry.* 1998;65:794-796.

48. Colebatch JG, Gandevia SC. The distribution of muscular weakness in upper motor neuron lesions affecting the arm. *Brain.* 1989;112:749-763.

49. Ross RT, Mathiesen R. Volitional and emotional supranuclear facial weakness. *N Engl J Med.* 1998;338:1515.

50. Sonstein WJ, LaSala PA, Michelsen WJ, Onesti ST. False localizing signs in upper cervical spinal cord compression. *Neurosurgery.* 1996;38:445-449.

51. Maynard FM, Bracken MB, Creasey G, et al. International standards for neurological and functional classification of spinal cord injury. *Spinal Cord.* 1997;35: 266-274.

52. Davenport RJ, Swingler RJ, Chancellor AM, Warlow CP. Avoiding false positive diagnoses of motor neuron disease: Lessons from the Scottish Motor Neuron Disease Register. *J Neurol Neurosurg Psychiatry.* 1996;60:147-151.

53. World Federation of Neurology Research Group on Neuromuscular Diseases. El Escorial World Federation of Neurology criteria for the diagnosis of amyotrophic lateral sclerosis. *J Neurol Sci.* 1994;124(Suppl):96-107.

54. Li TM, Alberman E, Day SJ, Swash M. Differential diagnosis of motoneurone disease from other neurological conditions. *Lancet.* 1986;2:731-733.

55. van Gijn J. The Babinski sign and the pyramidal syndrome. *J Neurol Neurosurg Psychiatry.* 1978;41:865-873.

56. Parkinson J. *An essay on the shaking palsy* (facsimile by Classics of Medicine library). Birmingham: Gryphon Editions; 1817.

57. Mulhearn RJ. The history of James Parkinson and his disease. *Austral N Zeal J Med.* 1971;1(Suppl 1):1-6.

58. Deuschl G, Bain P, Brin M. Consensus statement of the movement disorder society on tremor. *Mov Dis.* 1998;13(Suppl 3):2-23.

59. Findley LJ. Classification of tremors. *J Clin Neurophysiol.* 1996;13:122-132.

60. Karson CN, Burns RS, LeWitt PA, et al. Blink rates and disorders of movement. *Neurology.* 1984;34:677-678.

61. Bentivoglio AR, Bressman SB, Cassetta E, et al. Analysis of blink rate patterns in normal subjects. *Mov Dis.* 1997;12:1028-1034.

62. Klawans HL, Goodwin JA. Reversal of the glabellar reflex in Parkinsonism. *J Neurol Neurosurg Psychiatry.* 1969;32:423-427.

63. Shukla D. Blink rate as clinical indicator. *Neurology.* 1985;35:286.

64. Hughes AJ, Ben-Shlomo Y, Daniel SE, Lees AJ. What features improve the accuracy of clinical diagnosis in Parkinson's disease: A clinicopathologic study. *Neurology.* 1992;42:1142-1146.

65. Hughes AJ, Daniel SE, Ben-Shlomo Y, Lees AJ. The accuracy of diagnosis of parkinsonian syndromes in a specialist movement disorder service. *Brain.* 2002;125:861-870.

66. Hughes AJ, Daniel SE, Lees AJ. Improved accuracy of clinical diagnosis of Lewy body Parkinson's disease. *Neurology.* 2001;57:1497-1499.

67. Rajput SH, Rozdilsky B, Rajput A. Accuracy of clinical diagnosis in parkinsonism: A prospective study. *Can J Neurol Sci.* 1991;18:275-278.

68. Mark MH. Lumping and splitting the Parkinson plus syndromes: Dementia with Lewy bodies, multiple system atrophy, progressive supranuclear palsy, and cortical-basal ganglionic degeneration. *Neurol Clin.* 2001;19:607-627.

69. Wenning GK, Ben-Shlomo Y, Hughes A, et al. What clinical features are most useful to distinguish definite multiple system atrophy from Parkinson's disease? *J Neurol Neurosurg Psychiatry.* 2000;68:434-440.

70. Albanese A, Colosimo C, Bentivoglio AR, et al. Multiple system atrophy presenting as parkinsonism: Clinical features and diagnostic criteria. *J Neurol Neurosurg Psychiatry.* 1995;59:144-151.

71. Litvan I, Goetz CG, Jankovic J, et al. What is the accuracy of the clinical diagnosis of multiple system atrophy? A clinicopathologic study. *Arch Neurol.* 1997;54:937-944.

72. Litvan I, Jankovic J, Goetz C, et al. Accuracy of clinical criteria for the diagnosis of progressive supranuclear palsy (Steele-Richardson-Olszewski syndrome). *Neurology.* 1996;46:922-930.

73. Racette BA, Rundle M, Parsian A, Perlmutter JS. Evaluation of a screening questionnaire for genetic studies of Parkinson's disease. *Am J Med Genet.* 1999;88: 539-543.

74. Duarte J, Claveria LE, De Pedro-Cuesta J, et al. Screening Parkinson's disease: A validated questionnaire of high specificity and sensitivity. *Mov Dis.* 1995;10:643-649.

75. Hoehn MM, Yahr MD. Parkinsonism: Onset, progression, and mortality. *Neurology.* 1967;17:427-442.

58

Examination of the Sensory System

SIMPLE SENSATIONS

I. DEFINITIONS

There are four simple sensations: pain, temperature, touch, and vibration. These sensations are all called "simple," because their perception does not require a healthy contralateral cerebral cortex. Excepting the sense of vibration, the simple sensations have distinct sensory organs in the skin and, excepting touch, their pathways in the spinal cord are well defined.

Hypesthesia refers to a diminished ability to perceive a simple sensation; **anesthesia** refers to the complete inability to perceive a simple sensation. Although both "hypesthesia" and "anesthesia" originally referred only to the sensation of touch, many clinicians use the terms when reporting any of the simple sensations. **Hypalgesia** means there is a decreased sensitivity to painful stimuli; **analgesia,** a complete insensitivity. **Hyperpathia, hyperesthesia,** and **allodynia** all refer to an increased sensitivity to sensory stimuli, often with unpleasant qualities, although some experts restrict "hyperpathia" to increased sensitivity from *painful* stimuli and allodynia to discomfort from *tactile* stimuli.

II. TECHNIQUE

Which sensory tests to include in the physical examination depends on the clinical setting. For screening examinations in patients with no sensory complaints, testing only for touch on all four extremities usually suffices. For sensory complaints confined to one limb, testing for touch and pain sensation is usually performed, although testing for pain sensation has a better chance of detecting subtle radiculopathies and peripheral nerve disorders (see "Dermatomes").[1,2] For screening diabetic feet and limbs at risk for neuropathic ulcers and arthropathy, clinicians should use Semmes-Weinstein monofilaments (see Chapter 51). Finally, for any patients with sensory complaints involving large portions of a limb or the trunk, testing for all simple sensations is necessary to uncover "sensory dissociation" (i.e., perception of one modality but not another), which is an important clue to spinal cord disease (see "Sensory Syndromes" later in this chapter).

During sensory testing, the patient's perceptions are compared either with a known standard of normal sensation (e.g., Semmes-Weinstein monofilaments for tactile sensation and tuning fork tests for vibratory sensation), to the contralateral companion part of the patient's body, or to the clinician's own sense of what is normal, as gathered from previous experience.

A. TOUCH

The sensation of touch is usually tested qualitatively by stimulating the patient's skin lightly with a cotton wisp, piece of tissue paper, or the clinician's finger, or quantitatively by using Semmes-Weinstein monofilaments (see Chapter 51).

B. PAIN AND TEMPERATURE

The usual techniques for testing pain sensation are a safety pin bent at right angles or the sharp edge of a broken wooden applicator stick, both of which must be discarded after use to prevent the transmission of infection.[3] It is no longer permissible to use the built-in pin of many reflex hammers or the traditional tailor's pinwheel, because of the risk of transmitting infection.

The traditional test for temperature sensation uses tubes of warm and cold water, although testing the patient's ability to distinguish the cold stem of the tuning fork from the warmer index finger is much simpler.[4]

C. VIBRATION

Vibratory sensation is tested with a tuning fork (usually 128 Hz, less often 256 Hz). There is no compelling reason for using one tuning fork over the other, except that standards have been developed for the 128 Hz fork. Humans are most sensitive to vibration frequencies of 200 to 300 Hz and have difficulty consistently detecting frequencies below 100 Hz.[5,6] Traditionally, the tuning fork is applied against bony prominences, although this is based on the mistaken belief that bones contain the "vibration receptors"; vibratory sensation is just as good, or even better, over soft tissues without underlying bone (the clinician can easily demonstrate this by testing sensation on the abdominal wall).[7]

When a 128-Hz tuning fork is struck from a distance of 20 cm against the heel of the clinician's palm, a healthy 40-year-old person should perceive vibrations for at least 11 seconds when the stem of the fork is held against the lateral malleolus, and for at least 15 seconds when it is held against the ulnar styloid.[8] These values decrease 2 seconds for every decade of age greater than 40 years.

One disadvantage to vibratory testing is that the vibrating impulse is conducted away from the tuning fork, thus preventing precise definition of sensory boundaries in patients with peripheral nerve injuries.[7]

Rumpf introduced the tuning fork to bedside neurology in 1889.[9]

III. CLINICAL SIGNIFICANCE

A. TOUCH, PAIN, AND TEMPERATURE SENSATION

Abnormalities of the simple sensations define all important clinical sensory syndromes: peripheral nerve injury, radiculopathy, spinal cord syndromes, lateral medullary infarction, and thalamic and cerebral hemispheric syndromes (see "Sensory Syndromes"). No diagnostic test has proved superior to bedside examination. In patients with neuropathy, the clinician's bedside assessment of hypesthesia is a more specific predictor of fiber loss on nerve biopsy than automated touch-pressure esthesiometers.[10] In some ways, physical examination is even superior to nerve conduction testing, which evaluates only the larger myelinated peripheral nerve fibers, not the smaller unmyelinated fibers, which carry pain and temperature sensations and from which many uncomfortable sensory syndromes originate.[11]

Diabetic feet insensate to the 5.07 monofilament have increased risk of subsequent foot ulceration and amputation (see Chapter 51).[12–16]

B. VIBRATORY SENSATION

Vibratory sensation is often diminished in peripheral neuropathy and spinal cord disease but spared in disease confined to the cerebral cortex.[7] Although it is a highly developed sensation—Helen Keller could interpret speech by feeling the vibrations of the speaker's larynx, lips, and nose—it lacks distinct sense organs and its neuroanatomic pathways remain obscure.[7,17] Traditionally, it is associated with proprioception, because impulses from both sensations ascend in the posterior columns of the spinal cord, but there are many clinical examples of dissociation of vibratory and proprioceptive loss, both in peripheral neuropathy and spinal cord disease (see "Proprioception").[7,18]

C. HYPERPATHIA AND ALLODYNIA ARE NONSPECIFIC FINDINGS

Hyperpathia and allodynia occur in many different painful conditions, including peripheral neuropathy, brainstem infarction, and thalamic stroke; by themselves, they have no localizing value.[19,20]

PROPRIOCEPTION

I. DEFINITION

Proprioception allows individuals to detect joint motion and limb position when their eyes are closed.[21] Like most of the simple sensations, proprioception has distinct sense organs and ascending pathways in the spinal cord. Unlike simple sensations, however, full perception requires a healthy contralateral cerebral cortex; in this way, it resembles cortical sensations (see "Cortical Sensations").[22,23]

Sir Charles Bell originally called proprioception the "sixth sense." In 1906, Sherrington introduced the term "proprioception" to describe this sensation.[21,24]

II. TECHNIQUE

The conventional test of proprioception is to lightly hold the sides of the patient's finger or toe and bend it slowly up and down. The patient is asked to indicate any sensation of movement and the movement's direction. Because normal persons perceive motion much more easily than direction, a normal person may accurately indicate the presence of motion all of the time but indicate the wrong direction up to 10% of the time.[25] Normal individuals can detect 1 to 2 degrees of movement in most joints, the hips being the most sensitive.[25,26]

Another test of proprioception tests the ability to direct a limb to a given point, again with eyes closed. In one version, the clinician positions the patient's outstretched index finger on the clinician's own index finger. The patient then drops the arm to the side and attempts to find the previous position. Normal individuals consistently come within 5 cm of the target.[24]

Patients with severe proprioceptive loss depend on vision for balance and thus become very unstable when they close their eyes or walk in darkness. This dependence on vision forms the basis for another test of proprioceptive loss, "Romberg's sign," which is discussed fully in Chapter 5.

III. CLINICAL SIGNIFICANCE

Proprioceptive loss is common in peripheral neuropathy (e.g., diabetes mellitus), spinal cord disease (e.g., multiple sclerosis, B_{12} deficiency, tabes dorsalis), and severe hemispheric disease. In unilateral disease of the spinal cord (e.g., the Brown-Séquard syndrome), proprioception is lost on the side of weakness, opposite the side with pain and temperature loss (see "Sensory Syndromes"). In patients with strokes, proprioceptive loss indicates extensive damage and correlates with a poorer functional recovery and higher mortality.[27]

According to traditional teachings, a disproportionate loss of vibration sensation and proprioception (compared with pain and temperature sensation) occurs in diseases of the dorsal columns of the spinal cord (e.g., tabes dorsalis, multiple sclerosis, B_{12} deficiency) and some peripheral neuropathies (e.g., diabetic polyneuropathy). Although this teaching is true, most patients with these disorders also have abnormalities of pain and temperature sensation as well.[7,28]

CORTICAL SENSATIONS

I. DEFINITION

Cortical sensations are those sensations requiring higher integration and processing for them to be perceived properly. Consequently, perception of cortical sensations requires a healthy contralateral cerebral cortex. They may become abnormal in cerebral hemispheric disease, *even though* the simple sensations are preserved.

II. TECHNIQUE

Testing for cortical sensations has three requirements: (1) the patient's eyes are closed; (2) the patient lacks dementia; and, (3) most of the simple sensations, especially touch, are preserved. If the simple sensations are profoundly altered, as in severe peripheral neuropathy, no sensory information will reach the cerebral hemisphere and tests for cortical sensation become uninterpretable.

A. TWO-POINT DISCRIMINATION

Two-point discrimination is the ability to distinguish two compass points simultaneously applied to the skin. The normal minimal distance is 3 cm for the hand or foot and 0.6 cm for the fingertips.[18,22,29,30]

B. TACTILE RECOGNITION ("STEREOGNOSIS")

Tactile recognition is the ability to recognize common objects like a key, paper clip, coin, tweezers, or rubber ball placed in the hand. Normal individuals can name more than 90% of objects within 5 seconds or less.[31,32]

C. GRAPHESTHESIA

Graphesthesia is the ability to identify letters or numbers traced on the hand or foot. Normal individuals can easily recognize symbols 1 cm in height on the fingertips and 6 cm tall elsewhere.[22]

D. LOCALIZATION

Localization is the ability to accurately point to a spot on the body just touched by the clinician.

E. BILATERAL SIMULTANEOUS TACTILE STIMULATION

This tests the patient's ability to recognize that both sides of the body are being touched simultaneously. The term "tactile extinction" refers to the patient's consistent failure to detect the stimulus on one side of the body.[33]

F. APPRECIATION OF WEIGHTS

Appreciation of weights is the ability to perceive differences in weight between two objects, placed sequentially in the patient's hand. This test was used more often several decades ago than it is now.[34]

III. CLINICAL SIGNIFICANCE

Lesions of the posterior parietal lobe may preserve the simple sensations but eliminate proprioception and cortical sensations, the loss typically confined to just the contralateral distal parts of the limbs, sparing the face and trunk.[23,34-36]

It is important to note that cortical disease also may eliminate any or all of the simple sensations, especially if the lesion involves the anterior parietal lobe (postcentral gyrus) or deeper white matter.[7,23,34,37] These lesions often cause a dense sensory loss on the opposite side of the body, involving the trunk, limbs, and face, sometimes referred to as the "pseudothalamic syndrome" because of its resemblance to the sensory loss of thalamic disease (see "Sensory Syndromes").[23]

DERMATOMES

I. DEFINITION

Dermatomes define the area of skin innervated by a single nerve root or spinal segment. They are primarily used to determine whether the sensory loss on a limb corresponds to a single spinal segment, implying the lesion is of that nerve root (i.e., radiculopathy), and to assign the neurologic "level" to a spinal cord lesion.

II. DERIVATION OF THE DERMATOMAL MAPS

The original human dermatomal maps emerged from Sherrington's experiments with monkeys and Head's observations of patients with *Herpes zoster* infection.[2,38] These maps have been subsequently revised, based on several types of evidence collected during the last century, including neurosurgical observations (by Cushing, Foester, and Keegan), experiments injecting novocaine next to the nerve roots of medical student volunteers, and electrical stimulation of the skin while recording potentials at the nerve roots.[1,2,38–40] Differences among dermatomal maps, which are minor and primarily deal with how far proximally some limb dermatomes extend, probably reflect biologic variation and differences in experimental method (i.e., sensory loss from a herniated disc or novocaine injection is not necessarily the same as that from root resection).

III. TECHNIQUE

The dermatomal map in Fig. 58-1 is the international standard used for classifying patients with spinal cord injury (Table 58-1).[41] Two principles apply when evaluating the dermatomal pattern of sensory loss: (1) Contiguous dermatomes overlap, which means that damage to one nerve root may cause either no anesthesia or a sensory loss confined to a small area. These small areas, which are referred to as "signature zones," define the sensory level in patients with spinal cord disease.* (2) Tactile dermatomes are larger than pain dermatomes. This suggests that, when only one or two segments are affected, testing for pain sensibility is a more sensitive method of examination than testing for abnormal touch.[1,2]

---

*In sensory testing, as in motor testing, the neurologic "level" refers to the most caudal level with *normal* function, rather than the first level with abnormal function. For example, a patient with sensation in the nipple line, but none below it, has a "T4 sensory level."

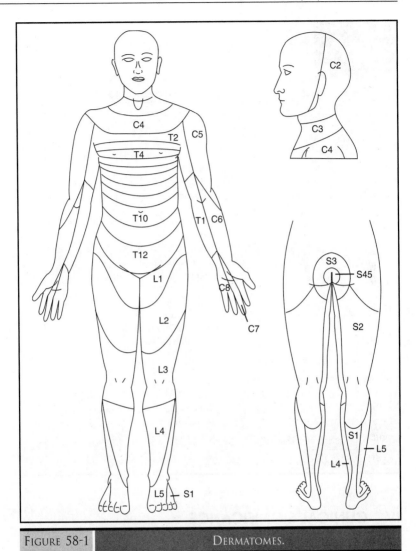

FIGURE 58-1   DERMATOMES.

This is the dermatome map recommended by the American Spinal Injury Association.[41] Note that the C2 dermatome includes the angle of the jaw and most of the ear. The precise boundaries of the S1 and S2 dermatomes are the most controversial.[39]

Table 58-1	Dermatomes and Their Signature Zones

Spinal Level	Signature Zone
Cervical	
C3	Supraclavicular fossa
C4	Top of acromioclavicular joint
C5	Lateral side of antecubital fossa
C6	Thumb
C7	Middle finger
C8	Little finger
Thoracic (selected levels)	
T1	Medial (ulnar) side of the antecubital fossa
T2	Apex of axilla
T4	Fourth intercostal space (nipple line)
T10	Tenth intercostal space (umbilicus)
T12	Inguinal ligament at midpoint
Lumbar	
L1	Half the distance between T12 and L2
L2	Mid-anterior thigh
L3	Medial femoral condyle
L4	Medial malleolus
L5	Dorsum of the foot at the third metatarsal phalangeal joint
Sacral	
S1	Lateral heel
S2	Popliteal fossa in the mid-line
S3	Ischial tuberosity
S4-5	Perianal level

Based on reference 41 and original work cited in text.

IV. CLINICAL SIGNIFICANCE

A. THE SENSORY LEVEL IN SPINAL CORD DISEASE

The patient's sensory level is often several segments *below* the actual level of the lesion in the spine (e.g., the patient with a T8 sensory level may have a lesion in the T3 segment of the spinal cord).*[42-45] There are two explanations for this

---

*During the first successful operation to remove a spinal tumor, in 1887, the surgeon's initial incision, which had been based on the patient's sensory level at T5, had to be revised upward twice before the tumor was found at the T2 level.[46]

phenomenon: one is that the organization of the ascending spinothalamic pathway (carrying pain and temperature sensation) makes the more lateral fibers carrying lower body sensations more vulnerable to external injury. Another is that the actual spinal lesion causes injury by compromising the cord's blood supply, thereby causing injury at a distant segment[42,43]

When the sensory and motor levels disagree, the motor level is a more reliable indicator of level of injury and future disability for the patient.[47] In some patients with spinal cord disease, the most accurate indicator of the spinal segment affected is the site of the patient's vertebral pain and tenderness or the level of the patient's radicular pain.[44,48]

B. DERMATOMAL LOSS IN RADICULOPATHY

The clinical significance of dermatomal sensory loss in disorders of the nerve roots is discussed in Chapter 60.

SENSORY SYNDROMES

I. TECHNIQUE

Figure 58-2 depicts the sensory loss of the important sensory syndromes. Sensory loss confined to a *portion* of a limb suggests injury to a peripheral nerve, plexus, or spinal root, subjects discussed in Chapter 60. When sensory loss involves *most of a limb* or the *trunk*, a systematic approach using the following questions defines the syndrome:

A. DOES THE SENSORY LOSS INVOLVE BOTH SIDES OF THE BODY?

Involvement of *both* sides indicates polyneuropathy or spinal cord disease. Involvement of *one* side indicates contralateral disease of the brainstem, thalamus, or cerebral cortex. In patients with pure hemisection of the spinal cord (i.e., Brown-Séquard syndrome), there is sensory loss on both sides of the body, although pain and temperature sensation is lost on the side *opposite to* the lesion and tactile sensation is lost on the side *of* the lesion.

B. IS THERE A SENSORY LEVEL?

A sensory level is a distinct border on the trunk, below which sensory testing is abnormal and above which it is normal. A sensory level indicates spinal cord disease, although the finding sometimes also occurs in lateral medullary infarction.[19,49–52]

C. IS THERE SENSORY DISSOCIATION?

Sensory dissociation is a disproportionate loss of one or more simple sensations with preservation of others. Loss of pain and temperature sensation with

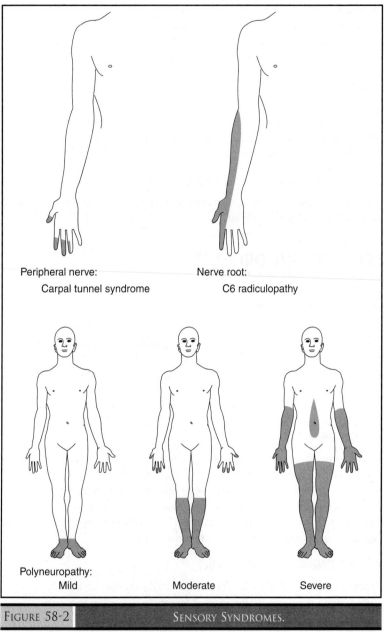

Peripheral nerve:
Carpal tunnel syndrome

Nerve root:
C6 radiculopathy

Polyneuropathy:
Mild   Moderate   Severe

FIGURE 58-2   SENSORY SYNDROMES.

In these figures, the gray shading indicates hypalgesia (loss of pain temperature sensation) and the arrows indicate limbs with significant accompanying weakness. In the Brown-Séquard syndrome (hemisection of the cord, *top row, right*), there is often diminished tactile sensation on the side of weakness and opposite the side with hypalgesia.

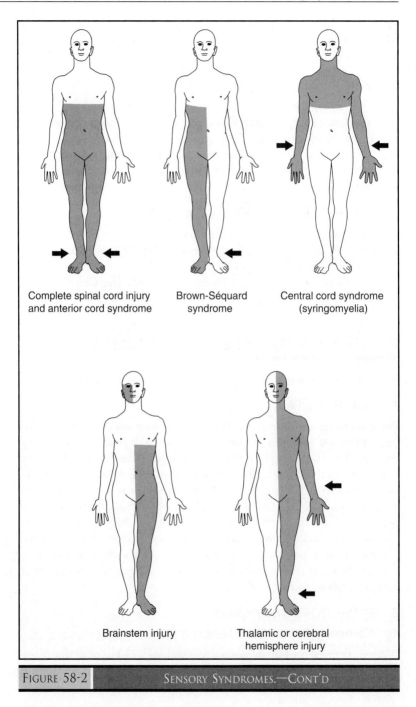

Complete spinal cord injury and anterior cord syndrome

Brown-Séquard syndrome

Central cord syndrome (syringomyelia)

Brainstem injury

Thalamic or cerebral hemisphere injury

FIGURE 58-2   SENSORY SYNDROMES.—CONT'D

preservation of touch and vibration sensation is a feature of some *incomplete* spinal cord syndromes (e.g., syringomyelia, spinal stroke, and Brown-Séquard syndrome).

D. IS THERE SENSORY LOSS ON THE FACE?

Sensory loss on the face indicates disease above the spinal cord, in the brainstem, thalamus, or cerebral hemispheres. In brainstem disease (e.g., lateral medullary syndrome), the sensory loss on the patient's face is *opposite* to the side of sensory loss on the body; in disease of the thalamus or cerebral hemisphere, the sensory loss on the face and body are on the *same* side.

E. ARE THERE ASSOCIATED NEUROLOGIC SIGNS?

Most disorders causing the sensory syndromes depicted in Fig. 58-2 also cause significant weakness (indicated by the arrows in Fig. 58-2), a major exception being the lateral medullary syndrome.

The presence of an associated **Horner's syndrome** (see Chapter 19 for definition) indicates disease of the ipsilateral brain stem or cervical spinal cord.[53]

II. DEFINITION OF THE SENSORY SYNDROMES

Peripheral nerve and spinal root disorders are discussed in Chapter 60.

A. POLYNEUROPATHY

Polyneuropathy is a bilateral "stocking-glove" sensory loss that spares the face (the sensory loss resembles the pattern of a stocking or glove because polyneuropathy affects all nerves of the same length equally). Because the sensory loss of polyneuropathy affects the longest nerves first, hypesthesia initially appears in the feet; later in the fingertips; and, only after extensive involvement of the arms and legs, the anterior trunk.[54] Atrophy of the small muscles of the feet and hands and absent ankle reflexes are common. Distal weakness may occur, but because the nerves to the foot dorsiflexors are longer than those to plantar flexors, patients with polyneuropathy have more trouble walking on their heels than on their toes (the opposite finding, trouble walking on toes but not on heels, suggests an alternative diagnosis).[55]

B. SPINAL CORD SYNDROMES

1. Complete Spinal Cord Lesion

A complete spinal cord lesion causes a sensory level with loss of all simple sensations below that level, weakness (tetraparesis or paraparesis), and urinary retention.

2. Incomplete Spinal Cord Lesions

a. Anterior Cord Syndrome

Spinal stroke, which may follow prolonged hypotension or trauma to the aorta, resembles the complete spinal cord lesion, except there is a disproportionate loss of pain and temperature sensation and relative sparing of touch and vibration, owing to the more vulnerable blood supply of the ventral cord.[56]

b. Brown-Séquard Syndrome

Brown-Séquard syndrome describes injury to half of the cord, causing *contralateral* loss of pain and temperature sensation but *ipsilateral* paralysis and diminished touch sensation.[53] Unilateral disease of the cervicothoracic region may involve the ascending sympathetic fibers and cause an ipsilateral Horner's syndrome.[53]

The pure Brown-Séquard syndrome is rare. Instead, most patients with unilateral disease of the spinal cord present with bilateral weakness and sensory loss, although the weakness is greatest on the side of the lesion and the hypalgesia is greatest opposite the lesion.[53]

c. Central Cord Syndrome

In syringomyelia (a central cord syndrome), the sensory loss typically involves one or both arms. Seventy-five percent of patients have atrophy and weakness of one or both hands or sternocleidomastoid muscles.[57,58]

C. LATERAL MEDULLARY INFARCTION ("WALLENBERG'S SYNDROME")

Lateral medullary infarction is a dramatic syndrome presenting with dizziness and causing sensory loss on opposite sides of face and body but no weakness (the lesion is ipsilateral to the facial analgesia). Common associated signs are diminished corneal reflex, ipsilateral limb ataxia, nystagmus, ipsilateral Horner's syndrome, gait ataxia, and ipsilateral palate weakness (Table 58-2).[49,51,59–63]

D. THALAMIC DISEASE

A lesion in the thalamus may cause loss of all simple sensations on the opposite side of the body, associated with hemiparesis, vertical gaze abnormalities, miosis, and aphasia.[37,64,65]

E. CEREBRAL HEMISPHERIC DISEASE

Cerebral hemispheral disease may cause a dense sensory loss and hemiparesis identical to thalamic disease ("pseudothalamic syndrome"),[23] or the selective loss of cortical sensations in the distal parts of the extremities (see "Cortical Sensations").

| Table 58-2 | Lateral Medullary Infarction (Wallenberg's Syndrome) |

Physical Finding	Frequency (%)*
Cranial nerves	
Diminished corneal reflex (V and VII)	91
Ipsilateral Horner's syndrome†	71–95
Ipsilateral face analgesia (V)	50–86
Nystagmus	56–100
Ipsilateral palate weakness (IX, X)	52–86
Ipsilateral facial weakness (VII)	21–43
Sensory	
Contralateral body analgesia	88
Coordination	
Ipsilateral limb ataxia	55–95
Gait ataxia	91

Data obtained from 290 patients from references 51, 59–63.
*Results are overall mean frequency or, if statistically heterogeneous, the range of values.
†Strictly speaking, Horner's syndrome does not involve cranial nerves, although it is discovered during examination of the pupils and eyelids.

REFERENCES

1. Inouye Y, Buchthal F. Segmental sensory innervation determined by potentials recorded from cervical spinal nerves. *Brain.* 1977;100:731-748.
2. Foester O. The dermatomes in man. *Brain.* 1933;56 part 1:1-39.
3. Finelli PF. Reflex hammer with built-in pin. *Neurology.* 1991;41:344.
4. DeMyer W. Pointers and pitfalls in the neurologic examination. *Sem Neurol.* 1998; 18:161-168.
5. Loefvenberg J, Johansson RS. Regional differences and interindividual variability in sensitivity to vibration in the glabrous skin of the human hand. *Brain Res.* 1984;301: 65-72.
6. Plumb CS, Meigs JW. Human vibration perception. *Arch Gen Psychiatry.* 1961;4: 611-614.
7. Fox JC, Klemperer WW. Vibratory sensibility: A quantitative study of its thresholds in nervous disorders. *Arch Neurol Psychiatry.* 1942;48:612-645.
8. De Michele G, Filla A, Coppola N, et al. Influence of age, gender, height and education on vibration sense: A study by tuning fork in 192 normal subjects. *J Neurol Sci.* 1991;105:155-158.
9. Pearce JMS. Early days of the tuning fork. *J Neurol Neurosurg Psychiatry.* 1998;65: 728, 733.

10. Dyck PJ, O'Brien PC, Bushek W, et al. Clinical vs. quantitative evaluation of cutaneous sensation. *Arch Neurol.* 1976;33:651-655.

11. Gilliat RW, Sears TA. Sensory nerve action potentials in patients with peripheral nerve lesions. *J Neurol Neurosurg Psychiatry.* 1958;21:109-118.

12. Rith-Najarian SJ, Stolusky T, Gohdes DM. Identifying diabetic patients at high risk for lower-extremity amputation in a primary health care setting: A prospective evaluation of simple screening criteria. *Diabetes Care.* 1992;15:1386-1389.

13. Boyko EJ, Ahroni JH, Stensel V, et al. A prospective study of risk factors for diabetic foot ulcer. The Seattle Diabetic Foot study. *Diabetes Care.* 1999;22:1036-1042.

14. Adler AI, Boyko EJ, Ahroni JH, Smith DG. Lower-extremity amputation in diabetes: The independent effects of peripheral vascular disease, sensory neuropathy, and foot ulcers. *Diabetes Care.* 1999;22:1029-1035.

15. Pham H, Armstrong DG, Harvey C, et al. Screening techniques to identify people at high risk for diabetic foot ulceration. *Diabetes Care.* 2000;23:606-611.

16. Abbott CA, Carrington AL, Ashe H, et al. The North-West diabetes Foot Care Study: Incidence of, and risk factors for, new diabetic foot ulceration in a community-based patient cohort. *Diabetic Med.* 2002;19:377-384.

17. Calne DB, Pallis CA. Vibratory sense: A critical review. *Brain.* 1966;89:723-746.

18. Renfrew S, Cavanagh D. The discrimination between pinching and pressing of the skin: The basis of a clinical test. *Brain.* 1954;77:305-313.

19. Soffin G, Feldman M, Bender MB. Alterations of sensory levels in vascular lesions of lateral medulla. *Arch Neurol.* 1968;18:178-190.

20. Archer AG, Watkins PJ, Thomas PK, et al. The natural history of acute painful neuropathy in diabetes mellitus. *J Neurol Neurosurg Psychiatry.* 1983;46:491-499.

21. McCloskey DI. Kinesthetic sensibility. *Physiol Review.* 1978;58:763-820.

22. Bender MB, Stacy C, Cohen J. Agraphesthesia: A disorder of directional cutaneous kinesthesia or a disorientation in cutaneous space. *J Neurol Sci.* 1982;53:531-555.

23. Bassetti C, Bogousslavsky J, Regli F. Sensory syndromes in parietal stroke. *Neurology.* 1993;43:1942-1949.

24. Cohen LA. Analysis of position sense in human shoulders. *J Neurophysiol.* 1957;21:550-568.

25. Laidlaw RW, Hamilton MA. A study of thresholds in apperception of passive movement among normal control subjects. *Bull Neurol Inst N Y.* 1937;6:268-273.

26. Laidlaw RW, Hamilton MA. The quantitative measurement of apperception of passive movement. *Bull Neurol Inst N Y.* 1937;6:145-153.

27. Smith DL, Akhtar AJ, Garraway WM. Proprioception and spatial neglect after stroke. *Age Ageing.* 1983;12:63-69.

28. Harati Y. Diabetic peripheral neuropathies. *Ann Intern Med.* 1987;107:546-559.

29. Gellman H, Gerlberman RH, Tan AM, Botte MJ. Carpal tunnel syndrome: An evaluation of the provocative diagnostic tests. *J Bone Joint Surg Am.* 1986;68A:735-737.

30. Buch-Jaeger N, Foucher G. Correlation of clinical signs with nerve conduction tests in the diagnosis of carpal tunnel syndrome. *J Hand Surg Br.* 1994;19B:720-724.

31. Dannenbaum RM, Jones LA. The assessment and treatment of patients who have sensory loss following cortical lesions. *J Hand Ther.* 1993;6:130-138.

32. Corkin S, Milner B, Rasmussen T. Somatosensory thresholds: Contrasting effects of postcentral-gyrus and posterior parietal-lobe excisions. *Arch Neurol.* 1970;23:41-58.

33. Schwartz AS, Marchok PL, Kreinick CJ, Flynn RE. The asymmetric lateralization of tactile extinction in patients with unilateral cerebral dysfunction. *Brain.* 1979; 102:669-684.

34. Holmes G. Disorders of sensation produced by cortical lesions. *Brain.* 1927;50: 413-427.

35. Pause M, Kunesch E, Binkofski F, Freund HJ. Sensorimotor disturbances in patients with lesions of the parietal cortex. *Brain.* 1989;112:1599-1625.

36. Derouesne C, Mas JL, Bolgert F, Castaigne P. Pure sensory stroke caused by a small cortical infarct in the middle cerebral artery territory. *Stroke.* 1984;15:660-662.

37. Kim JS. Pure sensory stroke: Clinical-radiological correlates of 21 cases. *Stroke.* 1992;23:983-987.

38. Wolf JK. *Segmental neurology: A guide to the examination and interpretation of sensory and motor function.* Baltimore: University Park Press; 1981.

39. Keegan JJ, Garrett FD. The segmental distribution of the cutaneous nerves in the limbs of man. *Anat Rec.* 1948;102:409-437.

40. Young JH. The revision of the dermatomes. *Aust N Z J Surg.* 1949;18:171-186.

41. Maynard FM, Bracken MB, Creasey G, et al. International standards for neurological and functional classification of spinal cord injury. *Spinal Cord.* 1997;35: 266-274.

42. Sonstein WJ, LaSala PA, Michelsen WJ, Onesti ST. False localizing signs in upper cervical spinal cord compression. *Neurosurgery.* 1996;38:445-449.

43. Jamieson DRS, Teasdale E, Willison HJ. False localising signs in the spinal cord. *Br Med J.* 1996;312:243-244.

44. Barron KD, Hirano A, Araki S, Terry RD. Experiences with metastatic neoplasms involving the spinal cord. *Neurology.* 1988;38:91-106.

45. Levack P, Graham J, Collie D, et al. Don't wait for a sensory level—Listen to the symptoms: A prospective audit of the delays in diagnosis of malignant cord compression. *Clin Oncol.* 2002;14:472-480.

46. Spillane JD. *The doctrine of the nerves: Chapters in the history of neurology.* Oxford: Oxford University Press; 1981.

47. Marino RJ, Rider-Foster D, Maissel G, Ditunno JF. Superiority of motor level over single neurological level in categorizing tetraplegia. *Paraplegia.* 1995;33:510-513.

48. Matsumoto M, Ishikawa M, Ishii K, et al. Usefulness of neurological examination for diagnosis of the affected level in patients with cervical compressive myelopathy: Prospective comparative study with radiological evaluation. *J Neurosurg Spine.* 2005; 2:535-539.

49. Matsumoto S, Okuda B, Imai T, Kameyama M. A sensory level on the trunk in lower lateral brainstem lesions. *Neurology.* 1988;38:1515-1519.
50. Currier RD, Giles CL, DeJong RN. Some comments on Wallenberg's lateral medullary syndrome. *Neurology.* 1961;11:778-791.
51. Kim JS. Pure lateral medullary infarction: Clinical-radiological correlation of 130 acute, consecutive patients. *Brain.* 2003;126:1864-1872.
52. Phan TG, Wijdicks EFM. A sensory level on the trunk and sparing the face from vertebral artery dissection: How much more subtle can we get? *J Neurol Neurosurg Psychiatry.* 1999;66:691-692.
53. Koehler PJ, Endtz LJ. The Brown-Sequard syndrome: True or false? *Arch Neurol.* 1986;43:921-924.
54. Waxman SG, Sabin TD. Diabetic truncal polyneuropathy. *Arch Neurol.* 1981;38:46-47.
55. Bourque PR, Dyck PJ. Selective calf weakness suggests intraspinal pathology, not peripheral neuropathy. *Arch Neurol.* 1990;47:79-80.
56. Silver JR, Buxton PH. Spinal stroke. *Brain.* 1974;97:539-550.
57. McIlroy WJ, Richardson JC. Syringomyelia: A clinical review of 75 cases. *Can Med Assoc J.* 1965;93:731-734.
58. Tashiro K, Fukazawa T, Mariwaka F, et al. Syringomyelic syndrome: Clinical features in 31 cases confirmed by CT myelography or magnetic resonance imaging. *J Neurol.* 1987;235:26-30.
59. Kim JS, Lee JH, Suh DC, Lee MC. Spectrum of lateral medullary syndrome: Correlation between clinical findings and magnetic resonance imaging in 33 subjects. *Stroke.* 1994;25:1405-1410.
60. Norrving B, Cronqvist S. Lateral medullary infarction: Prognosis in an unselected series. *Neurology.* 1991;41:244-248.
61. Peterman AF, Siekert RG. The lateral medullary (Wallenberg) syndrome: Clinical features and prognosis. *Med Clin North Am.* 1960;44:887-895.
62. Sacco RL, Freddo L, Bellow JA, et al. Wallenberg's lateral medullary syndrome: Clinical-magnetic resonance imaging correlations. *Arch Neurol.* 1993;50:609-614.
63. Fisher CM, Karnes WE, Kubik CS. Lateral medullary infarction: The pattern of vascular occlusion. *J Neuropathol Exper Neurol.* 1961;20:323-379.
64. Barraquer-Bordas L, Illa I, Escartin A, et al. Thalamic hemorrhage: A study of 23 patients with diagnosis by computed tomography. *Stroke.* 1981;12:524-527.
65. Walshe TM, Davis KR, Fisher CM. Thalamic hemorrhage: A computed tomographic-clinical correlation. *Neurology.* 1977;27:217-222.

Examination
of the Reflexes

Reflexes are involuntary contractions of muscles, induced by specific stimuli. In the neurologic examination, there are three types of reflexes: (1) muscle-stretch reflexes ("deep tendon" or "myotatic" reflexes), (2) cutaneous reflexes, and (3) primitive reflexes (or "release" reflexes). This chapter also discusses the Babinski response, which is an abnormal cutaneous reflex of the foot that appears in upper motor neuron disease.

REFLEX HAMMERS

I. TYPES OF REFLEX HAMMERS

Early in the history of reflex testing,* clinicians used various implements to elicit reflexes: The great British neurologist Gowers used the ulnar aspect of his

---

*Reflex testing became common after Erb and Westphal simultaneously discovered the value of muscle stretch reflexes in 1875.[1]

hand or his rigid stethoscope. Other clinicians were less selective, using paper weights, laboratory stands, or even table lamps.[2-4] In the late 1800s and early 1900s, many different reflex hammers were produced, some of which remain popular today.

A.   TAYLOR HAMMER

The Taylor hammer was developed in 1888 by J.M. Taylor, personal assistant to S. Weir Mitchell at the Philadelphia Orthopedic Hospital and Infirmary for Nervous Disease. This hammer has a tomahawk-shaped soft rubber hammer with a broad edge for percussing most tendons and a rounded point for reaching the biceps tendon or percussing muscles directly. The original handle ended in an open loop; the pointed end was added about 1920 for use in eliciting cutaneous reflexes.[4]

B.   QUEEN SQUARE HAMMER

The Queen Square hammer was developed by a Miss Wintle, a head nurse at the National Hospital for Nervous Diseases at Queen's Square, London, who for years made hammers from ring pessaries, solid brass wheels, and bamboo rods to sell to resident medical officers. This hammer has a rubber-lined disc attached to the end of a long rod, like a wheel on an axle.[2]

C.   BABINSKI HAMMER (OR "BABINSKI/RABINER" HAMMER)

This hammer has a handle that can be removed and attached either perpendicular or parallel to the disc-shaped head. Babinski's name probably reflects marketing more that innovation.[4]

D.   TROEMNER HAMMER

This hammer, the only one of the four that actually resembles a hammer, was made popular in this country by the Mayo Clinic, where the neurologist Woltman introduced it in 1927.[5]

II.   CLINICAL SIGNIFICANCE

No study has demonstrated any hammer to be superior to another, and selection depends more on personal preference and tradition. The Taylor is popular in America, the Queen Square in England, and the Troemner in continental Europe.[6] Some models (e.g., Babinski hammer) have built-in pins, designed for testing pain sensation and cutaneous reflexes. Because these pins could transmit infections, however, they should not be used.[7]

MUSCLE STRETCH REFLEXES

I. DEFINITION

Muscle stretch reflexes are involuntary contractions of muscles induced by a brisk stretch of the muscle. Muscle stretch reflexes are usually named after the muscle being tested (Table 59-1), the one notable exception being the Achilles or ankle jerk. Although these reflexes are often called "deep tendon reflexes," this name is a misnomer because tendons have little to do with the response, other than being responsible for mechanically transmitting the sudden stretch from the reflex hammer to the muscle spindle. In addition, some muscles with stretch reflexes have no tendons (e.g., "jaw jerk" of the masseter muscle).

Most healthy persons have the muscle stretch reflexes listed in Table 59-1.

II. TECHNIQUE

A. METHOD

The usual stimulus is a sharp tap with the reflex hammer on the muscle's tendon, near where the tendon inserts distally on bone. The Achilles reflex is also elicited sometimes by the plantar strike method, in which the reflex hammer strikes the clinician's hand, which is resting on the ball of the foot. In clinical studies of the Achilles reflex, both the plantar strike and tendon strike methods are equivalent.[19-21]

B. GRADING REFLEX AMPLITUDE

The most important observation during reflex examination is the reflex's amplitude. Unlike examination of motor strength, examination of reflexes lacks a

Table 59-1	Common Muscle Stretch Reflexes	
Name of Reflex	Peripheral Nerve	Spinal Level
Brachioradialis	Radial	C5-6
Biceps	Musculocutaneous	C5-6
Triceps	Radial	C7-8
Quadriceps (patellar)	Femoral	L2-L4
Achilles (ankle)	Tibial	S1

Based on references 8-18.

single universally accepted grading system. Proposed schemes range from S. Weir Mitchell's original 4 grades [4] to the Mayo Clinic's 9 grades.[22] A 5-point grading system (i.e., grades 0 through 4), reproduced in Table 59-2, is recommended by the National Institute of Neurological Disorders and Stroke.[23]

C. REINFORCEMENT: THE JENDRASSIK MANEUVER

According to the NINDS scale (see Table 59-2), grade 1 reflexes include reflexes brought out only during reinforcement, and grade 0 reflexes are those that are absent despite reinforcement. The most common method of reinforcing reflexes is the Jendrassik maneuver. In 1885, Erno Jendrassik reported that having the patient "hook together the flexed fingers of his right and left hands and pull them apart as strongly as possible" while the clinician taps on the tendon enhances the reflexes of normal patients.[2] Reflex enhancement with this maneuver persists as long as the patient is pulling apart the arms, up to 10 seconds in some studies.[24,25] In one study of normal elderly patients, the absent ankle jerk was made to appear 70% of the time using reinforcing maneuvers.[26]

III. CLINICAL SIGNIFICANCE

A. AMPLITUDE OF REFLEX

The amplitude of muscle stretch reflexes depends on the integrity of the lower and upper motor neurons innervating the reflex (see Fig. 57-2 in Chapter 57 for definition of lower and upper motor neurons). (1) The lower motor neurons of

Table 59-2	NINDS* Muscle Stretch Reflex Scale

Grade	Finding
0	Reflex absent
1	Reflex small, less than normal; includes a trace response or a response brought out only with reinforcement
2	Reflex in lower half of normal range
3	Reflex in upper half of normal range
4	Reflex enhanced, more than normal; includes clonus if present, which optionally can be noted in an added verbal description of the reflex

NINDS, National Institute of Neurological Disorders and Stroke, from reference 23.

a reflex are its peripheral nerve (second column in Table 59-1) and its spinal segment (third column in Table 59-1): disease at either of these locations *reduces* or *abolishes* the relevant reflex. (2) The upper motor neurons are the descending corticospinal pathways innervating the reflex: disease anywhere along this pathway (e.g., cerebral hemisphere, brainstem) *exaggerates* the reflex. (3) Disease of the *spinal cord*, where both upper and lower motor neurons reside, abolishes the reflex *at* the level of the lesion (lower motor neuron response) and exaggerates all reflexes from spinal levels *below* the level of the lesion (upper motor neuron response).

Nonetheless, absent or exaggerated reflexes, by themselves, do not signify neurologic disease.[27-29] For example, 6% to 50% of elderly persons without neurologic disease lack the ankle jerk bilaterally, despite the Jendrassik maneuver,[26,30] and a small percentage of normal individuals have generalized hyperreflexia.[27-29,31] Instead, the absent or exaggerated reflex is significant only when it is associated with one of the following clinical settings:

1. The absent reflex is associated with other findings of lower motor neuron disease (weakness, atrophy, fasciculations).
2. The exaggerated reflex is associated with other findings of upper motor neuron disease (i.e., weakness, spasticity, Babinski sign).
3. The reflex amplitude is asymmetric, which suggests either lower motor neuron disease of the side with the diminished reflex or upper motor neuron disease of the side with exaggerated reflex.
4. The reflex is unusually brisk compared with reflexes from a higher spinal level, which raises the possibility of spinal cord disease at some level of the spinal cord between the segments with exaggerated reflexes and those with diminished ones.

B. LOCALIZING VALUE OF DIMINISHED REFLEXES

In patients with nerve complaints of the arm or leg suggesting disorders of the cervical or lumbosacral nerve roots, the diminished reflex has important localizing value that indicates a lesion of the reflex's respective spinal root (see Table 59-1). A diminished biceps or brachioradialis reflex indicates C6 radiculopathy (likelihood ratio [LR] = 14.2),[16] a diminished triceps reflex indicates C7 radiculopathy* (LR = 3.0),[16,32] a diminished quadriceps reflex indicates L3 or L4 radiculopathy (LR = 8.7),[33-35] and a diminished Achilles reflex argues modestly for S1 radiculopathy (LR=2.9)[33-37] (see also Chapter 60).

---

*C6 and C7 radiculopathies are much more common than C5 or C8 radiculopathies (see Chapter 60).

C. ADDITIONAL FINDINGS IN THE HYPERREFLEXIC PATIENT

The physical finding of hyperreflexia has generated more eponyms in physical diagnosis than any other physical finding*, even though the basic pathophysiology for all exaggerated reflexes is the same (i.e., loss of corticospinal inhibition) and the reflexes differ only by which muscle is stretched and which method the clinician uses to stretch the muscle. Of the many findings that have been described in hyperreflexic patients, commonly recognized ones are finger flexion reflexes, jaw jerks, clonus, and "irradiating" reflexes.

1. Finger Flexion Reflexes (Introduced by Hoffman about 1900)

In a positive response, sudden stretching of the finger flexors causes the finger flexors to involuntarily contract (the finger flexion reflex, therefore, is no different from any other muscle stretch reflex). There are many ways to elicit this finding, each with its own eponym (e.g., Hoffman's sign, Finger Rossolimo sign, Troemner's sign, von Bechterew's reflex). One of these methods is described in Fig. 59-1. Like other exaggerated reflexes, finger flexion reflexes by themselves have little diagnostic value (i.e., they are detectable in 3% of healthy college students),[31] and, to be significant, they must accompany one of the settings described previously in "Amplitude of Reflex."

2. Jaw Jerk (Originally Described by Lewis in 1882)[39]

In a positive response, sudden stretching of the masseter muscle causes reflex contraction, moving the jaw briskly upward. With the patient's jaw slightly open, the clinician can elicit the reflex by tapping with a reflex hammer directly on the chin or on a tongue blade resting on the lower teeth or tongue. An exaggerated jaw jerk, sometimes appearing with clonus (see later), implies bilateral disease above the level of the pons (e.g., pseudobulbar palsy).[27] In patients with spastic tetraparesis, for example, an exaggerated jaw jerk excludes cervical cord disease and points to pyramidal tract disease above the pons.

3. Clonus

Clonus is a self-sustained, oscillating stretch reflex induced when the clinician briskly stretches a hyperreflexic muscle and then continues to apply stretching force to that muscle. Each time the muscle relaxes from the previous reflex contraction, the applied stretching force renews the reflex, setting up a rhythmic series of muscle contractions that continue as long as the tension is applied. These rhythmic oscillations ("clonus") are most easily elicited in the foot

---

*Dorland's Medical Dictionary lists 115 neurologic reflexes, 46 having eponyms.[38]

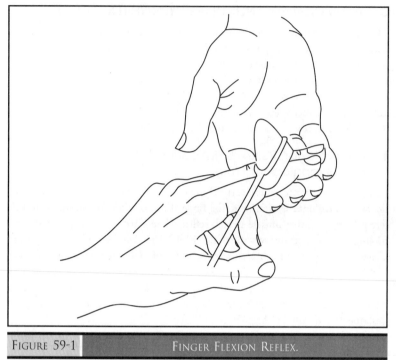

| FIGURE 59-1 | FINGER FLEXION REFLEX. |

After positioning the patient's hand in the supinated position with fingers slightly flexed, the clinician places his own index and middle fingers across the tips of the patient's fingers and taps them with the reflex hammer. Reflex contraction of the patient's finger flexor muscles is a positive response.

(usually with oscillations of 5–8 Hz), by briskly dorsiflexing the patient's ankle. Clonus also may be elicited in the quadriceps, finger flexors, jaw, and other muscles.

As expected mathematically, the frequency of clonus varies inversely with the length of the reflex path ($r = -0.80$, $p < .001$). Clonus of the wrist has a higher frequency than that of the ankle, simply because the nerves to the forearm are shorter than those to the calf.[40]

4. "Irradiation" of Reflexes

In some hyperreflexic patients, the blow of the reflex hammer is conducted mechanically through bone and tissues, where it may stretch hyperexcitable muscles at distant sites, thus producing additional, unexpected movements (e.g., "crossed adductor reflex").[28,41] Also, if this distant irradiation of a reflex is combined with paralysis of the reflex of interest, paradoxical movements or "inverted" reflexes may appear.

a. Crossed Adductor Reflex

Tapping on the medial femoral condyle, patella, or patellar tendon causes the contralateral adductor muscle to contract, moving the contralateral knee medially.[42]

b. Inverted Supinator Reflex

The "supinator reflex" is the brachioradialis reflex. Introduced by Babinski in 1910, this sign indicates spinal cord disease at the C5-6 level.[28,43,44] In a positive response, tapping on the brachioradialis muscle causes no flexion at the elbow but instead flexion of the fingers. The lesion at C5-6 eliminates the brachioradialis reflex (lower motor neuron) but exaggerates all reflexes below that level (upper motor neuron), including the finger flexion reflexes (C8), which are stimulated by mechanical conduction of the blow on the brachioradialis.

c. Inverted Knee Jerk[45]

The inverted knee jerk indicates spinal cord disease at the L2-4 level. In the positive response, attempts to elicit the knee jerk instead cause paradoxical knee flexion. Its two components are denervation of L2-4 (thus paralyzing the quadriceps jerk) and conduction of the blow to the muscle spindles of the hamstrings (innervated by the L5-S1 level and made hyperexcitable by the same lesion).

CUTANEOUS REFLEXES ("SUPERFICIAL" REFLEXES)

I. DEFINITION

Cutaneous reflexes are involuntary muscle contractions that follow stimulation of the skin surface by scratching, stroking, or pinching.

II. SUPERFICIAL ABDOMINAL REFLEX (T6 TO T11)

A. TECHNIQUE

In the superficial abdominal reflexes, stroking the skin of the abdomen causes the underlying abdominal wall muscle to contract, sometimes pulling the umbilicus toward the stimulus. The clinician usually tests one abdominal quadrant at a time using a side-to-side motion with a wooden applicator stick or the pointed end of the reflex hammer handle. The abdominal reflexes appear just as often whether the direction is medial-to-lateral or lateral-to-medial.[46]

B. CLINICAL SIGNIFICANCE

According to traditional teachings, superficial abdominal reflexes disappear with both upper and lower motor neuron disease. Their clinical value is slight, however, because they are also absent in about 20% of normal individuals, more so in the elderly.[46,47] Moreover, the observation of asymmetric reflexes or ones preserved only in the upper quadrants, patterns traditionally associated with neurologic disease, also are a common finding in healthy persons.[46-48]

III. BULBOCAVERNOSUS REFLEX (S2 TO S4)

A. TECHNIQUE

After positioning the patient in the lithotomy position, sudden manual compression of the glans penis or clitoris causes reflex contraction of the bulbocavernosus muscle and external anal sphincter. The reflex is detected either by palpating the skin behind the scrotum (bulbocavernosus muscle) or, more commonly, placing the index finger in the anal canal (external anal sphincter). Other effective stimuli are percussing the suprapubic area[49] or pulling the retention balloon of an indwelling Foley catheter against the bladder neck.[50]

B. CLINICAL SIGNIFICANCE

The bulbocavernosus reflex is one of the few ways to test the conus medullaris (distal end of the spinal cord) and the S2-S4 pelvic nerves (the only other bedside test of this region is testing sensation in the perineal, or "saddle" area).[50-52] Therefore, this reflex is particularly important in patients with urinary retention, which may be caused by disease of the pelvic nerves or cauda equina. In one study of consecutive patients referred for urodynamic studies,[50] most of whom had difficulty with urination, an *absent* reflex predicted disease in the S2-S4 segments only modestly in women (LR = 2.7) but much better in men (LR = 13.0). The modest accuracy of the sign in women may reflect damage to the pudendal nerve from prior childbirth or pelvic surgery.[50] In this study, the *presence* of a bulbocavernosus reflex was unhelpful: although the positive response is expected in patients with urinary retention from common disorders like prostate hypertrophy, it also is commonly found in incomplete lesions of the sacral nerves.

In spinal cord injury above the S2-S4 level (i.e., upper motor neuron lesion to S2-S4 segment), the bulbocavernosus reflex also disappears, but only temporarily for a period of 1 to 6 weeks.[50]

BABINSKI RESPONSE

I. DEFINITION

The Babinski response is an abnormal cutaneous reflex found in upper motor neuron disease affecting the muscles of the foot. In these patients, scratching the sole of the patient's foot causes an upward movement of the great toe, instead of the normal downward movement (Fig. 59-2). Much revered and much researched, this reflex was originally described by Babinski in 1896.[53,54] It goes by various names, including "Babinski response," "Babinski sign," "Babinski reflex," "up-going toe," and "extensor response."

In some patients with bilateral corticospinal tract disease, scratching the foot may even cause the contralateral great toe to move upward, a response termed "crossed dorsiflexion" or "crossed extensor" response.[53]

II. PATHOGENESIS

In response to painful stimuli applied to the lower limbs, most mammals rapidly withdraw that limb by flexing the hips and knees and dorsiflexing the feet and toes. This primitive reflex, the "flexion response," also occurs in human infants until the age of 1 or 2 years, after which the developing pyramidal tracts cause two important changes: (1) the flexion response becomes less brisk and (2) the toes no longer move upward, but instead moves downward because of the interval development of a normal plantar cutaneous reflex.[55] If pyramidal tract disease develops later in the person's life, the normal plantar cutaneous reflex disappears, and instead, painful stimulation of the foot causes the great toe to again move upward.

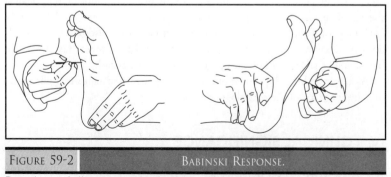

FIGURE 59-2	BABINSKI RESPONSE.

Drawing of the normal plantar cutaneous reflex (*left*) and the Babinski response (*right*), adapted from photographs taken by Babinski himself in 1900.[53]

The use of the term "extensor response" to describe the Babinski response is unfortunate and confusing: even though anatomists have always named the upward movement "extension" (e.g., great toe "extensor" muscle), physiologists have named the same upward movement "flexion" (e.g., the primitive "flexion response" discussed previously).

III. TECHNIQUE

A. ELICITING THE RESPONSE

Of the many ways to elicit this reflex,[56] a slow (i.e., 5 to 6 second) hockey-stick stroke beginning at the lateral plantar surface is best, using a wooden applicator stick, key, or pointed handle of the reflex hammer (see Fig. 59-2). This method is superior to other methods, including scratching the lateral sole, scratching below the lateral malleolus (Chaddock method), rubbing the anterior shin (Oppenheim method) or—the least effective stimulus—squeezing the calf (Gordon method).[57]

B. INTERPRETING THE RESPONSE

Helpful guidelines in assessing an equivocal toe response, based on careful electrodiagnostic studies and patient follow-up, are as follows: (1) The pathologic up-going toe results from contraction of the extensor hallucis longus muscle, whose tendon is conspicuous under the skin on top of the great toe.[58,59] Movement of the toe per se is not critical and may be prevented by joint disease. Moreover, the toe may seem to be upgoing—without contraction of the extensor hallucis longus muscle—when the ankle dorsiflexes or when the toe returns from an initial downward movement. (2) More than 90% of the time, the foot with the pathologic upgoing toe is weak or has difficulty with fine motor movements. An excellent test of fine motor movement is rapid foot tapping against the examiner's hand: normal persons accomplish 20 to 40 taps per 10 seconds. (3) The pathologic up-going toe coincides with a flexion response in the whole limb, which may be slight but is evident in the ipsilateral tensor fascia lata and hamstrings. (4) The pathologic up-going toe is reproducible.[55,60,61]

As Babinski himself pointed out, fanning of the toes is a normal phenomenon and not part of the pathologic response.[53,55]

IV. CLINICAL SIGNIFICANCE

A. ASSOCIATED CONDITIONS

The Babinski response is found in both destructive lesions of the pyramidal tracts (see Chapter 57) and in many metabolic disorders affecting these tracts, most of which are associated with altered mental status, such as seizures, meningitis, drug overdose, and renal and hepatic failure.[53]

B. FALSE-NEGATIVE RESPONSE

Patients may have pyramidal tract disease yet lack the up-going toe (i.e., false-negative response) because they have (1) spinal shock,[58] (2) a peroneal palsy denervating the muscles that dorsiflex the great toe (a common problem in bedridden patients because of pressure against the head of the fibula),[58] or (3) pyramidal tract disease sparing the muscles of the foot (e.g., upper motor neuron weakness is confined to the arm of that side).[62]

PRIMITIVE REFLEXES

I. DEFINITION

Primitive reflexes (or "release" reflexes) are a hodgepodge of reflexes that are normally present in infants but disappear during normal development of the central nervous system, only to reappear sometimes later in life when neurologic disease or aging removes (or "releases") the inhibiting influences of the central nervous system.[63] Among many primitive reflexes,[64] the more common ones are the palmomental reflex, glabellar reflex, grasp reflex, snout reflex, and suck reflex.

II. TECHNIQUE

A. PALMOMENTAL REFLEX

In this reflex, a key or other blunt object is used to apply an unpleasant stimulus to the patient's thenar eminence, stroking it briskly in a proximal to distal direction. A positive response is a brief contraction of the ipsilateral mentalis muscle, causing the ipsilateral lower lip to protrude, rise, or wrinkle.[65]

The wrinkle response at the corner of the mouth is probably the beginnings of a wince that would develop with more painful stimuli.[66] Theoretically, the stimulus could be applied anywhere on the skin of the patient's body, and in fact, descriptions of similar response after stimulation of the patient's arm, chest, trunk, sole of the foot, and tongue have all appeared.[66] The most sensitive area, however, is the thenar eminence.[67]

Marinesco and Radovici discovered the palmomental reflex in 1920.[66]

B. GLABELLAR REFLEX

The stimulus for the glabellar reflex is light taps with the finger or soft rubber reflex hammer, about two times per second, over the patient's glabella. Although most normal persons respond to this by blinking bilaterally, the blinking stops after the first few taps in normal individuals. Persistent blinking is a positive response, although there is no consensus whether habituation should be indefinite or just beyond a certain number of blinks (e.g., >4 successive blinks).

The glabellar reflex is sometimes called the "blink reflex" or "Myerson's reflex," although the original description was by Overend in 1896.[68]

C. GRASP REFLEX

In the grasp reflex, the clinician places his or her index and middle fingers over the thenar aspect of the patient's wrist and exerts pressure on the skin while withdrawing the fingers between the patient's thumb and index finger. In a positive response, the patient grasps the clinician's fingers, and the grasp progressively increases as the clinician attempts to withdraw.[64]

III. CLINICAL SIGNIFICANCE

A. GENERAL COMMENTS

Primitive reflexes are common findings in frontal lobe disease,[69] Parkinson's disease,[70-72] dementias,[73-77] and advanced human immunodeficiency virus (HIV) infection.[78] Other than the grasp reflex (see later), the precise neuroanatomic cause of these reflexes is unknown.

B. PALMOMENTAL REFLEX

The palmomental reflex is bilateral 38% to 75% of the time and unilateral 25% to 62% of the time.[79,80] The side of the reflex does not correlate with the side of the lesion.[65,79] In one study of 39 patients with a unilateral palmomental reflex, 44% had an ipsilateral cerebral hemispheric lesion, 36% a contralateral lesion, 10% bilateral lesions, and 10% no lesions.[80] In patients with Parkinson's disease, the palmomental reflex correlates with the degree of akinesia, and the reflex often disappears with the onset of levodopa-induced dyskinesias.[70]

C. GLABELLAR REFLEX

The afferent limb of the glabellar reflex is the trigeminal nerve, and the efferent limb is the facial nerve. Lesions of either nerve may interrupt the reflex (although in facial nerve palsy, the blinking continues on the sound side). This reflex is also a common finding in Parkinson's disease, and in these patients, the positive response may reverse after administration of levodopa.[71]

D. GRASP REFLEX

A positive grasp reflex is common in frontal lobe disease and, if both arms can be tested (i.e., no paralysis), the grasp reflex when present is usually bilateral.[69]

In patients with dementia, the sign correlates with more severe cognitive and functional impairment and greater loss of pyramidal cells in the frontal lobe.[73,74,77] Among patients admitted to a neurologic ward, a positive grasp reflex (defined as no habituation with three successive strokes) predicted discrete lesions in the frontal lobe or deep nuclei and subcortical white matter with a sensitivity of 13%, specificity 99% and positive LR of 20.2.[69]

E. PRIMITIVE REFLEXES AND NORMAL AGING

The palmomental and glabellar reflexes, but not the grasp reflex, also are described to occur in normal persons, although the reported frequencies from different studies vary widely.[75,76,78,81] The reported frequency for the palmomental sign in normal persons varies from 3% to 70%; that for the glabellar sign, from 3% to 33%.[70,76,78,81–84] A few of these "normal" persons with primitive reflexes undoubtedly have subclinical disease, as indicated by lesions in the basal ganglia or subcortical white matter on MRI imaging.[82] Others, however, have no evidence of neurologic disease; although, importantly, their findings differ from the pathologic response in two important ways: (1) the primitive reflex of patients without neurologic lesions is weak and fatigable, disappearing after the first few repetitive stimuli spaced evenly apart,[63] and (2) the primitive reflex of patients without neurologic lesions is an isolated finding. For example, less than 1% of normal persons have a positive palmomental reflex, if it is defined as persistence beyond 5 or more strokes of the thenar eminence.[67,70] In addition, even if the definition of a positive response includes fatigable primitive reflexes, less than 12% of normal persons have two primitive reflexes, and less than 2% have three or more primitive reflexes.[78,81,83–85]

REFERENCES

1. Louis ED. Erb and Westphal: Simultaneous discovery of the deep tendon reflexes. *Semin Neurol.* 2002;22:385-389.
2. Schiller F. The reflex hammer: In memoriam Robert Wartenberg (1887-1956). *Med Hist.* 1967;11:75-85.
3. Tyler KL, McHenry LC. Fragments of neurological history: The knee jerk and other tendon reflexes. *Neurology.* 1983;33:609-610.
4. Lanska DJ. The history of reflex hammers. *Neurology.* 1989;39:1542-1549.
5. Rooke ED. The Tromner hammer: A historical postscript. *Proc Mayo Clin.* 1960; 35:355-356.
6. Pryse-Phillips W. *Companion to clinical neurology.* Boston: Little, Brown and Company; 1995.
7. Finelli PF. Reflex hammer with built-in pin. *Neurology.* 1991;41:344.

8. Nieuwenhuys R. Bolk's studies of segmental anatomy. *Acta Morphol Neerl Scand.* 1975;13:7-33.

9. Wolf JK. *Segmental neurology: A guide to the examination and interpretation of sensory and motor function.* Baltimore: University Park Press; 1981.

10. Brendler SJ. The human cervical myotomes: Functional anatomy studied at operation. *J Neurosurg.* 1968;28:105-111.

11. Levin KH, Maggiano HJ, Wilbourn AJ. Cervical radiculopathies: Comparison of surgical and EMG localization of single-root lesions. *Neurology.* 1996;46:1022-1025.

12. Liguori R, Krarup C, Trojaborg W. Determination of the segmental sensory and motor innervation of lumbosacral spinal nerves. *Brain.* 1992;115:915-934.

13. Thage O. The myotomes L2-S2 in man. *Acta Neurol Scand.* 1965;41(Suppl 13):241-243.

14. Wilbourn AJ, Aminoff MJ. AAEM minimonograph 32: The electrodiagnostic examination in patients with radiculopathies. *Musc Nerv.* 1998;21:1612-1631.

15. Young JH. The revision of the dermatomes. *Aust N Z J Surg.* 1949;18:171-186.

16. Yoss RE, Corbin KB, MacCarty CS, Love JG. Significance of symptoms and signs in localization of involved root in cervical disk protrusion. *Neurology.* 1957;7:673-683.

17. Makin GJV, Brown WF, Ebers GC. C7 radiculopathy: Importance of scapular winging in clinical diagnosis. *J Neurol Neurosurg Psychiatry.* 1986;49:640-644.

18. Medical Research Council. *Aids to the examination of the peripheral nervous system.* London: Bailliere Tindall; 1986.

19. Schwartz RS, Morris JGL, Crimmins D, et al. A comparison of two methods of eliciting the ankle jerk. *Aust N Z J Med.* 1990;20:116-119.

20. O'Keeffe STO, Smith T, Valacio R, et al. A comparison of two techniques for ankle jerk assessment in elderly subjects. *Lancet.* 1994;344:1619-1620.

21. Clarke CE, Davies P, Wilson T, Nutbeam T. Comparison of the tendon and plantar strike methods of eliciting the ankle reflex. *J Neurol Neurosurg Psychiatry.* 2005;74:1351-1352.

22. Wiebers DO et al, editors. Members of the Mayo Clinic Department of Neurology. *Mayo Clinic examinations in neurology,* 7th ed. St. Louis: Mosby; 1998.

23. Hallett M. NINDS myotatic reflex scale. *Neurology.* 1993;43:2723.

24. Gassel MM, Diamantopoulos E. The Jendrassik maneuver. I. The pattern of reinforcement of monosynaptic reflexes in normal subjects and patients with spasticity or rigidity. *Neurology.* 1964;14:555-560.

25. Kawamura T, Watanabe S. Timing as a prominent factor of the Jandrassik manoeuvre on the H reflex. *J Neurol Neurosurg Psychiatry.* 1975;38:508-516.

26. Impallomeni M, Flynn MD, Kenny RA, et al. The elderly and their ankle jerks. *Lancet.* 1984;1:670-672.

27. Wartenberg R. Studies in reflexes: History, physiology, synthesis and nomenclature. I. *Arch Neurol Psychiatry.* 1944;51:113-133.

28. Wartenberg R. Studies in reflexes: History, physiology, synthesis and nomenclature. II. *Arch Neurol Psychiatry*. 1944;52:341-358.
29. Wartenberg R. Studies in reflexes: History, physiology, synthesis and nomenclature. III. *Arch Neurol Psychiatry*. 1944;52:359-382.
30. Bowditch MG, Sanderson P, Livesey JP. The significance of an absent ankle reflex. *J Bone Joint Surg Br*. 1996;78B:276-279.
31. Echols DH. The Hoffman sign: Its incidence in university students. *J Nerv Ment Dis*. 1936;84:427-431.
32. Lauder TD, Dillingham TR, Andary M, et al. Predicting electodiagnostic outcome in patients with upper limb symptoms: Are the history and physical examination helpful? *Arch Phys Med Rehabil*. 2000;81:436-441.
33. Kortelainen P, Puranen J, Koivisto E, Laehde S. Symptoms and signs of sciatica and their relation to the localization of the lumbar disc herniation. *Spine*. 1985;10:88-92.
34. Lauder TD, Dillingham TR, Andary M, et al. Effect of history and exam in predicting electrodiagnostic outcome among patients with suspected lumbosacral radiculopathy. *Am J Phys Med Rehabil*. 2000;79:60-68.
35. Portnoy HD, Ahmad M. Value of the neurological examination, electromyography and myelography in herniated lumbar disc. *Mich Med*. 1972;71:429-434.
36. Kerr RSC, Cadoux-Hudson TA, Adams CBT. The value of accurate clinical assessment in the surgical management of the lumbar disc protrusion. *J Neurol Neurosurg Psychiatry*. 1988;51:169-173.
37. Jensen OH. The level-diagnosis of a lower lumbar disc herniation: The value of sensibility and motor testing. *Clin Rheumatol*. 1987;6:564-569.
38. Friel JP, ed. *Dorland's illustrated medical dictionary*, 25th ed. Philadelphia: WB Saunders; 1974.
39. Lanska DJ. Morris James Lewis (1852-1928) and the description of the jaw jerk. *J Child Neurol*. 1991;6:235-236.
40. Iansek R. The effects of reflex path length on clonus frequency in spastic muscles. *J Neurol Neurosurg Psychiatry*. 1984;47:1122-1124.
41. Lance JW, DeGail P. Spread of phasic muscle reflexes in normal and spastic subjects. *J Neurol Neurosurg Psychiatry*. 1965;28:328-334.
42. Teasdall RD, van den Ende H. The crossed adductor reflex in humans: An EMG study. *Can J Neurol Sci*. 1981;8:81-85.
43. Estanol BV, Marin OSM. Mechanism of the inverted supinator reflex: A clinical and neurophysiological study. *J Neurol Neurosurg Psychiatry*. 1976;39:905-908.
44. Lance JW. Mechanism of the inverted supinator reflex. *J Neurol Neurosurg Psychiatry*. 1977;40:207.
45. Boyle RS, Shakir RA, Weir AI, McInnes A. Inverted knee jerk: A neglected localising sign in spinal cord disease. *J Neurol Neurosurg Psychiatry*. 1979;42:1005-1007.
46. Babu K, Kandasamy V, Thangavelu KS, Subrahmanyam M. Statistical approach to a neurological problem. *J Indian Med Assoc*. 1974;62:344-347, 358-349.

47. Madonick MJ. Statistical control studies in neurology. VIII. The cutaneous abdominal reflex. *Neurology.* 1957;7:459-465.

48. Yngve D. Abdominal reflexes. *J Ped Orthop.* 1997;17:105-108.

49. Hargrove GK, Bors E. The suprapubic abdominal reflex: A useful method to assess the function of the sacral reflex arcs. *J Urol.* 1972;107:243-244.

50. Blaivas JG, Zayed AAH, Labib KB. The bulbocavernosus reflex in urology: A prospective study of 299 patients. *J Urol.* 1981;126:197-199.

51. Bors E, Blinn KA. Bulbocavernosus reflex. *J Urol.* 1959;82:128-130.

52. Lapides J, Bobbitt JM. Diagnostic value of bulbocavernous reflex. *JAMA.* 1956;162:971-972.

53. van Gijn J. *The Babinski sign: A centenary.* Utrecht: Universiteit Utrecht; 1996.

54. Lance JW. The Babinski sign. *J Neurol Neurosurg Psychiatry.* 2002;73:360-362.

55. van Gijn J. The Babinski reflex. *Postgrad Med J.* 1995;71:645-648.

56. Goetz CG. History of the extensor plantar response: Babinski and Chaddock signs. *Semin Neurol.* 2002;22:391-398.

57. Dohrman GJ, Nowace WJ. The upgoing great toe: Optimal method of elicitation. *Lancet.* 1973;1:339-341.

58. Landau WM, Clare MH. The plantar reflex in man, with special reference to some conditions where the extensor response is unexpectedly absent. *Brain.* 1959;82:321-355.

59. van Gijn J. Babinski response: Stimulus and effector. *J Neurol Neurosurg Psychiatry.* 1975;38:180-186.

60. van Gijn J. The Babinski sign and the pyramidal syndrome. *J Neurol Neurosurg Psychiatry.* 1978;41:865-873.

61. van Gijn J. Equivocal plantar responses: A clinical and electromyographic study. *J Neurol Neurosurg Psychiatry.* 1976;39:275-282.

62. Fulton JF, Keller AD. *The sign of Babinski: A study of the evolution of cortical dominance in primates.* Springfield: Charles C. Thomas; 1932.

63. Vreeling FW, Jolles J, Verhey FRJ, Houx PJ. Primitive reflexes in healthy, adult volunteers and neurological patients: Methodological issues. *J Neurol.* 1993;240:495-504.

64. Schott JM, Rossor MN. The grasp and other primitive reflexes. *J Neurol Neurosurg Psychiatry.* 2003;74:558-560.

65. Owen G, Mulley GP. The palmomental reflex: A useful clinical sign? *J Neurol Neurosurg Psychiatry.* 2002;73:113-115.

66. Reis DJ, Sweden S. The palmomental reflex. *Arch Neurol.* 1961;4:486-498.

67. Marti-Vilalta JL, Graus F. The palmomental reflex: Clinical study of 300 cases. *Eur Neurol.* 1984;23:12-16.

68. Fine EJ, Sentz L, Soria E. The history of the blink reflex. *Neurology.* 1992;42:450-454.

69. De Renzi E, Barbieri C. The incidence of the grasp reflex following hemispheric lesion and its relation to frontal damage. *Brain.* 1992;115:293-313.

70. De Noordhout AM, Delwaide PJ. The palmomental reflex in Parkinson's disease: Comparisons with normal subjects and clinical relevance. *Arch Neurol.* 1988;45:425-427.

71. Klawans HL, Goodwin JA. Reversal of the glabellar reflex in Parkinsonism. *J Neurol Neurosurg Psychiatry.* 1969;32:423-427.

72. Brodsky H, Vuong KD, Thomas M, Jankovic J. Glabellar and palmomental reflexes in parkinsonian disorders. *Neurology.* 2004;63:1096-1098.

73. Forstl H, Burns A, Levy R, et al. Neurologic signs in Alzheimer's disease: Results of a prospective clinical and neuropathologic study. *Arch Neurol.* 1992;49:1038-1042.

74. Molloy DW, Clarnette RM, Mellroy WE, et al. Clinical significance of primitive reflexes in Alzheimer's disease. *J Am Geriatr Soc.* 1991;39:1160-1163.

75. Vreeling FW, Houx PJ, Jolles J, Verhey FRJ. Primitive reflexes in Alzheimer's disease and vascular dementia. *J Geriatr Psych Neurol.* 1995;8:111-117.

76. Hogan DB, Ebly EM. Primitive reflexes and dementia: Results from the Canadian study of health and aging. *Age Ageing.* 1995;24:375-381.

77. Burns A, Jacoby R, Levy R. Neurological signs in Alzheimer's disease. *Age Ageing.* 1991;20:45-51.

78. Tremont-Lukats IW, Teixeira GM, Hernandez DE. Primitive reflexes in a case-control study of patients with advanced human immunodeficiency virus type 1. *J Neurol.* 1999;246:540-543.

79. Whittle IR, Miller JD. Clinical usefulness of the palmomental reflex. *Med J Aust.* 1987;146:137-139.

80. Gotkine M, Haggiag S, Abramsky O, Biran I. Lack of hemispheric localizing value of the palmomental reflex. *Neurology.* 2005;64:1656.

81. Brown DL, Smith TL, Knepper LE. Evaluation of five primitive reflexes in 240 young adults. *Neurology.* 1998;51:322.

82. Kobayashi S, Yamaguchi S, Okada K, Yamashita K. Primitive reflexes and MRI findings, cerebral blood flow in normal elderly. *Gerontology.* 1990;36:199-205.

83. Isakov E, Sazgon L, Costeff H, et al. The diagnostic value of three common primitive reflexes. *Eur Neurol.* 1984;23:17-21.

84. Jacobs L, Gossman MD. Three primitive reflexes in normal adults. *Neurology.* 1980;30:184-188.

85. Di Legge S, Di Piero V, Altieri M, et al. Usefulness of primitive reflexes in demented and non-demented cerebrovascular patients in daily clinical practice. *Eur Neurol.* 2001;45:104-110.

Disorders of the Nerve Roots, Plexi, and Peripheral Nerves

I. INTRODUCTION

Nerve roots destined to innervate the limbs exit through vertebral foramina and intermingle in plexi (i.e., the brachial and lumbosacral plexi) before emerging as peripheral nerves that extend to the fingers and toes. Lesions anywhere along this pathway—from spinal nerve roots to the final peripheral nerve branch—produce combinations of pain, *lower* motor neuron weakness, and sensory loss.

A lesion in the nerve root is called radiculopathy; one in the plexus, plexopathy, and; one in the peripheral nerve, peripheral neuropathy. This chapter emphasizes how to distinguish these lesions in patients with nerve complaints of the arms or legs. Because the neuroanatomy of these lesions is complex, accurate diagnosis requires systematic examination of all the limb's muscles, sensation, and reflexes.

II. THE ARM

A. INTRODUCTION

In patients presenting with upper extremity nerve complaints, the most common neurologic diagnosis is carpal tunnel syndrome, followed by polyneuropathy, ulnar neuropathy, and cervical radiculopathy.[1-3] Other focal neuropathies and plexopathies are less common. Most cervical radiculopathies affect the C6 or C7 root.[4-7]

B. NEUROLOGIC FINDINGS

1. Motor

Most muscles of the arm are innervated by nerves from more than one spinal segment. Table 60-1 presents the relationship between the different peripheral

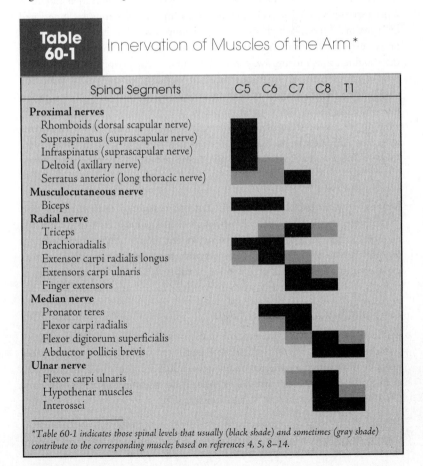

Table 60-1	Innervation of Muscles of the Arm*

Spinal Segments	C5	C6	C7	C8	T1
Proximal nerves					
Rhomboids (dorsal scapular nerve)					
Supraspinatus (suprascapular nerve)					
Infraspinatus (suprascapular nerve)					
Deltoid (axillary nerve)					
Serratus anterior (long thoracic nerve)					
Musculocutaneous nerve					
Biceps					
Radial nerve					
Triceps					
Brachioradialis					
Extensor carpi radialis longus					
Extensors carpi ulnaris					
Finger extensors					
Median nerve					
Pronator teres					
Flexor carpi radialis					
Flexor digitorum superficialis					
Abductor pollicis brevis					
Ulnar nerve					
Flexor carpi ulnaris					
Hypothenar muscles					
Interossei					

*Table 60-1 indicates those spinal levels that usually (black shade) and sometimes (gray shade) contribute to the corresponding muscle; based on references 4, 5, 8–14.

nerves (grouped in rows) and their corresponding spinal roots (in columns). The spinal levels listed in Table 60-1 are based on several lines of evidence, including Bolk's detailed dissection of a single human subject,[8,9] electrodiagnostic studies,[10,11] and bedside observations of patients with documented spinal root lesions.[5,12]

a.   Radiculopathy

Even though most muscles receive innervation from more than one spinal nerve root, injury to one root is usually sufficient to cause significant loss of power. The motor examination of radiculopathy has two characteristics: (1) Weakness affects two or more muscles from the same spinal segment but different peripheral nerves (i.e., all of the weak muscles are in the same *column* in Table 60-1). For example, a C6 radiculopathy may simultaneously weaken the elbow flexion (biceps muscle, musculocutaneous nerve) and wrist extension (radial and ulnar wrist extensors, radial nerve).[5] (2) Weakness may involve muscles innervated by "proximal nerves," which are listed in the top rows of Table 60-1. Proximal nerves originate from the nerve roots but then promptly innervate muscles of the shoulder, thus moving away from the course of the peripheral nerves of the arm. Therefore, if a muscle innervated by one of these nerves is weak in a patient with nerve complaints of the arm or hand, the lesion must be a proximal one near the nerve roots. A common example is the finding of scapular winging (i.e., weak serratus anterior muscle, long thoracic nerve) in a patient with arm pain and triceps weakness. Involvement of the serratus anterior points to the C7 root and away from the radial nerve or brachial plexus.[13]

b.   Brachial Plexopathy

Lesions of the brachial plexus cause simultaneous weakness of muscles from two or more adjacent spinal segments (i.e., adjacent *columns* in Table 60-1) and from two or more peripheral nerves. Brachial plexus lesions usually affect either the upper plexus (C5-6) as a group, causing weakness of the shoulder and upper arm but sparing all muscles of the hand, or the lower plexus (C7-T1) as a group, affecting all muscles of the hand but sparing those of the shoulder and upper arm.

c.   Peripheral Nerve Disorders

These lesions weaken two or more muscles from a *single* peripheral nerve (which may have different spinal segments) and spare muscles from other nerves. For example, a complete radial nerve injury weakens the brachioradialis muscle (C5-6)*, elbow extension (triceps, C7), wrist extension (wrist extensors, C6-7), and finger extension (finger extensors, C8).

---

*Testing elbow flexion with the forearm midway between supination and pronation reveals brachioradialis weakness.[14]

In Table 60-1, the muscles belonging to each peripheral nerve are listed in the order that their branches diverge from the main trunk. Therefore, a proximal lesion of the radial nerve in the axilla would cause the findings described in the previous paragraph, but a lesion of the radial nerve at the elbow, after the branch to the extensor carpi radialis longus, spares the triceps and brachioradialis but weakens more distal muscles (i.e., wrist and finger extensors).

Some peripheral nerve lesions can be recognized at a glance, such as the wrist drop of radial neuropathy and the "claw hand" appearance of ulnar neuropathy (Fig. 60-1). A callus over the hypothenar eminence in a patient with ulnar muscle weakness suggests damage to the deep branch of the ulnar nerve, caused by chronic pressure on the heel of the hand from bicycling or using a walker.[15,16]

2. Sensory Findings

Radiculopathy causes sensory loss in a dermatomal pattern (see Table 58-1 and Fig. 58-1 in Chapter 58). Brachial plexus lesions cause sensory loss from adjacent dermatomes. Peripheral nerve lesions cause the sensory loss described in

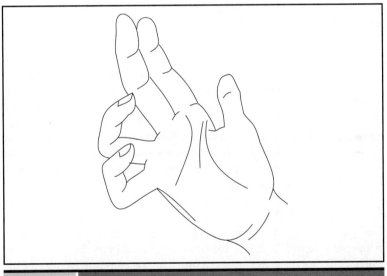

| FIGURE 60-1 | "CLAW HAND" OF ULNAR NERVE PALSY. |

All metacarpophalangeal joints are hyperextended because of paralysis of all interossei and unopposed action of finger extensors (radial nerve). The hyperextension is less prominent in the index and middle fingers because the lumbricals of these digits, innervated by the median nerve, act to flex the joint. Tethering from the flexor tendons causes all interphalangeal joints to flex.

| Table 60-2 | Sensory Branches of Peripheral Nerves of the Arm |

Nerve	Sensory Branches
Musculocutaneous nerve	Radial aspect forearm
Radial nerve	Dorsal arm and forearm
	Radial aspect dorsal hand
Median nerve	Radial palm
	First three digits and radial aspect ring finger
Ulnar nerve	Ulnar aspect of hand and digits

Table 60-2 (in Table 60-2, the branches are listed in proximal to distal order: therefore a proximal radial nerve lesion affects sensation of the posterior arm, forearm, *and* hand; one at the elbow affects only the dorsal hand).

One pure sensory syndrome of the arm is "cheiralgia paresthetica," from injury to the superficial branch of the radial nerve, usually because of too tight a wrist band or hand cuffs. Sensory findings are confined to the radial aspect of the dorsal hand.[17]

3. Reflexes

The three muscle stretch reflexes of the arm are the biceps (musculocutaneous nerve, C5-6), brachioradialis (radial nerve, C5-6), and triceps (radial nerve, C7-8).* Therefore, the finding of abnormal reflexes *excludes* both median and ulnar neuropathies and instead *argues for* radiculopathy or plexopathy. Radial nerve lesions usually spare the brachioradialis and triceps reflex because the branches to these muscles diverge from the main trunk proximally in the axilla, and most injuries to this nerve occur at a more distal point (e.g., humeral fracture or "Saturday night palsy").

4. Provocative Tests

One traditional test for cervical radiculopathy is "Spurling's test" or "neck compression test." In this test, the clinician turns and tilts the patient's head and neck toward the painful side and then adds a compressive force to the top of the head.[18] Aggravation of pain is a positive response. "Tinel's" and "Phalen's" signs, used traditionally to diagnose carpal tunnel syndrome, are discussed below.

---

*Even though weakness of the triceps may follow lesions in the C6 or C7 roots (C7 is most common; see Table 60-1), the absent triceps jerk usually results from C7 or C8 lesions.[5]

C. ADDITIONAL DIAGNOSTIC CLUES

1. The Clavicle

The brachial plexus lies just behind the clavicle. Therefore, additional physical findings in the supraclavicular space, such as mass, adenopathy, hemorrhage, or other evidence of trauma, suggest injury to the brachial plexus. Trauma *above* the clavicle injures roots; that *below* the clavicle injures peripheral nerves.

2. Horner's Syndrome (See Chapter 19)

An associated Horner's syndrome (i.e., ipsilateral small pupil and ptosis) indicates radiculopathy (C8-T1) or a lesion of the lower brachial plexus.

D. CLINICAL SIGNIFICANCE

1. Diagnosing Cervical Radiculopathy

EBM Box 60-1 presents the diagnostic accuracy of bedside examination for cervical radiculopathy, as applied to patients presenting with neck pain, arm pain, or both. In these patients, the most compelling arguments *for* radiculopathy are reduced biceps reflex (likelihood ratio [LR] = 9.1, see EBM Box 60-1), reduction of any arm reflex (i.e., biceps, brachioradialis, or triceps reflex, LR = 3.6), and a positive Spurling's test (LR = 3.6).[7,19] Findings arguing *against* radiculopathy are normal rotation of the neck (i.e., can rotate to affected side > 60°, LR = 0.2) and the absence of arm muscle weakness (LR = 0.4).

Despite its modest accuracy, however, Spurling's test should probably *not* be performed. In other studies of cervical radiculopathy, its sensitivity is only 9% to 16%,[20,21] and in patients with rheumatoid arthritis, cervical malformations, or metastatic disease, the test risks serious injury to the spine.

2. Localizing Cervical Radiculopathy

EBM Box 60-2 presents the diagnostic accuracy of the motor, sensory, and reflex examination in patients with known cervical radiculopathy, illustrating the accuracy of findings in predicting the exact level of the lesion. According to these LRs, the best indicator of C5 radiculopathy is weak elbow flexion (LR = 5.3). A diminished biceps or brachioradialis reflex (LR = 14.2), sensory loss affecting the thumb (LR = 8.5), and weak wrist extension (LR = 2.3) indicate C6 radiculopathy. Weak elbow extension (LR = 4.0) and a diminished triceps reflex (LR = 3.0) argue *for* C7 radiculopathy, whereas normal elbow extensor strength argues modestly *against* this diagnosis (LR = 0.4). Sensory loss affecting the little finger (LR = 41.4) and weak finger flexion (LR = 3.8) indicate C8 radiculopathy.

These LRs show that each of the indicator muscles discussed in Chapter 57 (i.e., elbow flexion for C5, wrist extension for C6, elbow extension for C7, and finger flexion for C8) predict the level involved (LRs = 2.3–5.3). The weaker

Box 60-1 · Diagnosing Cervical Radiculopathy in Patients with Neck and Arm Pain*

Finding[†]	Sensitivity (%)	Specificity (%)	Likelihood Ratio if Finding	
			Present	Absent
Motor examination				
Weakness of any arm muscle[6]	73	61	1.9	0.4
Sensory examination				
Reduced vibration or pinprick sensation in arm[6]	38	46	NS	NS
Reflex examination				
Reduced biceps reflex[6]	10	99	**9.1**	NS
Reduced brachioradialis reflex[6]	8	99	NS	NS
Reduced triceps reflex[6]	10	95	NS	NS
Reduced biceps, triceps or brachioradialis reflex[6]	21	94	**3.6**	0.8
Other tests				
Spurling's test[7,19]	30-50	84-93	**3.6**	0.7
Rotation of neck to involved side <60°[7]	89	48	1.7	**0.2**

NS, not significant; likelihood ratio (LR) if finding present = positive LR; LR if finding absent = negative LR.
*Diagnostic standard: For cervical radiculopathy, electromyography and nerve conduction studies.
†Definition of findings: For Spurling's test, see text.

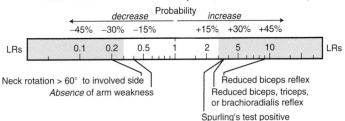

Localizing Cervical Radiculopathy*

Finding	Sensitivity (%)	Specificity (%)	Likelihood Ratio if Finding	
			Present	Absent
Motor examination				
Weak elbow flexion, detecting C5 radiculopathy[5]	83	84	**5.3**	NS
Weak wrist extension, detecting C6 radiculopathy[5]	37	84	2.3	NS
Weak elbow extension, detecting C7 radiculopathy[5]	65	84	**4.0**	0.4
Weak finger flexion, detecting C8 radiculopathy[5]	50	87	**3.8**	NS
Sensory examination				
Sensory loss affecting thumb, detecting C6 radiculopathy[5]	32	96	**8.5**	NS
Sensory loss affecting middle finger, detecting C7 radiculopathy[5]	5	98	NS	NS
Sensory loss affecting little finger, detecting C8 radiculopathy[5]	23	99	**41.4**	NS
Reflex examination				
Diminished biceps or brachioradialis reflex, detecting C6 radiculopathy[5]	53	96	**14.2**	0.5
Diminished triceps reflex, detecting C7 radiculopathy[5,6]	15-65	81-93	**3.0**	NS

NS, not significant; likelihood ratio (LR) if finding present = positive LR; LR if finding absent = negative LR.
Diagnostic standard: For level of radiculopathy, surgical findings[5] or electrodiagnosis.[6]

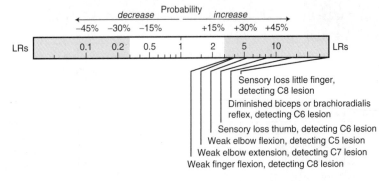

LOCALIZING CERVICAL RADICULOPATHY

a muscle is, the more significant its localizing value.[5] Also, although certain sensory findings are diagnostic (e.g., sensory loss affecting little finger of C8 radiculopathy, LR = 41.4), less than one in three patients with cervical radiculopathy have any sensory loss, and therefore the finding of *normal* sensation is never a compelling argument *against* cervical radiculopathy (i.e., negative LRs for all sensory findings are not significant).

Importantly, the LRs in EBM Box 60-2 apply only to patients with cervical radiculopathy. Patients with carpal tunnel syndrome may also develop hypesthesia of the thumb and those with ulnar neuropathy may develop hypesthesia of the little finger, although in these patients, the arm reflexes and arm and wrist strength are normal.

3. Plexopathy in Cancer Patients

If brachial plexopathy develops in a patient with cancer who has received radiation near the shoulder, the question arises whether the plexopathy is due to metastatic disease or radiation injury. Findings arguing for *metastatic* involvement are motor and sensory findings confined to C7-T1 (LR = 30.9) and Horner's syndrome (LR = 4.1). Findings arguing for *radiation* injury are motor and sensory findings confined to C5C6 (LR = 8.8) and lymphedema of the ipsilateral arm (LR = 4.9).[22]

4. Peripheral Nerve Injury: Diagnosis of Carpal Tunnel Syndrome

EBM Box 60-3 summarizes the diagnostic accuracy of findings for the most common peripheral neuropathy of the arm, carpal tunnel syndrome. According to this table, three findings argue modestly *for* carpal tunnel syndrome: diminished pain sensation in the distribution of the median nerve (LR = 3.1), a square wrist ratio (defined in footnote of EBM Box 60-3,

Box 60-3   Diagnosing Carpal Tunnel Syndrome*

Finding (Ref)[†]	Sensitivity (%)	Specificity (%)	Likelihood Ratio if Finding	
			Present	Absent
Hand diagram				
"Classic" or "probable"[23]	64	73	2.4	0.5
"Unlikely"[23]	4	...	**0.2**	...
Motor examination				
Weak thumb abduction[24,25]	63–66	62–66	1.8	0.5
Thenar atrophy[25–27]	4–28	82–99	NS	NS
Sensory examination (median distribution)				
Hypalgesia[24,26]	15–51	85–93	**3.1**	NS
Diminished 2-point discrimination[25,27,28]	6–32	64–99	NS	NS
Abnormal vibration sensation[25,28]	20–61	71–81	NS	NS
Diminished monofilament sensation[28,29]	59–98	15–59	NS	NS
Other tests				
Tinel's sign[24–28,30,31]	23–60	64–91	1.5	NS
Phalen's sign[24–28,30–33]	10–91	33–86	1.3	0.8
Pressure provocation test[24,28,32–34]	28–63	33–74	NS	NS
Square wrist ratio[24,35]	47–69	73–83	2.7	0.5
Flick sign[31,36]	37–93	74–96	NS	NS

NS, not significant; likelihood ratio (LR) if finding present = positive LR; LR if finding absent = negative LR.

*Diagnostic standard: For carpal tunnel syndrome, abnormal motor or sensory conduction within the carpal tunnel, measured by nerve conduction testing.

†Definition of findings: For hand diagram, see text; for all sensory findings, perception diminished in index finger compared with ipsilateral little finger (2-point discrimination used compass points separated by 4–6 mm, vibratory sensation used 126- or 256-Hz tuning fork, monofilament sensation abnormal if >2.83); for Tinel's sign, Phalen's sign, and pressure provocation test, the positive response is paresthesias in distribution of median nerve, although each test uses a different stimulus—tapping on the distal wrist crease over the median nerve (Tinel's sign), maximal wrist flexion for 60 seconds (Phalen's sign), and firm pressure with examiner's thumbs on palmar aspect of patient's distal wrist crease for 60 seconds (pressure provocation test)[37]; for square wrist ratio, antero-posterior dimension of wrist divided by medio-lateral dimension, measured with calipers at distal wrist crease, is ≥0.70[38]; and for Flick sign, on asking the patient, "What do you actually do with your hand(s) when the symptoms are at their worst?," the patient demonstrates a flicking movement of the wrist and hand, similar to that employed in shaking down a thermometer.[36]

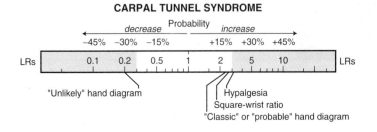

LR 2.7), and a "classic" or "probable" hand diagram (LR = 2.4)*. The most compelling finding arguing *against* carpal tunnel syndrome is an "unlikely" hand diagram (LR = 0.2). Several traditional tests such as Tinel's and Phalen's sign and other novel ones such as the pressure provocation and flick signs (defined in EBM Box 60-3), do not distinguish carpal tunnel syndrome from other common disorders causing hand dysesthesias (such as polyneuropathy, ulnar neuropathy, or radiculopathy, using electrodiagnosis as the diagnostic standard).[1,37]

III. THE LEG

A. INTRODUCTION

Among patients presenting with lower extremity nerve complaints, the most common neurologic diagnosis is by far lumbosacral radiculopathy, which almost always affects the L5 or S1 roots (each are affected with about the same frequency).[4,40–45]

B. NEUROLOGIC FINDINGS

1. Motor

Table 60-3 presents the innervation of the muscles of the leg, showing the relationship between different spinal roots (in columns) and the different peripheral nerves (grouped in rows).

---

*The Katz hand diagram is a self-administered diagram of the hand that depicts the patient's symptoms: the "classic" pattern depicts symptoms affecting at least two of digits 1, 2, or 3 but sparing the palm and dorsum of hand; the "probable" pattern is similar to the classic pattern, although palm symptoms are allowed; the "unlikely" pattern depicts symptoms not involving digits 1, 2, or 3.[23] Palm symptoms are not part of the "classic" pattern because the palmar cutaneous branch of the median nerve does not travel through the carpal tunnel.[39]

Table 60-3 Innervation of the Muscles of the Leg*

Spinal Segments	L2	L3	L4	L5	S1	S2
Proximal nerves						
Gluteus medius (gluteal nerves; internal rotation and abduction of hip)			■	■	▦	
Gluteus maximus (gluteal nerves; extension of hip)				▦	■	▦
Femoral nerve						
Iliopsoas	■	■	▦			
Quadriceps	▦	■	■			
Obturator nerve						
Thigh adductors	■	■	▦			
Sciatic nerve trunk[†]						
Hamstrings (knee flexion)				■	■	
Peroneal nerve[†]						
Tibialis anterior (dorsiflexion of ankle)			■	■		
Extensors of toes				■	▦	
Peroneal longus (eversion of ankle)				■	■	
Tibial nerve[†]						
Tibialis posterior (inversion of ankle)			■	■		
Gastrocnemius				▦	■	■
Flexor digitorum (curl toes)				▦	■	■

*Table 60-3 indicates those spinal levels that usually (black shade) and sometimes (gray shade) contribute to the corresponding muscle; based on references 4, 8, 9, 12, 14, 46, 47.
†The sciatic nerve trunk divides above the knee into the peroneal and tibial nerves. Therefore, lesions of the sciatic nerve trunk affect muscles of all three branches (see text).

a. Radiculopathy

Like radiculopathy of the arm, radiculopathy of the leg has two characteristics: (1) Weakness affects two or more muscles from the same spinal segment but different peripheral nerves (i.e., all muscles innervated by same *column* in Table 60-3). For example, an L5 radiculopathy may affect both the dorsiflexors of the foot and toes (peroneal nerve) and inversion of the foot (tibial nerve). (2) Weakness may involve "proximal nerves" to the glutei muscles (which cause characteristic abnormalities of the gait, i.e., either the gluteus maximus gait or Trendelenburg gait; see Chapter 5).

b. Lumbosacral Plexopathy

Unlike brachial plexus lesions, lumbosacral plexopathies tend to affect the entire leg (L2-S1) simultaneously, and discrete upper and lower plexus syndromes are rare.[48,49]

c. Peripheral Nerve Disorders

Peripheral nerve lesions weaken two or more muscles from a *single* peripheral nerve (which may belong to different spinal segments) and spare muscles from other nerves. For example, more than 85% of patients with foot drop because of peroneal nerve injury have weak ankle dorsiflexion (L4-5) and eversion (L5-S1) but preservation of inversion (i.e., same spinal segments but different nerve, the tibial nerve).[50]

The sciatic trunk divides into the peroneal and tibial nerves just above the knee. Therefore, lesions of the sciatic trunk may affect any of the muscles listed under "sciatic trunk," "peroneal nerve," and "tibial nerve" in Table 60-3. Most patients with sciatic neuropathy have either greater involvement of the peroneal division (75% of patients) or equal involvement of the peroneal and tibial divisions (20% of patients). A sciatic neuropathy with greater involvement of the tibial nerve muscles is uncommon.[51]

The finding of weakness predominantly of the proximal leg muscles argues against sciatic, peroneal, or tibial neuropathy because all of these nerves innervate muscles below the knee. Therefore, proximal weakness suggests femoral or obturator neuropathy; lumbosacral plexopathy or radiculopathy; or, if sensory findings are absent, muscle disease.

2. Sensory Findings

Radiculopathy causes sensory loss in a dermatomal pattern (see Table 58-1 and Fig. 58-1 in Chapter 58), peripheral nerve lesions causes the sensory loss described in Table 60-4, and lumbosacral plexopathies tend to affect the entire leg.

A pure sensory syndrome is "meralgia paresthetica," which consists of hypesthesia of the anterior and lateral thigh, usually caused by mechanical compression of the lateral femoral cutaneous nerve (e.g., obesity, pregnancy, or carpenter's belts).[52]

3. Reflexes

The two muscle stretch reflexes of the leg are the quadriceps reflex (femoral nerve, L2-L4) and Achilles reflex (tibial nerve, S1). The peroneal nerve does not contribute to the Achilles reflex. Consequently, in patients with foot drop, the finding of an asymmetrically diminished or absent ankle jerk argues *against* peroneal palsy and *for* sciatic neuropathy (87% have abnormal ankle jerk)[51] or lumbosacral radiculopathy (14%–48% have an abnormal ankle jerk).[12,40,44,53,54]

Table 60-4	Sensory Branches of Peripheral Nerves of the Leg
Nerve	**Sensory Branches**
Femoral nerve	Anterior thigh
	Medial calf
Obturator nerve	Medial thigh
Sciatic nerve trunk*	Posterior thigh
Peroneal nerve*	Lateral calf and dorsal foot
Tibial nerve*	Sole of foot

*The sciatic nerve trunk divides above the knee into the peroneal and tibial nerves. Therefore, lesions of the sciatic nerve trunk affect sensation from all three branches.

4. Provocative Tests

The "straight-leg raising" test is a traditional maneuver used to diagnose lumbosacral radiculopathy, which is usually caused by disc herniation. In the maneuver, the clinician lifts the extended leg of the supine patient, flexing the leg at the hip. In a positive response, the patient develops pain down the ipsilateral leg (if pain develops just in the hip or back, the test is considered negative). The "crossed straight-leg raising" maneuver consists of pain in the affected leg when the clinician lifts the contralateral healthy limb. The pathogenesis of the sign is believed to be stretching of the sciatic nerve and its nerve roots.[55]

A positive straight-leg raising test is sometimes called "Lasègue's sign," after the French clinician Charles Lasègue (1816–1883), although Lasègue never published a description of the sign. His student Forst described the maneuver in his 1881 doctoral thesis, crediting Lasègue. An earlier description of the sign was published by Yugoslavian physician Lazarevic, in 1880.[56–58]

C. CLINICAL SIGNIFICANCE

1. Lumbosacral Radiculopathy

EBM Boxes 60-4 and 60-5 review the diagnostic accuracy of the bedside examination in patients with nerve pain of one leg (i.e., "sciatica"). EBM Box 60-4 applies to all patients with sciatica. EBM Box 60-5 applies only to patients with known lumbosacral radiculopathy and addresses how accurately findings localize the level of the lesion.

In patients with sciatica, the findings arguing *for* disc herniation and lumbosacral radiculopathy* are calf wasting (LR = 5.2), weak ankle dorsiflexion

---

*A L4-5 disc compresses the L5 root and a L5-S1 disc compresses the S1 root.

Box 60-4   Diagnosing Lumbosacral Radiculopathy in Patients with Sciatica*

Finding (Ref)[†]	Sensitivity (%)	Specificity (%)	Likelihood Ratio if Finding	
			Present	Absent
Motor examination				
Weak ankle dorsiflexion[44]	54	89	**4.9**	0.5
Ipsilateral calf wasting[44]	29	94	**5.2**	0.8
Sensory examination				
Leg sensation abnormal[44,53,54]	16–50	62–86	NS	NS
Reflex examination				
Abnormal ankle jerk[44,53,54]	14–48	89–93	2.7	NS
Other tests				
Straight-leg raising maneuver[41,44,54,59-61]	64–98	11–61	1.3	**0.3**
Crossed straight-leg raising maneuver[44,59-62]	22–43	88–98	**3.4**	0.8

NS, not significant; likelihood ratio (LR) if finding present = positive LR; LR if finding absent = negative LR.

*Diagnostic standard: For lumbosacral radiculopathy, surgical findings,[41,44,59,60] electrodiagnosis,[53] or magnetic resonance imaging or computed tomography[54,61] indicating lumbosacral nerve root compression.

[†]Definition of findings: For ipsilateral calf wasting, maximum calf circumference at least 1 cm smaller than contralateral side[44]; for straight-leg raising maneuvers, flexion at hip of supine patient's leg, extended at the knee, causes radiating pain in affected leg (pain confined to back or hip is negative response); for crossed straight-leg raising maneuver, raising contralateral leg provokes pain in affected leg.

LUMBOSACRAL RADICULOPATHY

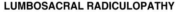

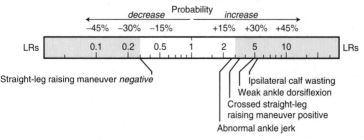

Localizing Lumbosacral Radiculopathy*

Box 60-5

Finding (Ref)[†]	Sensitivity (%)	Specificity (%)	Likelihood Ratio if Finding Present	Absent
Motor examination				
Weak knee extension, detecting L3 or L4 radiculopathy[53,63]	38–42	89	**3.7**	0.7
Weak hallux extension, detecting L5 radiculopathy[40,44,53]	12–61	54–91	1.6	NS
Weak ankle dorsiflexion, detecting L5 radiculopathy[44,64]	37–62	51–77	NS	NS
Weak ankle plantarflexion, detecting S1 radiculopathy[44,53]	26–45	75–99	NS	0.7
Ipsilateral calf wasting, detecting S1 radiculopathy[44]	43	82	2.4	0.7
Sensory examination				
Sensory loss L5 distribution, detecting L5 radiculopathy[40,44,64]	20–53	77–98	**3.1**	0.8
Sensory loss S1 distribution, detecting S1 radiculopathy[40,44,64]	32–49	70–90	2.4	0.7
Reflex examination				
Asymmetric quadriceps reflex, detecting L3 or L4 radiculopathy[40,53,65]	30–57	93–96	**8.7**	0.6
Asymmetric Achilles reflex, detecting S1 radiculopathy[40,44,53,64,65]	45–91	53–94	2.9	0.4

NS, not significant; likelihood ratio (LR) if finding present = positive LR; LR if finding absent = negative LR.
*Diagnostic standard: For level of radiculopathy, surgical findings and preoperative myelography,[40,44,64,65] myelography, magnetic resonance imaging,[63] or electrodiagnosis.[53]
†Definition of findings: For ipsilateral calf wasting, maximum calf circumference at least 1 cm smaller than contralateral side.[44]

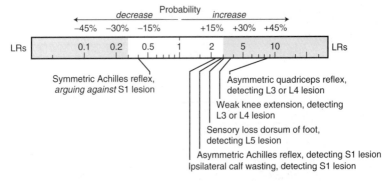

LOCALIZING LUMBOSACRAL RADICULOPATHY

Symmetric Achilles reflex, *arguing against* S1 lesion

Asymmetric quadriceps reflex, detecting L3 or L4 lesion

Weak knee extension, detecting L3 or L4 lesion

Sensory loss dorsum of foot, detecting L5 lesion

Asymmetric Achilles reflex, detecting S1 lesion

Ipsilateral calf wasting, detecting S1 lesion

(LR = 4.9), the *crossed* straight-leg raising maneuver (LR = 3.4), and the absent ankle jerk (LR = 2.7). A *negative* straight-leg raising maneuver argues *against* disc herniation (LR = 0.3).

In patients with sciatica and lumbosacral radiculopathy (see EBM Box 60-5), an abnormal quadriceps reflex (LR = 8.7) or weak knee extension (LR = 3.7) indicate the L3 or L4 level. The best test for L5 radiculopathy is a L5 sensory loss (dorsum of the foot; LR = 3.1). The best predictors for the S1 level are sensory loss in the S1 distribution (lateral heel, LR = 2.4), reduced Achilles reflex (LR = 2.9), and ipsilateral calf wasting (LR = 2.4).

2. Lumbosacral Plexopathy

a. Cancer Patients

In patients with known cancer and prior pelvic irradiation who present with lumbosacral plexopathy, findings confined to one leg argues for *recurrent tumor* (LR = 4.5) whereas findings in both legs argue for *radiation plexopathy* (LR = 7.5).[48]

b. Diabetic Amyotrophy [66–70]

Diabetic amyotrophy (or "diabetic proximal neuropathy") is a lumbosacral plexopathy of diabetic patients with presenting symptoms of weak thigh muscles and severe pain in the thighs or back, or both. The quadriceps, adductor and iliopsoas muscles are weak 100% of the time, and the glutei and hamstrings 50% of the time (all are proximal muscles). The weakness may be unilateral or bilateral, but it is always asymmetric. Sensation is normal (70% of the time) or diminished over the thigh (30% of the time). The quadriceps reflex is absent in 80% of patients.

Although patients with diabetes also develop femoral neuropathy,[71] femoral neuropathy affects only thigh flexion and knee extension and spares other proximal leg muscles.

REFERENCES

1. Haig AJ, Tzeng HM, LeBreck D. The value of electrodiagnosis consultation for patients with upper extremity nerve complaints: A prospective comparison with the history and physical examination. *Arch Phys Med Rehabil.* 1999;80:1273-1281.

2. Kothari MJ, Blakeslee MA, Reichwein R, Simmons Z, Logigian EL. Electrodiagnostic studies: Are they useful in clinical practice. *Arch Phys Med Rehabil.* 1998;79: 1510-1511.

3. Wainner RS, Fritz JM, Irrgang JJ, Delitto A, Allison S, Boninger ML. Development of a clinical prediction rule for the diagnosis of carpal tunnel syndrome. *Arch Phys Med Rehabil.* 2005;86:609-618.

4. Wilbourn AJ, Aminoff MJ. AAEM minimonograph 32: The electrodiagnostic examination in patients with radiculopathies. *Musc Nerv.* 1998;21:1612-1631.

5. Yoss RE, Corbin KB, MacCarty CS, Love JG. Significance of symptoms and signs in localization of involved root in cervical disk protrusion. *Neurology.* 1957;7:673-683.

6. Lauder TD, Dillingham TR, Andary M, et al. Predicting electodiagnostic outcome in patients with upper limb symptoms: Are the history and physical examination helpful? *Arch Phys Med Rehabil.* 2000;81:436-441.

7. Wainner RS, Fritz JM, Irrgang JJ, et al. Reliability and diagnostic accuracy of the clinical examination and patient self-report measures for cervical radiculopathy. *Spine.* 2003;28:52-63.

8. Nieuwenhuys R. Bolk's studies of segmental anatomy. *Acta Morphol Neerl Scand.* 1975;13:7-33.

9. Wolf JK. *Segmental neurology: A guide to the examination and interpretation of sensory and motor function.* Baltimore: University Park Press; 1981.

10. Brendler SJ. The human cervical myotomes: Functional anatomy studied at operation. *J Neurosurg.* 1968;28:105-111.

11. Levin KH, Maggiano HJ, Wilbourn AJ. Cervical radiculopathies: Comparison of surgical and EMG localization of single-root lesions. *Neurology.* 1996;46:1022-1025.

12. Young JH. The revision of the dermatomes. *Aust N Z J Surg.* 1949;18:171-186.

13. Makin GJV, Brown WF, Ebers GC. C7 radiculopathy: Importance of scapular winging in clinical diagnosis. *J Neurol Neurosurg Psychiatry.* 1986;49:640-644.

14. Medical Research Council. *Aids to the examination of the peripheral nervous system.* London: Bailliere Tindall; 1986.

15. Reid RI, Ashby MA. Ulnar nerve palsy and walking frames. *Br Med J.* 1982;285:778.

16. Maimaris C, Zadeh HG. Ulnar nerve compression in the cyclist's hand: Two case reports and review of the literature. *Br J Sports Med.* 1990;24:245-246.

17. Massey EW, Pleet AB. Handcuffs and cheiralgia paresthetica. *Neurology.* 1978;28:1312-1313.

18. Spurling RG, Scoville WB. Lateral rupture of the cervical intervertebral discs: A common cause of shoulder and arm pain. *Surg Gynecol Obstet.* 1944;78: 350-358.

19. Tong HC, Haig AJ, Yamakawa K. The Spurling test and cervical radiculopathy. *Spine*. 2002;27:156-159.

20. Viikari-Juntura E, Porras M, Laasonen EM. Validity of clinical tests in the diagnosis of root compression in cervical disc disease. *Spine*. 1989;14:253-257.

21. Lunsford LD, Bissonette DJ, Jannetta PJ, et al. Anterior surgery for cervical disc disease. Part 1. Treatment of lateral cervical disc herniation in 253 cases. *J Neurosurg*. 1980;53:1-11.

22. Kori SH, Foley KM, Posner JB. Brachial plexus lesions in patients with cancer: 100 cases. *Neurology*. 1981;31:45-50.

23. Katz JN, Stirrat C, Larson MG, et al. A self-administered hand symptom diagram in the diagnosis and epidemiologic study of carpal tunnel syndrome. *J Rheumatol*. 1990;17:1495-1498.

24. Kuhlman KA, Hennessey WJ. Sensitivity and specificity of carpal tunnel syndrome signs. *Am J Phys Med Rehabil*. 1997;76:451-457.

25. Gerr F, Letz R. The sensitivity and specificity of tests for carpal tunnel syndrome vary with the comparison subjects. *J Hand Surg Br*. 1998;23B:151-155.

26. Golding DH, Rose DM, Selvarajah K. Clinical tests for carpal tunnel syndrome: An evaluation. *Br J Rheumatol*. 1986;25:388-390.

27. Katz JN, Larson MG, Sabra A, et al. Carpal tunnel syndrome: Diagnostic utility of history and physical examination findings. *Ann Intern Med*. 1990;112:321-327.

28. Buch-Jaeger N, Foucher G. Correlation of clinical signs with nerve conduction tests in the diagnosis of carpal tunnel syndrome. *J Hand Surg Br*. 1994;19B:720-724.

29. Pagel KJ, Kaul MP, Dryden JD. Lack of utility of Semmes-Weinstein monofilament testing in suspected carpal tunnel syndrome. *Am J Phys Med Rehabil*. 2002; 81:597-600.

30. Heller L, Ring H, Costeff H, Solzi P. Evaluation of Tinel's and Phalen's signs in the diagnosis of the carpal tunnel syndrome. *Eur Neurol*. 1986;25:40-42.

31. Hansen PA, Micklesen P, Robinson LR. Clinical utility of the flick maneuver in diagnosing carpal tunnel syndrome. *Am J Phys Med Rehabil*. 2004;83:363-367.

32. Burke DT, Burke MAM, Bell R, et al. Subjective swelling: A new sign for carpal tunnel syndrome. *Am J Phys Med Rehabil*. 1999;78:504-508.

33. DeSmet L, Steenwerckx A, van den Bogaert G, et al. Value of clinical provocative tests in carpal tunnel syndrome. *Acta Orthop Belg*. 1995;61:177-182.

34. Kaul MP, Pagel KJ, Wheatley MJ, Dryden JD. Carpal compression test and pressure provocative test in veterans with median-distribution paresthesias. *Muscle Nerve*. 2001;24:107-111.

35. Radecki P. A gender specific wrist ratio and the likelihood of a median nerve abnormality at the carpal tunnel. *Am J Phys Med Rehabil*. 1988;67:157-162.

36. Pryse-Phillips WEM. Validation of a diagnostic sign in carpal tunnel syndrome. *J Neurol Neurosurg Psychiatry*. 1984;47:870-872.

37. D'Arcy C, McGee S. Does this patient have carpal tunnel syndrome? *JAMA*. 2000; 283:3110-3117.

38. Johnson EW, Gatens T, Poindexter D, Bowers D. Wrist dimensions: Correlation with median sensory latencies. *Arch Phys Med Rehabil.* 1983;64:556-557.

39. Lum PB, Kanaklamedala R. Conduction of the palmar cutaneous branch of the median nerve. *Arch Phys Med Rehabil.* 1986;67:805-806.

40. Kortelainen P, Puranen J, Koivisto E, Laehde S. Symptoms and signs of sciatica and their relation to the localization of the lumbar disc herniation. *Spine.* 1985;10: 88-92.

41. Kosteljanetz M, Espersen JO, Halaburt H, Miletic T. Predictive value of clinical and surgical findings in patients with lumbago-sciatica: A prospective study. I. *Acta Neurochir.* 1984;73:67-76.

42. Jonsson B, Stromqvist B. Symptoms and signs in degeneration of the lumbar spine: A prospective, consecutive study of 300 operated patients. *J Bone Joint Surg Br.* 1993;75B:381-385.

43. Supik LF, Broom MJ. Sciatic tension signs and lumbar disc herniation. *Spine.* 1994;19:1066-1069.

44. Kerr RSC, Cadoux-Hudson TA, Adams CBT. The value of accurate clinical assessment in the surgical management of the lumbar disc protrusion. *J Neurol Neurosurg Psychiatry.* 1988;51:169-173.

45. Hakelius A, Hindmarsh J. The comparative reliability of preoperative diagnostic methods in lumbar disc surgery. *Acta Orthop Scand.* 1972;43:234-238.

46. Liguori R, Krarup C, Trojaborg W. Determination of the segmental sensory and motor innervation of lumbosacral spinal nerves. *Brain.* 1992;115:915-934.

47. Thage O. The myotomes L2-S2 in man. *Acta Neurol Scand.* 1965;41(Suppl 13): 241-243.

48. Thomas JE, Cascino TL, Earle JD. Differential diagnosis between radiation and tumor plexopathy of the pelvis. *Neurology.* 1985;35:1-7.

49. Pettigrew LC, Glass JP, Maor M, Zornoza J. Diagnosis and treatment of lumbosacral plexopathies in patients with cancer. *Arch Neurol.* 1984;41:1282-1285.

50. Katirji MB, Wilbourn AJ. Common peroneal mononeuropathy: A clinical and electrophysiologic study of 116 lesions. *Neurology.* 1988;38:1723-1728.

51. Yuen EC, Olney RK, So YT. Sciatic neuropathy: Clinical and prognostic features in 73 patients. *Neurology.* 1994;44:1669-1674.

52. Massey EW. Sensory mononeuropathies. *Semin Neurol.* 1998;18:177-183.

53. Lauder TD, Dillingham TR, Andary M, et al. Effect of history and exam in predicting electrodiagnostic outcome among patients with suspected lumbosacral radiculopathy. *Am J Phys Med Rehabil.* 2000;79:60-68.

54. Vroomen PCAJ, De Krom MCTFM, Knottnerus JA. Consistency of history taking and physical examination in patients with suspected lumbar nerve root involvement. *Spine.* 2000;25:91-97.

55. Goddard MD, Reid JD. Movements induced by straight leg raising in the lumbosacral roots, nerves and plexus, and in the intrapelvic section of the sciatic nerve. *J Neurol Neurosurg Psychiatry.* 1965;28:12-18.

56. Pearce JMS. Lasegue's sign. *Lancet.* 1989;1:436.

57. Sugar O. Charles Lasegue and his 'considerations on sciatica'. *JAMA.* 1985;253: 1767-1768.

58. Dyck P. Lumbar nerve root: The enigmatic eponyms. *Spine.* 1984;9:3-5.

59. Kosteljanetz M, Bang F, Schmidt-Olsen S. The clinical significance of straight-leg raising (Lasegue's sign) in the diagnosis of prolapsed lumbar disc: Interobserver variation and correlation with surgical findings. *Spine.* 1988;13:393-395.

60. Spangfort EV. The lumbar disc herniation: A computer-aided analysis of 2504 operations. *Acta Orthop Scand.* 1972;(Suppl 142):1-95.

61. Poiraudeau S, Foltz V, Drape JL, et al. Value of the bell test and the hyperextension test for diagnosis in sciatica associated with disc herniation: Comparison with Lasegue's sign and the crossed Lasegue's sign. *Rheumatology.* 2001;40:460-466.

62. Hudgins WB. The crossed straight leg raising test: A diagnostic sign of herniated disc. *J Occup Med.* 1979;21:407-408.

63. Rainville J, Jouve C, Finno M, Limke J. Comparison of four tests of quadriceps strength in L3 or L4 radiculopathies. *Spine.* 2003;28:2466-2471.

64. Jensen OH. The level-diagnosis of a lower lumbar disc herniation: The value of sensibility and motor testing. *Clin Rheumatol.* 1987;6:564-569.

65. Portnoy HD, Ahmad M. Value of the neurological examination, electromyography and myelography in herniated lumbar disc. *Mich Med.* 1972;71:429-434.

66. Subramony SH, Wilbourn AJ. Diabetic proximal neuropathy: Clinical and electromyographic studies. *J Neurol Sci.* 1982;53:293-304.

67. Bastron JA, Thomas JE. Diabetic polyradiculopathy: Clinical and electromyographic findings in 105 patients. *Mayo Clin Proc.* 1981;56:725-732.

68. Chokroverty S, Reyes MG, Rubino FA, Tonaki H. The syndrome of diabetic amyotrophy. *Ann Neurol.* 1977;2:181-194.

69. Asbury AK. Proximal diabetic neuropathy. *Ann Neurol.* 1977;2:179-180.

70. Sander HW, Chokroverty S. Diabetic amyotrophy: Current concepts. *Semin Neurol.* 1996;16:173-178.

71. Fraser DM, Campbell IW, Ewing DJ, Clarke BF. Mononeuropathy in diabetes mellitus. *Diabetes.* 1979;28:96-101.

61

Coordination and Cerebellar Testing

I. INTRODUCTION

In the 1920s, after closely observing patients with cerebellar tumors and World War I soldiers with gunshot wounds to the posterior fossa, the British neurologist Gordon Holmes concluded that the following four physical signs were fundamental to cerebellar disease: ataxia, nystagmus, hypotonia, and dysarthria.[1-5]

II. THE FINDINGS

A. ATAXIA

Ataxia refers to incoordinated voluntary movements that lack the speed, smoothness, and appropriate direction seen in normal persons. Because the cerebellum's role is to organize and administer movement, testing for ataxia is possible only in patients with adequate motor strength (i.e., 4 or 5 on the MRC scale; see Chapter 57). Tests of ataxia include observation of the patient's gait (see Chapter 5), the finger-nose-finger test, heel-knee-shin test, and rapid alternating movements.

1. Finger-Nose-Finger Test

In this test, the seated patient takes the index finger of his outstretched hand and alternately touches his own nose and the clinician's index finger being held a couple of feet away. The patient with cerebellar disease may misjudge the range of movement (i.e., **dysmetria**), overshooting the target (i.e., **hypermetria**, as in missing the nose and slapping the hand into his own face) or undershooting the target (i.e., **hypometria**, as in stopping before reaching the clinician's finger). The patient's finger also may deviate from a smooth course, especially if the clinician shifts the target during the test. As the patient's finger approaches the target, an increasing side-to-side tremor may appear (i.e., **intention tremor** or "kinetic tremor," see Chapter 57).

2. Heel-Knee-Shin Test

In this test, the supine patient places the heel of one leg on the opposite knee and then slides it down the shin. Like the finger-to-nose test, a positive response may reveal any combination of ataxia, dysmetria, and intention tremor.

Decomposition of movement denotes an abnormal sequence of actions. For example, during the heel-knee-shin test, the patient may completely flex the hip before beginning to bend the knee, thus lifting the heel abnormally high in the air before lowering to complete the movement.[2]

3. Rapid Alternating Movements

Difficulty with rapid alternating movements is called **dysdiadochokinesia** (Babinski coined the original term "adiadochokinesis").[3] The usual test is rapid pronation and supination of the forearm, but other tasks such as clapping hands, tapping a table, or stamping the foot are just as adequate.[3] In all these tests, the movements of patients with cerebellar disease are slower and significantly more irregular in rhythm, range, and accuracy.

B. NYSTAGMUS

1. Definition

Nystagmus is an involuntary to-and-fro oscillation of the eyes. Nystagmus may be congenital or acquired, and the movements may affect both eyes ("bilateral") or just one eye ("unilateral"). Bilateral nystagmus may be "conjugate," which means both eyes have identical movements, or "dissociated," which implies separate movements. Nystagmus may be "pendular," which means the to- and fro-movements have the same velocity, or "rhythmic," which means the movement is slow in one direction and quick in the other (rhythmic nystagmus is usually called "jerk nystagmus"). Jerk nystagmus is named after the direction of the quick component (e.g., a "right conjugate jerk nystagmus"). Finally, the direction of the nystagmus may be horizontal, vertical, or rotatory.

2. Patterns of Nystagmus

Although nystagmus is a complicated subject that sometimes defies general principles,* several well-recognized patterns are described in the following sections.

a. Cerebellar Nystagmus

The most common nystagmus of cerebellar disease is a conjugate horizontal jerk nystagmus on lateral gaze (see Section III.A.2 below).

One rare type of nystagmus, "rebound nystagmus," has been described only in patients with cerebellar disease.[7-9] To test for this nystagmus, the patient first looks to one direction (say, to the right). In patients with a positive response, a brisk nystagmus with its fast component to the right appears. If the patient continues looking in this direction for about 20 seconds, the nystagmus fatigues and disappears (sometimes even reversing direction). The patient then returns his eyes to the primary position (i.e., straight ahead), and nystagmus to the left, not present initially, appears, although it fatigues over time. In these patients, the direction of the nystagmus in primary gaze can be reversed at will, depending on whether the patient looks first to the left or right.[7]

b. Nystagmus and Noncerebellar Disorders

Other useful patterns of nystagmus (not features of cerebellar disease) are optokinetic nystagmus (see Chapter 54), the nystagmus of internuclear ophthalmoplegia (see Chapter 55), and the nystagmus of vestibular disease (which is usually a conjugate rotatory jerk nystagmus).

3. Effect of Retinal Fixation

"Retinal fixation" means the patient is focusing his or her eyes on an object. Spontaneous nystagmus that diminishes during retinal fixation argues that the responsible lesion is located in the peripheral vestibular system; nystagmus that increases or remains unchanged during fixation argues that the lesion is in the central nervous system (i.e., brainstem or cerebellum). Neuro-ophthalmologists usually use electronystagmography to detect the effects of fixation (by comparing eye movements with eyes open with those with eyes closed), but general clinicians can accomplish the same during direct ophthalmoscopy: In a dimly lit

---

*One famous neuro-ophthalmologist once advised his students "never write on nystagmus, it will lead you nowhere."[6]

room, the clinician examines the optic disc of one eye and compares its movements as the patient fixes the opposite eye on a distant target with those when the patient's opposite eye is covered. If rhythmic movements of the optic disc first appear or worsen when the fixating eye is occluded, a peripheral vestibular disturbance is likely.[10]

C. HYPOTONIA (SEE CHAPTER 57)

The limbs of patients with cerebellar disease offer no resistance to passive displacement, sometimes resembling (in the words of Gordon Holmes) the "muscles of a person deeply under an anaesthetic, or of a corpse recently dead."[1] Holding the forearms vertically causes the wrist to bend to an angle much more acute than normal. Displacing the patient's outstretched arm downward causes abnormally wide and prolonged up-and-down oscillations, even when the patient is requested to resist such movements. Striking the patellar tendon causes pendular knee jerks, traditionally defined as three or more swings,[11] although, as already stated in Chapter 57, this threshold will have to be revised upward because many normal persons also demonstrate three or more swings.[12]

D. DYSARTHRIA

The speech of patients with cerebellar disease is slow, slurred, and irregular in volume and rhythm, findings that are collectively referred to as "dysarthria." In contrast to patients with aphasia, however, patients with dysarthria can name objects, repeat words, comprehend language, and speak sentences with words whose order makes sense.

III. CLINICAL SIGNIFICANCE

A. INDIVIDUAL FINDINGS

1. Ataxia

Ataxia of gait is the most common finding in all cerebellar syndromes (see later), and therefore, examination of the gait should be part of every patient with suspected cerebellar disease. Many patients with cerebellar disease have difficulty walking despite lacking all other findings of limb ataxia.

Simple measurements of the patient's dysdiadochokinesia—such as how quickly and accurately the patient can alternately tap two buttons spaced about 12 inches apart*—are accurate measures of ataxia that correlate well with other measures of disability.[13]

---

*Ninety percent of normal persons can accomplish at least 32 taps within 15 seconds, whereas 90% of patients with cerebellar ataxia cannot.[13]

2. Nystagmus

Seventy-five percent of cerebellar nystagmus is a conjugate horizontal jerk nystagmus that appears on lateral gaze (15% is a rotatory nystagmus and 10% a vertical nystagmus). Nonetheless, a horizontal jerk nystagmus is not specific for cerebellar disease and also occurs in peripheral vestibular disease and other central nervous system disorders. The direction of the jerk nystagmus has less localizing value than tests of ataxia (see Section B.1.a below).

The clinical utility of rebound nystagmus is limited because it is a late finding, and all patients described with the finding have had many other obvious cerebellar signs.[7,8]

3. Dysarthria

Dysarthria, the least common of the fundamental cerebellar signs (see later), appears more often with lesions of the left cerebellar hemisphere than with those of the right hemisphere.[14]

B. CEREBELLAR SYNDROMES

Most patients with cerebellar disease present with difficulty walking or headache, or both.[11,15] In adults, four cerebellar syndromes are common, each of which is characterized by a different distribution of the principal cerebellar signs.

1. Cerebellar Hemisphere Syndrome
a. Cerebellar Findings

Table 61-1 presents the physical findings of 444 patients with focal lesions (mostly tumors) confined to one hemisphere.[11,15] According to traditional teachings, cerebellar signs appear on the side of the body *ipsilateral* to the lesion. This teaching proved generally correct in the patients of Table 61-1, in whom signs of limb ataxia (i.e., dysmetria, intention tremor, dysdiadochokinesia) were unilateral 85% of the time, and, if unilateral, were on the side ipsilateral to the lesion 80% to 90% of the time. These patients also had more hypotonia on the side of the lesion and tended to fall toward the side of the lesion when walking.

Nystagmus has less localizing value. When present, nystagmus is unilateral in only 65% of patients, and in these, the direction of nystagmus points to the side of the lesion only 70% of the time.

b. Associated Findings

Despite having a lesion confined to the cerebellum, patients with structural cerebellar lesions may also have (1) cranial nerve findings (10%–20% of patients; usually of cranial nerves V, VI, VII, or VIII, ipsilateral to the side of the lesion 75% of the time[11,15]; (2) altered mental status (38% of patients, from compres-

Table 61-1	Unilateral Cerebellar Lesions*

Physical Finding[†]	Frequency (%)[‡]
Ataxia	
Gait ataxia	80–93
Limb ataxia	
Dysmetria	71–86
Intention tremor	29
Dysdiadochokinesia	47–69
Nystagmus	54–84
Hypotonia	76
Pendular knee jerks	37
Dysarthria	10–25

Data from 444 patients from references 11, 15.
*Diagnostic Standard: Clinical imaging, surgical findings, or postmortem examination.
†Definition of findings: See text.
‡Results are overall mean frequency or, if statistically heterogenous, the range of values.

sion of the brainstem or complicating hydrocephalus); (3) upper motor neuron signs such as hyperactive reflexes and Babinski's sign (28% of patients); and (4) papilledema (68% of patients).

In contrast, severe weakness and sensory disturbance are both uncommon, affecting only 4%.

2. Anterior Cerebellar Degeneration (Rostral Vermis Syndrome)[16]

In contrast to the cerebellar hemisphere syndrome, these patients have ataxia of gait (100%) and of both legs (88%) with relative sparing of the arms (only 16% of patients). Nystagmus and dysarthria also are much less frequent (9%, for both findings). This syndrome most often results from chronic alcohol ingestion.

3. Pancerebellar Syndrome

This syndrome causes the same signs listed in Table 61-1, but instead of being on one side of the body, the cerebellar signs are symmetric. Causes include drug intoxication (e.g., phenytoin), inherited disorders, and paraneoplastic syndromes.

4. Cerebellar Infarction

The physical signs of cerebellar infarction resemble those of the cerebellar hemisphere syndrome described previously, with three exceptions: In infarction, (1) all signs appear *abruptly*, (2) dysarthria is more prominent (44% of patients), and (3) weakness occurs more often (22% have hemiparesis; 24% have tetraparesis).[17-20] The two main arteries supplying the cerebellum are the superior cerebellar and posterior cerebellar arteries. An associated lateral medullary syndrome (see Table 58-2 in Chapter 58) suggests an infarct in the distribution of the posterior inferior cerebellar artery.[19,21]

REFERENCES

1. Holmes G. Clinical symptoms of cerebellar disease and their interpretation: Lecture 1. *Lancet.* 1922;1:1177-1182.

2. Holmes G. Clinical symptoms of cerebellar disease and their interpretation. Lecture 2. *Lancet.* 1922;1:1231-1237.

3. Holmes G. Clinical symptoms of cerebellar disease and their interpretation. Lecture 3. *Lancet.* 1922;2:59-65.

4. Holmes G. Clinical symptoms of cerebellar disease and their interpretation. Lecture 4. *Lancet.* 1922;2:111-115.

5. Fine EJ, Ionita CC, Lohr L. The history of the development of the cerebellar examination. *Semin Neurol.* 2002;22:374-384.

6. Wartenberg R. *Diagnostic tests in neurology: A selection for office use.* Chicago: Year Book Publishers, Inc; 1953.

7. Hood JD, Kayan A, Leech J. Rebound nystagmus. *Brain.* 1973;96:507-526.

8. Morales-Garcia C, Arriagada C, Cardenas JL, Otte J. Clinical significance of rebound nystagmus in neuro-otological diagnosis. *Ann Otol Rhinol Laryngol.* 1978;87(2 part 1):238-242.

9. Lin CY, Young YH. Clinical significance of rebound nystagmus. *Laryngoscope.* 1999;109:1803-1805.

10. Zee DS. Ophthalmoscopy in examination of patients with vestibular disorders. *Ann Neurol.* 1978;3:373-374.

11. Gilman S, Bloedel JR, Lechtenberg R. *Disorders of the cerebellum.* Philadelphia: F. A. Davis, Co; 1981.

12. Pickett JB, Tatum EJ. Pendular knee reflexes: A reliable sign of hypotonia? *Lancet.* 1984;2:236-237.

13. Notermans NC, van Dijk GW, van der Graff Y, et al. Measuring ataxia: quantification based on the standard neurological examination. *J Neurol Neurosurg Psychiatry.* 1994;57:22-26.

14. Lechtenberg R, Gilman S. Speech disorders in cerebellar disease. *Ann Neurol.* 1978;3:285-290.
15. Amici R, Avanzini G, Pacini L. *Cerebellar tumors: Clinical analysis and physiopathologic correlations.* Basel: S. Karger; 1976.
16. Victor M, Adams RD, Mancall EL. A restricted form of cerebellar cortical degeneration occurring in alcoholic patients. *Arch Neurol.* 1959;1:579-688.
17. Scotti G, Spinnler H, Sterzi R, Vallar G. Cerebellar softening. *Ann Neurol.* 1980;8:133-140.
18. Tohgi H, Takahashi S, Chiba K, Hirata Y. Cerebellar infarction: Clinical and neuroimaging analysis in 293 patients. *Stroke.* 1993;24:1697-1701.
19. Kase CS, Norrving B, Levine SR, et al. Cerebellar infarction: Clinical and anatomic observations in 66 cases. *Stroke.* 1993;24:76-83.
20. Sypert GW, Alvord EC. Cerebellar infarction: A clinicopathological study. *Arch Neurol.* 1975;32:357-363.
21. Amarenco P. The spectrum of cerebellar infarctions. *Neurology.* 1991;41:973-979.

62

Examination of Hysterical Neurologic Disorders

I. TRADITIONAL PHYSICAL FINDINGS OF HYSTERICAL DISEASE

Hysterical neurologic disorders (also called "nonorganic," "psychogenic," or "functional") occur commonly, accounting for 9% of admissions to a neurologic service, according in one study.[1] The traditional bedside findings that suggest functional disease are listed in the following sections.

A. FINDINGS WHOSE SEVERITY FLUCTUATES DURING THE EXAMINATION

Examples are the patient who falls suddenly while walking but catches himself or herself with knees and hips flexed, a position that requires considerable strength, or the patient whose stance is unstable until distracted by asking him or her to perform the finger-nose test.[2]

B. FINDINGS THAT DEFY NEUROANATOMIC EXPLANATION[3,4]

Findings that defy neuroanatomic explanation include **(1) hysterical hemianopia,** as in the patient who has right hemianopia with both eyes open or just the right eye open, but normal visual fields when just the left eye is open[5,6]; **(2) wrong-way tongue deviation,** that is, the tongue deviates away from the hemiparetic side (in cerebral hemispheric disease, the tongue deviates toward the hemiparetic side, see Chapter 56)[7]; and **(3) peripheral facial palsy and ipsilateral hemiparesis** (if a single lesion causes peripheral facial weakness and hemiparesis, the lesion is in the brainstem and the findings should be on opposite sides of the body).[8]

C. BIZARRE MOVEMENTS NOT NORMALLY SEEN IN ORGANIC DISEASE

Examples are the patient who drags the hemiparetic leg after him or her as if it were an inanimate object,[2,9] or the ataxic patient who sways dramatically without falling.[6]

D. FINDINGS ELICITED DURING SPECIAL TESTS

Findings elicited during special tests include **(1) optokinetic nystagmus** testing for functional blindness, because patients with intact vision cannot suppress this nystagmus (see Chapter 54), the presence of optokinetic nystagmus uncovers that the blindness is functional, and **(2) procedures that confuse the patient of sidedness,** such as a maneuver that mixes up the fingers to uncover hysterical hemianalgesia (Fig. 62-1).[10]

II. CLINICAL SIGNIFICANCE: CAVEATS TO THE DIAGNOSIS OF HYSTERICAL DISORDERS

Despite these traditional teachings, the clinician should be very reluctant to diagnose hysterical disease, primarily because many of these "nonorganic" findings, when subjected to serious study, also appear in patients with organic disease. For example, in studies of patients with known organic causes of their findings, 8% "split" their sensory findings precisely at the midline, up to 85% feel vibration less in numb areas, 48% have sensory findings that change between examinations or make no sense neuroanatomically, and 33% have "give-away" weakness.[11,12] All of these findings, at one point in time, have been presented as reliable markers of psychogenic disease.[13]

Rare disorders also will trip up the unwary clinician. For example, patients with the medial medullary syndrome also may point their tongue to the "wrong" side, and patients with advanced Huntington's disease are often regarded as having an hysterical gait when it is viewed in isolation.[9]

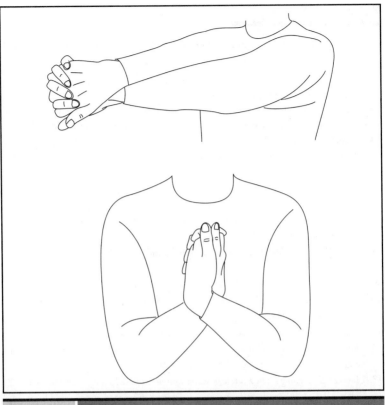

FIGURE 62-1   TEST FOR HYSTERICAL HEMIANALGESIA.

This test simply mixes up the fingers and confuses the body image. In the first step (*top row*), the patient's hands are pronated with the little fingers on top, the palms are outward, and fingers are interlocked. In the second step (*bottom row*), the hands are rotated downward, inward and upward, so the interlocked fingers are positioned in front of the chest. The clinician then repeats the sensory examination to determine if the patient is consistent in describing his sensory loss. In the final position, the fingertips end up on the same side of the body as their respective arms, and the thumbs (which are not interlocked) end up on the side opposite the fingers.

In clinical studies, 4% to 40% of patients given a diagnosis of hysterical neurologic disease are subsequently found to have a neurologic disease to account for the finding.[14–17] The diagnosis of hysterical illness, then, is often a diagnostic snare, best left to the experts who are paid to take on such risks.

REFERENCES

1. Lempert T, Dieterich M, Huppert D, Brandt T. Psychogenic disorders in neurology: Frequency and clinical spectrum. *Acta Neurol Scand.* 1990;82:335-340.
2. Lempert T, Brandt T, Dieterich M, Huppert D. How to identify psychogenic disorders of stance and gait. *J Neurol.* 1991;238:140-146.
3. Okun MS, Koehler PJ. Babinski's clinical differentiation of organic paralysis from hysterical paralysis: Effect on US neurology. *Arch Neurol.* 2004;61:778-783.
4. Koehler PJ, Okun MS. Important observations prior to the description of the Hoover sign. *Neurology.* 2004;63:1693-1697.
5. Keane JR. Hysterical hemianopia: The `missing half' field defect. *Arch Ophthalmol.* 1979;97:865-866.
6. Keane JR. Patterns of hysterical hemianopia. *Neurology.* 1998;51:1230-1231.
7. Keane JR. Wrong-way deviation of the tongue with hysterical hemiparesis. *Neurology.* 1986;36:1406-1407.
8. Keane JR. Hysterical hemiparesis accompanying Bell's palsy. *Neurology.* 1993;43:1619.
9. Keane JR. Hysterical gait disorders: 60 cases. *Neurology.* 1989;39:586-589.
10. Bowlus WE, Currier RD. A test for hysterical hemianalgesis. *N Engl J Med.* 1963;269:1253-1254.
11. Rolak LA. Psychogenic sensory loss. *J Nerv Ment Dis.* 1988;176:686-687.
12. Gould R, Miller BL, Goldberg MA, Benson DF. The validity of hysterical signs and symptoms. *J Nerv Ment Dis.* 1986;174:593-597.
13. Haerer AF. *DeJong's The neurologic examination.* Philadelphia: JB Lippincott; 1992.
14. Slater ETO, Glithero E. A follow-up of patients diagnosed as suffering from "hysteria." *J Psychosom Res.* 1965;9:9-13.
15. Couprie W, Wijdicks EFM, Rooijmans HGM, van Gijn J. Outcome in conversion disorder: A follow up study. *J Neurol Neurosurg Psychiatry.* 1995;58:750-752.
16. Mace CJ, Trimble MR. Ten-year prognosis of conversion disorder. *Br J Psychiatry.* 1996;169:282-288.
17. Crimlisk HL, Bhatia K, Cope H, et al. Slater revisited: 6 year follow up study of patients with medically unexplained motor symptoms. *BMJ.* 1998;316:582-586.

Likelihood Ratios and Their Confidence Intervals

A ppendix Table 1 displays the point estimates and 95% confidence intervals for all of the likelihood ratios presented in this book. Chapter 2 presents the methods used to obtain these estimates, and individual chapters define each physical finding and further discuss its significance.

Appendix Table 1 — Likelihood Ratios—Point Estimates and 95% Confidence Intervals

Finding	Positive LR (95% CI)	Negative LR (95% CI)
EBM Box 4-1 Dementia and delirium		
Abnormal clock drawing test	5.3 (2.5, 11.2)	0.5 (0.3, 0.7)
Mini-mental status, ≤23	8.1 (5.6, 11.6)	0.2 (0.1, 0.3)
Mini-mental status, ≤20	14.5 (6.8, 31.1)	...
Mini-mental status, 21–25	2.2 (1.6, 3.0)	...
Mini-mental status, ≥26	0.1 (0.1, 0.2)	...
Confusion assessment method, detecting delirium	10.3 (4.8, 21.9)	0.2 (0.1, 0.4)
Chapter 5 Stance and Gait		
Stops talking when walking, predicting falls	8.8 (2.1, 36.5)	0.6 (0.4, 0.8)
EBM Box 6-1 Hepatocellular jaundice		
Weight loss	0.8 (0.2, 3.2)	1.3 (0.5, 3.3)
Spider angiomata	4.7 (1.1, 22.4)	0.6 (0.5, 0.9)
Palmar erythema	9.8 (1.4, 67.6)	0.5 (0.4, 0.7)
Distended abdominal veins	17.5 (1.1, 277)	0.6 (0.5, 0.8)
Ascites	4.4 (1.1, 17.1)	0.6 (0.5, 0.8)
Palpable spleen	2.9 (1.2, 6.8)	0.7 (0.6, 0.9)
Palpable gallbladder	0.04 (0, 0.7)	1.4 (1.1, 1.9)
Palpable liver	0.9 (0.8, 1.1)	1.4 (0.6, 3.4)
Liver tenderness	1.4 (0.8, 2.6)	0.8 (0.7, 1.1)
EBM Box 6-2 Cirrhosis		
Spider angiomata	3.7 (2.0, 6.8)	0.6 (0.6, 0.7)
Palmar erythema	2.6 (1.4, 4.9)	0.7 (0.5, 0.9)
Jaundice	2.6 (1.9, 3.5)	0.8 (0.7, 0.9)
Dilated abdominal wall veins	5.4 (1.1, 25.3)	0.7 (0.6, 0.9)
Hepatomegaly	2.0 (1.4, 2.8)	0.6 (0.4, 0.8)
Palpable liver in epigastrium	2.6 (1.8, 3.8)	0.2 (0.1, 0.5)
Liver edge firm to palpation	2.7 (2.2, 3.3)	0.4 (0.3, 0.5)
Splenomegaly	2.3 (1.5, 3.6)	0.8 (0.7, 0.9)
Ascites	6.6 (3.6, 12.1)	0.8 (0.7, 0.8)
Peripheral edema	3.0 (1.9, 4.8)	0.7 (0.6, 0.9)
Encephalopathy	8.8 (3.3, 23.7)	0.9 (0.8, 1.0)
Chapter 7 Cyanosis		
Central cyanosis, detecting arterial deoxyhemoglobin level of ≥2.38 g/dL	7.4 (1.5, 36.8)	0.2 (0.1, 0.5)

Appendix Table 1   Likelihood Ratios—Point Estimates and 95% Confidence Intervals

Finding	Positive LR (95% CI)	Negative LR (95% CI)
EBM Box 8-1 Anemia		
Pallor at any site	4.1 (2.0, 8.7)	0.4 (0.3, 0.7)
Facial pallor	3.8 (2.5, 5.8)	0.6 (0.5, 0.7)
Nailbed pallor	3.9 (0.8, 18.6)	0.5 (0.4, 0.7)
Palmar pallor	5.6 (1.1, 29.1)	0.4 (0.4, 0.5)
Palmar crease pallor	7.9 (1.8, 35.3)	0.9 (0.9, 1.0)
Conjunctival pallor	4.7 (1.9, 11.5)	0.6 (0.4, 0.9)
Conjunctival rim pallor present	16.7 (2.2, 124.7)	...
Conjunctival rim pallor borderline	2.3 (1.5, 3.5)	...
Conjunctival rim pallor absent	0.6 (0.5, 0.8)	...
EBM Box 9-1 Hypovolemia		
Dry axilla	2.8 (1.4, 5.4)	0.6 (0.4, 1.0)
Dry mucous membranes of mouth and nose	2.0 (1.0, 4.0)	0.3 (0.1, 0.6)
Longitudinal furrows on tongue	2.0 (1.0, 4.0)	0.3 (0.1, 0.6)
Sunken eyes	3.4 (1.0, 12.2)	0.5 (0.3, 0.7)
Confusion	2.1 (0.8, 5.7)	0.6 (0.4, 1.0)
Weakness	2.3 (0.6, 8.6)	0.7 (0.5, 1.0)
Speech not clear or expressive	3.1 (0.9, 11.1)	0.5 (0.3, 0.8)
Chapter 10 Protein-Calorie Malnutrition and weight loss		
Alcoholism, predicting organic cause of weight loss	4.5 (1.1, 18.9)	0.8 (0.7, 1.0)
Cigarette smoking, predicting organic cause of weight loss	2.2 (1.1, 4.4)	0.6 (0.4, 0.9)
Prior psychiatric disease, predicting organic cause of weight loss	0.2 (0.1, 0.5)	1.8 (1.3, 2.5)
Abnormal initial physical examination, predicting organic cause of weight loss	20.3 (2.9, 142.8)	0.4 (0.3, 0.6)
Underestimation of weight loss, predicting organic cause	5.4 (2.0, 14.5)	0.6 (0.5, 0.8)
Overestimation of weight loss, predicting nonorganic cause	3.6 (2.0, 6.5)	0.4 (0.2, 0.6)
EBM Box 10-1 Protein-energy malnutrition		
Weight loss >10%	1.4 (1.1, 1.8)	0.9 (0.9, 1.0)
Low body weight	2.0 (1.4, 2.9)	0.9 (0.8, 1.0)
Upper arm circumference <85% predicted	2.5 (1.7, 3.6)	0.8 (0.7, 0.9)
Forearm circumference <85% predicted	3.2 (2.0, 5.1)	0.8 (0.6, 0.9)
Reduced grip strength	2.2 (1.7, 2.8)	0.4 (0.2, 0.6)

Continued

Appendix Table 1	Likelihood Ratios—Point Estimates and 95% Confidence Intervals—Cont'd	

Finding	Positive LR (95% CI)	Negative LR (95% CI)
Chapter 12 Cushing's Syndrome		
Clinically apparent osteoporosis, detecting Cushing's syndrome	17.6 (7.8, 39.4)	0.4 (0.3, 0.5)
Weight loss, detecting ectopic ACTH syndrome	20.0 (1.2, 340.8)	0.5 (0.2, 1.1)
Symptom duration <18 months, detecting ectopic ACTH syndrome	15.0 (3.2, 71.4)	0.1 (0, 1.0)
EBM Box 12-1 Cushing's syndrome		
Hypertension	2.3 (1.5, 3.7)	0.8 (0.6, 0.9)
Moon facies	1.6 (1.1, 2.5)	0.1 (0, 0.9)
Central obesity	3.0 (2.0, 4.4)	0.2 (0.1, 0.3)
Generalized obesity	0.1 (0, 0.2)	2.5 (2.1, 3.1)
Thin skinfold	115.6 (7.2, 1853.8)	0.2 (0.1, 0.6)
Plethora	2.7 (2.1, 3.5)	0.3 (0.1, 0.5)
Hirsutism, in women	1.7 (1.2, 2.5)	0.7 (0.5, 0.9)
Ecchymoses	4.5 (1.2, 16.4)	0.5 (0.4, 0.6)
Red or blue striae	1.9 (1.3, 2.7)	0.7 (0.6, 0.9)
Acne	2.2 (1.5, 3.2)	0.6 (0.5, 0.8)
Proximal muscle weakness	4.4 (1.0, 19.6)	0.4 (0.3, 0.6)
Edema	1.8 (1.1, 3.1)	0.7 (0.6, 0.9)
Chapter 13 Pulse Rate and Contour		
Pulsus paradoxus >12 mm Hg, detecting tamponade	5.9 (2.4, 14.3)	0.03 (0, 0.2)
Delayed carotid artery upstroke, detecting severe aortic stenosis	3.7 (2.5, 5.5)	0.4 (0.2, 0.9)
Hyperkinetic arterial pulse in mitral stenosis, detecting mitral regurgitation	14.2 (7.4, 27.2)	0.3 (0.2, 0.4)
EBM Box 13-1 Tachycardia		
Predicting mortality, trauma and hypotension	1.5 (1.4, 1.7)	0.2 (0.1, 0.5)
Predicting mortality, septic shock	2.0 (1.3, 3.3)	0.1 (0, 0.5)
Predicting mortality, pneumonia	2.1 (1.1, 3.8)	0.7 (0.5, 1.0)
Predicting mortality, myocardial infarction	3.0 (2.3, 4.0)	1.0 (0.9, 1.0)
Predicting complications, gallstone pancreatitis	6.8 (3.7, 12.5)	0.2 (0, 1.0)
Predicting mortality, pontine hemorrhage	25.4 (1.6, 395.3)	0.3 (0.2, 0.6)

Appendix Table 1
Likelihood Ratios—Point Estimates and 95% Confidence Intervals

Finding	Positive LR (95% CI)	Negative LR (95% CI)
EBM Box 13-2 Pulsus paradoxus and asthma		
Pulsus paradoxus >10 mm Hg, predicting severe asthma	2.7 (1.7, 4.3)	0.5 (0.4, 0.7)
Pulsus paradoxus >20 mm Hg, predicting severe asthma	8.2 (1.7, 40.3)	0.8 (0.7, 0.9)
Pulsus paradoxus >25 mm Hg, predicting severe asthma	22.6 (1.4, 363.2)	0.8 (0.8, 0.9)
EBM Box 13-3 Pulses and hypovolemic shock		
Carotid pulse present, detecting systolic blood press ≥60 mm Hg	1.2 (0.9, 1.8)	0.2 (0, 2.1)
Femoral pulse present, detecting systolic blood press ≥60 mm Hg	2.9 (1.1, 7.2)	0.1 (0, 0.5)
Radial pulse present, detecting systolic blood press ≥60 mm Hg	4.7 (0.7, 31.3)	0.5 (0.3, 0.9)
Chapter 14 Abnormalities of Pulse Rhythm		
Pounding sensation in neck, detecting intranodal reentrant tachycardia	350.7 (22.0, 5594)	0.1 (0, 0.2)
EBM Box 14-1 Atrioventricular dissociation		
Varying arterial pulse	2.1 (1.0, 4.4)	0.5 (0.3, 1.0)
Intermittent cannon A waves	3.8 (1.8, 8.2)	0.1 (0, 0.4)
Changing intensity of S_1	24.4 (1.5, 384.5)	0.4 (0.3, 0.7)
Chapter 15 Blood Pressure		
Mediastinal/aortic widening on CXR, detecting aortic dissection	2.0 (1.2, 3.4)	0.3 (0.2, 0.4)
Systolic blood pressure <100 mm Hg, detecting type A dissection	5.0 (1.8, 14.0)	0.9 (0.9, 1.0)
Murmur of aortic regurgitation, detecting type A dissection	5.0 (2.6, 9.8)	0.6 (0.5, 0.8)
Pulse deficit, detecting type A dissection	2.3 (1.6, 3.2)	0.9 (0.8, 1.0)
Detecting coarctation by physical examination	242.2 (89.3, 657)	0.2 (0.1, 0.4)
Proportional pulse pressure <0.25, detecting low cardiac index	6.9 (3.0, 15.8)	0.2 (0.1, 0.6)
Pulse pressure ≥80 mm Hg, detecting moderate-to-severe aortic regurgitation	10.9 (1.5, 77.1)	0.5 (0.2, 0.8)

Continued

| Appendix Table 1 | Likelihood Ratios—Point Estimates and 95% Confidence Intervals—Cont'd |

Finding	Positive LR (95% CI)	Negative LR (95% CI)
EBM Box 15-1 Hypotension		
Predicting mortality, intensive care unit	4.0 (3.6, 4.3)	0.8 (0.8, 0.9)
Predicting mortality, bacteremia	4.9 (4.2, 5.7)	0.6 (0.2, 1.4)
Predicting mortality, pneumonia	10.0 (5.6, 17.6)	0.8 (0.7, 1.0)
Predicting mortality, myocardial infarction	15.5 (12.2, 19.6)	0.7 (0.7, 0.7)
EBM Box 15-2 Aortic dissection		
Pulse deficit	6.0 (1.1, 32.5)	0.7 (0.5, 1.0)
Aortic regurgitation murmur	1.4 (0.9, 2.2)	0.9 (0.8, 1.0)
Focal neurologic signs	33.4 (2.0, 549)	0.9 (0.8, 1.0)
Combined findings, 0 predictors	0.1 (0, 0.2)	...
Combined findings, 1 predictor	0.5 (0.4, 0.8)	...
Combined findings, 2 predictors	5.3 (3.0, 9.4)	...
Combined findings, 3 predictors	65.8 (4.1, 1062)	...
EBM Box 15-3: Systolic blood pressure and impaired consciousness		
Systolic blood pressure <120 mm Hg, detecting structural brain lesion	0.1 (0.1, 0.2)	...
Systolic blood pressure 120–159 mm Hg, detecting structural brain lesion	1.2 (0.9, 1.6)	...
Systolic blood pressure ≥160 mm Hg, detecting structural brain lesion	10.4 (6.0, 18.2)	...
Chapter 16 Temperature		
WBC >15,000, detecting bacteremia	1.6 (1.2, 2.2)	0.8 (0.8, 0.9)
Bands >1,500, detecting bacteremia	2.6 (1.3, 5.1)	0.7 (0.6, 0.9)
Shaking chills, detecting bacteremia	1.8 (1.6, 2.1)	0.8 (0.7, 0.9)
Stepladder remittent fever, detecting typhoid fever	177.4 (11.1, 2842)	0.5 (0.4, 0.6)
EBM Box 16-1 Detection of fever		
Patient's report of fever	2.9 (1.1, 8.0)	0.3 (0.2, 0.5)
Patient's forehead abnormally warm	2.9 (2.5, 3.5)	0.3 (0.1, 0.6)
EBM Box 16-2 Detection of bacteremia		
Age 50 years or more	1.4 (1.2, 1.6)	0.3 (0.1, 0.8)
Renal failure	4.6 (2.6, 8.1)	0.8 (0.7, 0.9)
Hospitalization for trauma	3.0 (2.4, 3.8)	0.7 (0.3, 1.3)
Intravenous drug use	2.9 (1.1, 7.3)	1.0 (0.9, 1.0)
Previous stroke	2.8 (1.2, 6.2)	0.9 (0.8, 1.0)
Diabetes mellitus	1.5 (1.1, 2.1)	0.9 (0.9, 1.0)
Poor functional performance	3.6 (2.2, 5.9)	0.6 (0.4, 0.8)

Appendix Table 1 Likelihood Ratios—Point Estimates and 95% Confidence Intervals

Finding	Positive LR (95% CI)	Negative LR (95% CI)
Rapidly fatal disease (<1 mo)	2.7 (1.4, 5.2)	0.9 (0.9, 1.0)
Indwelling urinary catheter present	2.4 (1.2, 4.7)	0.8 (0.7, 1.0)
Central intravenous line present	2.0 (1.4, 2.8)	0.9 (0.8, 1.0)
Temperature ≥38.5°C	1.2 (1.1, 1.3)	0.5 (0.2, 1.0)
Tachycardia	1.2 (1.1, 1.4)	0.7 (0.6, 0.9)
Respiratory rate >20/min	0.9 (0.8, 1.1)	1.2 (0.8, 1.7)
Hypotension	2.6 (1.6, 4.4)	0.9 (0.9, 1.0)
Acute abdomen	1.7 (1.3, 2.3)	1.0 (0.9, 1.0)
Confusion or depressed sensorium	1.5 (1.3, 1.8)	0.9 (0.8, 1.0)
EBM Box 16-3 Extremes of temperature and prognosis		
Temperature >39°C, predicting mortality in pontine hemorrhage	23.7 (1.5, 371)	0.4 (0.2, 0.6)
Temperature <35.2°C, predicting death in heart failure	6.7 (2.7, 16.9)	0.7 (0.5, 1.0)
Temperature <36.1°C predicting death in pneumonia	3.5 (1.1, 10.9)	0.8 (0.5, 1.2)
Temperature <36.5°C, predicting death in bacteremia	3.3 (1.1, 10)	0.9 (0.8, 1.0)
Chapter 17 Respiratory Rate and Abnormal Breathing Patterns		
Asynchronous breathing, predicting hospital death or intubation	3.2 (1.3, 7.8)	0.5 (0.2, 1.0)
Paradoxical abdominal movements, detecting diaphragm weakness	3.2 (1.7, 5.9)	0.1 (0, 1.1)
Orthopnea, detecting low ventricular ejection fraction	2.7 (1.5, 4.9)	0.04 (0, 0.7)
EBM Box 17-1 Tachypnea		
Respiratory rate >24/min, predicting failure of weaning	2.9 (1.2, 7.1)	0.1 (0, 1.4)
Respiratory rate >27/min, predicting cardiopulmonary arrest	3.1 (1.9, 5.1)	0.6 (0.4, 0.7)
Respiratory rate >28/min, detecting pneumonia	2.0 (1.4, 2.8)	0.8 (0.7, 0.9)
Respiratory rate >30/min, predicting mortality in pneumonia	2.1 (1.7, 2.6)	0.6 (0.5, 0.8)
Chapter 19 The Pupils		
Asymmetric facial sweating in Horner's syndrome, detecting first or second order neuron lesion	2.4 (0.9, 6.1)	0.6 (0.4, 0.9)

Continued

Appendix Table 1	Likelihood Ratios—Point Estimates and 95% Confidence Intervals—Cont'd

Finding	Positive LR (95% CI)	Negative LR (95% CI)
EBM Box 19-1 Pupils		
Anisocoria > 1 mm, detecting intracranial structural lesion	9.0 (2.8, 28.8)	0.6 (0.5, 0.8)
Absent light reflex, detecting intracranial structural lesion	3.6 (2.3, 5.6)	0.2 (0.1, 0.4)
Post-topical cocaine anisocoria, detecting Horner's syndrome	96.8 (6.1, 1527.3)	0.1 (0, 0.1)
Dilation with topical hydroxyamphetamine, detecting 1st or 2nd order neuron lesion in Horner's syndrome	9.2 (2.0, 43.6)	0.2 (0.1, 0.3)
Anisocoria, detecting intraocular inflammation	6.5 (2.6, 16.3)	0.8 (0.8, 0.9)
Chapter 20 Diabetic Retinopathy		
Visual acuity 20/60 or worse, detecting diabetic retinopathy	1.2 (0.7, 2.3)	1.0 (0.9, 1.1)
EBM Box 20-1 Diabetic retinopathy		
Direct ophthalmoscopy through nondilated pupils, detecting diabetic retinopathy	6.2 (2.5, 14.9)	0.5 (0.3, 0.8)
Direct ophthalmoscopy through dilated pupils (general providers), detecting diabetic retinopathy	10.2 (6.0, 17.4)	0.4 (0.3, 0.5)
Direct ophthalmoscopy through dilated pupils (specialists), detecting diabetic retinopathy	18.6 (5.7, 61)	0.3 (0.2, 0.5)
EBM Box 21-1 Hearing tests		
Abnormal whispered voice test, detecting hearing loss	6.0 (4.4, 8.2)	0.03 (0, 0.3)
Rinne test, detecting conductive hearing loss	16.8 (13.8, 20.4)	0.2 (0.1, 0.8)
Weber test lateralizes to good ear, detecting neurosensory hearing loss	2.7 (1.2, 6.4)	0.5 (0.3, 1.1)
Weber test lateralizes to bad ear, detecting conductive hearing loss	6.4 (1.0, 43.3)	0.5 (0.3, 0.8)
Chapter 22 The Thyroid and Its Disorders		
Precise measurement of reflex time, hypothyroidism	18.7 (13.3, 26.3)	0.1 (0, 0.2)

Appendix Table 1   Likelihood Ratios—Point Estimates and 95% Confidence Intervals

Finding	Positive LR (95% CI)	Negative LR (95% CI)
EBM Box 22-1 Goiter		
No goiter, palpation or inspection	0.4 (0.3, 0.5)	...
Goiter by palpation, visible after neck extension	0.9 (0.4, 2.1)	...
Goiter, palpation and inspection in normal position	26.3 (5.2, 131.7)	...
EBM Box 22-2 Goiter, thyroid nodules, and carcinoma		
Goiter, vocal cord paralysis	45.2 (2.7, 762.1)	0.8 (0.6, 0.9)
Goiter, cervical adenopathy	13.4 (4.6, 39.2)	0.6 (0.4, 0.7)
Goiter, fixation to surrounding tissue	9.7 (4.5, 21.2)	0.4 (0.3, 0.6)
Goiter nodular (vs. diffuse)	1.5 (1.2, 1.9)	0.5 (0.3, 0.8)
Goiter, pyramidal lobe present	0.3 (0.1, 1.7)	1.1 (1.0, 1.2)
Thyroid nodule, vocal cord paralysis	12.0 (2.0, 70.5)	0.9 (0.8, 1.0)
Thyroid nodule, fixation to surrounding tissues	7.8 (3.3, 18.3)	0.8 (0.6, 1.0)
Thyroid nodule, cervical adenopathy	7.4 (2.9, 19.0)	0.7 (0.6, 0.9)
Thyroid nodule, diameter ≥4 cm	1.9 (1.4, 2.7)	0.5 (0.4, 0.7)
Thyroid nodule, very firm nodule	3.3 (0.4, 30.6)	1.0 (0.9, 1.0)
EBM Box 22-3 Hypothyroidism		
Cool and dry skin	4.7 (3.1, 7.1)	0.9 (0.8, 0.9)
Coarse skin	3.4 (1.4, 8.0)	0.7 (0.5, 0.9)
Cold palms	1.6 (1.0, 2.7)	0.8 (0.6, 1.1)
Dry palms	1.5 (1.0, 2.4)	0.8 (0.6, 1.1)
Periorbital puffiness	1.7 (0.7, 4.2)	0.6 (0.4, 0.8)
Puffiness of wrists	2.9 (1.7, 4.9)	0.7 (0.5, 0.9)
Hair loss of eyebrows	1.9 (1.1, 3.6)	0.8 (0.7, 1.0)
Pretibial edema	1.1 (0.9, 1.5)	0.7 (0.3, 1.6)
Hypothyroid speech	5.4 (2.7, 10.7)	0.7 (0.5, 0.9)
Slow pulse rate	4.1 (3.2, 5.3)	0.8 (0.7, 0.8)
Enlarged thyroid	2.8 (2.3, 3.4)	0.6 (0.6, 0.7)
Delayed ankle reflexes	3.4 (1.8, 6.4)	0.6 (0.4, 0.9)
Slow movements	1.0 (0.8, 1.2)	1.0 (0.3, 3.2)
Billewicz score less than −15 points	0.1 (0, 0.2)	...
Billewicz score −15 to +29 points	0.9 (0.4, 2.1)	...
Billewicz score +30 points or more	18.8 (1.2, 300.5)	...

Continued

Finding	Positive LR (95% CI)	Negative LR (95% CI)
EBM Box 22-4 Hyperthyroidism		
Pulse ≥90 beats/min	4.4 (3.8, 5.1)	0.2 (0.2, 0.3)
Skin moist and warm	6.7 (5.0, 9.1)	0.7 (0.7, 0.7)
Enlarged thyroid	2.3 (2.1, 2.5)	0.1 (0.1, 0.2)
Eyelid retraction	31.5 (16.6, 59.7)	0.7 (0.6, 0.7)
Eyelid lag	17.6 (9.2, 33.7)	0.8 (0.8, 0.8)
Fine finger tremor	11.4 (8.7, 14.8)	0.3 (0.3, 0.4)
Wayne index <11 points	0.04 (0, 0.3)	...
Wayne index 11–19 points	1.2 (0.7, 2.0)	...
Wayne index ≥20 points	18.2 (2.9, 113.5)	...
Chapter 23 Meninges		
Nuchal rigidity, detecting meningitis	3.0 (2.1, 4.2)	0.1 (0, 2.0)
EBM Box 23-1 Subarachnoid hemorrhage		
Neck stiffness	10.3 (5.2, 20.7)	0.4 (0.3, 0.7)
Neurologic findings not focal	5.9 (3.5, 9.9)	0.4 (0.2, 0.7)
Age ≤60 years	1.8 (1.4, 2.3)	0.3 (0.1, 0.8)
Seizures	2.2 (1.1, 4.5)	0.8 (0.6, 1.1)
Chapter 24 Peripheral Lymphadenopathy		
Pruritus, detecting serious disease	4.9 (1.8, 13.1)	0.9 (0.9, 1.0)
Sore throat, detecting serious disease	0.2 (0.1, 0.4)	1.4 (1.2, 1.6)
Epitrochlear nodes, detecting HIV seropositivity	4.5 (3.1, 6.7)	0.2 (0.1, 0.3)
EBM Box 24-1 Lymphadenopathy		
Male sex	1.3 (1.1, 1.6)	0.8 (0.7, 0.9)
Age 40 years or more	2.4 (1.7, 3.5)	0.4 (0.3, 0.6)
Weight loss	3.4 (2.2, 5.4)	0.8 (0.8, 0.9)
Fever	0.7 (0.5, 1.0)	1.1 (1.0, 1.2)
Head and neck nodes (excluding supraclavicular)	0.9 (0.8, 1.1)	1.1 (0.9, 1.2)
Supraclavicular nodes	3.2 (2.3, 4.3)	0.8 (0.7, 0.9)
Axillary nodes	0.8 (0.6, 0.9)	1.1 (1.0, 1.1)
Inguinal nodes	0.6 (0.4, 0.7)	1.1 (1.0, 1.1)
Epitrochlear nodes	0.7 (0.1, 7.6)	1.0 (1.0, 1.1)
Generalized lymphadenopathy	1.3 (0.6, 2.9)	1.0 (0.7, 1.4)
Lymph node size <4 cm^2	0.4 (0.3, 0.7)	...
Lymph node size 4–8.99 cm^2	2.0 (0.4, 9.2)	...
Lymph node size ≥9 cm^2	8.4 (2.1, 32.8)	...
Hard texture	3.2 (2.4, 4.3)	0.6 (0.4, 0.7)
Lymph node tenderness	0.4 (0.3, 0.6)	1.3 (1.1, 1.5)
Fixed lymph nodes	10.9 (2.0, 59.2)	0.7 (0.3, 1.3)

Appendix Table 1   Likelihood Ratios—Point Estimates and 95% Confidence Intervals

Finding	Positive LR (95% CI)	Negative LR (95% CI)
Rash	0.6 (0.3, 1.4)	1.0 (1.0, 1.1)
Palpable spleen	1.2 (0.6, 2.5)	1.0 (0.9, 1.0)
Palpable liver	1.2 (0.7, 1.9)	1.0 (0.9, 1.1)
Lymph node score −3 or less	0.04 (0, 0.2)	...
Lymph node score −2 or −1	0.1 (0, 0.3)	...
Lymph node score 0 to 4	1.1 (0.5, 2.3)	...
Lymph node score 5 or 6	5.1 (2.9, 8.8)	...
Lymph node score 7 or more	21.9 (2.7, 179.4)	...
Chapter 25 Inspection of the Chest		
Clubbing, detecting hypoxemia in cystic fibrosis	3.2 (1.7, 6.1)	0.1 (0.1, 0.3)
Absence of accessory muscle use, detecting normal diaphragmatic strength in amyotrophic lateral sclerosis	4.4 (1.7, 11.8)	0.2 (0, 2.6)
EBM Box 26-1 Percussion of the chest		
Conventional dullness, detecting pneumonia	3.0 (1.7, 5.2)	0.9 (0.8, 1.0)
Conventional dullness, detecting any abnormality	3.0 (1.4, 6.3)	0.9 (0.9, 1.0)
Hyperresonance, detecting chronic airflow obstruction	5.1 (1.7, 15.6)	0.7 (0.5, 1.0)
Diaphragm excursion < 2 cm, detecting chronic airflow obstruction	5.3 (0.8, 35.0)	0.9 (0.7, 1.1)
Auscultatory dullness, detecting any abnormality	1.7 (1.0, 3.0)	0.8 (0.6, 1.1)
Auscultatory dullness, detecting pleural fluid	18.6 (9.8, 35.2)	0.04 (0, 0.1)
Chapter 27 Auscultation of the Lungs		
Crackles, predicting 30-day mortality in patients with myocardial infarction	4.5 (3.9, 5.3)	0.7 (0.6, 0.8)
EBM Box 27-1 Breath sounds and vocal resonance		
Breath sound score ≤9, detecting chronic airflow obstruction	10.2 (4.6, 22.7)	...
Breath sound score 10–12, detecting chronic airflow obstruction	3.6 (1.4, 9.5)	...
Breath sound score 13–15, detecting chronic airflow obstruction	0.7 (0.3, 1.5)	...
Breath sound score, >15, detecting chronic airflow obstruction	0.1 (0, 0.3)	...

Continued

Appendix Table 1 — Likelihood Ratios—Point Estimates and 95% Confidence Intervals—Cont'd

Finding	Positive LR (95% CI)	Negative LR (95% CI)
Diminished breath sounds detecting pleural effusion in mechanically ventilated patients	4.3 (2.8, 6.5)	0.6 (0.5, 0.8)
Diminished breath sounds, detecting asthma during methacholine challenge	4.2 (1.9, 9.5)	0.3 (0.1, 0.6)
Diminished breath sounds, detecting pneumonia	2.3 (1.9, 2.8)	0.8 (0.7, 0.9)
Bronchial breath sounds, detecting pneumonia	3.3 (2.0, 5.6)	0.9 (0.8, 1.0)
Egophony, detecting pneumonia	4.1 (2.1, 7.8)	0.9 (0.9, 1.0)
EBM Box 27-2 Crackles and Wheezes		
Crackles, detecting pulmonary fibrosis in asbestos workers	5.9 (2.0, 17.2)	0.2 (0.1, 0.5)
Crackles, detecting left atrial pressure ≥12 mm Hg in patients with cardiomyopathy	3.4 (1.6, 7.2)	0.7 (0.6, 1.0)
Crackles, detecting myocardial infarction in patients with chest pain	2.1 (1.6, 2.8)	0.8 (0.7, 1.0)
Crackles, detecting pneumonia in patients with cough and fever	1.8 (1.2, 2.7)	0.8 (0.7, 0.9)
Early crackles, detecting obstructive disease	14.6 (3.0, 70)	0.4 (0.1, 1.4)
Early crackles, detecting severe obstruction	20.8 (3.0, 142.2)	0.1 (0, 0.4)
Unforced wheezes, detecting obstructive disease	2.8 (1.5, 5.0)	0.8 (0.7, 0.9)
Methacholine wheezes, detecting asthma	6.0 (1.5, 24.3)	0.6 (0.4, 0.9)
EBM Box 28-1 Ancillary tests		
Forced expiratory time <3 sec, detecting chronic airflow obstruction	0.2 (0.1, 0.3)	...
Forced expiratory time 3–9 sec, detecting chronic airflow obstruction	1.3 (0.5, 2.9)	...
Forced expiratory time ≥9 sec, detecting chronic airflow obstruction	4.1 (2.6, 6.4)	...
Snider test, detecting FEV_1 ≤1.6 L	9.6 (5.5, 16.6)	0.2 (0.1, 0.8)

Appendix Table 1 Likelihood Ratios—Point Estimates and 95% Confidence Intervals

Finding	Positive LR (95% CI)	Negative LR (95% CI)
Chapter 29 Pneumonia		
Absence of sore throat, detecting pneumonia	1.8 (1.3, 2.5)	0.7 (0.6, 0.9)
Absence of rhinorrhea, detecting pneumonia	2.2 (1.5, 3.2)	0.8 (0.7, 0.9)
EBM Box 29-1 Pneumonia		
Cachexia	4.0 (1.7, 9.6)	0.9 (0.8, 1.0)
Abnormal mental status	1.9 (1.2, 3.0)	0.9 (0.9, 1.0)
Temperature >37.8°C	2.0 (1.5, 2.6)	0.7 (0.6, 0.8)
Respiratory rate >28/min	2.0 (1.4, 2.8)	0.8 (0.7, 0.9)
Heart rate >100 beats/min	1.6 (1.4, 1.7)	0.8 (0.7, 0.9)
Percussion dullness	3.0 (1.7, 5.2)	0.9 (0.8, 1.0)
Diminished breath sounds	2.3 (1.9, 2.8)	0.8 (0.7, 0.9)
Bronchial breath sounds	3.3 (2.0, 5.6)	0.9 (0.8, 1.0)
Egophony	4.1 (2.1, 7.8)	0.9 (0.9, 1.0)
Crackles	1.8 (1.2, 2.7)	0.8 (0.7, 0.9)
Wheezes	0.8 (0.7, 0.9)	1.1 (1.0, 1.1)
Heckerling score, 0 or 1 finding	0.3 (0.2, 0.4)	...
Heckerling score, 2 or 3 findings	1.0 (0.9, 1.2)	...
Heckerling score, 4 or 5 findings	8.2 (5.8, 11.5)	...
EBM Box 29-2 Pneumonia and mortality		
Abnormal mental status	2.8 (2.1, 3.8)	0.6 (0.5, 0.7)
Respiratory rate >30/min	2.1 (1.7, 2.6)	0.6 (0.5, 0.8)
Systolic blood pressure <90 mm Hg	10.0 (5.6, 17.6)	0.8 (0.7, 1.0)
Heart rate >100 beats/min	2.1 (1.1, 3.8)	0.7 (0.5, 1.0)
Hypothermia	3.5 (1.1, 10.9)	0.8 (0.5, 1.2)
CURB score, 0 findings	0.3 (0.2, 0.5)	...
CURB score, 1 findings	0.9 (0.7, 1.3)	...
CURB score, 2 findings	1.9 (1.1, 3.5)	...
CURB score, 3 findings	4.7 (2.5, 8.9)	...
CURB score, 4 findings	10.2 (2.3, 44.9)	...
Chapter 30 Chronic Obstructive Lung Disease		
Early inspiratory crackles, detecting severe disease	20.8 (3.0, 142.2)	0.1 (0, 0.4)
EBM Box 30-1 Chronic obstructive lung disease		
Maximum laryngeal height ≤4 cm	3.6 (2.1, 6.0)	0.7 (0.6, 0.8)
Laryngeal descent >3 cm	0.9 (0.5, 1.4)	1.0 (0.9, 1.1)
Hoover's sign	4.2 (2.5, 7.0)	0.5 (0.4, 0.7)

Continued

Appendix Table 1	Likelihood Ratios—Point Estimates and 95% Confidence Intervals—Cont'd

Finding	Positive LR (95% CI)	Negative LR (95% CI)
Subxiphoid cardiac impulse	7.4 (2.0, 27.1)	0.9 (0.7, 1.1)
Absent cardiac dullness	11.8 (1.2, 121.4)	0.9 (0.7, 1.1)
Hyperresonance	5.1 (1.7, 15.6)	0.7 (0.5, 1.0)
Diaphragm excursion <2 cm	5.3 (0.8, 35.0)	0.9 (0.7, 1.1)
Breath sound score, ≤9	10.2 (4.6, 22.7)	...
Breath sound score 10–12	3.6 (1.4, 9.5)	...
Breath sound score 13–15	0.7 (0.3, 1.5)	...
Breath sound score, >15	0.1 (0, 0.3)	...
Early inspiratory crackles	14.6 (3.0, 70.0)	0.4 (0.1, 1.4)
Unforced wheezes	2.8 (1.5, 5.0)	0.8 (0.7, 0.9)
Forced expiratory time, <3 sec	0.2 (0.1, 0.3)	...
Forced expiratory time, 3–9 sec	1.3 (0.5, 2.9)	...
Forced expiratory time, ≥9 sec	4.1 (2.6, 6.4)	...
Combined findings, 2 of 3	25.7 (6.2, 105.5)	0.3 (0.2, 0.7)
Chapter 31 Pulmonary Embolism		
Sudden dyspnea	2.4 (2.0, 2.9)	0.3 (0.2, 0.3)
Hemoptysis	2.0 (1.4, 2.7)	1.0 (0.9, 1.0)
Syncope	2.0 (1.6, 2.5)	0.9 (0.8, 1.0)
Orthopnea	0.1 (0, 0.2)	1.1 (1.1, 1.1)
Pulse rate <90/min	0.3 (0.1, 0.8)	1.8 (1.3, 2.5)
Hypoxemia (pO_2 < 80 mm Hg)	1.2 (1.0, 1.4)	0.6 (0.3, 1.2)
Increased A-a gradient	1.1 (1.0, 1.2)	0.3 (0, 2.4)
EBM Box 31-1 Pulmonary embolism		
Temperature >38°C	0.4 (0.3, 0.7)	1.1 (1.0, 1.2)
Pulse >100/min	1.2 (0.9, 1.5)	0.9 (0.8, 1.1)
Respiratory rate >30/min	2.0 (1.5, 2.8)	0.9 (0.8, 0.9)
Systolic blood pressure ≤100 mm Hg	1.9 (1.1, 3.0)	1.0 (0.9, 1.0)
Cyanosis	1.0 (0.1, 8.3)	1.0 (0.9, 1.1)
Accessory muscle use	1.5 (0.6, 3.6)	0.9 (0.8, 1.1)
Crackles	1.2 (0.8, 1.7)	0.8 (0.5, 1.4)
Wheezes	0.2 (0.1, 0.4)	1.1 (1.1, 1.1)
Pleural friction rub	1.5 (0.6, 3.8)	1.0 (0.8, 1.1)
Elevated neck veins	0.8 (0.1, 6.3)	1.0 (0.9, 1.1)
Left parasternal heave	1.2 (0.1, 29.9)	1.0 (1.0, 1.0)
Loud P_2	1.1 (0.4, 3.1)	1.0 (0.8, 1.2)
New gallop (S_3 or S_4)	2.7 (1.0, 7.0)	0.8 (0.6, 1.0)
Chest wall tenderness	0.8 (0.6, 1.1)	1.1 (1.0, 1.1)
Unilateral calf pain or swelling	2.3 (1.8, 3.0)	0.9 (0.8, 1.0)
Wells score, low probability, 0–1 points	0.2 (0.1, 0.4)	...
Wells score, moderate probability, 2–6 points	1.7 (1.5, 2.0)	...

| **Appendix Table 1** | Likelihood Ratios—Point Estimates and 95% Confidence Intervals |

Finding	Positive LR (95% CI)	Negative LR (95% CI)
Wells score, high probability, 7 or more points	5.0 (2.5, 10)	...
Chapter 32 Inspection of the Neck Veins		
Catheter measurements of CVP ≥10 mm Hg, detecting pulmonary capillary wedge pressure ≥22 mm Hg	4.5 (3.6, 5.7)	0.3 (0.2, 0.3)
Intermittent cannon A waves, detecting atrioventricular dissociation	3.8 (1.8, 8.2)	0.1 (0, 0.4)
EBM Box 32-1 Inspection of neck veins		
Detecting measured CVP >8 cm H_2O	9.0 (3.7, 22.1)	0.2 (0, 1.5)
Detecting measured CVP >12 cm H_2O	10.4 (5.5, 19.9)	0.1 (0, 0.6)
Detecting elevated left heart diastolic pressures	3.9 (1.6, 9.4)	0.7 (0.5, 1.0)
Detecting low left ejection fraction	7.9 (2.8, 22.4)	0.9 (0.8, 1.0)
Predicting postoperative pulmonary edema	11.3 (5.0, 25.8)	0.8 (0.7, 1.0)
Predicting postoperative infarction or death	9.4 (4.0, 22.4)	0.8 (0.7, 1.0)
Abdominojugular test, detecting elevated left heart pressures	8.0 (2.1, 31.2)	0.3 (0.2, 0.6)
EBM Box 33-1 Percussion of the heart		
Dullness >10.5 cm from midsternal line, detecting cardiothoracic ratio >0.5	2.5 (1.8, 3.4)	0.05 (0, 0.3)
Dullness >10.5 cm from midsternal line, detecting increased left ventricular volume	1.4 (1.1, 1.7)	0.2 (0, 1.3)
Dullness extending beyond midclavicular line, detecting cardiothoracic ratio >0.5	2.4 (1.1, 5.2)	0.1 (0, 0.4)
EBM Box 34-1 Palpable apical impulse		
Supine apical impulse lateral to midclavicular line, detecting cardiothoracic ratio >0.5	3.4 (1.6, 7.3)	0.6 (0.5, 0.8)
Supine apical impulse lateral to midclavicular line, detecting low ejection fraction	10.1 (3.8, 26.6)	0.6 (0.5, 0.9)
Supine apical impulse lateral to midclavicular line, detecting increased ventricular volume	8.0 (1.9, 33.0)	0.7 (0.6, 0.9)

Continued

<table>
<tr><td>**Appendix Table 1**</td><td>Likelihood Ratios—Point Estimates and 95% Confidence Intervals—Cont'd</td></tr>
</table>

Finding	Positive LR (95% CI)	Negative LR (95% CI)
Supine apical impulse lateral to midclavicular line, detecting wedge pressure >12 mm Hg	5.8 (1.3, 26.0)	0.6 (0.4, 1.0)
Supine apical impulse >10 cm from midsternal line, detecting cardiothoracic ratio >0.5	4.3 (0.3, 70.8)	0.5 (0.3, 0.8)
Apical beat diameter ≥4 cm in lateral decubitus position, detecting increased ventricular volume	4.7 (2.1, 10.2)	0.4 (0.2, 1.0)
EBM Box 34-2 Abnormal palpable movements		
Hyperkinetic apical movement in mitral stenosis, detecting additional valvular lesion	11.2 (6.4, 19.5)	0.3 (0.2, 0.4)
Sustained apical movement, detecting severe aortic stenosis	4.1 (1.7, 10.1)	0.3 (0.1, 0.5)
Sustained apical movement, detecting moderate to severe aortic regurgitation	2.4 (1.4, 4.0)	0.1 (0, 0.9)
Sustained left lower parasternal movement, detecting right ventricular pressure ≥50 mm Hg	3.6 (1.4, 8.9)	0.4 (0.2, 0.7)
Palpable P_2, detecting pulmonary hypertension in patients with mitral stenosis	3.6 (1.5, 8.8)	0.05 (0, 0.8)
EBM Box 36-1 First and second heart sounds		
Changing intensity of S_1, detecting atrioventricular dissociation	24.4 (1.5, 384.5)	0.4 (0.3, 0.7)
Fixed wide splitting of S_2, detecting atrial septal defect	2.6 (1.6, 4.3)	0.1 (0, 0.8)
Paradoxic splitting of S_2, detecting significant aortic stenosis	2.4 (0.8, 7.0)	0.6 (0.2, 1.7)
Loud P_2, detecting pulmonary hypertension	1.2 (0.9, 1.5)	0.8 (0.3, 1.9)
Palpable P_2, detecting pulmonary hypertension	3.6 (1.5, 8.8)	0.05 (0, 0.8)
Chapter 37 The Third and Fourth Heart Sound		
S_3, detecting elevated filling pressure in mitral regurgitation	1.7 (1.0, 3.0)	0.7 (0.5, 0.9)
S_3, detecting depressed ejection fraction in mitral regurgitation	1.9 (1.2, 2.9)	0.6 (0.4, 0.9)

Appendix Table 1 — Likelihood Ratios—Point Estimates and 95% Confidence Intervals

Finding	Positive LR (95% CI)	Negative LR (95% CI)
S_3, detecting pulmonary capillary wedge pressure ≥ 12 mm Hg in aortic stenosis	2.3 (1.3, 4.0)	0.9 (0.8, 1.0)
S_3, detecting ejection fraction <50% in aortic stenosis	5.7 (2.7, 12.0)	0.8 (0.7, 0.9)
S_3, detecting regurgitant fraction $\geq 40\%$ in aortic regurgitation	5.9 (1.4, 25.3)	0.8 (0.7, 0.9)
S_3, detecting ejection fraction <50% in aortic regurgitation	8.3 (3.6, 19.2)	0.4 (0.2, 0.9)
EBM Box 37-1 Third and fourth heart sounds		
S_3, detecting ejection fraction <0.5	3.4 (2.6, 4.4)	0.7 (0.5, 0.9)
S_3, detecting ejection fraction <0.3	4.1 (2.3, 7.3)	0.3 (0.2, 0.5)
S_3, detecting elevated left heart filling pressures	5.7 (3.1, 10.3)	0.8 (0.7, 1.0)
S_3, detecting elevated BNP level	10.1 (4.2, 23.9)	0.5 (0.3, 0.8)
S_3, detecting myocardial infarction in patients with acute chest pain	3.2 (1.6, 6.5)	0.9 (0.8, 1.0)
S_3, predicting postoperative pulmonary edema	14.6 (5.7, 37.3)	0.8 (0.7, 1.0)
S_3, predicting postoperative infarction or death	8.0 (2.7, 23.4)	0.9 (0.8, 1.0)
S_4, predicting 5-year mortality after infarction	3.2 (1.3, 7.8)	0.8 (0.6, 1.1)
S_4, detecting elevated filling pressures	1.4 (0.8, 2.6)	0.6 (0.3, 1.4)
S_4, detecting severe aortic stenosis	0.9 (0.5, 1.9)	1.1 (0.6, 1.9)
EBM Box 39-1 Murmurs and valvular heart disease		
Abnormal heart examination, detecting valvular heart disease	18.3 (5.7, 59.3)	0.3 (0.2, 0.4)
Characteristic systolic murmur, detecting aortic stenosis	3.3 (2.8, 3.9)	0.1 (0, 0.1)
Characteristic systolic murmur, detecting mild mitral regurgitation or worse	5.4 (3.7, 8.1)	0.4 (0.2, 0.7)
Characteristic systolic murmur, detecting moderate-to-severe mitral regurgitation	3.3 (2.7, 4.1)	0.2 (0.1, 0.4)
Characteristic systolic murmur, detecting mild tricuspid regurgitation or worse	14.6 (4.5, 47.1)	0.8 (0.7, 0.9)

Continued

| Appendix Table 1 | Likelihood Ratios—Point Estimates and 95% Confidence Intervals—Cont'd | |

Finding	Positive LR (95% CI)	Negative LR (95% CI)
Characteristic systolic murmur, detecting moderate-to-severe tricuspid regurgitation	10.1 (5.8, 17.8)	0.4 (0.2, 0.7)
Characteristic systolic murmur, detecting ventricular septal defect	24.9 (8.6, 72.7)	0.1 (0, 1.4)
Characteristic systolic murmur, detecting mitral valve prolapse	12.1 (4.0, 36.4)	0.5 (0.2, 0.9)
Characteristic diastolic murmur, detecting mild aortic regurgitation or worse	9.9 (4.9, 20.0)	0.3 (0.2, 0.4)
Characteristic diastolic murmur detecting moderate-to-severe aortic regurgitation	4.3 (2.1, 8.6)	0.1 (0.1, 0.2)
Characteristic diastolic murmur, detecting pulmonary regurgitation	17.4 (3.6, 83.2)	0.9 (0.8, 1.0)
EBM Box 39-2 Systolic murmurs and maneuvers		
Louder during inspiration, detecting right-sided murmurs	7.8 (3.7, 16.7)	0.2 (0.1, 0.5)
Louder with Valsalva strain, detecting hypertrophic cardiomyopathy	14.0 (3.4, 57.4)	0.3 (0.1, 0.8)
Louder with squatting-to-standing, detecting hypertropic cardiomyopathy	6.0 (2.9, 12.3)	0.1 (0, 0.8)
Softer with standing-to-squatting, detecting hypertrophic cardiomyopathy	7.6 (2.5, 22.7)	0.1 (0, 0.4)
Softer with passive leg elevation, detecting hypertrophic cardiomyopathy	9.0 (3.5, 23.3)	0.1 (0, 0.7)
Softer with isometric hand grip, detecting hypertrophic cardiomyopathy	3.6 (2.0, 6.4)	0.1 (0, 0.9)
Louder with isometric hand grip, detecting mitral regurgitation or ventricular septal defect	5.8 (1.9, 17.3)	0.3 (0.2, 0.5)
Louder with transient arterial occlusion, detecting mitral regurgitation or ventricular septal defect	48.7 (3.1, 768.5)	0.2 (0.1, 0.5)

Appendix Table 1   Likelihood Ratios—Point Estimates and 95% Confidence Intervals

Finding	Positive LR (95% CI)	Negative LR (95% CI)
Softer with amyl nitrite inhalation, detecting mitral regurgitation or ventricular septal defect	10.5 (5.1, 21.5)	0.2 (0.1, 0.6)
Chapter 40 Aortic stenosis		
Calcification of aortic valve on chest radiography, detecting severe aortic stenosis	3.9 (2.1, 7.3)	0.5 (0.4, 0.7)
Left ventricular hypertrophy on electrocardiogram, detecting severe aortic stenosis	2.1 (1.7, 2.7)	0.5 (0.4, 0.6)
Delayed carotid upstroke, detecting moderate-to-severe aortic stenosis	13.1 (6.1, 27.8)	0.5 (0.4, 0.8)
A_2 reduced or absent, detecting moderate-to-severe aortic stenosis	10.7 (5.1, 22.4)	0.4 (0.3, 0.6)
Prolonged duration of murmur, detecting moderate-to-severe aortic stenosis	29.5 (9.6, 91.1)	0.3 (0.2, 0.4)
Late peaking murmur, detecting moderate-to-severe aortic stenosis	29.5 (9.6, 91.1)	0.3 (0.2, 0.4)
0–6 points, detecting moderate-to-severe aortic stenosis	0.2 (0.1, 0.4)	...
7–9 points, detecting moderate-to-severe aortic stenosis	2.7 (0.9, 8.1)	...
10–14 points, detecting moderate-to-severe aortic stenosis	10.6 (1.5, 73.3)	...
EBM Box 40-1 Characteristics of severe aortic stenosis		
Delayed carotid artery upstroke	3.7 (2.5, 5.5)	0.4 (0.2, 0.9)
Reduced carotid artery volume	2.3 (1.8, 2.9)	0.3 (0.2, 0.5)
Brachioradial delay	2.5 (1.4, 4.7)	0.04 (0, 0.7)
Sustained apical impulse	4.1 (1.7, 10.1)	0.3 (0.1, 0.5)
Apical-carotid delay	2.6 (1.4, 5.2)	0.05 (0, 0.7)
Absent A_2	4.5 (1.4, 14.1)	0.8 (0.7, 1.0)
Absent or diminished A_2	3.6 (2.6, 5.1)	0.4 (0.3, 0.6)
S_4 gallop	0.9 (0.5, 1.9)	1.1 (0.6, 1.9)
Late peaking murmur	4.4 (2.5, 7.6)	0.2 (0.1, 0.3)
Prolonged murmur	3.9 (2.1, 7.3)	0.2 (0.1, 0.5)
Murmur loudest over aortic area	1.8 (1.1, 2.9)	0.6 (0.4, 0.7)
Murmur transmits to neck	1.4 (1.1, 1.8)	0.1 (0, 0.8)

Continued

| Appendix Table 1 | Likelihood Ratios—Point Estimates and 95% Confidence Intervals—Cont'd | | |

Finding	Positive LR (95% CI)	Negative LR (95% CI)
EBM Box 41-1 Aortic regurgitation		
Characteristic diastolic murmur, detecting mild aortic regurgitation or worse	9.9 (4.9, 20.0)	0.3 (0.2, 0.4)
Characteristic diastolic murmur, detecting moderate-to-severe aortic regurgitation	4.3 (2.1, 8.6)	0.1 (0.1, 0.2)
Early diastolic murmur loudest at right sternum, detecting dilated aortic root or endocarditis	8.2 (5.0, 13.3)	0.7 (0.7, 0.8)
Early diastolic murmur softer with amyl nitrite inhalation, detecting aortic regurgitation (vs. Graham Steell murmur)	5.7 (0.5, 71.4)	0.1 (0, 0.3)
EBM Box 41-2 Moderate-to-severe aortic regurgitation		
Murmur grade 3 or louder	8.2 (2.2, 31.1)	0.6 (0.4, 0.9)
Diastolic blood pressure, >70 mm Hg	0.2 (0.1, 0.9)	...
Diastolic blood pressure, 51–70 mm Hg	1.1 (0.7, 1.7)	...
Diastolic blood pressure, ≤50 mm Hg	19.3 (2.7, 140.6)	...
Pulse pressure, <60 mm Hg	0.3 (0.1, 0.9)	...
Pulse pressure, 60–79 mm Hg	0.8 (0.2, 2.9)	...
Pulse pressure, ≥80 mm Hg	10.9 (1.5, 77.1)	...
Hill's test, <40 mm Hg	0.3 (0.2, 0.8)	...
Hill's test, 40–59 mm Hg	2.4 (0.6, 9.7)	...
Hill's test, ≥60 mm Hg	17.3 (1.1, 284.3)	...
Enlarged or sustained apical impulse	2.4 (1.4, 4.0)	0.1 (0, 0.9)
S_3 gallop	5.9 (1.4, 25.3)	0.8 (0.7, 0.9)
Duroziez's sign, femoral pistol shot, water hammer pulse	3.4 (0.4, 31.0)	0.7 (0.5, 0.9)
Chapter 42 Miscellaneous Heart Murmurs		
Characteristic systolic murmur, detecting mild mitral regurgitation or worse	5.4 (3.7, 8.1)	0.4 (0.2, 0.7)
Characteristic systolic murmur, detecting moderate-to-severe mitral regurgitation	3.3 (2.7, 4.1)	0.2 (0.1, 0.4)
Characteristic systolic murmur, detecting mitral valve prolapse	12.1 (4.0, 36.4)	0.5 (0.2, 0.9)
Characteristic systolic murmur, detecting mild tricuspid regurgitation or worse	14.6 (4.5, 47.1)	0.8 (0.7, 0.9)

Appendix Table 1   Likelihood Ratios—Point Estimates and 95% Confidence Intervals

Finding	Positive LR (95% CI)	Negative LR (95% CI)
CV wave >15 mm Hg, detecting moderate-to-severe tricuspid regurgitation	6.8 (3.4, 13.7)	0.6 (0.4, 0.8)
Characteristic diastolic murmur, detecting pulmonary regurgitation	17.4 (3.6, 83.2)	0.9 (0.8, 1.0)
Apical diastolic murmur, detecting mitral annular calcification	7.5 (2.3, 24.4)	0.9 (0.9, 1.0)
EBM Box 42-1 Severity of mitral and tricuspid regurgitation		
Murmur grade 3 or louder, detecting moderate-to-severe mitral regurgitation	4.4 (2.9, 6.7)	0.2 (0.1, 0.3)
S_3, detecting moderate-to-severe mitral regurgitation	4.4 (0.6, 31.8)	0.8 (0.7, 0.8)
Pulsatile liver, detecting moderate-to-severe tricuspid regurgitation	3.9 (1.4, 11.4)	0.8 (0.6, 1.0)
Systolic regurgitant venous waveform, detecting moderate-to-severe tricuspid regurgitation	1.5 (0.9, 2.5)	0.7 (0.5, 1.1)
EBM Box 42-2 Other cardiac findings in mitral stenosis		
Graham Steell murmur, detecting pulmonary hypertension	4.2 (1.1, 15.5)	0.4 (0.2, 0.9)
Hyperkinetic apical movement, detecting mitral regurgitation or aortic valve disease	11.2 (6.4, 19.5)	0.3 (0.2, 0.4)
Hyperkinetic arterial pulse, detecting mitral regurgitation	14.2 (7.4, 27.2)	0.3 (0.2, 0.4)
Chapter 43 Disorders of the Pericardium		
Pericardial rub in cancer patient, detecting idiopathic/radiation pericarditis	5.5 (1.4, 21.9)	0.4 (0.2, 0.9)
Pulsus paradoxus >12 mm Hg, detecting tamponade	5.9 (2.4, 14.3)	0.03 (0, 0.2)

Continued

Appendix Table 1 Likelihood Ratios—Point Estimates and 95% Confidence Intervals—Cont'd

Finding	Positive LR (95% CI)	Negative LR (95% CI)
Chapter 44 Congestive Heart Failure		
Crackles, detecting left atrial pressure ≥12 mm Hg in patients with cardiomyopathy	3.4 (1.6, 7.2)	0.7 (0.6, 1.0)
Pulse-amplitude ratio >0.7, detecting pulmonary capillary wedge pressure >15 mm Hg	18.2 (2.7, 123.4)	0.1 (0, 0.4)
S_3, detecting ejection fraction <0.3	4.1 (2.3, 7.3)	0.3 (0.2, 0.5)
Proportional pulse pressure <0.25, detecting low cardiac index	6.9 (3.0, 15.8)	0.2 (0.1, 0.6)
S_3, detecting consensus diagnosis of congestive heart failure	8.8 (4.4, 17.5)	0.8 (0.8, 0.9)
Elevated neck veins, detecting consensus diagnosis of congestive heart failure	4.3 (2.9, 6.4)	0.7 (0.6, 0.7)
EBM Box 44-1 Elevated left heart filling pressure		
Heart rate >100 beats/min	5.5 (1.3, 24.1)	0.9 (0.9, 1.0)
Abnormal Valsalva response	7.6 (1.7, 34.3)	0.1 (0, 0.8)
Crackles	1.6 (0.8, 2.9)	0.9 (0.9, 1.0)
Elevated jugular venous pressure	3.9 (1.6, 9.4)	0.7 (0.5, 1.0)
Abdominojugular test	8.0 (2.1, 31.2)	0.3 (0.2, 0.6)
Supine apical impulse lateral to MCL	5.8 (1.3, 26.0)	0.6 (0.4, 1.0)
S_3 gallop	5.7 (3.1, 10.3)	0.8 (0.7, 1.0)
S_4 gallop	1.4 (0.8, 2.6)	0.6 (0.3, 1.4)
Edema	1.4 (0.6, 3.2)	1.0 (0.9, 1.0)
EBM Box 44-2 Low ejection fraction		
Heart rate >100 beats/min	2.8 (1.3, 5.3)	0.8 (0.7, 1.0)
Abnormal Valsalva response	7.6 (4.9, 11.8)	0.3 (0.2, 0.4)
Crackles	1.7 (0.6, 4.6)	0.9 (0.8, 1.1)
Elevated neck veins	7.9 (2.8, 22.4)	0.9 (0.8, 1.0)
Supine apical impulse lateral to MCL	10.1 (3.8, 26.6)	0.6 (0.5, 0.9)
S_3 gallop	3.4 (2.6, 4.4)	0.7 (0.5, 0.9)
Murmur of mitral regurgitation	2.2 (0.9, 5.7)	0.8 (0.7, 1.0)
Hepatomegaly	0.9 (0.1, 9.4)	1.0 (0.9, 1.1)
Edema	1.5 (0.8, 2.9)	0.9 (0.9, 1.0)
Chapter 45 Coronary Artery Disease		
Pain radiating to left arm, detecting myocardial infarction	1.8 (1.1, 2.8)	0.7 (0.5, 1.1)
Pain radiating to right arm, detecting myocardial infarction	4.7 (1.9, 11.6)	0.8 (0.5, 1.1)

Appendix Table 1 Likelihood Ratios—Point Estimates and 95% Confidence Intervals

Finding	Positive LR (95% CI)	Negative LR (95% CI)
Elevated troponin T levels, detecting cardiac events in subsequent 30 days	6.1 (4.7, 7.9)	0.2 (0.1, 0.5)
EBM Box 45-1 Coronary artery disease		
Typical angina	5.8 (4.2, 7.8)	...
Atypical angina	1.2 (1.1, 1.3)	...
Nonanginal chest pain	0.1 (0.1, 0.2)	...
Pain duration >30 min	0.1 (0, 0.9)	1.2 (1, 1.3)
Associated dysphagia	0.2 (0.1, 0.8)	1.2 (1, 1.4)
Male sex	1.7 (1.6, 1.8)	0.3 (0.3, 0.4)
Age <30 years	0.1 (0, 1.1)	...
Age 30–49 years	0.6 (0.5, 0.7)	...
Age 50–70 years	1.3 (1.3, 1.4)	...
Age >70 years	2.6 (1.8, 4)	...
Prior myocardial infarction	3.8 (2.1, 6.8)	0.6 (0.5, 0.6)
Ear lobe crease	2.3 (1.3, 4.1)	0.6 (0.4, 0.8)
Arcus senilis	3.0 (1.02, 8.6)	0.7 (0.6, 0.8)
Chest wall tenderness	0.7 (0.4, 1.1)	1 (1, 1.1)
Ankle-to-arm pressure index <0.9	4.1 (1.02, 16.7)	0.8 (0.8, 0.9)
Laterally displaced apical impulse	13 (0.7, 228.3)	1 (0.9, 1)
Normal electrocardiogram	0.6 (0.3, 1.1)	1.2 (1, 1.6)
ST/T wave abnormalities	1.4 (1, 1.9)	0.9 (0.9, 1)
EBM Box 45-2 Myocardial infarction		
Male sex	1.3 (1.2, 1.4)	0.7 (0.7, 0.7)
Age <40 years	0.2 (0.1, 0.5)	...
Age 40–59 years	0.8 (0.6, 1.1)	...
Age ≥60 years	1.5 (1.4, 1.6)	...
Sharp pain	0.3 (0.2, 0.5)	1.3 (1.3, 1.4)
Pleuritic pain	0.2 (0.2, 0.3)	1.2 (1.2, 1.3)
Positional pain	0.3 (0.2, 0.5)	1.1 (1.1, 1.2)
Relief of pain with nitroglycerin	0.9 (0.8, 1.1)	1.1 (1, 1.2)
Chest wall tenderness	0.3 (0.2, 0.4)	1.3 (1.1, 1.4)
Diaphoretic appearance	2.9 (1.3, 6.6)	0.7 (0.6, 0.8)
Systolic blood pressure <100 mm Hg	3.6 (2, 6.5)	1 (0.9, 1)
Jugular venous distension	2.4 (1.4, 4.2)	0.9 (0.9, 1)
Pulmonary crackles	2.1 (1.6, 2.8)	0.8 (0.7, 1)
Third heart sound	3.2 (1.6, 6.5)	0.9 (0.8, 1)
Normal electrocardiogram	0.2 (0.1, 0.3)	1.5 (1.4, 1.6)
Nonspecific ST changes	0.2 (0.1, 0.6)	1.5 (0.9, 2.6)
ST elevation	22.0 (16.1, 30.3)	0.6 (0.6, 0.6)
ST depression	4.5 (3.5, 5.6)	0.8 (0.7, 0.9)
T-wave inversion	2.2 (1.8, 2.6)	0.9 (0.8, 1)

Continued

Finding	Positive LR (95% CI)	Negative LR (95% CI)
EBM Box 45-3 Predicting life-threatening complications in patients with acute chest pain		
"High" risk	8.7 (4.4, 17.1)	...
"Very low" risk	0.1 (0.1, 0.2)	...
Chapter 47 Palpation and Percussion of the Abdomen		
Pulsatile liver, detecting moderate-to-severe tricuspid regurgitation	3.9 (1.4, 11.4)	0.8 (0.6, 1.0)
Palpable spleen and adenopathy, detecting liver disease	0.04 (0, 0.6)	...
Palpable spleen and liver, detecting liver disease	2.7 (1.8, 3.9)	...
Massive splenomegaly, detecting hematologic disease	2.1 (1.1, 3.8)	...
EBM Box 47-1 Detection of enlarged liver and spleen		
Percussion span ≥10 cm in MCL, detecting enlarged liver	1.2 (1.0, 1.5)	0.5 (0.2, 1.7)
Palpable liver, detecting actual liver edge	233.7 (14.6, 3737)	0.5 (0.5, 0.6)
Palpable liver, detecting hepatomegaly	1.8 (1.5, 2.2)	0.6 (0.5, 0.8)
Palpable spleen, detecting splenomegaly	8.5 (6.2, 11.8)	0.5 (0.4, 0.7)
Positive spleen percussion sign (Castell's), detecting splenomegaly	1.7 (1.2, 2.2)	0.7 (0.5, 0.9)
Positive Nixon method, detecting splenomegaly	2.0 (1.2, 3.5)	0.7 (0.6, 0.9)
Traube's space dullness, detecting splenomegaly	2.1 (1.7, 2.6)	0.8 (0.6, 0.9)
EBM Box 47-2 Palpation of liver and spleen in various disorders		
Enlarged palpable liver, detecting cirrhosis	2.0 (1.4, 2.8)	0.6 (0.4, 0.8)
Palpable liver in epigastrium, detecting cirrhosis	2.6 (1.8, 3.8)	0.2 (0.1, 0.5)
Liver edge firm to palpation, detecting cirrhosis	2.7 (2.2, 3.3)	0.4 (0.3, 0.5)
Palpable liver in patients with jaundice, detecting hepatocellular disease (nonobstructive jaundice)	0.9 (0.8, 1.1)	1.4 (0.6, 3.4)
Liver tenderness in patients with jaundice, detecting hepatocellular disease (nonobstructive jaundice)	1.4 (0.8, 2.6)	0.8 (0.7, 1.1)

Appendix Table 1   Likelihood Ratios—Point Estimates and 95% Confidence Intervals

Finding	Positive LR (95% CI)	Negative LR (95% CI)
Palpable liver in patients with lymphadenopathy, detecting serious disease	1.2 (0.7, 1.9)	1.0 (0.9, 1.1)
Palpable spleen in returning travelers with fever, detecting malaria	6.6 (2.4, 17.9)	0.8 (0.7, 0.9)
Palpable spleen in patients with jaundice, detecting hepatocellular disease (nonobstructive jaundice)	2.9 (1.2, 6.8)	0.7 (0.6, 0.9)
Palpable spleen in patients with chronic liver disease, detecting cirrhosis	2.3 (1.5, 3.6)	0.8 (0.7, 0.9)
Palpable spleen in patients with lymphadenopathy, detecting serious disease	1.2 (0.6, 2.5)	1.0 (0.9, 1.0)
EBM Box 47-3 Gallbladder, bladder, and aorta		
Palpable gallbladder, detecting obstructed bile ducts	26.0 (1.5, 439.9)	0.7 (0.5, 0.9)
Palpable gallbladder, detecting malignant obstruction	2.6 (1.5, 4.6)	0.7 (0.6, 0.9)
Palpable bladder, detecting ≥400 mL or more urine in bladder	1.9 (1.4, 2.6)	0.3 (0.1, 0.7)
Expansile pulsation epigastrium, detecting abdominal aortic aneurysm	8.0 (4.2, 15.3)	0.6 (0.5, 0.7)
EBM Box 47-4 Ascites		
Bulging flanks	1.9 (1.4, 2.6)	0.4 (0.2, 0.6)
Edema	3.8 (2.2, 6.6)	0.2 (0, 0.6)
Flank dullness	1.8 (0.9, 3.4)	0.3 (0.1, 0.7)
Shifting dullness	2.3 (1.5, 3.5)	0.4 (0.2, 0.6)
Fluid wave	5.0 (2.5, 9.9)	0.5 (0.3, 0.7)
Chapter 48 Abdominal Pain and Tenderness		
Right lower quadrant tenderness, detecting appendicitis	3.0 (0.5, 17)	0.1 (0, 0.2)
Sonographic McBurney's point tenderness, detecting appendicitis	8.4 (2.9, 24.6)	0.1 (0.1, 0.3)
Sonographic Murphy's sign, detecting cholecystitis	9.9 (5.4, 18.3)	0.4 (0.3, 0.6)
Murphy's sign, detecting biliary tract sepsis in patients with pyogenic liver abscess	2.8 (1.1, 6.9)	0.8 (0.6, 1.0)

Continued

	Appendix Table 1	Likelihood Ratios—Point Estimates and 95% Confidence Intervals—Cont'd

Finding	Positive LR (95% CI)	Negative LR (95% CI)
Loin tenderness, detecting ureterolithiasis	27.7 (10.7, 71.9)	0.9 (0.8, 0.9)
Renal tenderness, detecting ureterolithiasis	3.6 (3.1, 4.1)	0.2 (0.1, 0.3)
Microscopic hematuria, detecting ureterolithiasis	73.1 (41.7, 128.1)	0.3 (0.2, 0.4)
Positive abdominal wall tenderness test in patient with chronic abdominal pain, predicting good response to local anesthetic injection	7.0 (3.4, 14.3)	0.2 (0.1, 0.5)
EBM Box 48-1 Acute abdominal pain, detecting peritonitis		
Guarding	2.6 (1.8, 3.9)	0.6 (0.5, 0.7)
Rigidity	3.9 (2.2, 6.7)	0.8 (0.7, 1.0)
Rebound tenderness	2.1 (1.7, 2.5)	0.5 (0.4, 0.6)
Percussion tenderness	2.4 (1.5, 3.9)	0.5 (0.3, 0.7)
Abnormal bowel sounds	2.2 (0.5, 9.7)	0.8 (0.7, 0.9)
Rectal tenderness	1.2 (1.0, 1.6)	0.9 (0.9, 1.0)
Positive abdominal wall tenderness test	0.1 (0, 0.7)	1.9 (0.9, 4.4)
Positive cough test	1.8 (1.4, 2.2)	0.4 (0.3, 0.5)
EBM Box 48-2 Acute right lower abdominal pain, detecting appendicitis		
Fever	1.5 (1.2, 1.8)	0.6 (0.4, 0.8)
Severe right lower quadrant tenderness	1.6 (0.7, 3.8)	0.2 (0.1, 0.3)
McBurney's point tenderness	3.4 (1.6, 7.2)	0.4 (0.2, 0.7)
Rovsing's sign	2.5 (1.4, 4.4)	0.7 (0.6, 0.8)
Rectal tenderness	1.1 (1.0, 1.2)	0.9 (0.9, 1.0)
Psoas sign	2.0 (1.2, 3.5)	0.9 (0.8, 1.0)
Obturator sign	1.4 (0.4, 4.5)	1.0 (0.9, 1.1)
EBM Box 48-3 Acute right upper abdominal pain, detecting cholecystitis		
Fever	1.1 (0.8, 1.7)	0.9 (0.8, 1.1)
Murphy's sign	1.9 (1.6, 2.4)	0.6 (0.4, 0.9)
Back tenderness	0.4 (0.3, 0.6)	2.0 (1.4, 3.0)
Right upper quadrant mass	0.8 (0.5, 1.2)	1.0 (1.0, 1.0)
EBM Box 48-4 Acute abdominal pain, detecting bowel obstruction		
Visible peristalsis	18.8 (4.3, 81.9)	0.9 (0.9, 1.0)
Distended abdomen	9.6 (5.0, 18.6)	0.4 (0.3, 0.5)
Guarding	1.0 (0.6, 1.7)	1.0 (0.7, 1.4)
Rigidity	1.2 (0.4, 3.6)	1.0 (0.9, 1.2)
Rebound tenderness	0.9 (0.7, 1.1)	1.1 (1.0, 1.2)

**Appendix
Table 1** Likelihood Ratios—Point Estimates
and 95% Confidence Intervals

Finding	Positive LR (95% CI)	Negative LR (95% CI)
Hyperactive bowel sounds	5.0 (2.4, 10.6)	0.6 (0.5, 0.8)
Abnormal bowel sounds	3.2 (1.7, 6.1)	0.4 (0.3, 0.5)
Rectal tenderness	0.9 (0.6, 1.5)	1.0 (1.0, 1.1)
EBM Box 48-5 Chronic upper abdominal pain		
Positive abdominal wall tenderness test, detecting visceral pain	0.1 (0.1, 0.3)	4.2 (2.2, 8.1)
Right upper quadrant tenderness, detecting cholelithiasis	1.1 (0.9, 1.4)	0.9 (0.7, 1.2)
Lower abdominal tenderness, detecting cholelithiasis	0.5 (0.3, 0.7)	1.4 (1.2, 1.6)
Epigastric tenderness, detecting positive upper endoscopy	0.9 (0.7, 1.3)	1.2 (0.6, 2.3)
Chapter 49 Auscultation of the Abdomen		
Abnormal bowel sounds, detecting small bowel obstruction	3.2 (1.7, 6.1)	0.4 (0.3, 0.5)
EBM Box 49-1 Auscultation of the abdomen		
Any abdominal bruit, detecting renovascular hypertension	5.6 (4.0, 7.7)	0.6 (0.5, 0.8)
Any abdominal bruit, detecting abdominal aortic aneurysm	2.0 (0.5, 8.6)	0.9 (0.8, 1.1)
Systolic/diastolic bruit, detecting renovascular hypertension	38.9 (9.5, 159.6)	0.6 (0.5, 0.7)
Chapter 50 Peripheral Vascular Disease		
Abnormal femoral pulse, detecting aortoiliac disease	31.0 (1.9, 500.6)	0.6 (0.5, 0.8)
Limb bruit, detecting arterial stenosis	3.2 (1.2, 8.7)	0.3 (0.1, 0.6)
Continuous femoral bruit, detecting arteriovenous fistula	80.8 (5.1, 1272.9)	0.04 (0, 0.6)
Expansile femoral pulsations, detecting false aneurysm	13.8 (3.6, 52.7)	0.1 (0, 0.3)
EBM Box 50-1 Peripheral vascular disease		
Wounds or sores on foot	7.0 (3.2, 15.6)	1.0 (1.0, 1.0)
Foot color abnormally pale, red, or blue	2.8 (2.4, 3.2)	0.7 (0.7, 0.8)
Atrophic skin	1.7 (1.2, 2.3)	0.7 (0.5, 1.0)
Absent lower limb hair	1.7 (1.2, 2.3)	0.7 (0.6, 1.0)
Foot asymmetrically cooler	6.1 (4.2, 8.9)	0.9 (0.9, 0.9)
Absent femoral pulse	6.1 (3.8, 10.0)	0.9 (0.9, 1.0)

Continued

Appendix Table 1	Likelihood Ratios—Point Estimates and 95% Confidence Intervals—Cont'd	
Finding	**Positive LR (95% CI)**	**Negative LR (95% CI)**
Absent posterior tibial and dorsalis pedis pulses	14.9 (3.3, 66.3)	0.3 (0.3, 0.4)
Limb bruit present	7.3 (3.6, 14.9)	0.7 (0.5, 0.9)
Capillary refill time ≥5 sec	1.9 (1.2, 3.2)	0.8 (0.7, 1.0)
Venous filling time >20 sec	3.6 (1.9, 6.8)	0.8 (0.7, 1.0)
EBM Box 51-1 The diabetic foot		
Unable to sense the 5.07 monofilament, detecting subsequent ulceration	2.4 (1.5, 3.7)	0.5 (0.4, 0.6)
Ulcer area >2 cm^2, detecting osteomyelitis	7.2 (1.1, 48.9)	0.5 (0.3, 0.8)
Positive probe test, detecting osteomyelitis	4.3 (1.7, 10.8)	0.4 (0.3, 0.6)
Ulcer depth >3 mm or bone exposed, detecting osteomyelitis	3.6 (1.3, 9.7)	0.2 (0.1, 0.5)
Erythema, swelling, purulence, detecting osteomyelitis	1.5 (0.5, 4.7)	0.8 (0.6, 1.3)
0 findings, detecting nonhealing wound at 20 weeks	0.5 (0.4, 0.5)	…
1 finding, detecting nonhealing wound at 20 weeks	0.8 (0.8, 0.8)	…
2 findings, detecting nonhealing wound at 20 weeks	1.8 (1.7, 1.8)	…
3 findings, detecting nonhealing wound at 20 weeks	3.5 (3.2, 3.8)	…
Chapter 52 Edema and Deep Vein Thrombosis		
Elevated neck veins, detecting measured CVP >8 cm H_2O	9.0 (3.7, 22.1)	0.2 (0, 1.5)
Active cancer, detecting deep vein thrombosis	2.9 (2.4, 3.6)	0.9 (0.8, 0.9)
Recent immobilization, detecting deep vein thrombosis	1.6 (1.3, 2.1)	0.9 (0.8, 0.9)
Recent surgery, detecting deep vein thrombosis	1.6 (1.3, 1.9)	0.9 (0.9, 1.0)
EBM Box 52-1 Deep vein thrombosis		
Any calf or ankle swelling	1.2 (1.1, 1.3)	0.7 (0.6, 0.8)
Asymmetric calf swelling, ≥2 cm difference	2.1 (1.8, 2.5)	0.5 (0.4, 0.7)
Swelling of entire leg	1.5 (1.2, 1.8)	0.8 (0.6, 0.9)
Superficial venous dilation	1.6 (1.4, 1.9)	0.9 (0.8, 0.9)

Appendix Table 1   Likelihood Ratios—Point Estimates and 95% Confidence Intervals

Finding	Positive LR (95% CI)	Negative LR (95% CI)
Erythema	1.0 (0.6, 1.7)	1.0 (0.8, 1.2)
Superficial thrombophlebitis	0.9 (0.2, 5.1)	1.0 (0.9, 1.1)
Tenderness	1.0 (1.0, 1.1)	1.0 (0.9, 1.1)
Asymmetric skin coolness	1.2 (0.6, 2.2)	0.9 (0.6, 1.4)
Asymmetric skin warmth	1.4 (1.2, 1.7)	0.7 (0.5, 1.2)
Palpable cord	1.1 (0.7, 1.6)	1.0 (0.9, 1.1)
Homans's sign	1.1 (0.9, 1.3)	1.0 (0.9, 1.1)
EBM Box 52-2 Wells score scheme		
Low pretest probability	0.2 (0.2, 0.3)	...
Moderate pretest probability	0.9 (0.7, 1.0)	...
High pretest probability	5.2 (3.2, 8.5)	...
Chapter 53 Examination of the Musculoskeletal System		
Valgus laxity in patients with knee injuries, detecting medial collateral ligament injury	146.5 (9.2, 2331)	0.2 (0.1, 0.3)
Examination for detection of posterior cruciate ligament injury	91.8 (18.2, 463.4)	0.1 (0, 1.4)
EBM Box 53-1 Shoulder pain		
Acromioclavicular joint tenderness, detecting acromioclavicular joint pain	1.1 (0.9, 1.3)	0.4 (0, 5.2)
Tenderness with compression of acromioclavicular joint, detecting acromioclavicular joint pain	1.6 (0.8, 3.0)	0.4 (0.2, 1.1)
Hawkin's impingement sign, detecting rotator cuff tendinitis	1.4 (1.1, 1.9)	0.3 (0.1, 0.6)
Neer's impingement sign, detecting rotator cuff tendinitis	1.3 (1.1, 1.6)	0.4 (0.3, 0.7)
Hawkin's or Neer's impingement sign, detecting rotator cuff tendinitis	1.6 (1.3, 2.0)	0.1 (0, 0.7)
Yergason's sign, detecting rotator cuff tendinitis	2.8 (1.2, 6.6)	0.7 (0.6, 0.9)
Painful arc, detecting rotator cuff tendinitis	1.7 (0.8, 3.6)	0.8 (0.7, 1.0)
Age ≤39 years, detecting rotator cuff tear	0.1 (0.1, 0.2)	...
Age 40-59 years, detecting rotator cuff tear	0.9 (0.7, 1.1)	...
Age ≥60 years, detecting rotator cuff tear	3.2 (2.4, 4.3)	...

Continued

<table>
<tr><td>**Appendix Table 1**</td><td>Likelihood Ratios—Point Estimates and 95% Confidence Intervals—Cont'd</td></tr>
</table>

Finding	Positive LR (95% CI)	Negative LR (95% CI)
Neer's impingement sign, detecting rotator cuff tear	1.5 (1.2, 2.0)	0.3 (0.1, 0.9)
Hawkin's impingement sign, detecting rotator cuff tear	1.7 (1.2, 2.3)	0.3 (0.1, 0.8)
Supraspinatus testing causes pain, detecting rotator cuff tear	1.5 (1.2, 2.0)	0.5 (0.2, 1.1)
Supraspinatus atrophy, detecting rotator cuff tear	2.0 (1.5, 2.7)	0.6 (0.5, 0.7)
Infraspinatus atrophy, detecting rotator cuff tear	2.0 (1.5, 2.7)	0.6 (0.5, 0.7)
Supraspinatus weakness, detecting rotator cuff tear	2.0 (1.7, 2.4)	0.5 (0.3, 0.7)
Infraspinatus weakness, detecting rotator cuff tear	1.8 (1.5, 2.2)	0.4 (0.3, 0.5)
Painful arc, detecting rotator cuff tear	1.1 (1.0, 1.1)	0.3 (0.1, 0.6)
Dropped arm test, detecting rotator cuff tear	5.0 (1.1, 22.2)	0.9 (0.9, 1.0)
Palpable tear, detecting rotator cuff tear	10.2 (1.3, 80.9)	0.1 (0, 0.2)
3 findings, detecting rotator cuff tear	48.0 (6.7, 344.4)	...
2 findings, detecting rotator cuff tear	4.9 (2.9, 8.3)	...
1 finding, detecting rotator cuff tear	0.9 (0.7, 1.1)	...
0 findings, detecting rotator cuff tear	0.02 (0, 0.1)	...
EBM Box 53-2 Diagnosis of osteoarthritis in patients with chronic knee pain		
Stiffness <30 min	3.0 (2.1, 4.4)	0.2 (0.1, 0.3)
Crepitus, passive motion	2.1 (1.7, 2.7)	0.2 (0.1, 0.3)
Bony enlargement	11.8 (4.9, 28.2)	0.5 (0.4, 0.6)
Palpable increase in temperature	0.3 (0.2, 0.5)	1.6 (1.4, 2.0)
Valgus deformity	1.4 (0.8, 2.4)	0.9 (0.8, 1.0)
Varus deformity	3.4 (1.6, 7.6)	0.8 (0.7, 0.9)
At least 3 out of 6 findings	3.1 (2.3, 4.1)	0.1 (0, 0.1)
EBM Box 53-3 Clinically significant knee fracture		
Age ≥55 years	3.0 (1.6, 5.3)	0.7 (0.5, 1.0)
Joint effusion	2.5 (2.0, 3.0)	0.5 (0.3, 0.7)
Ecchymosis	2.2 (0.9, 5.3)	0.9 (0.7, 1.1)
Limitation of knee flexion <90 degrees	2.9 (2.5, 3.4)	0.5 (0.4, 0.7)
Limitation of knee flexion <60 degrees	4.7 (3.8, 5.9)	0.6 (0.5, 0.7)
Isolated tenderness of patella	2.2 (1.6, 2.9)	0.8 (0.8, 0.9)
Tenderness at head of fibula	3.4 (2.5, 4.7)	0.9 (0.8, 1.0)

Appendix Table 1   Likelihood Ratios—Point Estimates and 95% Confidence Intervals

Finding	Positive LR (95% CI)	Negative LR (95% CI)
Inability to bear weight, immediately and in emergency department	3.6 (3.0, 4.3)	0.6 (0.5, 0.7)
Ottawa rule positive	1.7 (1.4, 2.1)	0.1 (0, 0.3)
EBM Box 53-4 Ligament and meniscal injuries		
Anterior drawer sign, detecting anterior cruciate ligament tear	11.5 (5.0, 26.2)	0.5 (0.4, 0.7)
Lachman's sign, detecting anterior cruciate ligament tear	17.0 (5.4, 53.1)	0.2 (0.1, 0.4)
Pivot shift sign, detecting anterior cruciate ligament tear	8.0 (3.5, 18.3)	0.8 (0.7, 1.0)
McMurray sign, detecting meniscal injury	8.2 (3.0, 22.5)	0.8 (0.7, 0.9)
Joint line tenderness, detecting meniscal injury	1.2 (1.0, 1.4)	0.7 (0.5, 1.0)
Block to full extension, detecting meniscal injury	3.2 (1.8, 5.9)	0.7 (0.5, 0.8)
EBM Box 53-5 Ankle and midfoot fracture		
Tenderness over posterior lateral malleolus, detecting ankle fracture	2.4 (1.9, 2.8)	0.4 (0.3, 0.5)
Tenderness over posterior medial malleolus, detecting ankle fracture	4.8 (2.6, 9.0)	0.6 (0.6, 0.7)
Inability to bear weight immediately after injury, detecting ankle fracture	2.6 (2.2, 3.1)	0.5 (0.4, 0.6)
Inability to bear weight 4 steps in the emergency room, detecting ankle fracture	2.5 (2.2, 2.8)	0.3 (0.2, 0.4)
Ottawa ankle rule, detecting ankle fracture	1.5 (1.2, 1.8)	0.1 (0, 0.2)
Tenderness at the base of the 5th metatarsal, detecting midfoot fracture	2.9 (2.5, 3.3)	0.1 (0.1, 0.2)
Tenderness of navicular bone, detecting midfoot fracture	0.4 (0.2, 0.9)	1.1 (1.0, 1.2)
Inability to bear weight immediately, detecting midfoot fracture	1.0 (0.5, 2.3)	1.0 (0.8, 1.3)
Inability to bear weight 4 steps in the emergency room, detecting midfoot fracture	1.1 (0.8, 1.4)	0.9 (0.8, 1.1)
Ottawa foot rule, detecting midfoot fracture	2.1 (1.3, 3.3)	0.1 (0, 0.2)

Continued

Appendix Table 1   Likelihood Ratios—Point Estimates and 95% Confidence Intervals—Cont'd

Finding	Positive LR (95% CI)	Negative LR (95% CI)
Chapter 54 Visual Field Testing		
Confrontational testing with red laser pointer, detecting anterior visual field defect	6.3 (3.4, 12.0)	0.3 (0.2, 0.5)
EBM Box 54-1 Visual field defects		
Anterior detects	6.1 (3.0, 12.4)	0.7 (0.6, 0.8)
Posterior defects	6.8 (2.6, 17.8)	0.4 (0.2, 0.8)
Asymmetric optokinetic nystagmus, detecting parietal lobe disease	5.7 (3.2, 10.1)	0.1 (0, 0.3)
Associated hemiparesis or aphasia, detecting parietal lobe disease	18.3 (6.0, 56.2)	0.1 (0, 0.7)
Chapter 56 Miscellaneous Cranial Nerves		
Hutchinson's sign, detecting ocular complications	3.5 (2.1, 5.8)	0.3 (0.1, 0.9)
EBM Box 56-1 Aspiration after stroke		
Abnormal voluntary cough	1.9 (1.3, 2.7)	0.6 (0.5, 0.7)
Dysphonia	1.3 (1.2, 1.5)	0.4 (0.3, 0.7)
Dysarthria	1.6 (1.2, 2.2)	0.5 (0.3, 0.8)
Drowsiness	3.4 (1.2, 9.5)	0.5 (0.3, 0.7)
Abnormal sensation face and tongue	0.5 (0.2, 1.2)	1.5 (0.9, 2.4)
Absent pharyngeal sensation	2.4 (1.6, 3.6)	0.03 (0, 0.5)
Tongue weakness	2.5 (0.7, 9.6)	0.6 (0.4, 0.9)
Bilateral cranial nerve signs	1.1 (0.8, 1.6)	0.8 (0.4, 1.6)
Abnormal gag reflex	1.5 (1.2, 1.8)	0.6 (0.4, 0.7)
Water swallow test	3.2 (2.1, 4.7)	0.4 (0.3, 0.5)
Oxygen desaturation 0–2 min after swallowing	3.1 (1.1, 8.6)	0.3 (0.2, 0.5)
Chapter 57 Examination of the Motor System: Approach to Weakness and Tremor		
Ipsilateral calf wasting in patients with sciatica, detecting disc herniation	5.2 (1.3, 20.8)	0.8 (0.6, 0.9)
Feet suddenly freeze in doorways, detecting Parkinson's disease	4.4 (1.5, 12.4)	0.7 (0.5, 1.0)
Voice progressively softer, detecting Parkinson's disease	3.2 (1.8, 5.8)	0.5 (0.1, 1.9)
Handwriting progressively smaller, detecting Parkinson's disease	2.7 (1.8, 4.0)	0.7 (0.3, 1.3)

Appendix Table 1 — Likelihood Ratios—Point Estimates and 95% Confidence Intervals

Finding	Positive LR (95% CI)	Negative LR (95% CI)
EBM Box 57-1 Unilateral cerebral hemispheric disease		
Arm rolling test	21.7 (6.3, 75)	0.3 (0.1, 1.1)
Pronator drift	10.3 (5.4, 19.6)	0.1 (0.1, 0.3)
Finger tapping test	6.6 (3.8, 11.6)	0.3 (0.2, 0.4)
Babinski response	19.0 (1.2, 297.8)	0.6 (0.4, 0.7)
Hyperreflexia	5.8 (3.2, 10.5)	0.4 (0.3, 0.5)
Hemianopia	12.5 (0.8, 199)	0.7 (0.6, 0.9)
Hemisensory disturbance	12.3 (0.8, 195.9)	0.7 (0.6, 0.9)
EBM Box 57-2 Suspected Parkinson's disease		
Prominent rigidity on initial examination, diagnosing Parkinson's disease	0.5 (0.4, 0.8)	1.6 (1.1, 2.4)
Tremor, diagnosing Parkinson's disease	1.3 (0.9, 1.7)	0.6 (0.4, 1.0)
Tremor-dominant disease, diagnosing Parkinson's disease	3.5 (0.5, 25.5)	0.9 (0.8, 1.0)
Signs are asymmetric, diagnosing Parkinson's disease	1.6 (1.0, 2.6)	0.7 (0.5, 0.9)
Bradykinesia, diagnosing Parkinson's disease	0.9 (0.8, 1.0)	3.7 (0.5, 27.9)
Tremor, bradykinesia, rigidity: 2/3 present, diagnosing Parkinson's disease	1.1 (1.0, 1.2)	0.2 (0, 1.7)
Tremor, bradykinesia, rigidity: 3/3 present, diagnosing Parkinson's disease	2.2 (1.2, 4.2)	0.5 (0.3, 0.7)
Tremor, bradykinesia, rigidity: 3/3 present, plus asymmetric and no atypical features, diagnosing Parkinson's disease	4.1 (1.7, 10.2)	0.4 (0.3, 0.6)
Good response to levodopa, diagnosing Parkinson's disease	1.8 (1.2, 2.8)	0.4 (0.2, 0.6)
Rapid progression, diagnosing multiple system atrophy	2.5 (1.6, 4.1)	0.6 (0.4, 0.8)
Absence of tremor, diagnosing multiple system atrophy	1.4 (1.0, 2.0)	0.7 (0.5, 1.1)
Speech and/or bulbar signs, diagnosing multiple system atrophy	4.1 (2.7, 6.1)	0.2 (0.1, 0.4)
Autonomic dysfunction, diagnosing multiple system atrophy	4.3 (2.3, 7.8)	0.3 (0.2, 0.4)
Cerebellar signs, diagnosing multiple system atrophy	9.5 (1.4, 64.7)	0.7 (0.5, 0.8)

Continued

Appendix Table 1
Likelihood Ratios—Point Estimates and 95% Confidence Intervals—Cont'd

Finding	Positive LR (95% CI)	Negative LR (95% CI)
Pyramidal signs, diagnosing multiple system atrophy	4.0 (1.2, 12.8)	0.7 (0.4, 1.0)
Dementia, diagnosing multiple system atrophy	0.3 (0.2, 0.6)	1.9 (1.5, 2.4)
Downgaze palsy and postural instability within first year of symptoms, diagnosing progressive supranuclear palsy	60 (3.7, 974.9)	0.5 (0.3, 0.7)
Chapter 59 Examination of the Reflexes		
Diminished biceps or brachioradialis reflex, detecting C6 radiculopathy	14.2 (4.3, 46.7)	0.5 (0.3, 0.8)
Diminished triceps reflex, detecting C7	3.0 (1.6, 5.6)	0.8 (0.7, 1.0)
Asymmetric quadriceps reflex, detecting L3-4 radiculopathy	8.7 (4.9, 15.5)	0.6 (0.5, 0.8)
Asymmetric Achilles reflex, detecting S1 radiculopathy	2.9 (1.8, 4.7)	0.4 (0.3, 0.6)
Absent bulbocavernosus reflex, detecting S2-S4 disease, men	13.0 (5.9, 28.9)	0.3 (0.2, 0.5)
Absent bulbocavernosus reflex, detecting S2-S4 disease, women	2.7 (1.6, 4.6)	0.6 (0.5, 0.9)
Grasp reflex, detecting frontal lobe or deep brain lesions	20.2 (4.8, 84.5)	0.9 (0.8, 0.9)
Chapter 60 Disorders of Nerve Roots, Plexi, and Peripheral Nerves		
Motor and sensory findings confined to C7-T1 in cancer patients with brachial plexopathy, detecting metastatic involvement	30.9 (2, 483.8)	0.3 (0.2, 0.5)
Horner's syndrome in cancer patients with brachial plexopathy, detecting metastatic involvement	4.1 (1.4, 12.2)	0.5 (0.3, 0.8)
Motor and sensory findings confined to C5-6 in cancer patients with brachial plexopathy, detecting radiation injury	8.8 (2.9, 26.4)	0.2 (0.1, 0.5)
Lymphedema of ipsilateral arm in cancer patients with brachial plexopathy, detecting radiation injury	4.9 (2.1, 11.6)	0.3 (0.2, 0.6)
Findings confined to one leg in cancer patients with lumbosacral plexopathy, detecting recurrent tumor	4.5 (1.8, 10.8)	0.1 (0, 0.4)

Appendix Table 1   Likelihood Ratios—Point Estimates and 95% Confidence Intervals

Finding	Positive LR (95% CI)	Negative LR (95% CI)
Findings affecting both legs in cancer patients with lumbosacral plexopathy, detecting radiation plexopathy	7.5 (2.5, 22.2)	0.2 (0.1, 0.5)
EBM Box 60-1 Diagnosing cervical radiculopathy in patients with neck and arm pain		
Weakness of any arm muscle	1.9 (1.4, 2.5)	0.4 (0.3, 0.6)
Reduced vibration or pinprick sensation in arm	0.7 (0.5, 1.0)	1.4 (1.0, 1.8)
Reduced biceps reflex	9.1 (1.2, 69.4)	0.9 (0.8, 1.0)
Reduced brachioradialis reflex	7.3 (0.9, 56.8)	0.9 (0.9, 1.0)
Reduced triceps reflex	2.3 (0.7, 7.0)	0.9 (0.9, 1.0)
Reduced biceps, triceps or brachioradialis reflex	3.6 (1.4, 9.2)	0.8 (0.7, 0.9)
Spurling's test	3.6 (2.1, 6.3)	0.7 (0.6, 0.9)
Rotation of neck to involved side <60 degrees	1.7 (1.3, 2.3)	0.2 (0.1, 0.9)
EBM Box 60-2 Localizing cervical radiculopathy		
Weak elbow flexion, detecting C5 radiculopathy	5.3 (2.7, 10.5)	0.2 (0, 2.5)
Weak wrist extension, detecting C6 radiculopathy	2.3 (1.1, 5.0)	0.8 (0.5, 1.1)
Weak elbow extension, detecting C7 radiculopathy	4.0 (1.8, 9.2)	0.4 (0.3, 0.6)
Weak finger flexion, detecting C8 radiculopathy	3.8 (1.7, 8.5)	0.6 (0.3, 1.1)
Sensory loss affecting thumb, detecting C6 radiculopathy	8.5 (2.3, 31.1)	0.7 (0.5, 1.0)
Sensory loss affecting middle finger, detecting C7 radiculopathy	3.2 (0.2, 60.1)	1.0 (0.9, 1.0)
Sensory loss affecting little finger, detecting C8 radiculopathy	41.4 (2.1, 807.3)	0.8 (0.6, 1.1)
Diminished biceps or brachioradialis reflex, detecting C6 radiculopathy	14.2 (4.3, 46.7)	0.5 (0.3, 0.8)
Diminished triceps reflex, detecting C7	3.0 (1.6, 5.6)	0.6 (0.3, 1.4)
EBM Box 60-3 Diagnosing carpal tunnel syndrome		
"Classic" or "probable" hand diagram	2.4 (1.6, 3.5)	0.5 (0.3, 0.7)
"Unlikely" hand diagram	0.2 (0, 0.7)	...
Weak thumb abduction	1.8 (1.4, 2.3)	0.5 (0.4, 0.7)
Thenar atrophy	1.6 (0.9, 2.8)	1.0 (0.9, 1.0)

Continued

<table>
<tr><th colspan="2">**Appendix Table 1**</th><th colspan="2">Likelihood Ratios—Point Estimates and 95% Confidence Intervals—Cont'd</th></tr>
</table>

Finding	Positive LR (95% CI)	Negative LR (95% CI)
Hypalgesia	3.1 (2.0, 5.1)	0.7 (0.5, 1.1)
Diminished 2-point discrimination	1.3 (0.6, 2.7)	1.0 (0.9, 1.1)
Abnormal vibration sensation	1.6 (0.8, 3.0)	0.8 (0.4, 1.3)
Diminished monofilament sensation	1.2 (1.0, 1.5)	0.4 (0.1, 2.0)
Tinel's sign	1.5 (1.1, 2.1)	0.8 (0.7, 1.0)
Phalen's sign	1.3 (1.2, 1.5)	0.8 (0.6, 0.9)
Pressure provocation test	1.0 (0.9, 1.2)	0.9 (0.8, 1.1)
Square wrist ratio	2.7 (2.2, 3.4)	0.5 (0.4, 0.8)
Flick sign	5.5 (0.4, 77.4)	0.3 (0, 2.8)
EBM Box 60-4 Diagnosing lumbosacral radiculopathy in patients with sciatica		
Weak ankle dorsiflexion	4.9 (1.9, 12.5)	0.5 (0.4, 0.7)
Ipsilateral calf wasting	5.2 (1.3, 20.8)	0.8 (0.6, 0.9)
Leg sensation abnormal	1.0 (0.7, 1.5)	1.0 (0.8, 1.1)
Abnormal ankle jerk	2.7 (1.6, 4.5)	0.8 (0.7, 1.0)
Straight-leg raising maneuver	1.3 (1.1, 1.6)	0.3 (0.2, 0.6)
Crossed straight-leg raising maneuver	3.4 (1.8, 6.4)	0.8 (0.7, 0.9)
EBM Box 60-5 Localizing lumbosacral radiculopathy		
Weak knee extension, detecting L3 or L4 radiculopathy	3.7 (1.9, 7.6)	0.7 (0.5, 0.8)
Weak hallux extension, detecting L5 radiculopathy	1.6 (1.3, 2.0)	0.8 (0.6, 1.0)
Weak ankle dorsiflexion, detecting L5 radiculopathy	1.3 (0.9, 1.8)	0.8 (0.6, 1.0)
Weak ankle plantarflexion, detecting S1 radiculopathy	4.8 (0.4, 60.4)	0.7 (0.6, 0.9)
Ipsilateral calf wasting, detecting S1 radiculopathy	2.4 (1.2, 4.7)	0.7 (0.5, 0.9)
Sensory loss L5 distribution, detecting L5 radiculopathy	3.1 (1.8, 5.6)	0.8 (0.7, 0.9)
Sensory loss S1 distribution, detecting S1 radiculopathy	2.4 (1.3, 4.2)	0.7 (0.6, 0.9)
Asymmetric quadriceps reflex, detecting L3-4 radiculopathy	8.7 (4.9, 15.5)	0.6 (0.5, 0.8)
Asymmetric Achilles reflex, detecting S1 radiculopathy	2.9 (1.8, 4.7)	0.4 (0.3, 0.6)

ACTH, adrenocorticotropic hormone; CXR, chest x-ray; WBC, white blood cell; HIV, human immunodeficiency virus; CVP, central venous pressure; BNP, B-type natriuretic peptide; MCL, midclavicular line.

Index

Note: Page numbers followed by the letter f refer to figures; page numbers followed by the letter t refer to tables and page numbers followed by the letter b refer to EBM boxes.